C0-ARE-569

THE UNIVERSAL
HOME DOCTOR

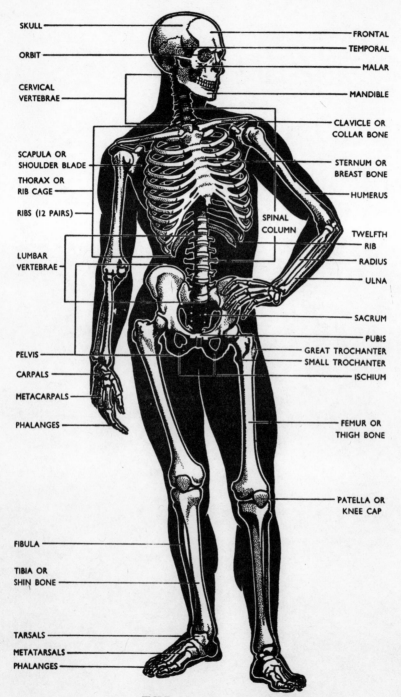

SKULL

ORBIT

CERVICAL
VERTEBRAE

SCAPULA OR
SHOULDER BLADE

THORAX OR
RIB CAGE

RIBS (12 PAIRS)

LUMBAR
VERTEBRAE

PELVIS

CARPALS

METACARPALS

PHALANGES

FIBULA

TIBIA OR
SHIN BONE

TARSALS

METATARSALS

PHALANGES

FRONTAL

TEMPORAL

MALAR

MANDIBLE

CLAVICLE OR
COLLAR BONE

STERNUM OR
BREAST BONE

HUMERUS

SPINAL
COLUMN

TWELFTH
RIB

RADIUS

ULNA

SACRUM

PUBIS

GREAT TROCHANTER

SMALL TROCHANTER

ISCHIUM

FEMUR OR
THIGH BONE

PATELLA OR
KNEE CAP

THE MALE SKELETON

THE UNIVERSAL

HOME

DOCTOR

Edited by

R. SCOTT STEVENSON

M.D., F.R.C.S.

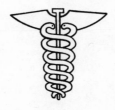

PRENTICE-HALL, INC.
Englewood Cliffs, N. J.
1965

ALL RIGHTS RESERVED. NO PART OF THIS BOOK
MAY BE REPRODUCED IN ANY FORM, BY MIMEO-
GRAPH OR ANY OTHER MEANS, WITHOUT PER-
MISSION IN WRITING FROM THE PUBLISHER.

Prentice-Hall, Inc.
Englewood Cliffs, New Jersey
U.S.A.

Library of Congress
Catalog Card Number: 65–14935

British Edition Published by
ODHAMS PRESS LIMITED
Long Acre, London, England

Second printing . . . . . . August, 1968

PRINTED IN THE UNITED STATES OF AMERICA

93898—B & P

INTRODUCTION

THIS book was designed to present to the reading public a short account of the principles of health, written in terms they would understand. The present edition has been extensively re-written and considerably shortened, with the original purpose borne in mind throughout. Although its concern is mainly with promoting health, the book contains sections dealing briefly with the structure (anatomy) and functions (physiology) of the body, and an outline of the causes, manifestations and treatment of disease. It contains practical advice on the management of sickness. It tells you what to do in a case of accident, poisoning or other emergency. It gives instructions on the steps to be taken in serious illness before the arrival of the doctor. So that the reader may make immediate and accurate reference, the subject matter has been arranged alphabetically with cross-references to subjects of related interest at the end of each entry.

Like other branches of science, medicine has grown during the present century from uncertain childhood into powerful adolescence. Much teaching that was accepted when this book first appeared has had to be discarded in the light of careful observation, experiment and deduction, which are the methods of science; but medicine remains, nevertheless, an art in so far as the term implies human skill. The doctor builds this skill on the foundation of his scientific training by long and constant practice. No book of reference can replace his advice, based as it is on acute observation, wide experience and rapid deduction. What it is hoped this book will do is to assist its readers in the recognition of the symptoms and signs of disease, so that they will neither consult their doctors too late, when delay would be harmful, nor pester him too often with trivial complaints, which could be dealt with at home.

When the causes of disease were unknown and effective treatment was, in consequence, rare it is scarcely surprising that methods of treatment were complex and varied, and their popularity depended more on the support of established authority than on proven merit. It has been a striking tendency in medicine of recent years that treatment has become simpler, and this change has been reflected in the pages of this book.

The boundaries of our knowledge of physiology have altered, as well as those of therapeutics. There is much that is unknown still about the functions of the body in health and still more about its behaviour in disease. The reader must bear in mind that it has often been necessary to be dogmatic for the sake of brevity and simplicity, when the facts have been far from brief or simple.

The discovery of penicillin by Sir Alexander Fleming in 1929 has now taken its place in the pages of history. The years which have elapsed since the war have witnessed much painstaking research into the products of the growth of moulds, and from this work has emerged a new and potent group of drugs which have been christened "antibiotics". These drugs, whose names like streptomycin, aureomycin, terramycin and chloramphenicol have become increasingly familiar, are active against a wide range of diseases, many of which were formerly without an effective answer. Synthetic penicillins have recently been produced in the laboratory, and found to be effective when taken by the mouth.

Much that is new has been learnt about the modes of action of the essential food substances known as vitamins and their numbers have been substantially increased. Surgery has made new strides forward, and greater accuracy in diagnosis has made possible remarkable reconstructive operations on the heart itself. The discovery of the so-called Rhesus blood groups has made it possible to anticipate severe anaemia in an infant before it is born, and has led to effective treatment in the form of prompt blood transfusion.

It is our hope that this book will provide a guide to help parents rear children with healthy bodies. It is their best life insurance. Mind and body are indivisible and disorder in one engenders disease in the other. The clear recognition of this relationship has given a new slant on some old diseases and has earned some reference in the text.

It is easy to glance through the pages of a book of this kind and imagine that one is the victim of all kinds of disease. If this is so, then the author has failed in his object. He has tried, not to foster morbid interest in disease, but to provide a guide to positive health—the key to a full and happy life.

THE EDITOR

CONTENTS

APPENDIX II

LIST OF PHOTOGRAPHS

THE UNIVERSAL
HOME DOCTOR

A BDOMEN. The trunk of the body is divided into two main compartments by a muscular diaphragm. Above the diaphragm is the chest or thorax, and below it is the belly, referred to in polite society as the abdomen. It is sometimes wrongly called the stomach, an error which frequently gives rise to confusion because the stomach is actually one of the many organs contained in the abdomen. The wall of the abdomen is made of muscle which allows the cavity to vary in size and shape with changes in the contained organs and with the movements of diaphragmatic respiration.

If we regard the diaphragm as the roof of the abdomen, then the floor will be the bony basin known as the pelvis which is formed by the fusion of the two hip-bones in front and by their union with the lower part of the spine behind. The muscular walls of the abdomen are attached behind to the spine, above to the lower margin of the ribs and below to the crests of the hip-bones.

The main artery of the body—the aorta —runs down the back of the abdomen closely applied to the spine and gives off branches throughout its length to supply all the organs in the belly. At the brim of the pelvis it divides into two branches destined to supply the lower limbs with blood. Surrounding the aorta is a network of nerves known as the solar plexus. The effect of a blow in the upper part of the belly, or *epigastrium,* such as occurs in boxing, is popularly regarded as due to transitory partial paralysis of the solar plexus.

Contents. The cavity of the abdomen is lined by a smooth membrane called the *peritoneum.* This membrane is reflected from the walls of the abdomen so as to provide a covering for all the enclosed *viscera* or organs. This will best be understood by imagining the way in which a partly inflated balloon forms a lining of rubber to cover a finger thrust towards its center. In this illustration, the finger represents one of the organs attached by its pedicle of connective tissue and blood vessels to the abdominal wall, and the balloon itself is the peritoneum. A small amount of serous fluid lies in the peritoneal cavity and protects the organs and the abdominal walls from friction.

The organs contained in the abdomen are described from the diaphragm downwards and their relationships are best understood by studying the diagrams. Closely applied to the diaphragm and with its main bulk lying to the right under the ribs is the *liver.* Hanging from the lower surface of the liver is a small bag in which bile produced by the liver is stored and concentrated before being poured into the duodenum. This is the *gall bladder.* The *stomach* lies towards the left side of the upper abdomen and crosses the midline to become continuous with a short loop of upper bowel known as the *duodenum.* Behind and to the left of the stomach is the *spleen.* The *pancreas,* or sweetbread, is a long gland firmly attached to the back of the abdomen. It extends from the loop of the duodenum across the abdomen to the spleen, and lies behind the stomach. Also attached to the back of the abdomen and lying on either side of the spine are the *kidneys.* Sitting on the upper poles of the kidneys are the *suprarenal glands,* or adrenals. In the bowl-shaped lower abdomen lie the *bladder* in front and the *rectum* or end bowel behind; and between them in the female sits the womb or *uterus.* The rest of the abdomen is filled with coils of bowel leading from the duodenum above to the rectum below. The long upper part of the bowel is the *small intestine,* and the shorter but stouter lower bowel is known as the large intestine or *colon,* and is divided for the purposes of description into ascending, transverse and descending parts.

Regions of Abdomen. For greater ease in describing the abdomen it is usual to divide it into regions. The area round the umbilicus or navel is called the *umbilical region.* Directly above it is the *epigastric region* or epigastrium, and below it the *hypogastric region.* To the right and left of the epigastrium are the *right* and *left hypochondriac regions.* At the sides of the umbilical region are the *right* and *left lumbar regions,* and below them the *right* and *left iliac regions.*

Abdominal Wall. This consists chiefly

1

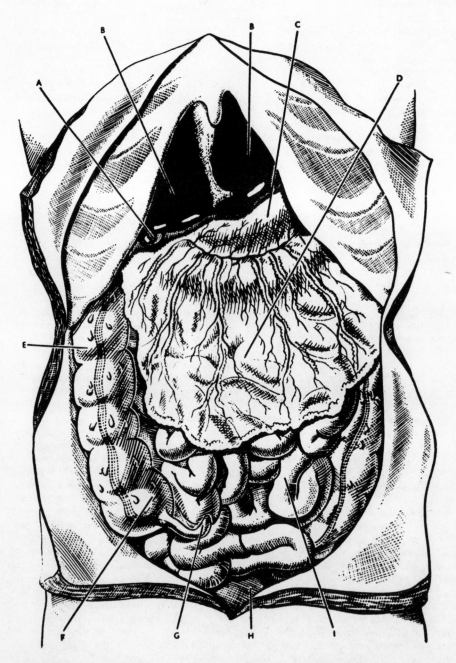

The Abdomen: A. *Gall Bladder;* B. *Liver;* C. *Stomach;* D. *Omentum covering the Intestine,*
E. *Colon (Large Intestine);* F. *Caecum;* G. *Appendix;* H. *Urinary Bladder.* I. *Small Intestine.*

2

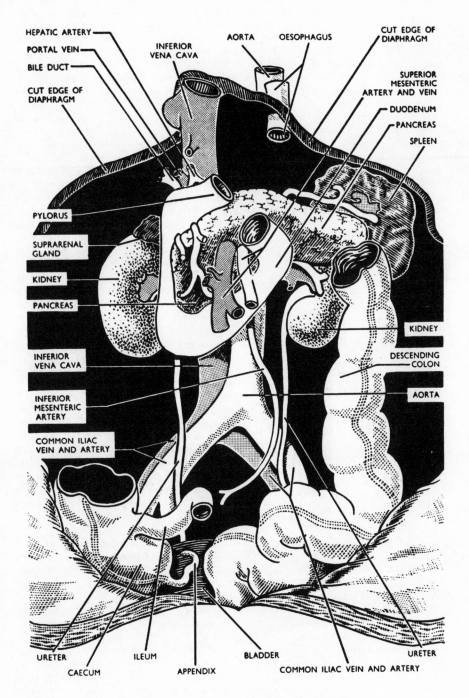

HEPATIC ARTERY
PORTAL VEIN
BILE DUCT
CUT EDGE OF DIAPHRAGM
INFERIOR VENA CAVA
AORTA
OESOPHAGUS
CUT EDGE OF DIAPHRAGM
SUPERIOR MESENTERIC ARTERY AND VEIN
DUODENUM
PANCREAS
SPLEEN
PYLORUS
SUPRARENAL GLAND
KIDNEY
PANCREAS
KIDNEY
DESCENDING COLON
INFERIOR VENA CAVA
AORTA
INFERIOR MESENTERIC ARTERY
COMMON ILIAC VEIN AND ARTERY
URETER
CAECUM
ILEUM
APPENDIX
BLADDER
COMMON ILIAC VEIN AND ARTERY
URETER

Posterior Abdominal Wall. (See ABDOMEN.)

3

of muscle and fat, and has the property of being very elastic, as may be seen from the way it is stretched by pregnancy or severe abdominal distension, and yet can regain its former size when the strain is relaxed. If the elasticity is lost through ill-health or neglect or overgrowth of fat, great discomfort may arise. It is important therefore to keep the muscles in tone through exercise. The abdominal wall has a number of weak spots in it. If the muscles are weakened from disuse, one or other of the organs contained in the abdominal cavity may break through one of these weak spots, thus causing the condition known as hernia (q.v.). This condition occurs in healthy people as an inherent weakness, but may arise as a result of some unwonted physical strain.

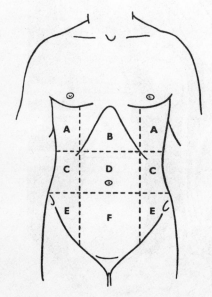

Abdomen, Divisions of: A. *Hypochondriac;* B. *Epigastric;* C. *Lumbar;* D. *Umbilical;* E. *Iliac;* F. *Hypogastric Regions.*

ABDOMINAL BELT. This is a special body belt for giving support to the abdominal muscles during pregnancy or in cases where the stomach muscles are weakened by illness or disuse.

ABDOMINAL INJURIES. *See* FIRST-AID SUPPLEMENT.

ABORTION. When the womb expels the developing ovum before the twelfth week of pregnancy, the event is called abortion. The word miscarriage is applied when this expulsion takes place between the twelfth and twenty-eighth week of pregnancy. After the twenty-eighth week the fetus or developing baby is said to have become "viable," which means that it is considered to have a fair chance of survival. Expulsion of the fetus after the twenty-eighth week before the expected date of delivery is referred to as "premature labor."

The commonest time at which these accidents occur is during the first twelve weeks of pregnancy. In the early months it is possible for abortion to pass unnoticed and be regarded in error as an unusually heavy period.

There are many known causes of abortion. Acute illness, such as pneumonia, or any of the infectious fevers in the mother may give rise to abortion. So may chronic maternal illness such as syphilis or tuberculosis. Where the mother has local disease or displacement of the womb, the developing ovum has a poor chance of survival. Direct injury to the abdomen may dislodge its slender attachments, and fright or shock may so interfere with its blood supply that it dies and is subsequently expelled. When from disease or interference with its blood supply the growing fetus dies, or when it is malformed from abnormal development, miscarriage follows. Some women have miscarriage after miscarriage, yet no cause can be discovered and they are described as having the "habit of abortion." In rare cases this may be due to deficiency of Vitamin E, but more commonly is the result of unbalanced secretions of the ductless glands which govern the whole course of pregnancy.

Doctors may have to induce abortion in cases where continued pregnancy would endanger the health or life of their patient, and this is referred to as "therapeutic abortion."

It is well known that drugs and instruments are sometimes used to procure abortion by those with little understanding of what they do. Such practices are criminal and result often in grave injuries from which the victim may well die. There is no known drug which will bring about abortion with any certainty except when given in such quantities as to endanger the life of the mother.

The cardinal symptom of abortion is bleeding. When bleeding occurs alone the abortion is described as "threatened," but when bleeding is accompanied by pain abortion is inevitable. The pain of abortion is due to contractions of the womb in the attempt to expel its contents and is of the same quality as the pain of labor.

A patient with a threatened abortion must go to bed immediately and stay there until two days after the bleeding has stopped. If pain and bleeding continue for more than a short time the doctor must be called. So must he be called if bleeding persists after the abortion is apparently complete, because this is usually due to fragments of membrane left behind remaining attached to the womb.

The prevention of abortion is directed to the cause, where the cause is apparent. Thus, maternal syphilis is treated and her displaced womb is corrected. In cases of habitual abortion where no cause is obvious it is usual to advise rest at those times when menstrual periods would be expected but for pregnancy. In occasional cases of this type, pregnancy can be carried to full term by the use of glandular extracts and Vitamin E.

The same care and attention are needed after abortion as after normal labor, because it may be just as tiring an experience and involve a considerable loss of blood. A short convalescent period is essential.

ABRASION. Abrasion is the term applied to a slight injury of the skin or mucous membrane. The most important thing is to keep the wound clean, and this is best done by applying a simple antiseptic lotion, such as boric acid lotion or iodine, and covering with a sterile dressing in order to prevent germs from entering.

ABSCESS. An abscess is a collection of pus, or matter. The center of an abscess is yellow in color, and is surrounded by a hot and painful area of hard, reddened flesh which is called the abscess wall, and which serves to keep the pus away from the healthy flesh.

Swelling is usually present and the pain of an abscess has a special throbbing quality. Abscesses are due to the invasion of the tissues by certain germs which have the property of stimulating pus-formation. The germ usually responsible for boils and abscesses under the skin is known as a *staphylococcus*. This germ is normally present on healthy skins and is the reason why untreated cuts so often turn septic. Some staphylococci, however, are unusually invasive and penetrate the skin through hair follicles and minute abrasions. It is these germs which are spread when some unfortunate people have crops of boils. If it is remembered that the pus from such boils is infectious, other members of the family can often be spared the discomfort of a similar visitation.

Some people seem to have a low resistance to invasion by these germs and treatment in these cases is often difficult. Patients with untreated diabetes and others who are ailing from some other cause may develop boils and abscesses.

Other abscesses are described under the headings, Breast Abscess, Gumboil, Psoas, Whitlow. (*See also* BONE; BRAIN; EAR; GLANDS; JOINTS; LIVER; LUNGS; RECTUM.)

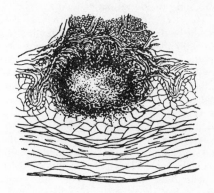

Abscess.

Cold Abscess. There is a form of chronic abscess which is due to the tubercle bacillus, and which is called a "cold abscess." It is of slow development and in the early stages may give rise to few or no symptoms. The usual signs of festering are not often present, but pus gathers slowly under the skin and its presence may be recognized from the fact that the skin pits on pressure, i.e., remains dented for a short time after it is pressed. If left to itself the pus may eventually break through the skin and drain away in the same way as acute abscesses. It is most frequently found in children and young people. If this type of abscess is suspected medical advice should always be sought, as there is usually underlying disease of deeper structures.

In the early stages nonoperative treatment is often tried, and a cure is sometimes obtained. The first essential of such treatment is absolute rest of the affected part for a very long period, even for several years. This rest is secured by means of splints and plaster of Paris bandages or jackets. The patient should live almost entirely in the open air on a generous diet which includes eggs, milk and butter in abundance. Cod-liver oil, or halibut-liver oil, taken daily, is most beneficial.

External Abscess. An external abscess is one which forms in the fleshy parts of the body, or in glands or the cellular tissue just under the skin. The original seat of infection being near the surface of the body, there is little resistance to the growing mass of suppuration, and the pus tracks outwards until the skin is forced to give way and provide an outlet for it.

The treatment of an external abscess should be directed towards maintaining the strength, and therefore the resisting powers, of the patient, and assisting the pus to come to the surface or to "point," as it is called. The patient should therefore rest and especially should keep the affected part at rest. If the temperature is raised, the resting should be done in bed.

Heat should be applied to speed up the full development of the abscess and because it relieves pain. This is best applied as dry heat from an infra-red lamp or, failing this, from a hot-water bottle. Hot fomentations or poultices are often used, but have the disadvantage of making the surrounding skin soggy, and promoting the development of satellite abscesses. Flax-seed meal is a convenient form of poultice. When the abscess begins to point, it should be opened. To leave the abscess to burst of its own accord only means a longer period of suffering for the patient, and the additional risk of septicemia or blood-poisoning. After the abscess has been opened with a carefully sterilized instrument—and this operation should be carried out by a doctor —special care should be taken to keep the

wound clean. The wound should be squeezed to expel as much pus as possible, and then the surrounding skin should be cleaned with a mild disinfectant. A dressing of boric acid in warm water, should be laid on the wound and covered with oiled silk. After the abscess has been opened no further poultices should be used, but antiseptic dressings applied. Both the sulphonamide drugs and penicillin are effective in discouraging the growth of staphylococci, and they may be prescribed by a doctor to abort a developing abscess or to assist in its healing. (*See also* BOILS; CARBUNCLE.)

Internal Abscess. An internal abscess is one which forms in one of the internal organs, such as the liver, kidneys or lungs, or in one of the passages through the body such as the bowels, the esophagus, the bladder, etc.

Internal abscesses are always a matter for the doctor and are often very serious. The earliest symptoms are a more or less localized pain of a throbbing nature, a general feeling of illness and a rise of temperature, with chills, headache and possibly fleeting pains in the limbs. These abscesses almost always require surgical treatment.

ABSORPTION. This means that one substance takes up another. The absorbent most often used in medicine is wood charcoal, which is given as a powder or in the form of lozenges or biscuits to absorb gases in the stomach or bowels, thus relieving flatulence. Charcoal has also been recommended as a means of removing the odor from foul ulcers.

ACARUS. This is the name applied to a mite which takes up its abode in the skin and is responsible for the skin disease known as the itch or scabies.

ACCIDENTS. Strictly speaking, an accident is something that occurs to a person without his expecting it and without his being able to prevent it at the time. The term includes injuries of all kinds, from a black eye to a fractured spine, some trivial and others fatal. A bruise is best treated by cold compresses, firmly applied; in the later stages, massage and gentle movements will prevent stiffness. A sprain requires firm bandaging of the affected joint and massage at an early stage; many so-called severe sprains are really fractures of a bone and should therefore be X-rayed to make certain. The treatment of a wound of any description should be directed, first, to stopping any bleeding, and second, to the application of sterile or at least clean dressings. (*See also* FIRST AID.) A fracture is usually discovered by the person injured being unable to lift the fractured limb, and on someone else trying to do so there is unnatural bending of the limb accompanied by severe pain. In the case of a fractured arm, the arm should be put in a sling, with the forearm at a right angle to the upper arm. When a leg is fractured it is best to bind the fractured leg by handkerchiefs, etc., to the uninjured one, using it as a splint. The fractured bone should be kept as much as possible in its natural position, to avoid its developing into a compound fracture through an end of a bone breaking through the skin. For burns and scalds, the best immediate dressing is a wet cloth wrung out of saline or bicarbonate of soda solution.

ACCLIMATIZATION. Becoming acclimatized means the process of becoming adapted to the climate of a country to which a person has removed. During the course of centuries human beings have naturally become suited to their surroundings, and any great change in their own particular environment is bound to cause great disturbance to their health, unless they take special care. For instance, when a Caribbean or African Negro goes to a temperate or cold country, he runs a much greater risk of getting tuberculosis, pneumonia, or bronchitis than does a white man who is accustomed to the cold climate. In the same way, a white man who goes abroad to a hot climate suffers more severely from malaria than a native who has always lived in the region. The process of acclimatization is always a slow one, and in cases where races of people have been forced to change their surroundings, it has always proved to be costly in human life. It may be said that this is one of nature's ways of eliminating the unfit.

ACCOMMODATION (OF EYE). When rays of light pass from one substance to another—for instance, from air into glass—they are bent from their direct line. This is well shown by putting a stick half its length into a pond, when it appears to be bent. Each substance has its own power of diverting rays of light, which is known as its *refractive power*. This is always the same for any given substance. One of the most important practical uses to which refractive power is put is in the use of *lenses* in eyeglasses, telescopes, microscopes, and other instruments. In the case of lenses, the refracted rays of light meet finally in a point called the "focus."

The eye in health has a changing refractive power; this is known as *accommodation*. If the eye is directed towards a distant object, the rays of light entering it should be focused exactly on the retina; and if the eye is turned towards an object a few inches off, as in reading, the elastic circular ligament in the center of which the lens is suspended is drawn together by the muscle, which allows the lens to become more globular. The lens therefore becomes a lens of higher power, and the diverging rays from a near object are still brought to a focus on the retina. The amount of power possessed by the eye of thus suiting itself for far and near objects is known as its range of accommodation.

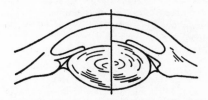

Accommodation of Eye: Showing Change in the Lens.

At the age of forty-five, the lens has lost much of its elasticity, though this change has been slowly going on through life, owing to the gradual sclerosis or hardening of the lens. By the age of sixty, though the lens may be quite clear, it is incapable of this accommodative change in shape. That is, it has now a constant refractive power such as a glass lens has, and its focus is for distant objects only. Consequently, a natural change with advancing years is that persons become unable to read, sew, or do other fine work without glasses, though for distant vision no such aid is necessary. This natural change is known as presbyopia (old-sightedness).

In addition to this, there are three errors

in the refractive power of the eye which may be present at birth, or come on early in life, or in the course of some disease, and persist through life. In these conditions, the movements of the lens are not always sufficient to focus rays of light accurately on the retina. They are known as astigmatism, hypermetropia, and myopia. (*See also* EYE; SIGHT, ERRORS IN; VISION.)

Spasm of Accommodation. This is often found in anyone with faulty accommodation, and is due to the habit of overcoming the fault by an involuntary over-usage of the muscle of the lens. The patient will complain, for instance, that after reading for some time, he cannot "focus" objects on the other side of the room; they look blurred and misty; but after a varying period the condition will pass off, and his distant vision be as good as before. Cases of severe spasm occur sometimes and are very distressing; in these there is always a nervous element.

The eyes are examined under a mydriatic (a drug which dilates the pupil, and is of great use to the oculist). It is then usual to prescribe drops of homatropin at bedtime. They "quiet down" the muscle and do not give rise to discomfort on the following day.

Correcting glasses are also ordered. At first great difficulty may be found in adapting the eyes to them (i.e., spasm occurs), but their use should be persevered with. After a short time they will be quite comfortable.

ACCOUCHEMENT. This is the French term for childbirth. A professional male attendant at childbirth is called an accoucheur and a professional female attendant an accoucheuse.

ACETABULUM. The acetabulum is a cup-shaped depression on each side of the pelvis, into which the head of the thigh bone (femur) fits.

ACETIC ACID. Acetic acid is the acid contained in vinegar. It is a colorless liquid and in its glacial form must not be taken internally. Vinegar is sometimes taken internally as a means of reducing stoutness. Whether it has the desired effect it would be difficult to say, but it would certainly be at the expense of good health. Glacial acetic acid is often applied to warts and corns, but great care should be taken

when using it for this purpose, as, owing to its burning action, it may cause irritation to the surrounding skin. Petroleum jelly should be smeared around the corn or wart in order to safeguard against any accident. Application of the acid should be made by a glass rod or by wrapping some cotton-wool around a match or orange-stick and dabbing immediately over the part. This should be carried out daily, but if any redness or irritation should occur, the applications must be stopped and not resumed until all symptoms have disappeared.

Dilute acetic acid is a 5 per cent solution of acetic acid. It may be given as an antidote to poisoning by alkalis such as strong ammonia, caustic potash or soda. Two or three tablespoonfuls should be given in a little water.

In cases of poisoning by strong acetic acid, the mouth is burnt, and the breath has an odor of vinegar. The treatment is to give chalk or whitewash in water immediately, and later white of egg or olive oil. No emetic should be given.

ACHE. This term is applied to any continuous or throbbing pain. It may occur in a variety of conditions. For instance, in rheumatism, it is not unusual for people to describe their symptoms as a "dull ache." In cases of abscess the pain may be of the throbbing variety.

ACHILLES TENDON. The Achilles tendon is the tendon at the back of the heel. It is so called after Achilles, one of the Greek leaders against the Trojans, about whom the story is told that his mother dipped him in the river Styx as a baby in order to make him invulnerable. Unfortunately, she had to hold him by some part of his body while she dipped him into the river. She therefore held him by the smallest possible place she could grip him by, which was the narrow part of the back of his heel. When he grew to manhood no spear or arrow could harm him, until one day his enemy, Paris, shot him in the back of the heel and thus killed him. The muscles of the calf of the leg are attached to the heel-bone by this tendon. It is the strongest tendon in the body and is not easily put out of order. If torn, it may require an operation to heal it. (*See also* HEEL.)

ACHONDROPLASIA. This is a peculiar disease affecting bones formed from cartilage which fail to develop to their usual size. The disease appears suddenly in an offspring of normal parents and thereafter that affected offspring will usually transmit the affection to his children. Delivery in achondroplasic women usually necessitates caesarian section (q.v.)

The commonest dwarf met in everyday life is an achondroplasic, and his appearance is familiar to everyone. The arms and legs are abnormally short, but the trunk and head are of normal size, the latter giving the impression of being larger than usual. The nose is ususally depressed at the bridge.

The general health is not affected and the subjects of achondroplasia are strong and of average intelligence. There is no means known of preventing its occurrence and no treatment is required. These people are found in all walks of life earning their livings in competition with people of normal stature. Many of them find their way into the circus ring or the music-hall stage, where their quaint acrobatics have a special charm.

The same condition occurs in dogs and its perpetuation is encouraged by inbreeding. The dachshund is a familiar example.

ACHYLIA GASTRICA. This is a deficiency of the normal gastric juice in the stomach.

ACID. This is a term generally applied to any substance which has a sour taste. In chemistry, substances which turn blue litmus paper red are called acids, and this property has been found to depend on the concentration of hydrogen ions. Substances which turn red litmus paper blue are called alkalis. It should be noted that many acids are poisonous and some are corrosive.

Treatment of Acid Poisoning. If strong corrosive acid is taken internally it produces a burning sensation in the mouth, throat, and stomach, and this is followed by severe pain. The patient should be given liberal doses of chalk, magnesia, baking soda, or whiting in water. The doctor should be called at once, but in the meantime *no* emetic should be given to the patient to cause vomiting. Demulcents, such as white of egg, olive oil, or arrow-root may be given. As the patient may

have difficulty in breathing, owing to irritation of the throat, cloths wrung out in hot water may be applied to relieve the pain. (*See also* FIRST-AID SUPPLEMENT.)

ACIDITY. This is commonly called "heartburn." It is a condition in which there is a sour or burning taste in the throat and at the back of the tongue, due to the welling up of acid fluid from the stomach into the mouth, together with an increased flow of saliva. It is one of the symptoms of dyspepsia and may result from hurried feeding or unsuitable food. It is usually relieved by taking alkalis by mouth. (*See also* ALKALI; HYPERCHLORHYDRIA.)

ACIDOSIS. This means a condition in which there is not enough alkali in the blood, with the result that the acids are present in too great a proportion.

Severe starvation leads to acidosis, and the faint but characteristic sweet smell which the acids impart to the breath and urine of a fasting person is supposed to have given rise in the olden days to the expression "the odor of sanctity."

Repeated vomiting, or any other interference with the normal ingestion of carbohydrate foods, leads to an abnormal breakdown of fats to supply the energy requirements of the body. This abnormal breakdown of fats occurs also in diabetes and is always accompanied by an increase in the acidity of the blood.

In order to prevent acidosis it is necessary to see that there is a sufficient supply of carbohydrate in the diet, and in the case of diabetes, insulin. Bicarbonate of soda should be taken several times a day, and glucose up to 2 oz. a day.

ACNE (Acne vulgaris). Acne, or "blackheads," is probably the most common form of chronic skin disease, and is most usual between the ages of sixteen and twenty-six. It is said to occur most often in dark males, but both sexes and all colorings are almost equally affected. It attacks certain definite areas of skin: the forehead, nose, and cheeks; the ear; the back of the neck; and the upper part of the body, both back and front. In rare cases, it covers the whole of the trunk and the limbs.

After thirty years of age it is very rare, but a disease resembling acne occurring after that age often signifies that the patient has been taking some drug, especially the iodides and bromides, or that his work brings him into contact with such irritating substances as tar, paraffin, or chlorine.

The essence of the disease is hyperkeratosis, or overgrowth of the horny layer of the skin. In the mouths of the sebaceous glands of the skin this overgrowth forms a *comedo,* which is a tiny black speck shaped like an elongated onion, and with its horny scales arranged in a similar way. The yellow material which can be squeezed out below this black speck is not really part of the comedo, but is oil which has been unable to get away. In this will be found the roots of a hair, a germ known as the *Bacillus acnes,* and several varieties of other germs, which add to the trouble. The comedo or "blackhead," as it is commonly called, does not get its color from dirt, but from the upper layers of the blackheads becoming dry and horny, and changing in color from oxidation.

Some of the blackheads become irritated, and papules or pimples are formed, which become inflamed. These go on until they form pustules, or tiny abscesses, which range in size from a pinhead to a pea. The number of these pimples depends to some extent on the health of the individual; the more rundown the patient, the greater the crop of pimples.

Sometimes a condition known as "hard acne" occurs. In this there is considerable thickening of the flesh beneath the skin, and abscesses begin to form. These show themselves as red, hard, painful lumps, sometimes half an inch across. They last for weeks or months, fester slowly, and leave a permanent scar.

The skin in acne becomes hardened and is oily, pale, and flabby from want of tone in the muscles of the skin.

Causes. The cause of acne is now generally considered to be the *Bacillus acnes,* which is always found in the comedones. This germ only flourishes in a greasy skin, and we find that sufferers from acne are those whose skin is abundant in natural oils. Among other causes are the increased activity of the skin and hair at the age of puberty, and the changes in the glands which occur at that time. Seborrhoea (dandruff) of the hair and skin (*See* Sebor-

rhoea) is very frequently found with acne, and many specialists believe that there is a definite connexion between the two diseases. The treatment of acne should therefore always include that of seborrhoea. Other contributory causes are defective general nutrition, constipation, anemia, and menstrual irregularities.

Treatment. The main factors in the cure of acne are time, attention to the general health, and perseverance with local treatment. Most cases, even if untreated, slowly clear up in the twenties; but few patients are willing to endure an unpleasant disease for years without some attempt at curing it. Also, the scars left may be disfiguring.

With regard to general treatment, the patient should attend most carefully to the rules of hygiene. He should take regular exercise in the open air, and eat plain but sufficient food, avoiding the rich, "fried-fat" type of diet, and having instead plenty of vegetables and fruit.

With regard to local treatment, one has always to remember the local symptoms of tough skin, greasiness, anemia, and flabbiness. One treatment, luckily, has an influence on all four, and that is the vigorous washing with plenty of soap accompanied by rubbing, which not only removes the grease and thickened horny layer, but by means of the friction with which it is applied, invigorates the blood supply and the muscles. Sulphur soap is generally recommended. This method of treatment is most conveniently carried out at night before going to bed. The simplest way of applying the soap is to make a very stiff lather (some people use a shaving-brush kept for the purpose), rub it very well in, and leave on until the skin begins to smart, then wash off with hot water. At first the patient can only stand a few minutes of the soap application, but the time can gradually be lengthened until he can leave the lather on for hours at a time, or even all night. On one evening a week petroleum jelly only should be used, to avoid too great an irritation of the skin.

Some authorities recommend steaming the face before beginning this treatment, so as to soften the blackheads, and then removing them by means of a comedo-extractor. This should be kept absolutely clean. The common practice of squeezing the comedo out with the nails should be given up; slight bruising is caused, and pustules form more readily in the damaged skin. A rubber sponge, used without soap, is good in some cases where the comedones are fairly loose.

After the face has been washed a sulphur lotion, of which there are endless varieties, should be applied on a cotton-wool swab.

If there are many blackheads, the soap treatment should be used more cautiously —though the skin, by virtue of its "horniness," is very tough in acne—and if too painful, calamine lotion should be used. This should be shaken, and painted on with a brush.

The effect of this treatment is to obtain a slow peeling of the horny layer, a removal of the comedones, and a healthy reaction of the skin by means of the massage. In very resistant cases, however, a more drastic method of peeling the skin with resorcin is employed, but should only be used under medical supervision. Resorcin of 30 to 50 per cent strength in zinc paste is applied at night, left on 30 to 50 minutes, or until "burning" occurs, then wiped off with cotton-wool dipped in olive oil. The face is then washed in the ordinary way, and cold cream is applied. This process should be repeated several times daily until the skin begins to peel, bringing with it the horny layer and many comedones. The patient must remain indoors during the whole of this treatment; but, in a bad case, it "does more in a week than a milder treatment would accomplish in two months." After peeling is complete, a soothing ointment is applied. The treatment may need to be repeated once or twice before a satisfactory result is obtained.

There are far too many variations of these older methods of treatment to give in detail, but the above may be taken as a fair sample. Among newer methods, the use of X-ray, light treatment, or a judicious mixture of the two is becoming more and more popular. They are used to produce an artificial inflammation of the skin —the X-ray having the stronger effect and being especially useful in cases of "hard acne" in much the same way as with the resorcin paste. These methods are often best used after a preliminary medical treat-ment, for if they, especially X-rays, are used before any other kind of procedure it is not uncommon for the disease to become worse for the time being. General improvement, however, occurs after a short period, so that no anxiety need be felt by the patient. Vitamin D is said to have a good effect on acne, and irradiated ergosterol (obtainable under various patented names) internally is said to be helpful; penicillin, also, is sometimes beneficial.

ACNE ROSACEA. *See* ROSACEA.

ACONITE. Aconite, aconitine, and their preparations, are obtained from the roots of *Aconitum Napellus* or monkshood. They produce local anesthesia of the skin. Care should be taken that they do not come into contact with any mucous membrane or broken skin. They are used in the form of an ointment, but much more frequently as a liniment for relieving the pain of muscle strains. Poisoning by aconite is dealt with in the first-aid supplement.

ACQUIRED CHARACTERISTICS. Acquired characteristics of body and mind are those which are not born in us and which develop as a result of our up-bringing. (*See also* ENVIRONMENT.)

ACRIFLAVINE. This is also called flavine, and is a comparatively new antiseptic which is powerful in character, but quite harmless. It is bright yellow when mixed with water. Acriflavine is frequently used as a 1/1000 solution in normal saline as an antiseptic for wounds. It develops its antiseptic action slowly, but that action is not impeded by the presence of serum, as is the case with many antiseptics.

ACROMEGALY. The red-staining cells of the front part of the pituitary gland secrete into the circulation a growth-promoting hormone known as *somatotrophin*. This hormone or "chemical messenger" regulates the rate of growth of all the body tissues. Sometimes as a result of tumors or overgrowth of the pituitary gland this hormone is produced in excess of normal requirements. If this occurs in childhood or adolescence, the result is a giant. After the age of twenty-one, however, most of the bones are incapable of further growth and excess of somatotrophin gives rise to the condition called *acromegaly*. Thus there is a selective overgrowth of the bones of the face, the lower jaw in particular; the hands and feet, which in early adult life continue to grow, develop to an unnatural size; and the spine increases in length though without increasing stature by becoming hunched. The skin becomes thick and coarse. The muscles, like all other tissues, take part in this remarkable overgrowth though to a lesser extent, and in fact these people belie their terrifying appearance and are often surprisingly weak. Those cases due to a tumor of the pituitary gland may develop symptoms from pressure on nearby structures. Thus we find that vision may be disturbed as a result of pressure on the optic nerves and headaches may occur. Later it is not uncommon to find signs indicating diminished function of the gland, and this is brought about by

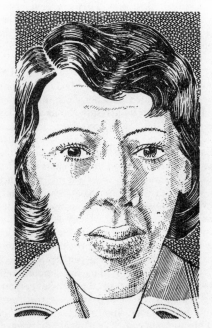

The Facial Appearance in Acromegaly.

the growing tumor compressing and destroying the normal part.

Treatment. Where there are signs of underactivity of the pituitary, it is possible to cure these by injection of a suitably chosen gland extract.

X-rays have been used to bombard the gland from several directions, with shrinkage of the tumor.

When X-rays fail, it has been found pos-sible to remove the gland by surgical operation, though this is never lightly undertaken. (*See also* Brain; Ductless Glands.)

ACROMION. The acromion is a bony projection of the shoulder blade or scapula. Frequently this is injured by a fall, but more often the collarbone which is a attached to it is broken through the force of the blow.

ACTH. Corticotropin, a pituitary hormone, which controls the secretion of adrenal hormones, such as hydrocortisone. (*See also* Cortisone.)

ACUTE. If an illness begins suddenly and gets quickly worse with pronounced symptoms, which in a few days or even hours are at their height, the illness is called *acute*. Diseases are described as acute, subacute (more gradual than acute), and chronic where the condition remains for a period of weeks or months in a stationary condition without becoming either acute or cured). (*See also* Disease.)

ADAM'S APPLE. The lump seen under the skin in the front of the throat is commonly known as the Adam's apple. It is really the most prominent cartilage of the larynx, and is much larger in men than in women. (*See also* Larynx.)

ADDISON'S DISEASE. Addison's disease is a rare condition named after the English physician who first described it—Thomas Addison, a north-countryman of humble parentage who became one of a group of brilliant physicians attached to the staff of Guy's Hospital in London during the middle of the nineteenth century.

The condition is due to some alteration in the function of the suprarenal glands, which fail to produce their internal secretions in sufficient amount to maintain health. This is often the effect of tuberculosis on the glands.

The disease usually comes on gradually with increasing mental and physical weakness, usually worse after periods of activity. At the same time, the color of the skin deepens to a darker shade of brown or even to slate gray. The appetite becomes poor and weight is lost. At times there are attacks of sickness and diarrhea, and at these times weakness may be profound. The blood pressure is low, and without treatment the disease generally continues down-hill, with periods of improvement and other periods when it is worse.

Treatment. It has been shown that the primary disorder which occurs as a result of deficient working of the suprarenal gland is in the regulation of the level of salt in the blood. In consequence, it has been found that many cases can be kept well by increasing their intake of salt by mouth. More severe cases need to have their deficiency replaced by injection of cortisone, made from the suprarenal cortex of animals. A substance, *desoxycortone acetate,* or, more conveniently, DCA, has been made by chemists in the laboratory and will often control the disease when given by injection or implanted in the form of pellets into the abdominal wall. (*See also* ADRENAL; DUCTLESS GLANDS.)

ADDUCTOR. Muscles which move the structures to which they are attached towards the middle line of the body are called adductor muscles.

ADENITIS. This term means inflammation of a gland. Inflammation of the lymph glands of the neck is common and often due to unhealthy tonsils.

ADENOIDS. Behind the uvula and higher up, quite out of sight except when looked for with a special mirror on the end of a long handle, lies a mass of tissue which is called the nasopharyngeal tonsil. A swollen condition of this is known as adenoids. It is composed of the same tissue as the ordinary tonsils, and is normally present in young children, but it should not be so large and swollen that it blocks the back of the nose and interferes with breathing. Infected adenoids are a common cause of deafness and of inflammations of the ear in children. A child with adenoids usually has a characteristic look, with open mouth, long face, narrow nose, prominent front teeth, high, arched roof of the mouth, and flat chest. But in the early stages of the condition, some of these features may not be present, and the adenoids may only be detected on examination by a doctor.

Treatment. There is no doubt that the best treatment for adenoids is removal by operation, which is only a slight affair, and the child's health nearly always improves at once. Whether the tonsils should always be removed at the same time is another matter: under the age of five it is not usually advised nowadays, unless there are enlarged glands in the neck.

ADHESIONS. By adhesions are meant the undesirable attachment that occur in a joint or between internal organs after injury or inflammation. Any joint which has been injured is very apt to become stiff and limited in its range of movement. To prevent adhesions, massage and movements of the joint are begun at an early stage in treatment. If the joint does become set, to get back its range of movement the adhesions may have to be forcibly broken down under an anesthetic.

The inflammatory type of adhesion occurs mostly in the abdomen or lungs and may follow an operation or inflammatory disease, but in some cases they seem to arise as a separate disease. They are not dangerous in themselves, but may cause great inconvenience by obstructing the working of the organ to which they are attached. In the abdomen they may cause strangulation of the bowel or may upset the working of the stomach.

Treatment. If the condition is very distressing it may be necessary to cut the adhesions by surgical operation, but as they are apt to recur, it is as well to try nonsurgical treatment such as massage and electricity.

ADHESIVE PLASTER. This is better known as adhesive tape and is chiefly used for holding dressings in position over a wound. The tape is applied and held in position for a moment, the heat of the body usually causing it to stick and hold fast. If the adhesive is difficult to remove, benzine on a pledget of cotton will greatly aid its detachment. A quick tearing off, sometimes recommended, is unnecessary and unwise. Adhesive plaster should be avoided when dressing septic wounds as it promotes a soggy condition of the skin in which germs readily gain foothold. Similarly, bandages are better dressings for hairy parts and safer for those with sensitive skins.

ADIPOSE TISSUE. Adipose tissue is another name for fatty tissue, the cells of which contain fat globules. (*See also* OBESITY.)

ADIPOSIS DOLOROSA. This is also described as Dercum's disease, and is characterized by the formation of soft painful nodules or swellings of fat throughout the body. It is a very rare condition, but sometimes occurs in women after middle age. Treatment is not very satisfactory, but injections of pituitrin may prove helpful.

ADOLESCENCE. Adolescence or "growing up" in boys usually lasts about ten years, from the age of fifteen to about twenty-five. This is the most critical time in the life of a man, as it is during these years that his character is formed and the basis for his conduct during the rest of his life takes shape. It is a stage which is full of difficulties, and one which demands sympathy and understanding on the part of parents.

The term puberty is given to the age at which a boy becomes capable of being a father. The age varies between twelve and seventeen years, but in temperate climates it is usually around the age of fifteen. The most obvious outward sign of this change is the breaking of the voice, which begins to assume its bass character after a very embarrassing period of intermittent squeakiness. Hair also begins to make its appearance on the face and pubis. The internal activities which are going on in the body at this period are very important ones. The reproductive organs undergo considerable development and become very sensitive to mental and physical stimulus. The sexual instincts begin to show themselves, and the instinct for fatherhood, which is one of the strongest instincts in nature, is unconsciously being aroused. It is at this period that the proper teaching of the meaning of sex should be carried out. The question of whether a boy should be told or not should never arise. It is the duty of every parent or guardian to advise a boy to the best of his ability on all matters connected with sex. It is much better for the boy to learn of these matters in a clean and wholesome manner. There is no doubt that ignorance or the acquisition of knowledge from misinformed companions has caused a great deal of unhappiness in many ways. The nobler instincts should be appealed to, and the proper care of the body and self-control should be emphasized. At this stage in a boy's life there is usually the desire to prove his manhood and stand well in the eyes of his friends. The perils which beset a growing boy are all recognized, and a little helpful guidance, especially from a man, may do much to clear up mental worries and launch the boy into successful manhood.

Adolescence, in Girls. Just as the age of puberty and adolescence plays an important part in the life of a boy, so it is of no less importance in that of a girl. The age at which puberty commences varies between the eleventh and seventeenth year. Adolescence, by which we mean the time in which the girl is growing into the adult woman, usually ends about the twenty-first year, but may go on until the twenty-fifth.

During this period the tissues of the growing girl undergo very rapid changes and assist in the development of her bony framework. This often accounts for the characteristic lankiness and "growing pains" which are noticed at this time. Among the most evident changes are those which occur in the shape of the pelvis. The hip-bones tend to widen and become more curved. The breasts enlarge. The young girl is rapidly developing into a young woman with increasing interest in her own appearance. Not only does the complexion seem to take on an added freshness, but the hair becomes brighter and the eyes develop a new beauty of expression.

Knowing that all these changes are taking place inwardly as well as outwardly, the mother should be ever watchful to see that the young girl does not overtire herself by doing too much either physically or mentally. The bones while they are in this stage of development are very soft, and irreparable damage may take place through careless habits. Many slight deformities have had their origin in allowing the adolescent girl to lean forward on her elbows instead of sitting upright, or from the habit of continually standing on one leg. These little alterations in shape may interfere with the functions of the pelvis in later life.

The periods of menstruation should commence about this time, and should normally occur about once a month. There is a wide variation in the amount and duration, but it should not be accompanied by much pain or distress. A little discomfort and transient depression are the rule at period time and need occasion no anxiety. Much pain, or complete cessation of periods, should be a reason for seeking medical advice.

The mental and moral outlook during the period of adolescence is usually developing rapidly in the growing girl. Her doubts and anxieties are numerous, and it is at this time that a mother should show her greatest sympathy and understanding and prepare her for the important part she may be called upon to play later on in life.

ADRENAL. The word adrenal means "near to the kidney" and is commonly used to denote the suprarenal glands, which are two small bodies placed at the upper ends of the kidneys. The juices which they produce, and which are released into the blood as it passes through them, are essential to life.

The adrenals are composed of two parts, the *cortex* and the *medulla*. The cortex is absolutely necessary to life, and its destruction leads to the disease called Addison's disease (q.v.). The secretion produced by the medulla is called adrenalin, and preparations of it are among the most useful drugs we possess.

At least twenty-eight different crystalline compounds have been isolated from the suprarenal cortex and their chemical compositions determined. Their functions are not yet fully determined, but include: (1) the regulation of the levels of various salts in the blood and tissues; (2) the control of the working capacity of muscles; (3) the provision of a mechanism for resistance to stresses imposed on the body by the toxins of germs, cold, shock, and

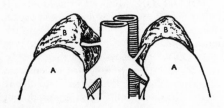

Adrenals or Suprarenal Glands: A. *Kidneys;* B. *Adrenals.*

so on. It is to the last group that cortisone and hydrocortisone, which are dealt with in a separate heading, belong.

Overactivity of the suprarenals in children leads to precocious sexual development, which frequently results, in the case of girls, in premature menstruation, and in the case of boys, in unusual muscular development. In women there may be an excessive growth of hair on the face and body and the appearance may become masculine, with a deepening of the voice. The bearded lady of the fair-ground booths is a classical example of this disorder. (*See also* DUCTLESS GLANDS.)

ADRENALIN OR ADRENALINE. This is the name of a preparation containing the chemical produced by the adrenal inner medulla. It is used to arrest bleeding when it can be applied locally— for example, to the sockets of teeth after extraction, or to the bleeding-point in the nose for nose-bleeding. It is also used to increase the blood pressure in diseases where the circulation is poor, and is of great value in the treatment of urticaria, hay fever, and asthma. It is given by hypodermic injection in cases of shock and collapse, and there is no other drug known which is so successful in restarting a heart which has stopped beating and in counteracting the effects of chloroform.

ADULT. An adult is a person of mature or legal age. The age of legal responsibility in most states is twenty-one, though in many states a person is allowed to drive an automobile or contract marriage at an earlier age.

ADULTERATION. This term is applied to the addition to an article of food of any substance is not naturally present which may or may not be harmful to the health of the consumer. Milk may be adulterated by the addition of water, and this may be very injurious in cases of infant feeding. The addition of any preservative or coloring matter to milk is now regulated by the Food and Drug Administration.

Chemicals are very often added to preserve certain foods. The law demands that the public should be notified by a label on the articles so preserved.

AEROBIC. Aerobic means requiring oxygen or air to live. This term is applied to microbes which require oxygen. Those that do not grow in oxygen are called anaerobic. There are some microbes that are able to grow without oxygen, though they make use of it when present; others grow in its presence, but flourish best without it.

AEROPHAGY. "Air-swallowing," the taking in and swallowing of air. This is a bad habit usually found in nervous patients and of which they are unaware. The patient constantly swallows air and then belches it up again, a habit which can be very disagreeable to those who have to live with him. Occasionally, however, aerophagy may be due to disease of the stomach, such as dilatation of the stomach. In air-swallowing due to nervous causes, the patient should have the matter carefully explained to him and should realize that by resisting all desire to bring up wind he will speedily break himself of the habit. (*See also* FLATULENCE.)

AFEBRILE. Afebrile means without fever.

AFFERENT. This term means carrying towards the center. Nerves which convey sensation towards the central nervous system are afferent nerves. The same term is applied to blood vessels, such as the arteries, which convey blood to the tissues.

AFTERBIRTH. This is the popular name for the placenta, cord, and membranes by which the unborn child is attached to the womb. The placenta comes away a little time after the birth of the child, and it is of the greatest importance that the whole of these membranes should be expelled from the womb. In cases where a portion has been left behind, bleeding persists, and the fragment forms a nucleus on which germs may multiply and infect the mother. (*See also* CHILDBIRTH; LABOR.)

AFTER-PAINS. Following a first labor, no pain is experienced when contractions of the womb occur, but after second or subsequent labors these contractions are felt during the first two or three days and are known as afterpains. These contractions are necessary to expel the blood-clots and debris that collect in the womb after delivery. The return of the womb to normal is usually quicker in those cases in which the mother breast-feeds her baby.

AGE CHANGES. Much depends on the amount of wear and tear a person has undergone throughout life, but despite this fact, there are changes in the body which must occur inevitably. After middle age, the ravages of time have left their mark on all the organs of the body, and the blood supply becomes poorer. The various glands which provide the internal juices upon which the working of the body depends become less active as life goes on.

The teeth show very marked changes in old age, usually resulting in their loss. The joints also are greatly affected and often become painful and less mobile. The diet in old age should be as simple as possible, and the needful amount of food becomes much less after the age of forty. In extreme old age a very small amount of food and sleep suffices.

The body may either lose weight or become fatter. Another change which takes place in old age is in the hair, which usually becomes white and may fall out. The mind loses its capacity for grasping details, and in very old age enters a state of second childishness when it is concerned only with the satisfaction of material wants. (*See also* DEGENERATION.)

AGGLUTINATION. The joining together of blood corpuscles or bacteria is called agglutination. Agglutinins are substances occurring in the blood of a person or an animal suffering from a disease caused by microbes and which are capable of causing the clumping together of the microbes peculiar to that disease. This is exemplified in the *Widal reaction,* which is the test for typhoid fever. The addition of a few drops of a recent culture of the microbe *Bacillus Typhoidus* to the blood of a typhoid fever patient causes agglutination of the microbes, thereby proving that the case is one of typhoid fever.

AGITATION. Medically speaking, agitation means mental disturbance or excitement, restlessness. It is derived from the Latin *agito,* I stir. (*See also* EMOTION.)

AGONY. Persons may say they are "in agony" when they are suffering violent pain or extreme anguish. The phrase "the agony of the death-struggle" is often used, but is a theatrical phrase with little meaning.

AGORAPHOBIA. This term is applied to an exaggerated and unhealthy fear of open places or spaces. The word literally means "fear of a market place." (*See also* CLAUSTROPHOBIA.)

AGRANULOCYTOSIS. Agranulocytosis is a disorder of the bonemarrow whereby it fails to manufacture enough granular white blood cells. The condition is recognized by microscopic examination of a specimen of blood when it is found that these granular leucocytes are either absent altogether or present only in scanty numbers. Since it is the function of these cells to protect the body from invasion by germs, it is scarcely surprising that widespread infections occur in their absence. Thus in agranulocytosis we find inflammation and ulceration of the mouth and throat and sometimes in the vagina and rectum. Symptoms are usually sudden; the temperature is raised and the patient is very ill.

Treatment. It is fortunate that this disorder of bone marrow is usually transient and treatment aims at tiding the patient over until the marrow is restored to normal function. This is achieved by setting up a barrier against bacterial invasion with injections of penicillin and replacing the deficient blood by transfusion. Several drugs are known which are able to stimulate the bone marrow to fresh efforts, and these are often prescribed. Pentnucleotide by injection is perhaps the best known of these drugs, but pyridoxine and folic acid also possess the power to stimulate marrow activity.

Sometimes this condition arises from excessive radiation, but more commonly is due to certain drugs used medicinally. Amidopyrine was formerly used as a cure for headaches but has been abandoned owing to the frequency with which it causes agranulocytosis. The sulphonamide drugs are known to have this effect and should only be used under medical direction. Thiouracil, a drug used in the treatment of thyroid disorders, gold salts, and butazolidin all may possess this depressing effect on bone marrow.

AGRAPHIA. This is a condition in which the patient is unable to express ideas in writing. In certain forms of this trouble, the patient may be able to write, but what he has written conveys no meaning whatever. Sometimes the patient may be quite unable to copy writing, but be perfectly able to write from dictation, while another form is loss of capacity to write from dictation.

AGUE. An old-fashioned name for malarial fever, in which there are severe chills and sweatings and which recur at regular intervals. (*See also* MALARIA.)

AILING CHILDREN. What a difference there is between the strong, noisy, boisterous, healthy child, brimful of energy and high spirits, and his sickly and ailing brother or sister! The little mite may be suffering from anything or nothing. It may be a child who has had a bad start in life, perhaps having been born before time, or perhaps having severe illnesses such as measles or scarlet fever at an early age. Often that early weakness will be grown out of and the child will later on be as strong as the others; or it may be that the infant has been born with some defect which will always be a handicap or has suffered from some disease such as rheumatic fever, tuberculosis or typhoid fever, which will leave it weak in after life. Whether the cause is permanent or temporary, however, the ailing child should never be neglected. Treatment in early life may turn the weakling into a strong man or woman, or, if this is not possible, may prevent him from becoming a permanent invalid.

It is often a fact that the parents who are accustomed to the child and see it every day may be the last people to notice when it begins to go downhill, and attention may be drawn to the child's condition first of all by some relative who sees it after an interval, or by the neighbors or the school-teacher. Then the mother will remember that of late it has been listless, not playing with the others as it used to do. Perhaps it has taken to merely "picking" at its food, or it may have begun to crave for unusual things to eat, such as pickles or a lot of sweets. It may have grown thin or it may have grown fat, colorless, and flabby. Its nature may have altered and it may have become nervy, fidgety, bad-tempered and inclined to cry on the slightest provocation; or it may have become heavy, sluggish, and stupid. There may be nervous upsets such as bed-wetting, sleeplessness, or night terrors. Furred tongue, bad or sweet-smelling breath, a large, round, sticking-out stomach—all are symptoms of health that is not quite as good as it should be. If any of these things are noticed to last for any length of time in a child, it should be taken to the private or school doctor to be examined. "A stitch in time saves nine" is very true of health. Adenoids may cause deformities in the nose and chest that will not mend if they are left too late. A tuberculous joint has a very good chance of getting strong enough to be useful if treated at an early stage. An unstable nervous system may be toned up so that hysteria and neurasthenia are avoided in later life. A little prevention is worth a lot of cure.

AILUROPHOBIA. An unnatural fear of cats. This is different from the easily understandable dislike of the domestic cat found in people who get asthma when they are in the same room as a cat.

AIR. The air or atmosphere consists of a mixture of gases: 77 parts of nitrogen, 23 parts of oxygen and a trace of carbon dioxide. It also contains traces of ammonia, argon, nitrites, and organic matter, as well as a varying amount of water vapor. The purest air is to be found on the tops of mountains or far out at sea. In towns the air is always polluted by gases given off from factories, incinerators, cars, buses, and tobacco smoking, and these, and bad ventilation, encourage the growth and spread of germs which produce disease.

The air is laden with particles of dust which contain specks of coal-dust, hairs, pollen, splinters of wood and many other substances, all of which may be injurious to the lungs. When polluted air is constantly being breathed, especially if there is an excess of silica dust such as occurs in coal mines, an inflammatory condition of the lungs called silicosis may result.

AIR CUSHION. An air cushion is usually made of soft rubber, and can be inflated to any degree required. The round air-cushion with a hole in the middle is the most useful in cases where a patient requires support without disturbance to a wound.

AIR HUNGER. Difficulty of breathing or dyspnoea when a person gasps for breath is referred to as air hunger, and is often due to heart disease. (*See also* DYSPNOEA.)

AIR SICKNESS. This shows itself by sweating, pallor, nausea and vomiting, and usually occurs when in the air, but may develop after a flight has been completed. It is of the same nature as seasickness and is due to an upset of the balancing apparatus of the semicircular canals and the eyes; it is best treated by taking a hyoscine preparation or an antihistamine drug, an hour before flying. Tightening the safety belt and keeping the eyes on a distant point help to overcome it. (*See also* ANOXAEMIA.)

AIR-SWALLOWING. *See* AEROPHAGY.

ALBINISM. Albinism is a condition in which a person or animal is born without the usual coloring matter in the skin. The hair is quite white and the eyes are pink.

ALBUMIN. Albumin is the chief substance found in the tissues of human beings. It contains carbon, hydrogen, nitrogen, oxygen, and sulphur. The white of an egg (called albumen) is largely composed of albumin.

ALBUMINURIA. When albumin, which is an important substance present in the human tissues, appears in excess in the urine, the patient is said to have albuminuria. Its appearance may mean very little if it is temporary and due to faults of the diet or to a feverish condition, but it is also a symptom of disease of the kidneys, and its presence should always lead to a thorough investigation. In pregnant women especially, the presence of albuminuria should always be looked upon as a warning that there may be a danger of the serious condition known as eclampsia or "fits" arising, and for this reason the urine should be regularly examined during pregnancy.

Albuminuria occurs without any apparent reason in children, but they usually grow out of it. There may also be a considerable amount of albumin present in the urine of athletes directly after strenuous exercise. This has no significance.

Many cases of albuminuria are first discovered when the patient submits to examination for life insurance, to which it is usually a bar, owing to the serious outlook regarding a long life for the person with a chronic kidney disease such as Bright's disease (q.v.).

ALCOHOL. The "alcohol" which is commonly referred to is one of a large group of chemical substances known as the alcohol group. Many of these are produced by the fermentation of sugary fluids, ethyl alcohol (alcohol) being much the most important. A simpler member of the same series is methyl alcohol, which is obtained by distilling wood, and is called wood alcohol, or wood spirit. It has similar actions to alcohol, but in human beings is apt to produce fatal and serious results from a single dose. Blindness is frequently caused in this manner.

If a sugary solution is fermented with yeast, as is done in the making of beer and wine, the fermentation continues until the sugar is practically exhausted or until the percentage of alcohol in it has risen to about 12 per cent, at which strength the yeast becomes inactive. This means that any natural fermented liquor contains a dilute solution of alcohol. Wine which is maturing may be a little more concentrated. Further distillation of such a solution of alcohol by the proper method results in the production of pure or rectified spirit (90 per cent), which in turn may be entirely freed from the remaining water and *absolute* alcohol is obtained. Distillation of fermented liquors is the essential feature of the production of strong liquors such as whisky, brandy, rum, gin, or vodka. The flavor depends upon the presence of various other substances which are present together with the alcohol.

When it is pure, alcohol is a colorless liquid with a very faint and fleeting odor.

Effects on Man. In dealing with the action of any drug on living tissues, its strength at the point at which it acts is very important. Strong alcohol used locally on any particular spot is capable of producing great irritation and damage. This property may, however, be used for hardening the skin, and also as an antiseptic, since it will kill bacteria. The drinking of strong liquors is liable to lead to damage of the delicate lining of the stomach unless this be protected by the presence within it of other liquids or solid food. It is also associated with a violent burning sensation both in the mouth and in the gullet, as well as in the stomach. This may vary from the pleasant warming sensation which makes for good fellowship to a severe pain. Different individuals vary considerably in the way they are affected by strong liquors. The ability to tolerate alcohol or to "hold one's liquor" may be lost during or after an illness.

The local irritation caused by drinking strong liquor leads to changes in the body which may not appear to have any connection with it, such as the raising of the blood pressure or the quickening of the rate of breathing. The administration of alcoholic stimulants is thus frequently useful in attacks of fainting, where both the blood pressure and the breathing are impaired. Other irritants, such as smelling salts (sal volatile), serve equally well.

Drinking dilute alcohol induces a feeling of warmth and well-being, and a marked flushing of the face. Not infrequently, gas contained in the stomach is released and allowed to escape by the mouth. These combined actions are known as a carminative effect, and alcohol is sometimes prescribed to secure this effect.

Alcohol in the stomach also causes an abundant production of the gastric, or digestive juices, which property is valuable in cases where these juices are scanty and poor owing to fatigue, exhaustion, general weakness, or excitement. Strong solutions, however, may diminish the juices and should not be taken on an empty stomach.

Alcohol is rapidly absorbed into the bloodstream, and in addition it is unusual in that it passes very readily from the stomach itself into the bloodstream, since most substances are absorbed from the intestine. Substances dissolved in alcohol are also absorbed more quickly than normal. In the bloodstream it is rapidly carried to all parts of the body and is almost entirely consumed, by being burnt up into energy, this taking place chiefly in the muscles. Alcohol is like sugar in that the tissues may consume it without any preliminary change.

Alcohol supplies energy to the body and may thus be considered a food. Unlike other foods, such as sugar, alcohol must be used at once and cannot be stored. In a starving animal which is drawing on its resources of fat or other tissues in order to live, alcohol can save this tissue by supplying the necessary energy. It is extremely easily made use of by the body, even more easily than sugar, but it cannot be stored. The high calorific value of alcohol increases the need of the body for Vitamin B and symptoms of Vitamin B deficiency not infrequently develop in those living exclusively on a diet of whisky and soda.

Since it is very rapidly absorbed, it can

be used without the expenditure of any energy by the body itself; it is valuable therefore in states of great exhaustion, associated with starvation, and in diseases in which the digestion of food is greatly impaired. The addition of alcohol to an otherwise generous diet leads to the conservation of the other food, and in consequence an increase of weight. It is thus used together with strong sugary solutions to fatten thin people; especially popular is the drinking of stout for this purpose. Alcohol only supplies energy to the body, and as this requires many other things in order to function properly, the use of alcohol in place of natural food may lead to a virtual starvation and consequently to grave damage. This is one of the chief causes of ill-health in persons taking large doses of alcohol, and is probably more important than the presence of the alcohol itself. Only a litle alcohol (2 per cent) escapes being used up by the tissues, unless excessive quantities are taken. Moreover, the tissues learn to burn it at a more rapid rate, and thus tolerance is obtained. In healthy people this tolerance may be very large, but is less in sickness.

When alcohol is present in the bloodstream it tends to accumulate more rapidly in fatty tissues, which are well supplied with blood, than elsewhere. Its greatest effect is noticed on nerve tissue, and as the largest collection of nerve tissue is usually situated in the brain, alcohol produces its chief effects there, which are to delay and diminish its response to stimuli. This action is termed *depressant*. Roughly speaking, alcohol depresses the nervous system in a descending order, the more lately acquired faculties being more easily disturbed than the older ones. To this it must be added that alcohol, in common with other drugs, especially picks out that part of the brain which may be weak, either by inheritance, disease, damage, or fatigue. It is untrue to say that alcohol depresses the highest faculties first, since these are not necessarily the same as those most lately acquired. Where education has been continuous and beneficial this might be true; but where, however, the process of education has been interrupted, this may actually be the reverse.

One must take the action of alcohol on the brain to be a gradual undermining of its educational processes, those very recently acquired, or only weakly established (the actual time involved in the learning is most important) being wiped out first. Thus some people who are quite nice when sober, have their social manners removed by alcohol, and under its influence behave badly. On the other hand, those possessing a sound continuous education, and who have continued their moral and mental development without break in their later life's work, gaining good control over themselves, never become really objectionable in their behavior, apart from an increasing stupidity and lethargy.

"Taking wine like gentlemen" is a phrase which has a real meaning. Unstable folk, who because of undue sensitiveness have become reserved and shy, may lose this control in the early stages of the depressing action of alcohol, and may therefore appear to become greatly stimulated. Such people are dangerously affected by alcohol, since this loss of control is associated with a feeling of greatly increased powers. They are in consequence very liable to form the habit of using alcohol for this purpose, and thus become drunkards. Others who are tired and worried by business affairs get the fatigued part of their brain depressed, and in consequence they become relatively cheerful under the influence of quite small doses of alcohol. In this class alcohol may be a real service provided that it is taken in strict moderation and under suitable circumstances, in that it allows an overtired brain to rest in such a way that the untired body may obtain some healthful exercise.

Alcohol is often regarded as a stimulant, and at first sight a superficial study seems to support this view. Very careful observations, however, have shown that from the very commencement of its action some control over the working of the body becomes slackened, especially of the finer perceptions, both of a mental and a muscular nature. Its stimulant effect therefore, can be likened to the removal of control of the mental brakes. In those people where the brakes have not been well-developed, or are over-strained by shock or worry, their removal may take place quite early, and the person becomes excessively excited. In others the brakes are paralyzed along with the rest of the mental processes and they become sleepy and stupid. A further conclusion of the greatest importance is, that while the removal of the brakes may be harmless, or even beneficial, as on an occasion such as a convivial banquet, it may be very dangerous in anyone who is doing something which requires continuous and accurate judgment. In such persons as drivers of any sort of vehicles, workers amongst machinery, and so on, the loosening of the control over the nerves and muscles due to alcohol will be fraught with great danger. For this reason one of the Scandinavian countries forbids anyone driving a public conveyance or motor-car to take any alcohol for several hours beforehand. This prohibition, as can be seen, rests on a sound scientific basis.

It is often stated that alcohol shortens life, and leads to the degeneration of the race. Statistics show without doubt that heavy drinkers up to the age of seventy have a poorer expectation of life than the rest of the population. Over this age they appear to have a much better one. On the other hand moderate drinkers appear to have a slightly greater expectation of life at all age periods up to seventy, as compared with total abstainers. From these very recent studies it is safe to conclude that alcohol in moderate amounts has no effect at all on the duration of life, either beneficial or otherwise.

It is believed that alcohol predisposes to disease, especially infection, and it is well known that alcoholics formerly died when attacked by pneumonia. The probable explanation is that alcoholics do not take sufficient care of themselves, especially in regard to what they eat, and that they become in consequence of this more prone to illness.

Effects on Appearance. Alcohol in any strength has certain definite effects on the appearance. It is not the purpose of this article to discuss the remote effects of chronic alcoholism, the terrible mental and bodily changes which inevitably occur, but to indicate the first alterations produced by even a small quantity consumed regularly.

Alcohol has a definitely harmful effect on the complexion. The pleasant feeling of warmth it gives to the skin is caused by distension of the blood vessels; if these are frequently stimulated they appear to become tired, and remain distended, thus causing an unbecoming permanent flush. Accompanying this, the overfeeding of the skin associated with the excessive blood supply causes an increased working of the oil-glands and the sweat-glands, and also leads to thickening of the skin. So that in addition to redness, the skin becomes coarse and greasy, with marked pores, which no amount of make-up will effectually conceal. The eyes lose their clear, healthy look (they, too, have an increased blood supply), and become dull and bleared.

Alcohol, because it is a rapidly and easily digested food, rapidly adds to the weight of the body. It produces fat inside and out. Add to these changes the look of mental dullness so often seen, even at this stage, and it will be admitted that the appearance will not be improved by its regular and immoderate use.

ALCOHOLIC NEURITIS. *See* MULTIPLE NEURITIS.

ALCOHOLIC POISONING. A very large dose of alcohol leads to such depression of the nervous system that finally the vital centers controlling the breathing, the beating of the heart, and the rate of the blood in the blood vessels fail, and the person may die. An intravenous injection of thiamine (Vitamin B_1) should be given at once by a doctor. Death may take place also as a consequence of the exposure and loss of body heat in those cases where the intoxication has taken place out of doors. In these cases, pneumonia is a common end. Occasionally the breathing of vomited material, due to person lying on the back, may cause death.

Chronic Alcoholic Poisoning. It is generally recognized that the habitual consumption of excessive amounts of alcohol is due to some failure or imperfect development of the mind. In simple cases, drinking alcohol is a method of temporarily escaping reality. Constant running away from reality, or failure to adjust oneself to the circumstances of one's life, together with the presence of a drug which constantly lowers the vitality, especially when the mode of living is imperfect, leads in many cases to complete mental and physical breakdown. In physically weakly people, large continued doses of alcohol lead to an early failure of some function necessary to life, and death results.

ALIMENTARY CANAL. This is the passage through which food passes from the mouth to the anus or lower opening of the bowel. Its parts are called, in the order in which they occur, the mouth, pharynx, esophagus (or gullet), the stomach and pylorus, duodenum, jejunum, ileum (small intestine), caecum and appendix, colon (large intestine), the rectum and anus.

ALKALI. This term is derived from an Arabic word meaning soda-ash. When an alkali comes in contact with an acid substance, the two unite and neutralize each other; in other words, they form a salt substance which is neither alkaline nor acid. This principle is embodied in the treatment of dyspepsia and peptic ulcer. In these cases a weak alkali such as bicarbonate of soda or magnesia is given to neutralize the acid gastric juice, with effective relief of pain.

ALKALINE POISONING. Strong alkalis such as caustic soda, strong ammonia, etc., act as very corrosive poisons. Emetics should not be given, as the act of vomiting would only increase the irritation of the throat. While the doctor is being called, the patient may be given a small quantity of lemon juice or vinegar, in about half a glass of water. This may be followed by milk, white of egg beaten up with a little water, barley-water, arrowroot or olive oil. To relieve pain in the abdomen and throat, hot fomentations should be administered and the patient should be kept as warm as possible. (*See also* FIRST-AID SUPPLEMENT.)

ALKALOID Alkaloids are substances, extracted from plants, which have a powerful action. They are alkalis and are nearly all bitter to the taste. Some of our most powerful and useful drugs are alkaloids. A few of the more common ones are aconite, obtained from monkshood, atropine from deadly night-shade, cocaine from coca leaves, digitalin from foxglove, ergotin from rye, morphia, heroin, and codeine from poppies, nicotine from tobacco, quinine from cinchona bark, and strychnine from nux vomica seeds.

ALLERGY. This means "altered reaction," and is best described as an abnormal sensitivity or idiosyncrasy in certain individuals to some substance, food, or material. The substance producing "allergy" is usually a protein, and is known as an allergen. Its manifestations, such as swelling, itching, and bodily discomfort, are often brought about by a particular article of food, the most common being fish, eggs, milk, and wheat. If, for example, after a meal all of the participants become ill, something was probably wrong with the food; but if only one person becomes ill, with all eating the same food, something was probably wrong with that individual. In the first case, the condition is food-poisoning; in the second case, food *allergy*. But allergy is not necessarily associated only with a disposition to being upset by certain foods. Hay fever, in which the person is upset by the irritation of certain pollens—timothy grass being the most common—is a form of allergy; and so is asthma which, however, may often be brought on by certain articles of food; one person may get an attack of asthma from the same food from which another allergic person may get an attack of hives (urticaria). The real cause of allergy is still obscure, but it can be controlled by the avoidance of the upsetting articles of food, and by injections of adrenaline, ephedrine, or peptone. Antihistamine drugs, such as phenergan and benadryl, are often effective in controlling alergic reactions, though they are more effective in hay fever and urticaria than in asthma. (*See also* ANAPHYLAXIS; ASTHMA.)

ALMOND. Almonds are among the most nutritious members of the nut family and contain a large percentage of highly digestible fat, as well as protein and carbohydrate. One great objection—shared with most nuts—is the large amount of cellulose they contain, which makes careful chewing necessary. The bitter almond contains an oil which is quite distinct from the oil obtained from sweet almonds. Ordinary almond oil is a very pleasant substance and is often used in ointments. The oil of bitter almonds is used in small quantities as a flavoring in cakes and confectionery. Prussic acid is produced from the oil of bitter almonds.

Bitter Almond Poisoning. The patient

should be roused by dashing cold water on his face and chest. An emetic of mustard and water should be given. If the breathing is difficult, artificial respiration should be started. Some stimulant, such as brandy or whisky, may be given, and the patient should be kept warm with hot-water bottles and the doctor called for. (*See also* ARTIFICIAL RESPIRATION; EMETIC.)

ALOES. Aloes is one of the most popular drugs used for the purpose of purging the bowels. It is included in many patent medicines and pills, acts chiefly on the lower bowel, and is useful in the treatment of chronic constipation. It is not a suitable drug to give to pregnant women, as it has been known to produce abortion. It is, indeed, popularly thought among many ignorant women that all they have to do to procure abortion in the first months of pregnancy is to take stiff and purging doses of aloes. This is, of course, mere folly. If a pregnant woman is healthy, aloes will only make her miserable and uncomfortable, to the detriment of her health. Aloes alone causes severe griping pains, so it is often used in combination with some such drug as belladonna.

ALOPECIA AREATA. This is the term given to the development of small rounded areas of baldness on the scalp. These sometimes increase in size and run together until the whole scalp appears absolutely hairless. The cause of this disease is not definitely known and its course is unpredictable. Recovery is usually slow, and in elderly persons, will probably take a longer time.

Treatment. All forms of treatment aim at stimulating the scalp in some way or another. The scalp should be kept thoroughly clean and sulphur ointment should be rubbed in every night. Other remedies are turpentine, vinegar and paraffin oil. It should be remembered that the rubbing necessary for the application of these remedies is probably the most important part of the cure. Applications of ultraviolet rays have sometimes proved of great benefit. (*See also* BALDNESS.)

ALTITUDE. By altitude is meant the height of a place above the level of the sea, which is the standard by which height is measured, since the sea is the one thing which is the same height all over the world. Consumptives often travel to Arizona or

New Mexico for treatment, and their recovery is frequently attributed to the lightness and purity of the air in that part of the country. In actual fact, however, climate is now regard as less important than proper treatment with modern medicines such as isoniazid and streptomycin, together with hygienic and dietetic measures. Nowhere is height so important to health as in very hot countries such as India and the Malay States. In these countries there are hill stations high up in the mountains to which people from colder climates can go every year for a period of respite from the great heat which is not natural to them.

The pressure of oxygen in the atmosphere at altitudes more than 14,000 ft. is insufficient to support life for long. Aircrews and mountaineers working above this level need added oxygen from a cylinder. Accidents in aircraft have occurred from failure to observe this simple rule. Neglect of it leads to mental disturbances, fits, and paralysis.

ALUM. Alum is an astringent formerly used in a throat paint. Powdered alum applied to a cut will often stop bleeding. One or two teaspoonfuls dissolved in a pint of hot water may be used as a vaginal douche in cases of leucorrhoea or "whites." A solution of alum is useful to destroy slugs, snails, and their eggs without harming the plants.

ALVEOLAR ABSCESS. *See* GUMBOIL.

ALVEOLUS. The bony socket in which the tooth is fixed is known as an alveolus. A gumboil is known as an alveolar abscess and is usually due to a decayed tooth.

AMAUROSIS. This is the technical name for part or total blindness. (*See also* BLINDNESS.)

AMBLYOPIA. For centuries the term amblyopia has been used to mean defective vision for which there is no recognizable cause in any part of the eye. It has been described as a "disease in which the patient sees nothing and the physician sees nothing."

The term amblyopia, though loosely employed, is convenient to describe cases in which the ophthalmoscopic changes are insufficient to account for the symptoms.

The causes suggested are very numerous,

the most important being (excluding diseases of the eye and neighboring parts) toxins such as tobacco and lead, and defective development. In toxic amblyopia, the poison may be introduced from without, or manufactured in the body. Tobacco and lead are by far the most important in the first group, though quinine, sodium salicylate, morphia, and other drugs are sometimes the cause. Body toxins, which cause more passing and less characteristic symptoms, are chiefly uremia; migraine caused by digestive disorders; and, more rarely, fevers, such as malaria. (*See also* BLINDNESS; DEFECTIVE VISION.)

AMENORRHOEA. This means the absence of the "courses" or menstrual flow during the period of life in which they should be present. (*See also* MENSTRUATION.)

AMMONIA. A strong, colorless, pungent gas which is very easily dissolved in water. Preparations of ammonia are used extensively in medicine as heart stimulants and gastric stimulants. It is also useful in bronchitis. Aromatic spirit of ammonia or *sal volatile* is used in many forms of smelling salts. Household ammonia is used for domestic purposes, but it should on no account be taken internally. Ammonia is a very good application in cases of insect bites or stings.

Ammonia Poisoning. Ammonia acts as a corrosive poison and breathing its vapour has been known to cause death. The air passages become inflamed and great difficulty in breathing may result as a consequence. No emetic should be given. Lime juice or vinegar in half a glass of water followed by bland substances such as milk, eggwhite, arrowroot, or olive oil may be administered. The patient should be kept warm and the doctor called for.

AMNESIA. This is the medical name for loss of memory. The condition calls for psychological treatment.

AMNION. The amnion is the bag or sac in which the foetus or unborn child is enclosed. It contains one or two pints of fluid in which the child floats.

AMOEBA. This is a single-celled, colorless, jelly-like germ found in the sea and in fresh waters. This single cell represents one of the simplest forms of animal life,

and as such may be regarded as the original ancestor of man.

An amoeba is responsible for a disabling inflammation of the gut in tropical countries, known as amoebic dysentery.

AMPOULE. An ampoule is a small, sealed glass capsule. Ampoules are used for holding small measured quantities of drugs, vaccines, or serums sterile and ready for use.

AMPUTATION. By amputation is meant the cutting off of a limb or other part of the body. Amputations have been called the last resort of the surgeon, and are never carried out nowadays unless the surgeon has found himself unable to cure the disease which makes the amputation necessary. Amputations are much less common today, except in time of war, than they were a generation or two ago. In performing an amputation a surgeon always preserves as much of the limb as he can, but at the same time he must consider how to make the stump as suitable as possible for having an artificial limb fitted. (*See also* ARTIFICIAL LIMBS.)

AMYL NITRITE. This is a clear, yellowish liquid, with a penetrating odor. When given by inhalation it is rapidly absorbed and produces relaxation of the muscular walls of arteries. It relieves Angina of Effort (*see* ANGINA PECTORIS) by dilating the coronary arteries which supply the heart with blood. Amyl nitrite is usually supplied in small capsules which can conveniently be carried and used by crushing in a handkerchief when necessary. (*See also* ANGINA PECTORIS.)

AMYLOID DISEASE. This name is given to a condition in which a starch-like substance is found in the tissues owing to disease.

The process affects the tissues of the blood vessels of various organs, especially the liver, spleen, kidneys and bowels, and is associated with chronic suppuration in the body. Another name for this condition is lardaceous disease. (*See also* NEPHRITIS.)

ANALGESIA. By analgesia is meant insensibility to pain. A remedy that relieves or deadens pain is called an analgesic. (For a description of various analgesics *see also* ANESTHESIA.)

ANEMIA. Anemia may mean a deficiency of blood as a whole in the body, or it may be a deficiency of the number of red cells in the blood, or of the red-coloring matter (hemoglobin) of the blood.

Anemia may be local, e.g., affecting a small portion of the body only, when it is known as *ischemia,* or it may be general throughout the whole system when it is divided into two main types—*primary anemia* and *secondary anemia.* A primary anemia is one for which there is no obvious cause, while a secondary anemia is one for which a cause can be found. Anemia may be due to a failure to manufacture enough blood, to increased use of it in the body, or to loss by bleeding.

General pallor is not necessarily an indication of anemia. The Latin races are paler than the Anglo-Saxons. People who work with lead, such as painters, and addicts of drugs such as morphia may all have a permanently pale skin, but it does not follow that they are anemic.

Local Anemia or Ischemia. All the tissues of the body are supplied with blood which is pumped round from the heart. The supply to the various parts can be regulated by the contractions of the arteries according to the needs of the parts. Under certain conditions it may happen that too much blood enters one area so that other parts suffer from a shortage. This occurs in a state of shock, when the blood remains in the smaller blood vessels of the abdomen and the brain may have too little blood, with the result that the individual becomes unconscious. Another form of local anemia is seen in Raynaud's disease, in which the walls of the arteries of the extremities, e.g., the fingers and toes, contract and do not allow the blood to enter the parts. (*See also* RAYNAUD'S DISEASE.)

Symptoms of Anemia. Perhaps the earliest complaint is a feeling of "being out of sorts" or tiredness. Relatives or friends may notice an increasing pallor. Later it is found that jobs which were formerly done with ease leave the patient a trifle breathless. Sometimes there is discomfort in the upper abdomen, or indigestion, and on rising from a chair the patient may have to hold on for a moment until a transient dizziness passes off. Complaint is often made of palpitations and pulsation in the neck, which is really just awareness of a rapidly beating heart.

Menstruation is either more free than normal or very scanty. Any small scratch or cut may be difficult to stop bleeding. The defective supply of blood in the brain often results in a kind of neurasthenia; the patient worries over trifles, sudden noises make him jump, he is unable to concentrate or to stand prolonged mental or physical strain.

Chlorosis. This is a special type of iron-deficiency anemia occurring in adolescent girls. The skin may assume a characteristic greenish complexion, which is most marked in brunettes. The body as a rule is well nourished, and this, together with the peculiar complexion, forms a characteristic picture. Owing to the change in the mode of living among women, the disease is now a rare one.

Causes of Anemia. The causes of anemia have been fairly completely worked out so that fewer and fewer cases are labelled as "primary anemias." Roughly, cases can be divided into two main groups—those in which there is excessive loss or destruction of blood, and those in which there is defective blood formation. In the first group belong those who have obviously lost blood from injury, childbirth, or piles. In some cases the loss of blood takes place silently, as from a bleeding peptic ulcer. Sometimes blood undergoes destruction while still in the circulation. This occurs in malaria and in an inborn weakness of the red cells called acholuric jaundice.

In the group due to defective blood formation, many cases are the result of inability to absorb the materials necessary for the manufacture of hemoglobin. Iron is the most important of these materials, and some people seem to be unable to absorb it properly from their gut. This deficiency can always be replaced by providing an excess of available iron in the form of pills. Green vegetables and meat normally provide enough iron to supply our needs. Falure to absorb a complex chemical substance known as Vitamin B_{12}, which is the active principle of extracts of liver, causes pernicious anemia.

Last of all are a few cases due to failure of the bone marrow to produce red cells.

This type of anemia is known as aplastic anemia and may be due to drugs or infections. More rarely, it is without determinable cause.

Treatment of Anemia. Clearly a careful analysis of the cause is the best guide to treatment. Bleeding must be stopped and the blood replaced if necessary by transfusion. General hygiene is important; proper ventilation of the bedroom at night, so that the air breathed out is not allowed to accumulate. Clothing should be sufficient for warmth, but should not be excessive. Meals must be regular and no food must be taken between meals. The amount of sleep required by the patient depends on the severity of her case; where there is any failure of the circulation, the patient should remain in bed altogether, until these symptoms disappear. Where there are signs of mental irritability, some sedative, such as bromide or aspirin, may be necessary at first. Later on exercises, which must be graduated and should always stop before producing fatigue, are very useful, since they assist the circulation generally. The exercises increase the activity of the skin and tone up the whole body generally. (*See also* SUPPLEMENT ON ATHLETICS AND REMEDIAL EXERCISES.)

Drug Treatment of Anemia. Iron-deficiency anemia is treated by giving one of many active preparations of iron by mouth. Ferrous sulphate is probably the best preparation and is dispensed in pills and capsules. The daily dose needed to effect a cure is 9 grains. An excellent form is as Blaud's pills, which are not a patent medicine, but an old and valuable formula. They are given in large doses, up to 45 grains a day. Iron and ammonium citrate is also valuable, up to 90 grains a day being given. It is most important to go on taking the iron for at least three months, and if necessary to resume it afterwards in smaller doses as recurrences are so common.

Colloidal forms of iron suitably prepared, injected daily for a dozen times or so into the bloodstream, will often cure the anemia for several months.

In the case of children it is necessary to accustom them to the iron gradually, giving iron and ammonium citrate in small, increasing doses; it can be given in milk. Infants are said to be better with traces of copper and manganese with the iron. The child should have plenty of fresh air and plain food such as milk, eggs, butter, and oatmeal.

ANEMIA, PERNICIOUS. This serious disease is described in a separate article under the heading PERNICIOUS ANEMIA.

ANESTHESIA. By anesthesia is meant the state of unconsciousness or insensibility to pain to which patients are reduced before a surgeon performs an operation on them. It may not be necessary to render the patient completely unconscious if only a small part of the body is to be dealt with, such as a finger or the opening of a boil, so that anesthetics are divided into the two classes, *general* and *local,* according to whether the whole body is to be rendered insensible or only a small part.

Until about halfway through the last century operations were performed on conscious patients and there are many old accounts of how dreadful this must have been, several strong men being sometimes required to hold the agonized patient down on the table while the operator continued with his job. Many cases there were too of absolute heroism where operations were borne without flinching which must have entailed pain so great that none could contemplate enduring it nowadays. It was not possible, of course (before the discovery of modern anesthetics), to perform any of the delicate operations on vital organs that are now possible. Surgery was mostly a matter of cutting off limbs, "cutting for stone," bleeding, and a sort of digging out of tumours. Naturally, all sorts of ways were tried to deaden the pain by stupefying the patient. The ancient Greeks used nepenthe, and hyssop was offered to Christ on the Cross. Preparations of opium and hashish and similar drugs were tried, and often the patients were operated on when "dead drunk." At a later period hypnotism was tried and was occasionally successful.

At the beginning of the nineteenth century, Sir Humphry Davy, the great scientist, discovered that he could anesthetize himself with nitrous oxide ("laughing gas"), but his discovery was not made any use of until fifty years later. In 1846, W. T. G. Morton first used ether in Boston, Mass., and in 1847 Sir James Simpson discovered the anesthetic use of chloroform at Edinburgh. It was not, however, until Simpson administered chloroform to Queen Victoria at one of her confinements that general anesthesia received the approval that made it so universal as it is today.

The drugs chiefly used today for general anesthetics by the inhalation method are halothaneurthoxygen, and nitrous oxide, commonly called "gas" or ether. Each will be mentioned in a short paragraph, but whatever the anesthetic drug used, the effects and method of giving it are much the same. There is first a semiconscious state in which the patient feels the world swirling around him and in which he may talk, sing or laugh. With a skilled anesthetist this only lasts a very short time, perhaps only seconds, and it is quite unnecessary for people to worry themselves, as they frequently do, by thinking that they may behave in an unseemly fashion or use had language that they would not use in daily life. As far as the patient is concerned, it is the usual experience for him to hear the anesthetist say when he is commencing to give the anesthetic some such phrase as "breathe deeply please," and then to know no more at all until some time after the operation is safely over and he is comfortably back in bed. In the matter of taking an anesthetic well, the patient can help the doctor considerably by overcoming his dread beforehand and going to the operation with a quiet mind. It is only reasonable to suppose that the patient who enters the operation theater with a contented and resigned mind will be easier to anesthetize than the patient who gives way to panic at the last moment and struggles against efforts to give him the anesthetic which will relieve him of his pain. In this connection it may be pointed out that when a death occurs while a patient is under an anesthetic the law requires that there shall be an inquest, and inquests are reported in the newspapers, but no mention is made of the thousands of persons who undergo operations and survive the anesthetic. Far more people are killed by accidents in the streets than by anesthetics, and sensible people do not go through life dreading they will be killed every time they venture to cross the road.

Nitrous Oxide. Also known as laughing gas, this is used for short operations, such as the extraction of teeth, as it enables the patients to lose and regain consciousness in a very short time. The patient feels quite well after the operation and is able to walk home. It is chiefly used for dental work and other short operations. It has great advantages since it rarely causes vomiting, and there is no need for the patient to be watched for a long time afterwards. Nitrous oxide is a gas with practically no smell. It is sold in cylinders in liquid form, and by turning on the tap it is set free as a gas. It is then passed into a rubber bag and from this container is passed to a suitable mask or face-piece, and then to the patient.

An "ordinary" anesthetic consists in giving the patient just enough gas to make him unconscious for about a minute. The mask is then removed entirely from the patient's face and the small operation is performed before the patient recovers consciousness. In some cases a condition of analgesia—in which the patient is not quite unconscious but does not feel pain—may be present for a good deal longer.

Ethyl Chloride. This substance deserves to be specially mentioned. It is a fluid which can be carried about in glass tubes. It turns into vapor very easily, but unfortunately has an unpleasant smell, which can, however, be disguised to a certain extent by adding to it a scent such as eau-de-Cologne. Ethyl chloride was formerly used for short operations such as the removal of adenoids in children, and was used to add to the effect of nitrous oxide in adults, in cases where the latter gas is not sufficient by itself.

Chloroform. Chloroform is a sweet-smelling fluid. When it is used by itself it must be mixed with air. It can also be used together with nitrous oxide or ether. In children there may sometimes be a delayed harmful effect on the liver, though the danger of this may be lessened by giving the patient glucose before the operation.

Ether. Ether has become more popular than chloroform for general use because it is supposed to be safer. It stimulates the heart and causes the blood pressure to rise, whereas chloroform depresses the heart and lowers the blood pressure. It is, however, more irritating to the lungs and has a less pleasant smell than chloroform.

Pentothal. This is usually given by injection into a vein, and can be used along with most other anesthetics, such as gas and oxygen.

Trilene (trichloroethylene). This resembles chloroform, but is much safer, and is usually given mixed with gas and oxygen.

Fluothane (halothane). This is non-explosive, reduces blood pressure, does not affect the heart, and gives good muscle relaxation. It is, however, rather expensive.

Muscle relaxants. These are used in order to bring about muscular relaxation in the patient, without deep anesthesia, so that consciousness returns early. The most popular are Tubarine (a curare preparation) and Scoline (suxamethonium), which are given by intravenous injection.

Intubation. In many operations, when gas and oxygen is administered (usually along with another anesthetic, such as trilene) the anesthetist prefers to give it by means of a rubber tube passed down the nose or mouth into the windpipe, after the patient has been put to sleep. This is safe, harmless, and helpful alike to the patient and to the surgeon.

Premedication. This means the giving of drugs for various purposes before an operation. One of the commonest drugs to be given before an operation is atropine, which diminishes the saliva in the mouth and prevents irritation of the lungs. Other drugs, such as morphine derivatives (Npeutopon, Demeral and Dilaudid) and scopolamine, are used before the operation to quiet the patient's mind and prevent any feeling of dread of the anesthetic. The barbiturates Nembutal and Seconal are also used in this way. It is usual to make the patients go to sleep in their beds by this means, so that they do not know of the journey to the operating theater and do not wake up or remember anything until several hours after everything is over.

The first attempts to achieve this were by injecting a mixture of ether and olive oil into the bowel. This caused the patient to go to sleep in bed, and if necessary a small amount of ether was given in the usual way during the operation. Other drugs given thus are paraldehyde and, more recently, avertin (or bromethol), which is of German origin and has proved very successful in general use. The advantages of this method are that the patient is not frightened before-hand and will sleep for a longer time afterwards and so will feel less pain. There is less vomiting after the operation and less of the general anesthetic is required during the operation.

There are, however, several disadvantages. More nursing will be required after the operation, since the patient takes longer to become conscious. He will not be able to clear his throat and lungs by coughing or spitting, and great care must be taken lest too much of other sedative drugs is given afterwards. It is often necessary to give morphia after these anesthetics, as they tend to make the patients more excited than the ordinary general anesthetic. The harmful effects on the lungs and liver are the same as with general anesthetics taken by the old inhaling methods.

Local Anesthesia. The main difference between local anesthesia or analgesia and general anesthesia is that in a local anesthetic only a portion of the body is rendered insensitive to pain, and the patient remains conscious. Large operations can be performed under a local anesthetic when the patient's heart is in a bad condition.

Drugs Used. Of the drugs used for local anethetics, cocaine is the best known, though nowadays it is only applied for operations on the eyes, nose or throat, and never injected, because of the serious effect it may have on the general health if used in this way for larger operations; also because of the fact that it goes bad very easily. Several new preparations have therefore been introduced which are used in the same way as cocaine, but have not its disadvantages. It is sufficient here merely to give the names of some of them, as for example, Nupercaine Kylocaine, Neppercaine and Benzocaine and Procaine. Quinine-and-urea-hydrochloride is found useful when prolonged anesthesia is desired, as its effects may last several days.

To obtain the effect of deadening the part to be operated on, these drugs are injected into the flesh of the part, or into or near the nerves which supply the part with the power of feeling, or they may be rubbed on, painted or sprayed on to the surface.

Another way of deadening pain in a

small area is to freeze the skin of the part with a freezing mixture which is sprayed on to it. This deadens sensation for only a very brief time and is useful for opening small abscesses and similar short operations. Ethyl chloride is the drug generally used for this freezing.

Spinal Anesthesia. Sometimes the anesthetic drug is injected straight into the spinal canal in the backbone, thus temporarily destroying all feeling below this point; the patient has usually been given a narcotic or stupefying drug such as morphia or scopolamine some time beforehand to help to obtain the deadening effect. These spinal anesthetics are used for large operations on the lower body which take a long time and would otherwise require a long general anesthetic and cause the patient a lot of shock.

Anesthesia and Analgesia in Childbirth. Birth is always looked upon as a natural function, but the pain which now accompanies it is probably one of the penalties of civilization. The biblical teaching that pain and travail are associated with childbirth may to some extent account for the fact that so little attention has been paid to this in the past. When Sir James Simpson, of Edinburgh, endeavored to bring relief to women in labor, his strongest opponents were those who brought out ecclesiastical dogma in argument.

Suffering such as is often felt during childbirth will cause exhaustion, which is the chief cause of delay in the birth and the most frequent cause for forceps having to be used. The results of exhaustion may be shock, faintness, bleeding, and perhaps even blood poisoning. The main difficulties to be met are that the pains of labor are prolonged for several hours, and that there are two lives to be considered, while the effects of drugs upon the unborn child are practically unknown.

Twilight Sleep. In order to carry out the proper procedure for twilight sleep, the patient should be put to bed in a darkened and soundproof room. If the room cannot be made completely dark, a bandage should be placed over the patient's eyes. The ears should be plugged so that no noises from the outside are allowed to disturb her and the nurses must walk in rubber-soled shoes. Small doses of scopolamine should be given as long as the patient is still able to recognize familiar objects handed to her, and repeated until a state of amnesia or loss of memory is reached. The object of this treatment is that the patient shall have no recollection of anything that takes place while she is in labor or while the child is actually being born.

This method of relieving pain in childbirth has been largely discarded because the drug scopolamine in the doses needed to produce amnesia depresses the breathing of the newborn infant.

Gas. Gas in the form of nitrous oxide and air or oxygen is often given to relieve labor pains, and it does not seem to have any ill-effects on either the mother or the child. Its only disadvantage is that a somewhat cumbersome piece of apparatus is needed for its safe administration.

Chloroform. Chloroform is a very satisfactory anesthetic and can be used as soon as the patient feels the labor pains beginning. Small doses of chloroform are now being put up into ampoules so that anyone can use it when necessary without fear of taking an overdose.

Trilene. This is used a great deal and is safer than chloroform; it seems to have less effect on the child and does not in any way interfere with the normal processes of childbirth.

Many of the aftereffects of an anesthetic can be avoided if it is given properly, but though nausea and vomiting may occur, they are not serious.

Treatment of Vomiting. If the patient vomits after an anesthetic he should be turned over to the right side. Strong black coffee may be given by mouth.

The "pernicious" type of vomiting, characteristic of delayed chloroform poisoning, is serious; it is treated by means of injections of glucose and insulin.

ANESTHESIA OF THE SKIN. By anesthesia is meant loss of feeling—that is, loss of sensation—in any part.

Anesthesia of the skin is always due to some damage to the nerves which supply the skin at that point, since it is through the nerves that we feel at all. This damage may be permanent, and feeling may never be recovered, as in some nervous diseases. In leprosy, the first thing that the unfortunate victim may notice is that in places he cannot feel even fire, if it is placed on his skin. A temporary loss of sensation in the skin may be due to some slight accident which has jarred the nerve but not destroyed it, or may be due to something rubbed on to the skin to deaden it, or a "freezing" mixture.

By carefully considering the areas of the skin that are insensitive, it is possible to discover which nerves are at fault. When the nerves corresponding to those areas are found to be in a healthy condition it is probable that the anesthesia is due to hysteria, in which disease there are often areas on the skin which are so insensitive that a pin may even be stuck into them. These hysterical areas appear to have no relation to the areas which are supplied by particular nerves. For instance, it is not uncommon to find what is called the "glove and stocking" form of anesthesia, in which the area which is insensitive is exactly that covered by the gloves and stockings and stops exactly where they end in a sharp line. In hysteria there are also patches of insensitiveness which may be found anywhere on the body. These patches have often been described in the old accounts of the trials of so-called witches, and unfortunately for the poor women who were accused of being witches, it was thought that the patches were the mark of the Devil.

Treatment must be that of the disease which causes the condition.

ANALYSIS. By analysis is meant the separation of anything that is made up of several different things into those different substances which compose it. Clinical analysis of a disease means a thorough examination of the symptoms and course a disease is running in order to discover the nature and cause of the disease. Chemical analysis is the splitting up of a mixture into the different drugs that compose it. A chemical analysis of milk will discover the proportion of fat, water, etc., present in the given sample. In the treatment called psychoanalysis, which is sometimes used for certain mental conditions, the contents of the mind as represented by thoughts, dreams, etc., are analyzed, and this process is called the "analysis" of the patient.

ANAPHYLAXIS. Anaphylaxis is a state in which an individual is so sensitive to certain substances that they constitute a poison for him, whereas they are harmless for other persons. Everyone knows someone who cannot touch fish, must not eat eggs, or gets a rash when he eats strawberries. Sometimes these people are born anaphylactic to the particular thing which disagrees with them, but sometimes the condition comes on after the nervous system has been subjected to some severe shock or strain. In women, anaphylaxis may develop after the birth of a child, for instance. A common beginning of anaphylaxis is when a serum or vaccine is being

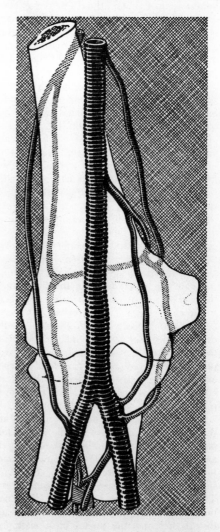

Arterial Anastomosis around the Elbow.

taken in continually increasing doses and suddenly one dose makes the patient violently ill for a short period, and any further dose would cause a similar or worse attack; the patient has become anaphylactic to the serum. Anaphylaxis is part of the condition known as allergy, and the article on allergy should be read by anyone interested in the subject.

ANASARCA. Anasarca is another name for dropsy, or the accumulation of fluid in the tissues of the body. To detect its presence press firmly with the finger on the skin. If the depression made by the finger takes some time to fill up, dropsy is present.

ANASTOMOSIS. The junction between two blood vessels arising from different roots is called an anastomosis. When the parent trunk is obstructed, the onus of carrying on the circulation falls on these communicating branches. Sometimes it is necessary to establish a new channel of communication between two organs or two distinct parts of the same organ. This also is an anastomosis. An example of this is when one part of the bowel is removed because of disease and the two sound parts on either side of it are joined to each other. (*See also* ARTERY.)

ANATOMY. By the term anatomy is meant the study of the structure of the human body. The knowledge of anatomy which we have today has been gained during hundreds of years of painstaking dissection, and the amount of knowledge that has been thus acquired is indeed vast.

In the science of anatomy the various systems of the body are grouped under the following headings: Osteology, the skeleton or bony parts of the body; Arthrology, the articulations or joints; Myology, the muscles; Angiology, the vascular system including the heart, blood vessels, lymphatic vessels and lymph glands; Neurology, the study of the nervous system; and Splanchnology, the description of the viscera or organs of the body, the breathing apparatus, the digestive system and the genito-urinary organs.

ANDROGEN. Androgen is an extract of the tissue of the testicle. The drug testosterone is a synthetic androgen which is prepared in laboratories. It is employed chiefly in cases of delayed sexual development or injury or disease of the testicle. The drug is used in women for controlling excessive bleeding at periods and sometimes to improve thickening of the breast tissue.

ANDROPHOBIA. This means fear or dislike of the male sex.

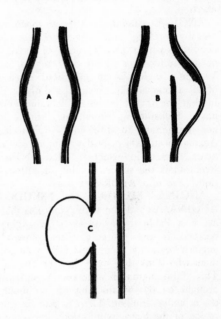

Aneurism: A. *Fusiform;* B. *Dissecting;* C. *Saccular.*

ANEURISM. An aneurism is an abnormal swelling of an artery. An external aneurism or aneurism of limb may be the result of an accident, and if it can be reached it may be treated surgically. The most serious form of aneurism is that of the aorta, or large artery, into which the blood from the heart is pumped. The most common cause of this is syphilis. It usually occurs in persons over thirty, and men are more frequently attacked than women.

The symptoms of aneurism are very variable, but there may be pain, faintness, swelling of the face, neck, arms or hands, breathlessness on exertion and even coughing and bringing up of blood. The throbbing of the aneurism may be visible on the chest.

Treatment. The treatment of aneurism is always a matter for a doctor. Some aneurisms become cut off by hardened clotting and cause no more trouble; others run a long course up to twenty years and enable the patient to carry on with limited activity. The treatment should begin with some months in bed with treatment of the various symptoms, and when the patient is allowed up again, he must avoid all violent exertion.

ANGINA. Angina is a term meaning literally, choking, and is used to describe conditions where there is a sense of choking or of suffocation. Fibrinous angina or Vincent's angina is an infectious disease of the throat closely resembling diphtheria in that the throat becomes ulcerated and has a foul-smelling membrane, but it is not dangerous to life like diphtheria. Angina pectoris or cardiac angina is a heart disease in which a characteristic symptom is the sudden feeling of suffocation. (*See also* ANGINA PECTORIS.)

ANGINA MINOR, or PSEUDO-ANGINA. A condition with symptoms that are very liable to be mistaken for angina pectoris is the cause of great mental anguish to many men, especially younger men, who think they have the true angina. This "false angina" is a nervous complaint brought on by oversmoking or too much tea or coffee-drinking. There is pain in the region of the heart, palpitation, and sometimes pain down the left arm. Emotion brings on the attacks, and they are as common in women as in men. The condition is mild and unimportant, and can easily be overcome by cutting down smoking and coffee-drinking, and toning up the nervous system. Unfortunately, many people do not believe their doctors and continue to suffer the mental anguish of thinking that they have angina pectoris.

ANGINA PECTORIS. Angina pectoris (breast pang) is a disease affecting the heart and is due to narrowing of the arteries which supply the heart with blood, a process which accompanies advancing years. Women rarely suffer from it, and manual laborers are not often attacked. It is more common in those whose life is one of stress and strain. Worry seems to be an active factor in causing it, and it has been called the doctor's disease beause it is very common in the medical profession. The typical sufferers from angina pectoris are business men or shopkeepers, leading lives of strain and fond of good living. It is to some extent hereditary.

Symptoms. The symptoms depend upon the severity of the attack. In the mildest form there may be only a feeling of tension or discomfort, which may grow to positive pain, deep in the region of the breastbone. The pain is constantly brought on by effort and relieved by a period of rest. Thus we find that grandfather, though able to walk uphill quite well, is brought to a stop constantly at the same point by his anginal pain. After a short rest he can carry on. This discomfort often follows emotional upset. It may be present on rising to speak in public, but soon passes off.

In a "high-pressure" life, a man may feel this tension in the breast for weeks without any pain, or without being able to pin it down to any one spot. It disappears after a night's rest, and may disappear entirely when the "harness" is taken off. John Hunter, the famous surgeon who was afflicted with this disease, used to say that his life was in the hands of any rascal who chose to worry him.

An Attack of Angina Pectoris. As stated previously, an attack is usually brought on by emotion or exertion, an angry scene at a meeting, or a "late for the train" rush to the station. The person is seized with a pain in the region of the heart and a feeling of tightness as if the chest had been seized in a vice. He remains motionless on a bench or against some such support as a wall. Pains sometimes shoot down his left arm and there may be numbness of the fingers and round about the heart. The face grows pale and ashen, and often a profuse sweat breaks out. The attacks last from a few seconds to a minute or two after which the patient finds himself relieved of his pain, straightens himself up, and proceeds on his way. He may feel exhausted and shaken for some time. The term angina pectoris is used when the attack of cardiac pain is of short duration and, unlike coronary thrombosis, causes no lasting damage to the heart.

Treatment. When a man has had an attack of true angina he must realize that the time has come to "go slow." If he can retire from business he should do so, keeping a small interest in it if he would be happier that way, but not an interest which would involve him in any heavy responsibility.

Angina pectoris is a warning by Nature that life must be slackened down, because the machinery is wearing thin. Recently, removal of the thyroid gland by operation has been performed successfully for angina pectoris in a number of cases, because this had the effect of slowing down the metabolism or working of the body. The question of diet has become one of great importance to the sufferer. If he is to continue living comfortably, he must smoke and drink in strict moderation and avoid overeating. He will not want to indulge in violent exercise, but he should live on the level as much as possible and avoid going up and down stairs as much as he can. If he takes care of himself he will probably live comfortably for years.

The pain of angina pectoris is rapidly relieved by the drug called nitroglycerin which acts by dilating the coronary vessels. It can be taken quite freely and has no harmful side-effects. Sufferers from angina pectoris should carry tablets of this around with them in their pockets and use it when they feel an attack coming on. Amyl nitrite, which used to be the favorite remedy and, indeed, acts more quickly, often has upsetting side-effects; but no treatment is as effective as the "quiet life" and the avoidance of those situations which are known to bring on an attack. (*See also* Coronary Thrombosis.)

ANGIOMA. This is the medical term for a tumor or swelling which consists of a mass of any kind of blood vessel. The form of angioma which is most common is a birthmark or naevus.

ANGIONEUROTIC EDEMA, or GIANT URTICARIA. In spite of its somewhat long name this is a fairly common complaint which ranges in severity from a mere discomfort to a serious upset of the general health. The chief feature of the condition is the sudden appearance of swellings in the skin, or the tissues under the skin. These swellings come up suddenly and are hot, red and intensely irritable for a short time; then they subside and disappear just as quickly as they came. In a more severe form there may be swelling

internally in the membranes which line the different organs of the body, and for the time being a serious condition may be caused by pressure of the swellings and the blocking of swollen passages. The most alarming swelling is that of the throat. When this occurs the larynx may swell so rapidly and to such an extent, that the patient is in danger of suffocation. The lips may swell to such an extent that the mouth cannot be opened or the hands and feet may be so swollen that the fingers and toes cannot be bent.

The causes of angioneurotic edema are not definitely known. In many cases it is hereditary and runs in families where other diseases of the class called "allergic diseases," such as hay fever and asthma, are found. In these cases the complaint usually causes no trouble beyond the liability to swell about the face and limbs and parts where there is pressure by the clothes, etc. In other cases the condition first appears after shock or childbirth; it often occurs together with urticaria, the condition which is popularly known as "hives."

Treatment. Immediate treatment is important and, if a doctor is at hand, he will immediately inject adrenalin, or peptone and ephedrine into the muscular tissue of the body. This injection usually has a remarkable effect in stopping the attack from becoming a bad one. The general treatment follows the same lines as the treatment of other allergic states. The general health must be looked to, foci of infection must be sought out and attended to. In chronic cases, long courses of injections of peptone may be of material benefit. Glucose, calcium, and ephedrine taken by mouth are all useful in certain cases. Very frequent attacks are treated by giving antihistamine drugs such as Benadryl by mouth over long periods. A long vacation may help to clear up the condition, which in the nonhereditary varieties will usually wear itself out in from one to three years' time. (*See also* Allergy.)

ANIMAL HEAT. The temperature— the heat of the body—is one of several guides to a person's condition, and it is taken with a thermometer.

Clearly marked on the thermometer are figures giving the temperature of a person in ordinary health, for it has been found that we all, in health, register pretty much the same irrespective of the temperature of the surroundings. This normal temperature is known as *animal heat.*

When a boy comes in from a game of football with the perspiration streaming from him, he is giving off some of his body heat in a perfectly natural way through the pores of the skin. We are meant to relieve unusual heat by perspiring.

All over the skin are millions of minute sweat glands; on the inner part of our hands we have nearly three thousand of them to one square inch. Some of the natural heat of the body escapes that way.

Fat for Heat. We must eat to live, and to keep up our natural body heat we need certain foods. One of these is fat. Every explorer knows this; people who live in intensely cold climates make a habit of eating fat, and we should remember in the cold weather to arrange for fat in some form in the daily menu.

Clothes do not *give* warmth to the body, though they help to *keep it in.* So airmen, and other people who are exposed to unusual cold, wear insulated coats, and most of us wear more or thicker clothing in winter.

ANIMALS AS DISEASE CARRIERS. Quite a few diseases, especially skin diseases, are caught by human beings from domestic animals. Favus, a skin disease very much like ringworm, is sometimes conveyed to children by cats. Glanders is an infectious disease which chiefly affects the glands, eyes and noses of horses, but persons who handle them are liable to contract the disease.

No less important is it to remember that the family cat is very well qualified to act as a "carrier" of infectious diseases. In its various prowlings and hobnobbings with other cats, it is very liable to pick up all sorts of microbes. Diphtheria and some other infectious diseases have been known to owe their onset to the handling of these pets. Tuberculosis is greatly spread through the medium of infected meat and milk, and scarlet fever and diphtheria may also be contracted from certain diseases of the cow. Rats are instrumental in carrying bubonic plague, as well as many other diseases. Mice carry a form of meningitis

which can be transmitted to man. Dogs carry the virus causing hydrophobia and are also known to infect man with tapeworm cysts and the germ of a rare illness called canicola fever. The risk of infection from household pets is small in the U.S., and the most dangerous carrier of disease in our midst is our fellow man.

ANKLE. The ankle is the joint where the bones of the leg meet the bones of the foot. It is a joint of the hinge variety, and allows two movements: the raising of the foot and the lowering of the foot. The movement of raising the foot is called *dorsiflexion,* and the movement of lowering the foot *plantarflexion.* When a person is standing erect the foot should be at right angles to the leg.

The ankle joint is formed by the lower ends of the bones of the leg, which are called the tibia and fibula, and the anklebone, or talus, as it is called. Underneath the anklebone lies the heelbone, or calcaneum, and in front of it the five tarsal bones which form the instep or tarsus. The blood supply of the foot is by way of the anterior tibial artery, which can be felt in the midline of the front of the ankle, and is thereafter called the dorsal artery of the foot (*dorsalis pedis*), and the posterior tibial artery (plantar arteries) which can be felt below the inner side of the ankle.

The ankle is surrounded by ligaments which connect the surface of the lower end of the tibia to the anklebone. Other ligaments bind the anklebone to the heel and bones of the foot.

The ankle joint is a very powerful joint, and is not often dislocated, but it is the most frequently sprained joint in the body. It is very often the site of synovitis or watery swelling, and disease or injury may lead to ankylosis or severe stiffening of the ankle joint.

Injuries. The ankle joint, which has to support the entire weight of the body, is necessarily a very strong joint and is strongly supported by ligaments. It is not therefore easy to dislocate it, though dislocation sometimes does occur, most often in cases where there is a smashed bone as well. The treatment is a matter for a skilled surgeon, as the joint very easily becomes stiffened and rigid and a permanent limp and weakness may sometimes result. A less severe form of dislocation and fracture at the ankle is that known as Pott's fracture, where the fibula is fractured at its lower end, the ligaments of the ankle joint are torn, and the foot is bent in an outward and backward direction. This may happen by some accident such as slipping off the pavement, or landing after a jump with the feet turned out. It may not incapacitate the individual at the time, but may be regarded as only a severe sprain until X-ray examination shows the true situation. In another fracture of the ankle called Dupuytren's fracture, the two legbones, the tibia and fibula, may be separated and the anklebone may be pushed up between them.

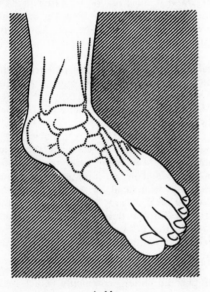

Ankle.

Sprained Ankle. Although fractures and dislocations of the ankle are comparatively rare, there is no joint which is so easily and so frequently sprained. A sudden turning of the foot may be enough to cause a sprain, which is a tear of a whole or part of the ligament at the side of the ankle. The symptoms are intense pain, marked swelling and discoloration, but the joint can still be freely moved. A firm bandage should be applied and kept on for forty-eight hours, after which massage may be started and the joint kept strapped in the intervals. In a slight case the patient may begin to put weight on the foot after a few days, provided that the ankle is well strapped and a strong shoe is worn.

ANKYLOSIS. This is the name given to the stiffness of the joints which is sometimes found after an accident or disease. Sometimes the stiffness may be due to adhesions or tough bands which have formed, or to the shortening of ligaments and muscles, in which case the joint will still be able to move, though its movements are limited. More rarely the bones forming the joint have grown together and in such cases no movement is possible.

ANKYLOSTOMIASIS. This is the medical name for hookworm disease or miner's anemia. The condition is described under HOOKWORM DISEASE.

ANODYNE. An anodyne is a medicine that gives relief from pain.

ANOPHELES. Anopheles is the species of mosquito which carries malaria, the disease which is such a scourge in tropical countries. Like other sorts of mosquitoes they only breed where there is marshy ground or stagnant water, and even a bucket of water kept handy in case of fire may become a breeding spot unless it is kept carefully covered over. Mosquitoes very rarely fly far from their breeding places, and the anopheles is no exception to this rule; they may, however, be blown by the wind over a considerable range. The female insect may lay anything from 50 to 400 eggs, and she requires blood to feed them on. (*See also* MOSQUITO.)

ANOSMIA. This is the name given to the condition in which the sense of smell is lost. This happens sometimes for a few days after influenza and as a result of injuries of the skull. Very rarely the sense is permanently lost.

ANOXEMIA. This is due to lack of oxygen in the blood. Oxygen is one of the gases of which the air is made up, and it is necessary to keep the body in health. The body obtains oxygen by breathing air into the lungs and separating the oxygen from the other parts of the air which are then breathed out again, while the oxygen is taken up into the bloodstream and distributed throughout the body in a manner which is described in the article on the circulation of the blood. Lack of oxygen in the blood occurs in diseases where the breathing is out of order, such as pneumonia, or when a person is high up in mountains or in an airplane or balloon. The condition is then called mountain-sickness or airsickness. (*See also* AIRSICKNESS; MOUNTAIN-SICKNESS.)

ANT BITE. Ant bites are not a matter of great importance in the U.S., but they are sometimes seen, perhaps when a person has been foolish enough to sleep on the ground in the neighborhood of an ant hill. There may then be troublesome little red and itchy bites which should be treated by bathing with some alkaline solution such as bicarbonate of soda, and otherwise treated like midge or mosquito bites. (*See also* BITES AND STINGS.)

ANTACID. An antacid is any substance which counteracts or neutralizes acidity. Any alkali substance is an antacid. (*See also* ACIDOSIS; ALKALI.)

ANTENATAL CARE. For the normal and healthy woman, the months before her baby is born should be a time of physical well-being and happy preparation; but in too many cases this is not so, and the expectant mother is harassed with discomforts and ailments which very often could be avoided or relieved. In some cases she drifts into more serious conditions, which may even cause her to lose her own or her baby's life. At the beginning of the present century, more than 150 babies out of every 1,000 were doomed to be born dead or to die shortly afterwards, and four or five mothers out of every 1,000 died in childbirth. Today the situation with regard to infant life has improved until there are fewer than 30 deaths from every 1,000 births, and the death-rate among mothers has also declined sharply.

The decline in the infant mortality rate can be directly traced to improved conditions of living and the facilities that are now provided for the care and instruction of expectant mothers.

The chief difficulty which has to be overcome is that of getting the expectant mothers to consult their doctors or attend motherhood classes. This is often due to shyness, but in many cases it is due to the ignorance of the young woman as to what lies before her, and how she should do her duty to herself and her unborn child. Often the young woman is not encouraged to go seek information by the older women who advise her. They say that nature will do all that is required. Childbirth is a natural process, and the normal woman who lives a normal life does come through the experience with little strain; but some women are not normal, and if the condition from which they suffer is discovered in time a great deal of future suffering may be spared.

Every woman should have herself examined as soon as she knows that she is pregnant. Any abnormality or deformity will then be discovered, and she will be told how to conduct her life and look after her health in the way best suited to her; and it must not be forgotten that for the nine months before birth the mother's health is the baby's health. (*See also* CHILDBIRTH; PREGNANCY.)

ANTERIOR. This term is used medically to describe any organ or part of the body that is in front of any other part. The opposite of this term is posterior.

ANTERIOR POLIOMYELITIS. *See* INFANTILE PARALYSIS.

ANTHELMINTIC. Any drug which is used to kill intestinal worms is called an anthelmintic. In many cases the parasites are not killed in the intestines, but are so violently stimulated or stupefied by the drug that they are swept away by the usual castor-oil purge, which is administered after an anthelmintic is given. Examples of anthelmintics are Thymol and Antepar.

ANTHRACOSIS. Anthracosis, a variety of pneumoconiosis, commonly called coal-miner's lung, is a disease of the lungs arising from the continuous breathing of air containing particles of silica found in some coal seams. The disease is growing less prevalent, and with better ventilation of coalmines, the adoption of wet drilling or direct exhausts to the drills, and, if the circumstances require it, the use of respirators, the disease would become a rarity. The lung becomes black in appearance and tough in texture. The chief symptom is breathlessness, and cough. The patient must be removed from mine-dust permanently, and should take particular care to avoid chills or anything which would lead to catarrhal colds and bronchitis. Any exertion which causes breathlessness should be avoided.

ANTHRAX. This is an acute infectious disease due to a germ called the *Bacillus anthracis*. It is common in eastern Europe and Asia amongst animals, such as sheep, cattle and horses. Human beings become infected on the skin by handling imported hides or by using infected shaving brushes which are usually made from horsehair. The lung variety of anthrax results from inhaling bacilli in the handling of wool (wool-sorter's disease), and possibly the intestinal form is due to eating infected meat.

Infection occurs usually through a bruise or cut in the skin, and the incubation period is sometimes less than twenty-four hours. The first thing that is noticed is a small red pimple which quickly becomes inflamed and angry-looking. This may at first be mistaken for an ordinary boil or septic spot, but the appearances quickly become very characteristic in anthrax. The pimple becomes encircled by small whitish blisters, and in a day or two black slough or dead matter may appear in the center. The neighboring glands are usually enlarged and the temperature may be anything from normal to about 103 deg. F. If the case is treated efficiently within a day or so of its onset the hope of recovery is very good, but in severe cases death may occur within a week. The sore should not be opened, as this increases the risk of blood-poisoning.

Treatment. Injections of special serum may be given. A course of one of the sulphonamide drugs will rapidly and effectively control the infection. Penicillin by injection may also be used. (*See also* ANTIBODIES; SERUM.)

ANTHROPOLOGY. Anthropology is the science of the nature of man and his social habits.

ANTIBIOTICS. These are substances derived from nature which prevent the growth and reproduction of germs. The meaning of the term has been narrowed to include only those substances produced by molds. The first of these antibacterial substances, penicillin, was discovered by Alexander Fleming in 1929, and their use

in medicine is a more recent development still. Since penicillin was first used by injection to cure disease due to germs in man, research into the products of the growth of molds has progressed rapidly. The physician is now armed with a host of effective new drugs, and their numbers are swelling as the years pass. Penicillin, though lethal to many germs, is practically harmless to the tissues of man, but many of the newer antibiotics are not so and their usage has to be tempered by discretion. Streptomycin is such a substance.

Included among the newer antibiotics are terramycin, aureomycin, and chloramphenicol. The last of these was the first to be manufactured in the laboratory from simpler substances. Recently certain penicillins have also been produced in the laboratory, which are effective when given by the mouth. The individual drugs of this group are dealt with in separate sections. (*See also* AUREOMYCIN; CHLORAMPHENICOL; PENICILLIN; STREPTOMYCIN; TERRAMYCIN.)

ANTIBODIES. Diseases are most often caused by the invasion of the body by swarms of germs or bacteria, which rapidly increase in number. The body, however, has the power to produce other substances in the blood and tissues which destroy these bacteria and neutralize the poisons which they manufacture in the blood. These other substances are called antibodies and antitoxins. When a sufficient number of antibodies has been produced in the blood to deal with the bacteria and get the upper hand of them, the person will recover from the disease or will become immune to it. This is the principle at the root of vaccination and inoculation against disease. By injecting the bacteria or their poisons into the blood of a person when he is well and healthy, his blood will be enabled to produce a supply of antibodies which will protect him from the germs of the disease when he becomes infected with it, and he will either not have it at all or will have it in a much milder form than he would if his blood did not already contain antibodies. (*See also* ANTITOXIN; IMMUNITY.)

ANTIDIPHTHERIC SERUM. This serum is prepared by artificially infecting a horse with diphtheria. It contains the substances which the blood produces to neutralize the poisons formed by the germs of diphtheria. It should always be injected as soon as signs of diphtheria appear, otherwise the patient will have a poorer chance of recovery. It is given also to people who have been in contact with the case to try to prevent their developing the disease. So necessary is this serum that fresh supplies of it are kept ready for immediate use in an emergency.

ANTIDOTE. An antidote is any substance which prevents or counteracts the action of a poison. As the quick administration of an antidote may save the life of a person who has taken poison either accidentally or on purpose, it is the duty of every adult to know at least some of the common antidotes, and a list of them should be kept handy in every household, factory and office. Coffee, made very strong, acts as an antidote in opium poisoning and cases where the patient tends to become drowsy. Strong tea acts in the same way in morphia poisoning. Acids are antidotes to alkalis and, similarly, alkalis are antidotes to acids. For quick reference, a list of poisons and their antidotes is given under the heading POISONS in the FIRST-AID SUPPLEMENT.

ANTIMONY. Antimony is a metal possessing a bluish-white shiny appearance. In medicine it is chiefly used in the treatment of syphilis and in certain diseases caused by parasites such as bilharzia.

Poisoning by Antimony. In cases of poisoning by antimony the patient should be made to vomit by giving an emetic of a tablespoonful of mustard, or salt, in half a tumblerful of warm water. Strong tea should then be given, and the patient should be fed on milk and white of egg. He should be kept warm by putting hot-water bottles at his feet and sides.

ANTIPHLOGISTIC. An agent or substance which reduces or subdues inflammation or fever is called antiphlogistic. Pastes such as Antiphlogistine are now widely used instead of poultices to reduce inflammation. (*See also* KAOLIN.)

ANTIPYRETIC. This is a drug which is used for lowering the temperature. The most important antipyretics are phenacetin and antipyrine. Cold, such as a cold bath, or sponging, or the application of ice packs, is the method which was formerly used a great deal for lowering the temperature in cases of fever. Fever or high temperature is normally a beneficial reaction on the part of the body and represents its attempt to resist invasion by germs or parasites. To help the body to overcome infection, e.g., by giving quinine in cases of malaria, or sulphamezathine in pneumonia, is to remove the need for fever. These are the best antipyretics, and cold sponges are better reserved for the occasional case with a dangerously high temperature (105 deg. F. or more).

ANTISEPTICS. An antiseptic is a substance which is used to prevent the growth of germs; a disinfectant is a drug which is used to kill them. It is important to know the difference between the two, because a drug which is disinfectant in certain circumstances will, in other circumstances, act only as an antiseptic. Certain antiseptics, such as carbolic acid, etc., lose much of their power through having to be well diluted with some other substance. Carbolic acid, if used alone for any length of time, would cause great damage to the tissues and thus defeat its own ends.

This antiseptic is used a great deal as a deodorant and disinfectant for drains, bedpans, soiled linen, and surgical instruments. A dilute carbolic lotion is used to wash wounds and keep them antiseptic. Carbolic gauze and carbolic lint preparations are also sometimes used for dressing wounds.

Formaldehyde is a powerful disinfectant, but it is not much used in surgery because it tends to retard healing. The vapor from formaldehyde is recommended for disinfecting sickrooms after illness. It does not destroy colored materials nor damage books or pictures.

Preparations of iodine are used a great deal to prevent infection in cuts and abrasions. Iodine and glycerin is used as a throat paint in cases of tonsillitis.

Hydrogen peroxide is perhaps one of the most well-known antiseptics. It is beneficial in its action on suppurating wounds; the effect of the gas bubbles helps to remove much of the pus. It is invaluable in aiding the removal of dressings which are sticking to a wound. The dressing should be well soaked in a warm solution of peroxide of hydrogen and it will then come away more readily. This antiseptic makes an excellent mouthwash and deodorant, and also helps to keep the teeth clean and white. It is used in hair coloring preparations, as it possesses strong bleaching properties.

Potassium permanganate can be used as a mouthwash or gargle, a solution of 1 in 500 if the mouth condition is foul. In cases of gonorrhoea and in uterine diseases, a solution of 1 in 1,000 may be used as a douche. This drug is used a great deal as a deodorant for drains, etc.

Boric acid makes an excellent mild antiseptic and is largely used to keep wounds, ulcers, and sores clean and sweet.

Many of the new antibiotic drugs are useful locally as antiseptics as well as being given internally.

There are numerous reliable proprietary ones, such as Micrin, Cepacol and Listerine, to be had.

Antiseptic surgery. This was first introduced by Lord Lister when he was Professor of Surgery at Glasgow in the year 1867, and since then the method has developed into aseptic surgery, in which germs are *prevented* and not merely killed off when present. At a modern operation every instrument, dressing and the operating table is aseptic, and the nurses and the surgeons and the surrounding atmosphere are all rendered as aseptic as possible. In this way the treatment of surgical wounds becomes a comparatively slight affair, in comparison with former days when death from sepsis was the rule, rather than the exception. (*See also* ASEPSIS.)

ANTISPASMODIC. Antispasmodics are drugs which relieve colic or spasms These drugs include the narcotic drugs such as belladonna and opium, and carminative drugs such as sal volatile, etc. In severe colic, the spasmodic pains may be relieved by the application of a hot-water bottle to the abdomen.

ANTITOXIN. An antitoxin is a substance formed in the blood to protect the body against an invasion of germs. It neutralizes or combats the poisons produced by the germ, but the antitoxin for any particular disease will only neutralize the toxin or poison of that disease. For example, the antitoxin for diphtheria will have no effect against the toxin for lockjaw.

ANTRUM. The antrum is the largest

of the sinuses or spaces filled with air in connection with the nose, and lies within the upper jaw. The opening into the nose is situated high up in the antrum, and is thus badly placed for drainage. When, therefore, the antrum becomes infected, either from the nose through influenza or a similar cause, or from an abscess at the root of a tooth in the upper jaw, it is difficult for the infection to clear up naturally, and the antrum usually has to be drained surgically, either by having a small cannula passed into it, or by an operation under local or general anesthetic. A one-sided nasal discharge makes a doctor suspicious that the antrum is infected, and sometimes there is an unpleasant smell in the nose; it may be necessary to have the nasal sinuses X-rayed for confirmation of the diagnosis. (*See also* SINUS.)

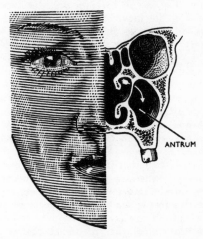

Antrum.

ANUS. The opening at the lower end of the rectum, or lowest part of the large bowel, is known as the anus. In certain cases an opening may have to be made from the lower bowel to the outside at some point above the normal anus; this is termed an artificial anus or colostomy. Imperforate anus is the term applied to complete absence of the natural opening which is found sometimes in newborn babies; in such cases a surgical operation is necessary. Fissure, fistula, piles, abscess, pruritus, prolapse, and stricture are conditions which occur in the region of the anus.

ANXIETY. Anxiety is a state of nervous tension brought about by fear. This is a normal reaction to many situations encountered in our passage through life. Thus sickness, exposure to physical danger, or the threat of insecurity in our jobs give rise in normal people to a feeling of anxiety. The extent and duration of this anxiety is to some extent related to the imaginativeness of the individual; some people will always foresee danger before it arrives, always meeting trouble half way—the worriers of this world. It is normal for anxiety to disappear as soon as the cause is removed. When a state of morbid anxiety exists for no obvious cause, then such a person is said to be suffering from an *anxiety state.* Now a mental state of fear, as is well known to us all, is accompanied by certain unpleasant bodily sensations. The mouth becomes dry, the hands tremble, the heart races and we may be sick or have diarrhea; we are unable to sleep when we go to bed and our head aches with the sense of tension. We are irritable and unable to concentrate and have a sickening pain over the heart. All of these symptoms may be complained of in *anxiety state,* or one only may be singled out and have attention focused on it, yet the anxiety which caused it may be overlooked.

It is found that people are reluctant to confess to a feeling of fear as it is thought that thereby they lower their prestige. It is for this reason, and because the cause of the state of anxiety may have been long since forgotten, that the mind prefers a physical explanation of such bodily symptoms. It is important, however, that sufferers from this disorder should have some insight into the mechanism whereby their symptoms arise, since only by understanding are they able to root out the original causes. These often go back to the misty days of early childhood when the habit of anxiety was acquired in the background of an unhappy home. Such deep-rooted anxiety states may be well-nigh impossible to treat and are the cause of much ill-health and loss of working capacity. It is every parent's duty to see that his children do not lack a sense of security, and a show of fear must be a signal for sympathetic searching for a cause. In this way it may be possible to spare the rising generation from one of the scourges of our own.

AORTA. The aorta is the largest artery of the body. It is the chief of the vessels which carry blood, after it has been mixed with oxygen, to the tissues of the body. It begins at the left side of the heart and extends downwards and backwards, keeping to the left of the backbone until it enters the abdominal cavity through a special opening in the diaphragm. In the abdomen it divides into two branches called the right and left *common iliac arteries.* In its course it is called by several different names. It begins as the *ascending aorta,* which gives off the *right and left coronary arteries* which supply the heart. The second portion of the aorta is called the *arch of the aorta.* It curves upwards, backwards and to the left behind the breastbone, and joins on the *descending aorta.* The branches of the arch of the aorta are given off from the top of the arch and are called the *innominate,* the *left common carotid* and the *left subclavian.* The descending aorta divides into two portions, the *thoracic* and the *abdominal aortas.* The thoracic aorta has many branches to the chest.

The main artery of the lower body is the *abdominal aorta,* which supplies the abdomen and the organs contained in it with blood. It is a continuation of the *aorta* through the diaphragm into the abdomen, where it lies in front of the backbone, and behind the duodenum and coils of the small intestine. It descends as far as the fourth lumbar vertebra, where it divides and finishes its course as the two *common iliac arteries.* The branches of the abdominal aorta are numerous and important. They are divided into three sets: the *visceral* branches which directly supply the organs; the *parietal* branches which supply the diaphragm, and the intercostal and sacral regions; and the *terminal* branches composed of the two common iliac arteries which pass down the groins and carry the blood-supply to the lower limbs. (*See also* ARTERY; HEART.)

A.P.C. TABLETS. These tablets, as their initials suggest, contain Aspirin, Phenacetin and Caffeine. They are justifiably popular for the relief of discomfort in the early stages of a cold and for trivial headaches.

The caffeine is a mental stimulant and combats the depressing effect of the other drugs given alone. They can be bought from any druggist in tablets weighing 7½ grains, and one or two will suffice.

APERIENT. Drugs or substances which produce a mildly purgative action on the intestine and lead to two or three soft motions of the bowels daily are called aperients or laxatives. The most useful drug in this class is cascara in some form. It has a very bitter taste, but can be had in small sugar-coated pills of various strengths, in a sweetened liquid form called cascara evacuent, or, if a purge is required, as cascara sagrada. A great advantage of cascara is that gradually increasing doses are not required, and the drug can be left off when no longer necessary without any bad effects. Various forms of health salts taken in a tumbler of water before breakfast make a very pleasant aperient.

Where the bowel needs a lubricant, liquid paraffin is of great benefit and is obtainable in a great variety of forms. Vegetable laxatives such as psyllium seed jelly preparations and preparations of agar-agar, a seaweed found in Japan, are very useful for long-continued use. With many people fresh fruit juice or an increase of fruit and vegetable in the diet is an adequate aperient.

APEX. The summit or top of anything. When applied to the lungs, the apex of the lung is the top part behind the border of the first rib. The apex-beat of the heart is the beat of the heart felt between the fifth and sixth ribs, about 3½ in. from the middle of the breastbone. The apex-beat may alter its situation in cases of enlargement of the heart and other conditions.

APHASIA. Aphasia is a defect in, or loss of, the power of expressing ideas by speech, writing or signs, or of understanding what is spoken or written. It is due to injury or disease of certain parts of the brain. These special parts of the brain which control speech are known as the speech centers, and in right-handed people they are usually situated on the left side of the brain, while in those who are left-handed they are generally found on the right side. The speech centers can be most easily explained by following the education of a child. The child first hears sounds,

which after a time he associates with certain objects. Next, he ceases to be content to hear sounds, but wants to produce them. He succeeds in doing so by developing a part of his brain which is connected with movements of the tongue and lips (the "motor" speech center). If this part of the brain becomes injured or diseased, the patient is unable to speak intelligibly and the defect is called motor aphasia.

When the child learns to read and write, further centers are developed. First, written or printed characters have to be recognized; that needs one center—the "seeing" speech center. Afterwards they have to be reproduced; that needs another center—the "writing" speech center—which is developed in another part of the brain, close to that part of the brain which controls the movements of the hands. Further education makes even better communication between these various centers necessary. For example, in order to write from dictation, a message has to be sent from that part of the brain which deals with hearing, to the seeing speech center and from there to the writing speech center. In order that a child may be able to read aloud, a message must travel from the seeing speech center, first to the hearing center, and then to the motor speech center. Thus, according to which center is diseased or damaged, so will the type of aphasia vary. If the seeing center is destroyed, then written language, though seen, conveys no meaning, and the patient is said to suffer from word-blindness. Motor aphasia has already been mentioned. If the hearing center is damaged, the patient cannot understand what is said to him, a condition which is called word-deafness; but these conditions are uncommon.

Treatment for word deafness and for word blindness is by a method of constant repetition. In the first case the patient is educated in the pronunciation of words which he understands in written or printed form, his eyes following the words as he associates the sounds with them. In the second case the patient learns to ally the sounds with which he is familiar to the written symbols, repeating the sounds as he writes, first in printed letters, then in script.

All these centers are situated close

together in the brain, so that any disease which is progressive, like a tumor, will in the end destroy all the speech centers, although the way in which the speech defect first appears may enable the doctor to tell exactly where the tumor is growing. The commonest cause of aphasia is a stroke or accident to one of the blood vessels of the brain. Some speech disorder is the usual legacy of a stroke affecting the left side of the brain, but a large degree of recovery usually takes place. (*See also* APOPLEXY; BRAIN; NERVOUS SYSTEM.)

APHONIA. Aphonia means loss of the power of speech. The most usual cause of loss of voice is inflammation of the vocal cords, due to over-use or misuse of the voice. Voicelessness may also be due to paralysis and sometimes to hysteria. (*See also* HYSTERIA.)

APOMORPHINE. Apomorphine is made from morphine. It is the most powerful emetic known, and is largely used in the treatment of cases of poisoning. It is given by injection under the skin, and produces rapid and violent vomiting. It can be used in cases where emetics taken by mouth into the stomach would not act, and it has the advantage of not irritating the stomach.

APONEUOROSIS. Aponeuorosis is a particular sort of tough, sheet-like tendon which is attached to muscles, or encloses and binds down to muscles.

APLOPLEXY or STROKE. A loss of consciousness with some paralysis, which is due to a sudden interference with the blood supply of part of the brain, is known as apoplexy. It occurs most commonly in elderly people, in whom the arteries of the brain are inelastic, so that the blood tends to clot in them, thus cutting off the supply of blood from certain areas of the brain; or the walls of the arteries may be so weakened that they become fragile and burst, giving rise to hemorrhage. In younger people, in middle life syphilis plays an important part in producing apoplexy, as this disease causes certain changes in the blood vessels, which promote clotting of the blood in them.

Apoplexy in people under forty is rare, but it may occur in one of two ways. In disease of the valves of the heart, sometimes a small piece of clot on one of the valves becomes broken off and is carried round in the blood circulation until it reaches a tiny vessel in the brain, where, unable to pass any farther, it lodges, thus blocking the opening of the vessel so that no blood is able to pass along it. This cuts off the blood supply from an area of the brain, but in time the lodged clot contracts, and the pathway for the blood is clear again. That is why in this form almost complete recovery is the rule unless the clot is a very large one, or the vessel in which it has lodged is itself unhealthy.

A few unfortunate people have arteries inside their skulls with thinner walls than usual at particular points, where the arteries divide into smaller and again smaller branches. Gradually the arteries become stretched at these points and may give way. The person who has had such a stroke may survive several attacks, but, if the cause is recognized, will usually need a surgical operation designed to promote clotting and healing in the weakened blood vessel.

It must, however, be emphasized that this type of stroke in young people is rare, compared with the type seen in the elderly from blood clotting in an artery, or from bursting of a weakened vessel. The common type, that due to clotting of the blood, most frequently occurs when the apoplexy happens during sleep or under conditions of quiet. The history is often that the patient went to bed feeling extra tired, and next morning woke up and found that he was paralyzed down one or other side. The exact symptoms and signs of such an apoplexy will depend on which artery has become obstructed, but a certain artery which supplies one particular region of the brain is nearly always affected, and when this area of the brain is deprived of its blood supply, paralysis of the opposite side of the body occurs. If the left side of the brain is damaged, then most probably speech will be lost, at least temporarily, as this side of the brain controls speech, but if the right side of the brain has suffered, then speech will be preserved.

When apoplexy is due to blood clotting and not to bleeding from a burst vessel, unconsciousness may be only slight, and the patient may recover consciousness within a few hours. Where bleeding has occurred, unconsciousness is much more severe; it is prolonged, and the patient very often passes into a coma from which he may not awaken. Although the patient is breathing noisily and hurriedly and puffing out his cheeks, it can readily be seen that on the side of the paralysis the cheek is less puffed out at each breath than it is on the sound side. And even though a patient be deeply unconscious it is possible to show that the limbs on the paralyzed side when raised, and allowed to fall again, do so "all of a piece," in a more lifeless manner than upon the sound side.

A good deal of recovery in the paralyzed limbs may take place from an apoplexy due to clotting of the blood in the vessels. The outlook for complete recovery depends on many factors, especially on the condition of the blood vessels and heart. Re-education of the paralyzed limbs as regards movements is of the utmost importance, and the patient should be urged to try to move his paralyzed limbs as much as possible, as soon as he is completely conscious. There is no fear that by moving the limbs he will bring on another stroke. Many patients who have had one stroke caused by clotting of the blood in a vessel go for many years without another. The best preventive measure against a stroke in those who are known to have bad arteries is moderation in all things: in diet, alcohol, physical and mental exercise.

APOTHECARIES' WEIGHTS AND MEASURES.

This is a system of weights and measures used in the making-up of medicines. The troy pound of 5,760 grains is the standard; it is subdivided into 12 ounces of 480 gains each. The ounce is subdivided into 8 drachms or drams, the drachm into 3 scruples, and the scruple into 20 grains. For fluid measure, the quart of 32 fluid ounces is subdivided into 2 pints, the pint into 16 fluid ounces, the ounce into 8 fluid drachms or drams, and the fluid drachm into 60 minims.

Apothecaries' Weight.

```
   20 =    1
   60 =    3 =  1
  480 =   24 =  8 =  1
5,760 =  288 = 96 = 12 = 1
```

Apothecaries' Measure.

```
    60 =      1
   480 =      8 =    1
 7,680 =    128 =   16 = 1
61,440 =  1,024 =  128 = 8 = 1
```

For domestic use the measures given below may prove a valuable help.

A teaspoonful is a bit over a fluid dram.

A dessertspoonful is about two fluid drams.

A tablespoonful is about half a fluid ounce.

A wineglassful is about one and a half to two fluid ounces.

A teacupful is about five fluid ounces.

A waterglassful is about eight fluid ounces.

A tumblerful is about eleven fluid ounces.

APPENDICITIS. This term describes an inflammation of the appendix, a small worm-like projection from the caecum, or blind end of the commencement of the large intestine. The cause of appendicitis is not definitely known. In most cases it appears to be due to invasion of germs, such as streptococci, etc., which enter the appendix from the intestine, or in other cases it may be due to germs from a distant source of infection, such as the tonsils or teeth. Germs from the latter source are blood-borne, i.e., they travel in the bloodstream from some distant part of the body to the appendix. Some cases are said to be due to internal obstruction of the appendix by lumps of hardened feces, pits and skins of fruit, thread-worms in masses, and swallowed foreign bodies. In one such case a gold link of a bracelet was found neatly tucked away inside the appendix. It is on the whole a disease of youth and middle-age; males are attacked slightly oftener than women, and it is more common among civilized races.

Appendicitis is a disease which comes on in definite attacks with, usually, a pain-free interval between them. In the typical attack the patient has been out of sorts for some days and begins to complain of attacks of pain of a griping character in the right side of the abdomen or round the umbilicus (navel). On walking the pain may be of a stabbing nature and be felt in the right groin. There may be vomiting, constipation, or diarrhea. The temperature rises and the pulse is rapid. There is a well-marked tenderness in the region known as McBurney's point. To find this point for oneself, place the thumb of the right hand on the umbilicus and the little finger on the point the of the hip; if the middle finger is now pressed down it should be approximately in the region of McBurney's point. An appendix which is acutely inflamed should always be removed, as the condition rarely cures itself, and the results of neglect are serious. After repeated attacks the appendix may become gangrenous, and each attack will add to the number of adhesions in the abdomen and the severity of the operation for its removal.

In an acute attack of appendicitis the patient is obviously very ill and in great pain, and no time should be lost in sending for the doctor. *No laxative should be given* as is sometimes done under the impression that the case is one of colic due to constipation. Nowadays immediate operation is advised when the condition has been present for less than forty-eight hours, but when it has been present for several days, operationis often deferred as an abscess may have started to form.

Appendicitis is favorably influenced by penicillin, but still usually requires operation.

APPENDIX. The vermiform appendix, or appendix as it is more usually called, is a relic which has no definite use in human beings. In animals such as the rabbit or horse, which feed entirely upon vegetarian matter, it is large and appears to be of some importance, whereas in meat-eating animals like the lion and tiger, it is even more minute and shrivelled up than in human beings who live on a mixed diet of flesh and vegetables. In shape it is tubular, attached at one end to the caecum, into which it has a small opening which is protected by a valve. The other end swings free, but is usually adherent to the caecum or some part of the lining of the abdomen. In length appendices vary from 1 to 10 in., the average being 3 or 4 in. in length. The position in which the appendix lies varies also. About half the number point straight upwards and lie either behind the caecum and ascending colon, or to the

right of them. This is called the retrocaecal position. Others run upwards and inwards, pointing towards the spleen, and others again, known as the pelvic appendix, hang straight downwards from the caecum into the pelvis. The length and position of the appendix exert a considerable influence upon its liability to infection, and on the symptoms and signs when it is inflamed. (*See also* APPENDICITIS; INTESTINE.)

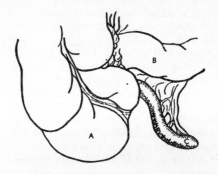

A. *Caecum;* B. *Ascending Colon;* C. *Appendix.*

APPETITE. Everyone who enjoys good health should be blessed with a good appetite. The sight and smell of food very often increases the flow of the gastric juices within the body, thus giving an added zest to the appetite. In the same way, a meal badly cooked and served will often have the effect of taking away the appetite altogether.

When the health is normal and the body is functioning well, it is proper to follow your fancy in the choice of foods. The body generally knows what is good for it and what it can deal with. It is only when the body is physically out of order that the appetite becomes poor and the normal diet no longer suitable. Among the more common causes of loss of appetite are constipation, too little exercise, and the abuse of alcohol or tobacco.

In people who lead a sedentary life it is not to be expected that the appetite should be as hearty as in those who work out of doors. A brisk walk before meals will increase the appetite and probably make food taste twice as good.

Sometimes an unusually good appetite may be a symptom of gastric catarrh, and, in cases of duodenal ulcer, pain is always most severe when the patient is hungry. This symptom is known as "hunger pain" and it is usually relieved by the taking of food. In acute fevers the appetite disappears altogether, and it is usually poor in tuberculosis and anemia.

Some believe that much can be done to improve the appetite by the taking of "bitters." Substances such as gentian and quassia are very often used to increase the appetite and aid digestion. Their action tends to increase the flow of saliva and gastic juices. Some people have the pleasant habit of indulging in cocktail before meals. This not only increases the appetite, but when taken in the company of other people, tends to brighten the mental outlook and produce a feeling of well-being which should accompany the function of eating; but it is harmful for the young.

ARACHNOID MEMBRANE. This is the delicate membrane covering the brain, so called because of its resemblance to a spider's web. (*See also* BRAIN.)

AREOLA. The brownish area of skin surrounding the nipple of the breast is known as the areola. During pregnancy a second areola occurs, surrounding this. Areolar tissue is the medical name for any loose tissue that lies beneath the skin, and which goes to fill up all the odd corners of the body. (*See also* BREAST; NIPPLE.)

ARGYRIA. (Greek: argyros, silver). This condition consists of the staining of the skin and insides of the eyelids as a result of prolonged use of, or exposure to, silver. Any silver preparations, especially silver nitrate, applied as drops; or the use of silver internally in disease; or the prolonged administration of argyrol; or exposure in the course of work to some salts of silver, will produce the condition. The color is a greenish or brownish grey, and in the eye the lower part is seen to be more stained than the upper. All these conditions were formerly far more common than at present, though staining of the conjunctiva is still fairly frequently seen. It is permanent, and no treatment affects it in the least.

A form of temporary staining of the conjunctiva may be mentioned here: that caused by a particle of "lead" from an eyebrow pencil entering the eye. This may cause serious trouble, even to loss of the sight. (*See also* EYE.)

ARGYROL. Argyrol is a silver proteinate containing 20 to 25 per cent of silver. It was formerly used a great deal as a 10 per cent watery solution in the treatment of eye and nose and throat affections.

ARM. The arm is properly the upper extremity from the shoulder to the wrist, but the part from the elbow to the wrist is sometimes called the forearm. The bones of the arm are the humerus, the large bone in the upper arm, and the ulna and radius in the forearm. The humerus consists of the long shaft and a head and end. The head is well rounded and fits snugly into the concave end of the scapula, or shoulder blade, forming a ball-and-socket joint at the shoulder. At the elbow, which will be described separately, the humerus connects up with the radius, on the outer or thumb side of the limb, and the ulna on the inside. These two bones touch at the upper and lower ends, but curve slightly away from each other in between. The arm is moved by muscles coming from the shoulder blade, the collarbone, and the main trunk of the body. The blood supply is conveyed to the arm by the brachial, radial, and ulnar arteries. (*See also* ELBOW; WRIST.)

ARMPIT. The armpit or axilla is the space between the upper part of the wall of the chest and the upper part of the arm. The important nerves and blood-vessels going to the arm are near the surface in the armpit, so it is a dangerous part to injure. Care must be taken, too, that where crutches are used they are well padded and do not press unduly in the armpit, or paralysis of the nerves of the arm may occur, a condition which is known as *crutch palsy*. The glands of the armpit are liable to abscesses (axillary abscess) which may be very troublesome to heal. It must not be forgotten, too, that the glands of the armpit enlarge in cases of chronic inflammation or cancer of the breast, and should they be found to be enlarged should be seen by a doctor. It is very important to attend carefully to the cleanliness of the armpit, as sweat is profuse there, and if unattended to may cause an unpleasant odor. Deodorants of various kinds are used by many men and women as a routine part of their daily toilet.

AROMATIC. This term is applied to substances having a fragrant, spicy taste and odor. They include cinnamon, ginger, peppermint, aniseed. Many aromatics are used to flavor medicines, but in addition, they are useful in the treatment of indigestion.

ARRHYTHMIA. This is absence of rhythm, or irregularity of the heart's beat. Irregularity of the heart's action occurs in health, particularly in the young, and need occasion on anxiety. Among the elderly, the presence of irregularity may signify a disorder of the heart, especially with a rapid and irregular pulse. Healthy adults may occasionally be aware of a transient irregularity of no importance.

ARROWROOT. Arrowroot is a variety of starch derived from *Maranta arundinacea* of the West Indies, southern United States, etc. When cooked it is a very popular food for invalids. It should be supplemented by milk and eggs, and other ingredients if necessary. A dessertspoonful of arrowroot should be placed in a teacup and thoroughly mixed with a small quantity of milk or cold water till quite smooth. Then add by degrees half a pint of boiling milk, continually stirring the mixture. Sugar may be added, or a teaspoonful of brandy, or it may be flavoured with lemon peel if desired. (*See also* SUPPLEMENT ON DIET AND INVALID COOKERY.)

ARSENIC. Arsenic is a brittle, crystalline metal which, in various forms, is used a great deal in medicine. As it is a highly poisonous substance, it should never be taken internally except under medical supervision. This drug is contained in many preparations sold for agricultural purposes, such as sheepdip, weed-killers, and insect-destroyers, and many deaths have occurred through the careless handling of these preparations.

In medicine it is given internally as a tonic, and it is used in the treatment of syphilis and chronic skin diseases. One peculiarity of arsenic is that it may be found many years after death in the bodies of those who have taken it during life.

Poisoning by Arsenic. Cases sometimes occur in which a patient who has been given arsenic as a medicine may show slight symptoms of poisoning. These are nausea, slight vomiting, loss of appetite, abdominal pain, and mild diarrhea. The eyes and nose may water and there may be headache. These symptoms often occur in workers who handle arsenic in the manufacture of various articles, especially wallpapers and fabrics. Long-continued use of arsenic may cause peripheral neuritis, the chief symptoms of which are paralysis of the muscles of the limbs accompanied by darting pains and rapid muscular wasting.

In cases of acute poisoning, the onset of symptoms is very rapid. Vomiting occurs and is brown in color and often streaked with blood. There is profuse diarrhea and severe abdominal pain. The throat feels parched and burning; there may be cramp in the calves. The skin usually becomes cold and clammy, the pulse becomes feeble, and the patient dies of collapse.

Treatment. This consists of washing out the stomach thoroughly, and emetics should be given. Large amounts of magnesia should be administered or large doses of castor-oil and water. The patient should be kept as warm as possible with hot blankets, and hot-water bottles to the feet and abdomen; hot coffee may be given.

ARTERIOSCLEROSIS. The term means hardening of the arteries. In late middle life, or early old age, the elastic walls of the arteries, which are chiefly composed of muscle, begin to wear out. In order to repair the elastic, as it were, fresh muscle is formed in the walls of the arteries, but this muscle is of an inferior quality to that which the individual was born with, and it soon breaks down (or degenerates, as it is termed), leaving the walls of the arteries weaker than before. Most of the symptoms of arteriosclerosis are due either to thickening of the walls of the arteries in the various organs of the body or to bursting of a blood vessel, the final result in many cases of the weakened wall. Whether a person suffers from arteriosclerosis or not depends on many factors, but there is no doubt that the most important one is the quality of the arteries he inherits. If the muscular walls are of good quality in the first place, it is likely that unless he commits grave excesses in the way of eating and drinking while taking insufficient exercise, or is the victim of some kidney trouble, he will escape all but the mildest symptoms of the condition. If on the other hand, there is a family history of bad arteries, several members of the family having died of strokes or of kidney trouble, care is necessary from youth upwards to avoid overeating, hard drinking, and excessive smoking. The muscular wall of the heart shares in the general thickening of the arteries and many symptoms are due to this cause. The symptoms of this disorder are variable, and many of the minor discomforts of advancing years are its consequence. It is often associated with a raised blood pressure. Headache may be complained of, and giddiness, a full feeling in the head, and noises in the ears are very common symptoms. In many cases, patients complain that they are unable to walk more than a few steps in comfort, not because their legs have no power, but on account of the severe cramps they get in the legs after taking a few paces. These cramps are due to the muscles of the legs getting insufficient blood to carry out their work owing to narrowing of the arteries.

More severe symptoms may show themselves in the form of diminution of vision and shortness of breath on very slight exertion. The desire to pass water frequently at night increases. These people are liable to burst a blood vessel in the brain, giving rise to one form of apoplexy, or to failure of the kidneys to carry out their proper functions. The heart is called upon to work harder to maintain the flow of blood against the resistance of the hardened arteries, and it too may show signs of failure.

Treatment. The treatment of the condition, while it obviously cannot restore the lost elasticity of the arteries, can do much to rid the patient of his troublesome symptoms. Moderation in food and drink is essential and a meatless diet is recommended. Spirits and heavy wines are not allowable, and heavy beers are decidedly bad for such patients, but light wines are permissible. Regular exercise of not too strenuous a nature is advisable, walking being one which is often neglected. It is important to ensure regular action of the bowels. A mild dose of salts has much to recommend it. Patients with arteriosclerosis

should be kept as free from worry as possible, in bad cases should be urged to "take things easy" as there is always a risk of worry or anger bringing on hemorrhage into the brain. (*See also* ANGINA.)

ARTERY. The arteries are the tubular vessels which convey the blood from the heart to the tissues. They are composed of three coats: the outer coat is of fibrous tissue amongst which are elastic fibers; the middle coat is composed of muscular fibers; and the inner coat is the lining membrane. The arterial system of the body has been compared to a tree, the trunk of which is the main artery called the aorta, whilst the smaller arteries branch off at intervals to the different limbs and organs of the body. They, in their turn, have smaller arteries branching off them. The aorta being the largest and therefore the most important artery, is buried deeply in the middle line of the body. The joining together of two arteries is called an anastomosis (q.v.). The aorta and its dependent arteries convey the blood from the lungs to the tissues of the body and are called the arteries of the systemic circulation. The pulmonary artery conveys the impure blood to the lungs to be mixed with oxygen, and is the main artery of the pulmonary system. The main arteries of the body are the aorta, the pulmonary, the innominate, right and left subclavian, common carotid, axiliary, brachial, radial ulnar, iliac, femoral, anterior and posterior tibial. These are described under their separate headings.

The cutting of an artery gives rise to profuse and dangerous bleeding, with bright red blood. Arteries themselves are liable to become hardened in various ways and to lose their elasticity. This condition is known as arteriosclerosis (q.v.). It is usually accompanied by the condition known as "high blood pressure," and renders them liable to break.

ARTHRITIS. Inflammation of a joint is called arthritis. Sometimes this inflammation is due to direct invasion of the joint by the germs of disease such as happens after penetrating injuries. Sometimes germs are carried by the blood stream and settle in a joint: this is how tuberculous joints arise. The degenerative changes of old age pick out certain joints, just as they do all the other tissues of the body, and give rise to a type of arthritis known as osteo-arthritis. Rheumatoid arthritis is a common form of arthritis and its cause is not fully understood in spite of intensive research. (*See also* GOUT; RHEUMATOID ARTHRITIS; SPONDYLITIS DEFORMANS; STILL'S DISEASE.)

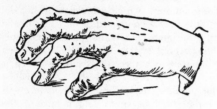

Arthritis, showing arthritic joints of finger.

ARTICULATE. The ordinary meaning of the word articulation is to speak distinctly and clearly. In medical language it means the joining up of joints. An articulated skeleton, such as we see in museums, is one that has been prepared and so arranged as to leave free movement of all the joints.

ARTIFICIAL LIMBS. An artificial limb is, as its name implies, an apparatus designed to replace a limb which has been cut off, either by accident, or by operation because of disease. To be useful the artificial limb must be able to reproduce as far as possible the working of the natural limb. It must fit comfortably and firmly so that there is no unnessary pain, or any interference with the other parts of the body. It must be light in weight, but strong enough to bear the weight which will be put on it, if it is a leg. If it is an arm it must be able to grasp objects in various ways and hold them for a long time if necessary. Such has been the advance in technical skill that a useful comfortable limb can be obtained by almost everyone who needs it.

Duralumin. Artificial limbs are usually made of wood, plastic or metal, or of a mixture of these materials. Until recently wood was found the lighter material, but now a metal has been discovered which combines the strength of steel with the light weight of aluminium. This metal is called *duralumin* and is an alloy of aluminium and other metals. Its discovery has revolutionized the artificial limb industry, and has made the all-metal limb, with its superior advantages, a very satisfactory article. It is possible to hammer metal to fit, which cannot be done with wood. The metal leg is several times lighter than the wooden one and is also much stronger. Duralumin legs will not rust or tarnish and are not affected by seawater.

Artificial legs. A good artificial metal limb should only weight about 3 lb. The ankle can be made either flexible or stiff, and the limb is made so that if a part breaks it can be replaced. The movements of a natural leg are copied so that by a powerful elastic strap the knee bends into the sitting position when required. A spring is introduced into the ankle part of the limb so that there is a slight spring in the step as there is in the natural walk. Artificial legs are so successful nowadays that when the wearer gets used to his apparatus he can walk and sit down in the normal manner and can even play games as energetic as tennis.

Artificial arms and hands. In the case of the arms and hands it is more difficult to make up for the intricate movements which the fingers and hand are capable of, but the thumb can be separated from the rest of the fingers by means of a strap passing round the back part of the shoulders. A "hunching" movement of the shoulder will pull on the strap and thus open and close the joint of the thumb. For craftsmen, it is possible to have different varieties of artificial hands most suitable for their particular trade, such as a good "holding" hand for metalwork, and so on.

Schools for the re-education of limbs. It was Napoleon who first ordered the establishment of special schools for individuals who had had a limb amputated, but it was not until after the First World War that any real progress was made. The schools occupy themselves with the training of limbs where it is not possible to wear artificial substitutes, and in cases where artificial limbs are worn, they help the individual to obtain best use of them, and advise him in the choice of occupation. Where a right-handed individual loses his right hand, he is taught to use the left, and to use the artificial hand on the other side for holding purposes. This re-education usually takes from three to four weeks.

Sensations in amputated limbs. A curious thing that happens after a limb has been lost is that the patient may for several months, or even for years, have the feeling that the limb is still present, and may feel that he has the power of moving and bending it. These people also continue to feel sensations that were formerly present, such as painful feelings in the fingers or toes. These feelings are hallucinations—that is, there have no real origin in fact, but are present only in the mind—and are due to irritation of the nerve endings in the fleshy part of the stump. They are dangerous, however, besides being painful, because they appear so real to the individual that he may try to walk on a leg that is not there, and accidents from this cause are not uncommon.

Fortunately these sensations are not usually permanent, and disappear more rapidly if re-education of the stump is undertaken. They rarely last after work has been begun again.

ARTIFICIAL PNEUMOTHORAX. This term describes the injection of air into the pleural cavity, in order to collapse the lung and so rest and heal it, when it

is affected by tuberculosis. (*See also* TUBERCULOSIS.)

ARTIFICIAL RESPIRATION. Artificial respiration means artificial breathing and has to be used in cases where the heart is beating but the breathing has stopped. In cases of accident and drowning the heart goes on beating for a short time after the actual breathing has stopped, and in most cases, if artificial respiration can be employed at once, the heart will continue beating and the breathing will be restored. For this reason it is very desirable that all able-bodied adults who mix much among their fellow men should have a working knowledge of one or other of the means of performing artificial respiration.

Artificial respiration tries to imitate as far as possible the movements of natural breathing, and the following are the best-known methods of doing this.

Schäfer's Method. This is still a method of use, especially if there is only one first-aider available. However, if familiar with mouth to mouth resuscitation, this latter method is strongly preferred.

Place the patient on the ground, face downwards, with a coat or cushion under the lower half of the chest. Turn the

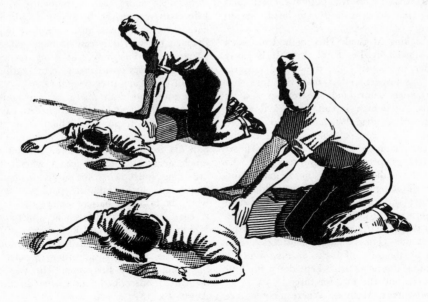

Artificial Respiration: Schäfer's Method.

49

patient's face sidewards in such a way that the nose and mouth are clear of any obstruction such as sand if it is on the beach. Kneel astride of the patient or to one side facing his head. Place the hands on the lower part of the patient's back on each side at a level of the lowest ribs. In this position press down on the ribs, using the full weight of the body in the downward pressing movement. Air and water (if the case is one of drowning) will then gush from the patient's mouth. Repeat this movement twelve or fifteen times a minute and continue for at least half an hour keeping the hands in position all the time; if other competent people come up they may take turns. In this method no attempt is made to imitate the indrawing movements of breath-taking, only those of expelling air, the lungs themselves do the rest by expanding again naturally and of their own accord.

Holger Nielsen Method. In this method, which is said to be even more efficient, the patient is also placed in the prone position, with one cheek resting on his hands. The operator kneels in front, facing the patient's head, and places his hands on the patient's back below the shoulder blades, with his fingers spread out. He bends forward and brings his weight to bear steadily on the patient's chest, and pulls his arms towards his head, ten to twelve times per minute.

Rocking Method. This method has been introduced by Dr. F. C. Eve. It is easily and conveniently carried out and requires far less physical effort than Schäfer's, but it requires some kind of stretcher and an object on which it can be rocked at an angle of 45 deg. When the head is tilted down the organs of the abdomen fall on to the diaphragm and compress the heart and lungs, producing expiration; with the feet down the organs in the abdomen pull the diaphragm back into the abdominal cavity; the chest cavity is enlarged and inspiration results. Even a completely toneless diaphragm responds to these mechanical forces. The rocking should be carried out at the rate of eight or nine times a minute, the head being kept down for four seconds and the feet for three.

Silvester's Method. Where helpers are available Silvester's method is a useful one. The patient lies on his back in this method. With the patient on his face, first repeat a few minutes of Schäfer's method to free the lungs of air and water. Then turn the patient on his back with a support under his shoulders, a roll of clothing being sufficient. If a slight incline, with the patient's head lower than his feet, can be arranged, so much the better. To keep the throat clear the tongue must be pulled forward out of the mouth, and it may be necessary for someone to hold it there by means of a cloth or forceps if they are at hand.

Kneel at the patient's head, and grasp his arms at the wrists. Draw them upwards and outwards above his head, keeping them there while two can be counted; this represents "breathing in." Next bend the patient's elbows, let them down and press them into the patient's chest while two can be counted. This imitates "breathing out." Repeat the two movements alternately at the rate of fifteen series to the minute. The patient's feet are better to be held steady by another helper, and the tongue must be kept from falling back in the mouth and thus blocking the throat.

As soon as the patient begins to breathe of his own accord, stop all the movements, but be ready to begin again if the breathing stops once more, as it frequently does. Efforts to restore the breathing should be carried on for at least an hour before hope is given up, and if it can be managed, an even longer time may still bring success. There are cases on record where breathing has started again after several hours.

In most hospitals there is a machine known as the "iron lung," designed to carry out artificial respiration which must be kept up for long stretches at a time. The patients for whom it is useful are not so much accident cases as cases where the breathing fails owing to paralysis of the diaphragm, as in infantile paralysis. The whole body of the patient except the head is enclosed in this "life-saving machine." It may be necessary, and in fact very often is necessary, to practice artificial respiration on a newborn baby, in order to start it breathing for the first time. The way to do this is described under the heading ASPHYXIA. (*See also* p. 574.)

Mouth-to-Mouth Method, a new method,

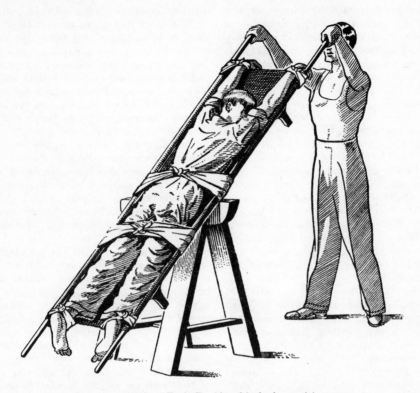

Artificial Respiration: Eve's Rocking Method, requiring apparatus.

which involves laying the patient on the ground, head back, chin up.

Kneel at the side of the head, pinch the nostrils shut with your fingers, seal the patient's mouth with yours, and blow gently to inflate the lungs. When the chest rises, remove the mouth. Do 10 times a minute. (*See also* FIRST AID SUPPLEMENT.)

ARTIFICIAL SUNLIGHT. For a full account of treatment by artificial sunlight and its different rays, ultraviolet, etc., *see* LIGHT TREATMENT.

ASCARIS. This is a species of parasitic worm which inhabits the intestine of most animals. The *ascaris lumbricoides,* or the roundworm, is a variety which is found in the intestine of animals and man, especially young children. (*See also* WORM.)

ASCHHEIM-ZONDEK TEST. This is a very exact test for pregnancy, depending on a substance found in the urine of the pregnant woman, probably derived from the placenta.

ASCITES. This is the name given to the collection of fluid in the abdomen in dropsy. This fluid is nonpurulent, that is, it does not contain pus. It is generally the result of heart or kidney failure or cirrhosis of the liver, but may also be found in diseases such as tuberculosis, cancer, aneurism, or thrombosis.

The patient with ascites complains of enlarged belly, with a heavy feeling and discomfort. The legs swell and the patient is breathless and perhaps has palpitations.

Not more than a pint and a half of fluids should be taken in the day, and an attempt should be made to increase the amount of urine passed, medicines employed for this purpose being called *diuretics*. Salt should be left out of the food as much as possible. In extreme cases of ascites it may be necessary to have the abdomen "tapped" as it is called, and the fluid drawn off. (*See also* DIURETICS; EDEMA.)

ASEPSIS. This term means the state of wounds in which there is no pus and which, therefore, are free from harmful bacteria. The term aseptic surgery is applied to the modern method of surgery which aims at preventing bacteria from entering wounds and setting up infection.

It is not so very long ago that many people who had had surgical operations suffered from—and frequently died from—a mysterious kind of fever which was common in those days. Three out of four people used to die from it after major operations, and for want of a better name it was known as "hospital gangrene." This unaccountable disease was a puzzle to the whole medical profession and doctors were warned to get their patients out of hospital wards as quickly as possible after operation. Indeed, people were frightened of going into hospitals at all for fear they would not come out alive.

Nobody knew the cause of this fatal malady. Some thought it was the old buildings of those days which had bad drainage, or no drainage at all; others attributed it to overcrowding, lack of fresh air and other defects. Florence Nightingale, who experienced its ravages in the hospitals of the Crimea, referred to it as a "special hospital disease."

It was Joseph Lister (later Lord Lister) who found and attacked the real cause—germs entering the wound after operation—and who laid the foundation stone of aseptic surgery as we know it today.

Lister at first attempted to prevent the entry of germs into the wound by means of his famous carbolic spray, and out of this pioneer work has grown what we know as modern hospital methods of "surgical cleanliness." He would not have recognized the modern operating theater with its rounded corners and enamelled walls, the shaving and painting of the patient's skin, covering with sterilized towels, the careful washing of the surgeon's and nurses' hands, and the wearing of rubber gloves, sterilized overalls, caps and masks—all with the object of keeping the wound free from germs—as the direct outcome of his work.

Lister's great work would not have been possible had it not been for Louis Pasteur, the great French scientist, who formulated the germ theory of putre-faction. He showed that germs caused fermentation, and Lister, by the analogy of fermentation

with inflammation, suspected, and eventually proved, that germs were in fact the cause of inflammation and sepsis.

The study of asepsis has gone a long way since Lister first employed his crude carbolic spray. Antiseptics of various kinds have been developed in the search for one which would destroy bacteria and yet not damage the tissues of the body. While they have not, perhaps, been too successful in killing the bacteria actually present in wounds, they have been invaluable for purposes of sterilizing instruments and infected matter outside the body. But asepsis essentially aims at keeping wounds free from invasion by bacteria rather than destroying bacteria when present. (*See also* ANTISEPTICS.)

ASPHYXIA or SUFFOCATION. Asphyxia is a state produced when air is prevented for any reason from entering the lungs.

The air passages which may be concerned are the nose, the pharynx or back of the mouth, the larynx, the windpipe (trachea) and the bronchial tubes. Anything which prevents the free passage of air in these tubes will cause asphyxia.

The condition may be accidental, as in drowning; when objects such as food, tin whistles, etc., are accidentally drawn into the larynx; or it may be due to disease. The most common cause formerly was diphtheria, which causes a membrane to grow at the back of the throat. This membrane may extend downwards to the vocal cords where the airway is narrowest, and restrict the passage of air still further till cyanosis or intense blueness occurs, and finally asphyxia. A large goiter or swelling in the neck may press on the windpipe and narrow it; in fact, any tumor growing outside the windpipe or bronchial tubes may narrow them and may finally result in suffocation.

The condition of necessity is quickly over, since it must either be relieved or the patient dies. At first there is intense blueness of the mucous membranes and skin; marked swelling of all the veins and the eyes stick out. There will be convulsive movements of the chest, which will make it clear to the most unpracticed eye that the patient is struggling to breathe past some obstruction. If the obstruction is not relieved, these movements become less marked and gradually cease; the congestion of the veins diminishes as the circulation fails, the blueness gives way to a greyish pallor, and life ceases altogether.

Asphyxia lasting for more than about five or six minutes will possibly be followed by permanent damage to the brain.

Causes. Accidental asphyxia may arise from the following causes:—

(1) Obstruction of the air-passages as in drowning, strangulation, choking or swelling of the throat due to the sting of a poisonous insect.

(2) Inhalation of poisonous gases or fumes such as household gas or the exhaust of an automobile.

(3) Mechanical pressure, such as strangling.

Treatment. Treatment of asphyxia will clearly depend upon the cause. Some of the more common causes, together with the measures that should be taken to restore respiration, are given below.

DROWNING. Complete and prolonged immersion in water causes death, which is called "death by drowning." Always try to resuscitate persons who are rescued, for breathing can often be started again by artificial respiration (q.v.).

CHOKING. The cause is generally a piece of crust, or similar object, that has "gone the wrong way," or, in children, it may be a candy or a marble. Loosen the collar, if any, lean the affected person forward and thump him hard between the shoulders. A child may be held upside down and thumped. If this fails, introduce a finger into the mouth and try to reach the obstruction. This will at least produce a severe retch and cough which may suffice to dislodge the offending object. If these measures are unavailing, send for a doctor without further delay.

SWELLING OF THE THROAT. If the patient is breathing, give ice to suck or cold water to drink, and call the doctor urgently.

STRANGULATION. In a case of hanging, act promptly. Grasp the lower limbs and lift so as to reduce the tension on the rope. If alone do not go for help, but try to cut or loosen the rope and get the body down. Then free the neck, loosen any tight clothing and perform artificial respiration.

SUFFOCATION BY SMOKE, GASES OR FUMES. The would-be rescuer must protect himself by tying a wet handkerchief, folded diagonally, across the bridge of his nose so that it hangs down over his mouth. Crawl swiftly along the floor and drag the affected person out. If the person is heavy, or if he has to be dragged a considerable distance, tie his wrists together with a handkerchief, kneel astride his body facing his head, and with his arms looped over your neck, crawl along the floor on hands and knees, dragging his body between your legs. Loosen the clothing and, if breathing has ceased, perform artificial respiration.

"BLUE ASPHYXIA" IN THE NEWBORN. This is characterized by a blue color and a strongly beating heart. It is usually due to an obstructed airway, or it may be due to a narcotic drug previously administered to the mother—e.g., chloroform, morphia, etc.

The treatment is first to clear the air passages with a suction pump and then to start artificial respiration, being careful not to injure the infant's chest. If possible, a mixture of carbon dioxide and oxygen should be given by a tube down the throat. If the lungs are healthy, normal breathing is rapidly established again.

"WHITE ASPHYXIA" IN THE NEWBORN. This is characterized by pallor, muscular weakness, and a feeble circulation. It is really a condition of heart failure, and the treatment must be gentle. The infant must be kept warm and should be given the carbon dioxide oxygen mixture as above. Failure to respond to this usually denotes severe damage in the brain of the child.

ASPIRATION. This term is applied to the act of sucking up or sucking in. It is a method used for withdrawing fluid from a cavity such as the chest, etc. An aspirator is the name given to the apparatus which is used for drawing off fluids by suction.

ASPIRIN. Acetylsalicylic acid is more commonly known as aspirin. It is beneficial in cases of rheumatism in which it relieves pain and promotes sweating. One or two tablets taken before going to bed often ensure a good night's sleep. It is useful in cases of influenza, headaches and neuralgia. In influenza, 5 to 15 grains taken at bedtime will often induce perspiration, and allay fever. Children should not be given more than from ½ to 5 grains. Some people cannot take aspirin as it causes palpitation, and it is inadvisable for people suffering from heart disease to take this drug in large doses. Aspirin should never be taken in large continuous doses, as it has a very depressing effect; about 15 grains should be the largest dose taken, the usual tablet containing 5 grains.

ASTHMA. An affection characterized by spasmodic attacks of breathlessness and coughing and a feeling of suffocation and tightness in the chest. It is due to spasm of the rings of muscle which surround the finer air tubes, and this effect is produced by several different causal factors.

(1) **Allergy.** Allergic diseases are diseases which run in families. One member of the family may have asthma, another hay fever, another urticaria (hives), and another certain types of eczema, all of which are different manifestations of various forms of allergy. For instance, in asthmatic patients certain things which would not affect another person act as irritants to them and bring on an attack of asthma; one man may get asthma at the seaside and another among the mountains; the breathing of grass pollen or the dust of feathers; the eating of shellfish, fish, strawberries, eggs, milk, aspirin tablets, etc., are all examples of the diversity of things that may cause asthma. It is interesting to note, too, that the proximity of certain domestic animals may cause attacks. The cat and horse are fairly common examples. Horsehair mattresses, down pillows and grass baskets and various furs are also frequent unsuspected causes.

(2) **Infection.** Some cases of asthma are due to infection in the lungs or air-passages. The most frequent of these causes is to be found in affections of the nose and throat, such as nasal polypi.

(3) **Emotional Upset.** Mental influences such as emotion, fatigue, anxiety, or even the picture of some article which causes asthma such as flowers, a cat, etc., may be sufficient to start an attack.

As has been said previously, asthma runs in families, and men are more often attacked than women. It usually shows itself first in childhood or early manhood. The attacks very often come on in the middle of the night after the patient has been sound asleep. He is in great distress and may get up and go to an open window in search of air. A bad attack of asthma is always very distressing to the onlookers. The patient's face becomes pale and drawn with an anxious expression. His lips may be blue, his breathing is short and jerky, and he may look as if he were going to die, but, fortunately, he never does. Asthma is not a fatal disease, however troublesome it may be.

Attacks may last for two hours or even longer, and usually finish with a fit of coughing and the bringing up of sputum. The patient will probably be so exhausted that he will drop asleep and for the next two or three days he may continue to breathe in a wheezy, labored fashion.

In children the asthmatic attacks may cease for no apparent reason, but the child will still be allergic, and must not receive serum treatment for any other disease without first having ascertained how he is likely to react to it.

Treatment. At the first symptom an adrenalin injection under the skin may stop the attack at once. As skilled attention is not usually at hand when an attack begins, it is as well for an asthmatic to find out between times what drugs agree with him and have something always within reach in tablet form, such as tablets of ephedrine sulphate, which give great relief to many people. A strong cup of coffee helps others. People liable to frequent attacks need to take regular doses of ephedrine or aminophyline by mouth. 1/500 adrenalin solution, when finely atomized, is readily absorbed from the air-passages, and many patients get instant relief from inhalation of one of the many patent preparations on the market. This method avoids the unpleasantness of frequent injections. The patient must avoid those emotional situations which he has learned give rise to an attack. Sometimes it is possible to determine what the patient is sensitive to, and thus he may be able to avoid contact with it. When attacks occur frequently at night, the patient should sleep on a foam rubber mattress with a pillow of kapok or foam rubber. The bedroom should be as bare of furnishings as possible. (*See also* ALLERGY.)

ASTIGMATISM. This is described under the heading, SIGHT, ERRORS IN.

ASTRAGALUS. *See* TALUS.

ASTRINGENT. Any drug or substance which produces dryness of the tissues is called an astringent. An astringent is used to arrest bleeding, diarrhea, etc.

The number of astringents is fairly large, and among the more well-known ones are vinegar or acetic acid, alum, tannic acid, silver nitrate, copper sulphate, and adrenalin.

ATAXIA. Ataxia or ataxy is a nervous disorder in which the patient is unable to control his movements. In other words, he is unable to walk without staggering or swaying. Each separate muscle may be in perfect working order and quite efficient, but the patient loses his sense of co-ordination and is therefore unable to produce the necessary action required for walking. In some forms of ataxia there is an hereditary tendency and it may occur in several members of a family, and sometimes in several generations of the same family.

Ataxia is a very common symptom of many nervous diseases and may be quite temporary and unimportant, as in cases of hysteria, etc. The ataxic walk is very characteristic, and is often confused with the walk of a drunken man. The patient walks with his legs rather wide apart, and the feet are thrown out in rather an aimless fashion. There is usually difficulty and stumbling in the effort to lift the feet up steps, and when the patient is standing still he places his feet wide apart in order to balance himself better. Much can be done to re-educate and train a patient to make the best use of his limbs, but it takes time, and patience and perseverence are required. (*See also* TABES DORSALIS.)

ATHEROMA. Atheroma is the term applied to hardening of the arteries, due to inflammatory or degenerative changes in their coverings. Atheroma, which is a form of arteriosclerosis, is usually associated with high blood pressure (*See also* ARTERIOSCLEROSIS.)

ATHLETE'S FOOT. This is a common fungus infection of the feet. It is usually acquired by walking barefoot on a wet bathroom floor which has been infected by a previous occupant. It causes a mild scaliness between the toes, especially the outer three. It is always worse when the feet are sweaty, after, say, a long walk, when the affected clefts become red, sodden and painful. It may spread to the sides of the feet, the groin, and the hands.

Treatment. The feet must be washed and *dried* with special care every morning and evening. Socks must be changed daily and a dusting-powder of Desenex be used. At night Sopronal ointment should be applied after washing. In place of these, there is a wider range of equally effective preparations extensively advertised, but it must be remembered that no treatment will work if the rules of foot hygiene are disregarded.

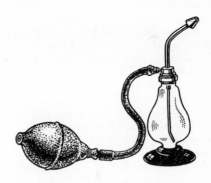

Atomizer.

ATOMIZER. An atomizer is an instrument for transforming a liquid into a fine spray and for projecting the spray as required.

ATROPHY. When there is a wasting of the tissues of the body or when the tissues diminish in bulk, this process is termed atrophy. It takes place in old age, where the reparative capacity of the tissues is greatly diminished. Muscular atrophy may set in by the inability of a patient to move his limbs for himself. This may be lessened by massage or stimulation by electricity.

General wasting often occurs in children who are being starved from insufficient or improper feeding. Rickets, syphilis, and tuberculosis, as well as many other serious diseases, generally give rise to wasting, especially in young children (*See also* EMACIATION.)

ATROPHY (SENILE) OF THE SKIN. The skin, like all other parts of the body, undergoes changes as we pass from middle to old age. It not only receives less nourishment, but can deal with less. Its glands become inactive, and the skin itself becomes dry, thin, and "poor." Its elasticity also goes and with it the power of accommodating itself to the size and shape of the parts underneath, so that it becomes loose and wrinkled.

Treatment. Grease in some form is the best treatment; it not only relieves the itching, but counteracts the dryness and scurfiness of the skin. If the patient can digest fats readily, he should take plenty in the diet in addition, to increase the fat layer under the skin. Itching is often worse in very thin old people than in the well-covered. Externally, almond-oil, cold cream, and petroleum jelly are all good; but it should be remembered that the skin has its likes and dislikes for grease in different forms. If one form of grease does not suit it the patient should be encouraged to try another till he discovers one that does suit him. A hot bath at night is often very helpful, followed by the ointment. For use in the daytime, a lotion is more convenient.

ATROPINE. This is a drug obtained from the plant, *Atropa belladonna,* more commonly known as deadly nightshade.

Given internally or by hypodermic injection, atropine lessens the perspiration and stops the flow of saliva in the mouth. It is often injected to relieve bronchial spasm, whooping cough, and asthma. It is effective in relieving the pain of colic.

Atropine acts on the nerve endings in the muscles of the eye. If it is dropped into the eye, or given by mouth, the pupil of the eye dilates to a very marked degree; this fact is made use of when examining the eyes. Belladonna is one of the favorite remedies for bed-wetting, as children do not suffer from any ill effects from this drug.

Poisoning by Atropine. Poisoning often occurs as the result of eating the leaves of the deadly nightshade plant or through having an overdose of the drug. The mouth and throat will become dry and difficulty will be experienced in swallowing. The pupil will be dilated and the vision may become confused; the skin will feel very dry. If the dose has been a large one, the symptoms will appear quickly and the pulse rate may increase rapidly. The patient may become giddy and stagger when he walks, and a rash may appear on the skin. Later, the patient may become delirious and death may take place from failure of the breathing. Treatment consists of emetics or washing out the stomach. Artificial respiration should be employed if necessary and the patient should be kept warm with hot-water bottles. Strong coffee may be given later.

AUDITORY or ACOUSTIC NERVE. This is the eighth cranial nerve and is the nerve of hearing and balance. It comes out from underneath the brain and goes through a little opening in the skull to the internal ear. This analyzes the sounds brought to it by the external ear and sends on the messages to the brain by the auditory nerve.

AURA. This word literally means a breath, and it is applied to the slight warning symptoms which go before an attack of epilepsy. The "aura" may appear in various ways. Sometimes the patient is warned by a peculiar taste in the mouth or an itching on some part of the body, or the warning may be a mental one. (*See also* EPILEPSY.)

AUREOMYCIN. The discovery of penicillin led to a widespread search for similar substances capable of destroying germs in the human body. It has been discovered that *streptomyces aureofaciens,* a mold growing in the soil, produces such an "antibiotic" substance which is curative over a remarkable range of diseases. This substance has been called aureomycin. Unlike the other antibiotics, it can be absorbed in effective concentrations when given by mouth, and avoids the disadvantage of requiring repeated injection. It has been shown to be curative in nearly all the common varieties of pneumonia, in gonorrhea, and in meningococcal meningitis. Perhaps most remarkable of all, it will cure certain diseases caused by viruses, those minute disease agents which cannot be seen with an ordinary microscope. It will cure psittacosis, hitherto untreatable.

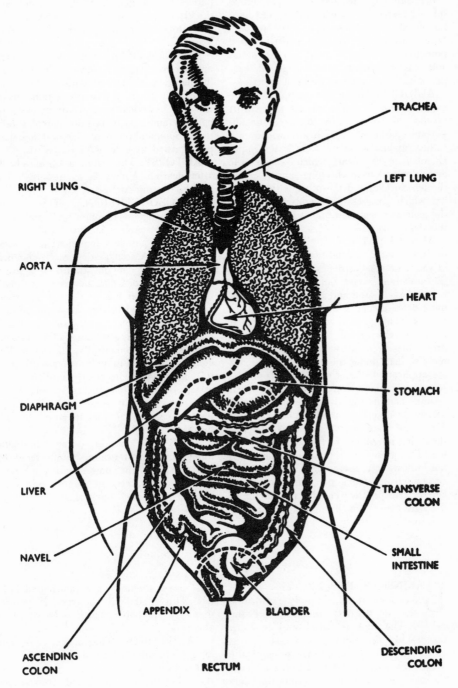

TRACHEA

LEFT LUNG

RIGHT LUNG

AORTA

HEART

DIAPHRAGM

STOMACH

LIVER

TRANSVERSE
COLON

NAVEL

SMALL
INTESTINE

APPENDIX

BLADDER

ASCENDING
COLON

DESCENDING
COLON

RECTUM

Organs of the Body (Male).

Aureomycin has been shown to have an effect on the tiny germs called *rickettsia* which cause typhus and Rocky Mountain spotted fever against which there has been no effective treatment up to the present. It is thus obvious that this drug has a potentially enormous field of usefulness and has the double advantage of easy administration and few harmful effects.

AURICLE. This name is applied to the expanded portion or pinna of the ear. It is also the term given to two very important parts of the heart which are rather ear-like in shape. One is the upper chamber of the heart which receives the arterial blood from the lungs and is called the left auricle, and the other is the chamber which receives the venous blood from the general circulation and is known as the the right auricle.

AUSCULTATION. This is a method of finding out the conditions and functions of various organs of the body by the sounds they themselves give out. The stethoscope is now largely used and it is able to furnish more definite conclusions for diagnosis.

An advantage of the stethoscope is that it enables the doctor to study the sounds proceeding from very small areas, much more so than under the method of immediate application of the ear. Apart from the sounds which the heart valves make when opening and closing, there are other sounds which are described as murmurs or bruits. There are many varieties of murmurs and they each have their own place and meaning. The presence of these murmurs does not indicate any disease of the heart unless certain changes take place in their character. Long practice enables the doctor to distinguish between the normal and abnormal sounds.

AUTOGENOUS VACCINE. An autogenous vaccine is one made from the patient's own germs. Stock vaccines are usually made from germs grown in the laboratory. (*See also* GERM; IMMUNITY; VACCINE.)

AUTOMATISM. This is the term applied to that state in which persons go through various actions without the mind controlling them. Automatic actions occur in some hysterical patients or in cases of epilepsy and also in certain mental conditions. Somnambulism or sleepwalking may be regarded as a form of automatism.

AUTOPSY. The examination of a body after death is known as an autopsy. (*See also* POST-MORTEM.)

AUTOSUGGESTION. This term means to suggest to one's self, and as a method of treatment in illness which exists only in the patient's imagination it is of great value. Autosuggestion received much attention early in the twentieth century from the work of Coué, a French physician.

Autosuggestion has proved of a certain value, when used in the way Coué recommended, in sleeplessness, where the cause is mental anxiety or stress. The patient repeats, quite mechanically, the words "I'm going to sleep, I'm going to sleep," in a soft monotonous whisper, until he falls asleep. After a few nights it becomes a habit to repeat this phrase and often sleeplessness can be completely cured by this means.

AVERTIN. Avertin is an anesthetic fluid, of German origin, administered by injection into the bowel and used with considerable success in surgery and midwifery. (*See also* ANESTHESIA.)

B **ABINSKI'S REFLEX.** This is the name given to a simply performed test to discover the state of the nerves. The foot is bared and a sharp object—like the point of a pin—is drawn along the sole. In a normal state of the nerves the toes would bend down towards the sole, but in certain nervous disorders the big toe bends upwards and the other toes spread themselves in fan-shaped fashion. This action of the toes is natural in very young babies, but in older people is abnormal.

BACILLURIA. The presence of any kind of bacillus or germ in the urine is called bacilluria. The germ may get into the urine through the blood, from which it passes to the kidney and then to the bladder, or it may enter at the urethra below and spread upward. The finding of bacilluria always signifies infections somewhere in the urinary tract, either alone or as part of a widespread infection such as typhoid fever.

The symptoms and treatment of bacilluria are dealt with under the sections on CYSTITIS and PYELITIS.

BACILLUS. Certain types of germs or microbes which are shaped like little rods are termed bacilli, which is the plural of bacillus. A great number of diseases owe their origin to bacilli in some form or another, for instance, tuberculosis, meningitis, anthrax, diphtheria, typhoid fever, dysentery, and many others. The cultivation of certain bacilli plays a very important part in the processes of wine making; they are also responsible for the rotting which takes place in dead animal matter. (*See also* GERM.)

BACK. The back consists of the spinal column or backbone with the back parts of the ribs and of the haunch-bones and sacrum, with the muscular tissue which binds these bones together. The muscles of the back are very powerful and have to support the head, as well as move the upper and lower limbs. The *trapezius* is a large triangular sheet of muscle connecting the arm with the spinal column. It stretches from the back of the neck to the middle of the back. The *latissimus dorsi* is the corresponding triangular sheet of muscle in the lower back, attaching to the lower limbs. The *levator anguli scapulae* is a band of muscle proceeding from the neck to the shoulder which helps to raise the arm. The *rhomboideus major* and *rhomboideus minor* assist in the act of breathing and turning the back from side to side. These are the most important muscles of the back, but there are many more.

A well-developed muscular back can be bent almost to the floor backwards and forwards and sideways, but because of its great supply of muscular tissue it is very frequently the seat of muscular pains. Strains and twists are of frequent occurrence also. Diseases and injuries of the spinal column are not uncommon. A theory is held by people who call themselves *chiropractors* that most disease is due to pressure on the nerves of the spinal column owing to displacements of the *vertebrae* or small bones of the spinal column. Such a belief has little foundation in observed fact. (*See also* BACKBONE.)

BACKACHE. Many people have an aching pain in the back without being able to state any reason for it. Pain, stiffness or tenderness in the back is a symptom encountered in a number of different diseases. An early symptom of smallpox is severe aching in the back, and there is always a certain amount of backache in fevers. In meningitis, or brain fever, backache may be severe. This is often accompanied by stiffness at the back of the neck. In rheumatism, chronic or acute, there may be much pain and stiffness. Pain in the back about the level of the waist may be due to spinal disease or kidney trouble.

Any severe pain in the muscles of the back is often loosely described as "lumbago." When this occurs suddenly during a heavy lifting strain and is followed by spread of pain down the leg, it is often due to rupture of the nucleus of the fibrous pad which lies between the vertebrae—so-called "slipped disk." If this painful and disabling condition does not respond to rest in bed, an operation to remove the offending nucleus may be needed. Many obscure backaches have been found to be due to a piece of fat becoming nipped between the fibres of a muscle.

In women, pain in the back is so common that women have been divided into two classes, "those with backaches and those without them." In some cases the pain may be due to a disorder of the reproductive organs. In such cases the pain is usually felt low down in the back and relief may sometimes be had from surgical operation. There are, however, many women who suffer from pain in the small of the back without any sign of disease and who are otherwise perfectly well. It is usually worse when the woman is tired, and before and during menstruation. Rest, especially lying down, is the only way of relieving the pain, but it does not cure it. This form of backache is very often due to weakness of the muscles of the back which is turn is probably due to insufficient exercise. Persistent backache is a signal for seeking medical advice.

BACKBONE. The backbone is the popular name for the spinal column or vertebral column, the strong supporting column of bone which stretches from the head to the bottom of the back and has the shoulder bones, the ribs and the haunch bones attached to it. In the normal adult who is standing erect, the spinal column curves slightly in four parts. Beginning at the head it curves slightly out, then in a sweeping curve inwards under the shoulders, out over the haunches and in at the end of the spine. Other curves are developed by bad posture when the backbone is in a flexible state due to youth or illness. These abnormal curvatures are called *lordosis, kyphosis,* and *scoliosis.* The spinal column is composed of thirty-three small bones, called *vertebrae,* which are joined together by cartilage and ligaments. Each vertebra has a hole through it, through which the spinal cord runs for the whole length of the spine. The thirty-three vertebrae are divided into groups of cervical, thoracic, lumbar, sacral, and coccygeal vertebrae. From the head downwards there are seven cervical vertebrae, twelve thoracic, five lumbar, five sacral, and four coccygeal vertebrae. The cervical, thoracic, and lumbar vertebrae are separate bones, but the sacral and coccygeal vertebrae are joined together to form bones called the sacrum and the coccyx.

The spaces between the vertebrae are filled with elastic tissue which acts as a buffer from shock, so that a severe blow on either end of the spine, such as would be caused by sitting down suddenly on something hard or being hit violently on the top of the head, does not fracture the spine, as it certainly would if the spine were composed of solid bone.

The spinal cord inside the backbone is very strongly protected from injury, and dislocations of vertebrae are very rare. Fracture of the backbone only occurs as the result of great violence, such as being run over by a heavy vehicle, or crushed under a heavy load. If a fracture does occur, however, it is a very serious matter, because of the damage which will most likely be done at the time of the accident to the spinal cord, which may lead to paralysis. The backbone is liable to be attacked by tuberculosis and other bone diseases, and also by abnormal curvatures. (*See also* Spinal Curvature.)

BACTERIA. This is the medical name for germs. Other names are microbes or micro-organisms. These are described under the heading Germ.

BAGASSOSIS. Bagassosis is an acute fever, with bronchitis and pneumonia, caused in workers who shred sugar-cane from which the sugar has been extracted (bagasse).

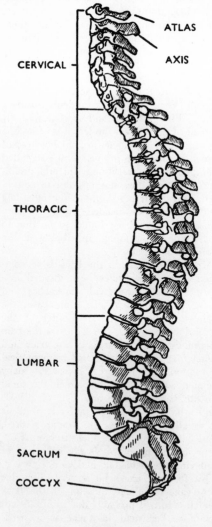

ATLAS

AXIS

CERVICAL

THORACIC

LUMBAR

SACRUM

COCCYX

Backbone.

BAKERS' ITCH. This is a kind of eczema which breaks out in the form of small blisters which afterwards burst and discharge a clear, watery fluid or "weep" as it is called. This form of itch is due to acquired sensitivity to flour and occurs in allergic subjects. The disease is very hard to get rid of, and some workers may have to change their job. (*See also* DER-MATITIS).

BALANITIS. This is the name given to inflammation of the head of the penis, or organ of reproduction in the male. Lack of cleanliness is often the cause of the complaint. The foreskin should be drawn back and the part washed carefully. In some cases it might be better if the operation of circumcision, or cutting short of a too long foreskin, were performed, thus allowing the part to be kept clean more easily.

BALDNESS. The question of the relation between the general health and baldness is a much discussed one, but there can be no doubt that there is a close relationship between the two. The loss of hair in old age shows that this is so. Loss of color and thinking of the individual hairs almost always start about the age of the forty. Premature or early baldness is generally the result of a diseased state of the scalp. Dandruff and greasiness are signals to be looked out for and promptly treated when they appear, if baldness is to be avoided. In dry seborrhea (scurf), a disease which is described later, dandruff is usually present in excessive quantities and is flaky in character; in the greasy form of the disease, the dandruff sticks closely to the scalp and makes the hair appear limp and moist.

Scurf. Scurf usually makes its appearance long before it becomes troublesome enough to attract attention. It attacks the scalp gradually and may go on for years. The condition is caused by a germ which is infectious, and is usually spread by hairbrushes, combs, hats, towels, and the like.

Premature baldness. This is much more common in men than in women. In men, thinning of the hair generally begins on the crown of the head, but in some cases the hair recedes from the temples, leaving the crown of the head well covered. Temporary loss of hair often occurs

owing to certain diseases, and a change of climate, especially if it is to a warm one, will sometimes account for it. During the summer months many people find that their hair becomes noticeably thinner. This is of course a natural process, the same as the molting of the coats of animals in summer.

Complete baldness. In cases of typhoid fever and scarlet fever or severe measles, people have been known to become completely bald, and in some wasting diseases, such as tuberculosis, the hair may also fall out. In any form of illness it is usual to find the hair losing its glossiness and becoming thin and easily broken. It is generally the rule that the hair will return to its normal state once health is restored.

Treatment. To increase the growth of the hair the general health must be carefully attended to. Once the body is in perfect health, the hair will naturally improve in glossiness and growth. To treat a diseased condition of the scalp, absolute cleanliness is the first and most important step. Dandruff is a condition which may take a long time to get rid of and in which patience and perseverance play a large part if it is ever to be overcome. The head should be washed with a pure soap, such as the ordinary liquid green soap which is obtainable in bottles quite cheaply from any druggist. It should be rinsed thoroughly with repeated fresh waters. This should be done every other day in the case of a man or short-haired woman, or at least twice a week even if the hair is long and difficult to wash and dry. After washing, rub in, and repeat daily, an ointment made up of 25 grains of salicylic acid to 1 ounce of petroleum jelly. This ointment should be rubbed into the scalp for about ten minutes, not merely plastered on the scalp. It should be remembered that by vigorously rubbing the scalp the blood supply is brought to the surface, and this acts as an important part of the cure. Stimulating the scalp by the use of electricity is also very helpful, and most hairdressers have the apparatus for carrying out this treatment, but it is rather expensive. Treatment by mercury-vapor lamps is said to have had some wonderful results in baldness.

Baldness which occurs in patches is

medically termed *alopecia areata,* and will be found under its own heading.

Baldness may be due to an abnormal state of the roots of the hair which is present from birth, and is usually found in other members of the same family. Nothing much can be done for them and they usually have to wear wigs.

BALSAM. Balsams are oily, pleasant-smelling substances which are obtained from the stems of certain trees and plants. Sometimes they flow out of the plant naturally, but usually they have to be obtained by making a slit in the stem or leaves of the plant and collecting the juice which oozes out. A balsam, generally speaking, is a mixture of oils, resins, and acids.

Friar's Balsam. As its name suggests, this was discovered by the friars many hundreds of years ago and is the balsam which is best known. Its medical name is compound tincture of benzoin. Benzoin or Gum Benjamin is a resin obtained from a plant which grows in tropical countries, and to make Friar's Balsam it is mixed with other ingredients. It is used as a dressing for wounds and sores of all sorts, and as an antiseptic. As well as these uses, it is very popular in cases of bronchitis and sore throat, or severe cold in the head. It may be swallowed in doses of a teaspoonful to loosen a cough and help to bring up expectoration, but more often it is used as an inhalant. One or two teaspoonfuls are put in a pint jug of hot water and the patient puts a towel over his head and the jug and breathes in the steam. Alternatively, an inhaler may be used. If this is done every two or three hours. stuffy heads and sore throats and chests will be made much more comfortable.

BANDAGES AND BANDAGING. There are two chief varieties of bandage, the *triangular* and the *roller.* They are generally made of calico, bleached or unbleached, or of white cotton sheeting. Linen is an excellent material for the purpose, but too costly.

In first-aid work, the triangular bandage is far the more commonly used. It is made by cutting diagonally across a piece of material from 36 to 42 in. square. Two triangular bandages are thus formed measuring 36 to 42 in. along the sides and 50 to 60 in. along the base.

The parts of a triangular bandage are the point or apex, the base, the two sides, and the two ends.

A *broad-fold* bandage is made from a triangular bandage by bringing the point to the center of the base and folding again.

A *narrow-fold* bandage is made from a broad-fold bandage by folding once more.

There are two methods of folding a bandage for packing: (*a*) Make a narrow-fold bandage and bring the two ends together to the center. Do the same again and then double the bandage upon itself to form a compact oblong. The bandage can be rapidly undone and is ready folded for use. (*b*) Spread out the bandage on a flat surface. Fold one end over to lie on the other, thus forming a triangle half the size of the original.The center of the original base is now the apex and the original apex is one of the new ends. Fold the original apex over to the new apex and also the new ends, thus forming a square. Fold this over to form an oblong and once again to make a small square.

Always tie the ends of a triangular bandage with a square or reef knot. A granny knot is not safe and should never be used.

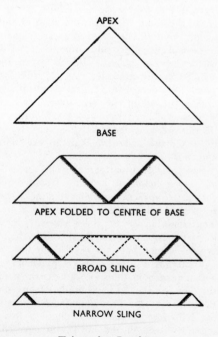

Triangular Bandage.

Place the knot so that it does not press into or chafe the patient. If it is likely to be uncomfortable, place a pad between it and the patient's skin. When a knot is completed, the ends should be tucked out of sight. If a knot is not practicable, large safety pins are used to secure the bandage. (*See also* KNOTS.)

Triangular Bandages

(*a*) **Large Arm Sling.** This is used to support the forearm. Pass one end of the bandage over the shoulder on the normal side and round the back of the neck. Bring it down nearly to the level of the breast on the injured side. Slip the apex of the bandage across the front of the body and behind the elbow of the injured arm. Bend the elbow and lay the fore-arm over the middle of the bandage. Bring up the lower end and tie just below the collarbone. Now bring forward the apex from behind the elbow and fix with two safety pins.

It is advisable to adjust the large arm sling so that the fingernails of the supported hand are just visible beyond the edge of the sling. From their appearance the state of the circulation in the injured limb can be judged. If the nails show a bluish tinge, denoting constricted circulation, the position of the hand may need to be changed

or the sling dispensed with to free the circulation.

(*b*) **Narrow Arm Sling.** This bandage supports the wrist, leaving the elbow free. It is used for a fracture of the upper arm, and for minor injuries to the hand or shoulder.

Pass a broad-fold bandage over the sound shoulder, behind the neck and down nearly to breast-level on the injured side. Bend the elbow so that the forearm is at right angles to the upperarm. Place wrist over the middle of the bandage so that half the little finger extends beyond the edge of the bandage. Carry the second end up to the first and tie just below the collarbone on the injured side.

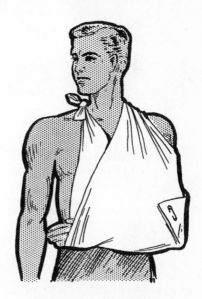

Triangular Bandaging: final stage.

(*c*) **St. John's Sling.** This bandage supports the arm and keeps it close to the side. For an injury on the *right* side proceed as follows. If the injury is on the *left* side, substitute "left" for "right."

1. Fold the patient's right forearm flat across his chest, fingers pointing to his left shoulder.

2. Take an unfolded triangular bandage with its apex in your left hand and one end in your right. Lay it over the patient's forearm, the end on his left shoulder, the apex well beyond his right elbow.

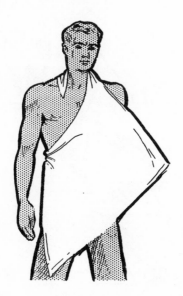

Triangular Bandaging: First stage of sling for fractured fore-arm.

3. Tuck the base of the bandage well in under the hand and forearm, supporting the elbow meanwhile. Bring the lower end across the patient's back, up over the left shoulder to the front and tie the ends.

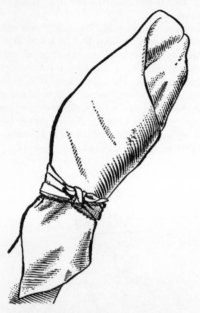

Hand Bandage:
half finished.

4. Hold away the side of the bandage lying on the forearm and tuck the apex well in between the forearm and the side you hold. This produces a fold which you bring round behind the arm and pin securely to the bandage where it runs up the back.

There are many simple ways of improvising a sling. Take two handkerchiefs. Tie one loosely round the neck. With the other make a sling, the ends being tied in the loop formed by the first handkerchief. This will give a sling of the necessary length; or simply support the hand well inside the buttoned coat. This is more effective if the sleeve is pinned to the coat as well. A third method is to turn up the lower edge of the coat and pin it near the lapel.

Bandage for the Hand. Spread out a triangular bandage on a flat surface and fold a hem along its base. Place the open hand on the bandage, palm downwards, the wrist on the hem. Fold back the apex

over the back of the hand and wrist. Cross over the ends and pass them round and round the wrist, finally tying them over the back of the wrist. Now fold back the apex over the knot towards the fingers and pin it.

Bandage for the Wrist. Place the hand palm downwards over the center of a narrow-fold bandage. Pick up the ends and bring them round the hand, leaving the thumb clear. Cross them over the back of the hand and round and round the wrist and lower forearm. Tie off on the back of the forearm.

Bandages on the Elbow. Fold a 3-in. hem along the base of a bandage. Bend the injured elbow and lay the middle of the hem on the back of the forearm folded side inwards and the point of the bandage reaching up the back of the upper arm. Cross the ends in front of the elbow then round and round the back of the arm above the elbow. Tie them behind, turn down the point to hide the knot, and pin it to the bandage.

Bandage for the Shoulder. To keep a dressing on top of the shoulder. Two bandages are needed. Fold a 3-in. hem along the base of the first bandage. Place its center-hem inwards, against the upper

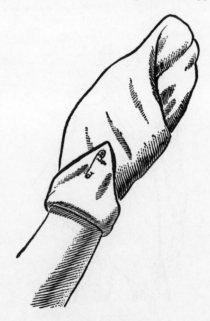

Hand Bandage:
final stage.

arm, the apex running up the side of the neck to the ear. Pass the ends round and round the arm and tie. With the other bandage apply a narrow arm sling with the knot on top of the apex of the first bandage. Draw up the apex and fold it down neatly over the knot and pin securely to keep the whole thing in place.

Bandage for the Whole Foot. To keep a dressing on the foot. Fold a 2-in. hem along the base of a triangular bandage. Place the foot in the center of the bandage, the toes pointing to the apex. Fold back the apex over the toes and instep and leave it pointing up the front of the ankle. Gather up the ends so that the heel is covered and cross them over the instep. Take them round behind the ankle, cross them and bring them forward again. Tie them in front. (If the bandage is too long, pass the ends once round the sole of the foot before tying off.) Draw up the apex, fold it over and pin it to the bandage above the instep.

Bandage for the Ankle. When treating an injured ankle, place the center of a narrow-fold bandage against the sole of the foot. Bring up the ends and cross them over the top of the foot. Pass them round behind the ankle, cross them and bring them forward. Cross them again and down round the sole of the foot. Continue until the ends are short and tie them off where convenient.

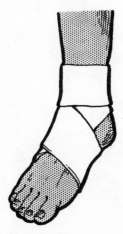

Elastic Bandage for Ankle.

Bandage for the Knee. Fold a 2-in. hem along the base of the bandage. Place the

apex in front of the middle of the thigh and the center of the base just below the kneecap. Cross the ends behind the knee. Then bring them round to the front and tie above the knee. Pull up the apex to smooth out the bandage. Fold it over the knot and pin.

Bandage for the Hip. To keep a dressing in position on the hip, two bandages are needed. With the first, make a narrow-fold bandage and tie it round the patient just below the rim of the haunch bone (pelvis), with the knot on the outer side of the affected hip. Lay the second bandage on the hip and pass the apex under the knot of the first bandage. Draw it up for about 4 in. Fold the base of the second bandage inwards in a 2-in. hem and pass the ends horizontally in and round the thigh, and round and out again. Tie them on the outside. Pull up the apex to smooth out the bandage. Turn it down over the knot and pin in position.

Bandage for Chest and Abdomen. Spread an open triangular bandage over the chest and abdomen, the base lying across the chest and the apex pointing down. Pass the ends under the armpits, behind the body and tie. Spread a second bandage similarly, but with the base lying across the lower abdomen and the apex pointing to the chin. Tuck the apex in under the first bandage and pin it there. Pass the ends round the patient and tie behind. Turn up the apex of the first bandage and pin it. *N.B.*—The foregoing is an emergency bandage to be replaced later by the orthodox "many-tailed" bandage.

Bandage for the Chest. Used to keep a dressing on the chest. Stand in front of the patient and place an open triangular bandage on his chest. Push the apex well over the shoulder on the dressed side. Fold the base over inwards in a 3-in. hem. Bring the ends round behind the back and tie them vertically below the apex. One end will be longer than the other. Carry it up and tie to the apex on top of the shoulder.

Bandage for the Back. This is applied in the same way as the bandage for the chest, except that the patient stands with his back, not his front, towards the dresser.

Bandage for the Scalp. Used to keep a

dressing on top of the head. Lay an open triangular bandage on top of the patient's head, so that the apex hangs down over the nape of the neck. Fold a hem about 2 in. wide in the base, so that it lies above the eyebrows. Go behind the patient and draw back the ends, so that they pass just above the ears. Cross them over and pass them to the front again. Tie neatly in the center of the forehead. Gently pull down the apex until the bandage is smooth, then turn it up and pin on top of the head.

Bandage for the Eye. Place the center of a narrow-fold bandage over the dressing on the eye. Carry one end round below the ear on the injured side and the other end over the top of the head on the un-injured side. Cross the ends at the back of the head, bring them forward again and tie off over the injured eye.

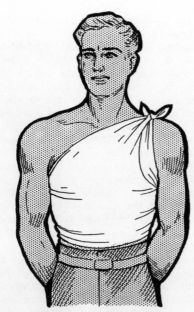

Bandaging Chest: front view.

Roller Bandages

Roller bandages are strips of material rolled into firm cylinders for easy application. They are usually some yards in length and of various widths suitable for different parts of the body as shown below.

	Width	Length
Fingers	½–1 in.	1–1½ yd.
Arms	2–2½ in.	3–6 yd.
Head	2–2½ in.	3–6 yd.
Legs	3–3½ in.	6–8 yd.
Trunk	4–6 in.	6–8 yd.

When a roller bandage is ready for use, the roll is called the "head" and the loose end the "tail."

These bandages may be rolled by hand, but can be more quickly and efficiently rolled by machine.

When rolled up, the free end should always be secured by a safety pin; this ensures a pin being to hand to fasten the bandage when needed.

The principal uses of a roller bandage are:

1. To retain dressings or splints in position.
2. To support a sprained or dislocated joint, when the patient begins to use it again, and to prevent swelling.
3. To treat or prevent varicose veins.
4. To drive the blood to a different part of the body, as is done by bandaging limbs in extreme collapse from hemorrhage.
5. To prevent hemorrhage after operations.

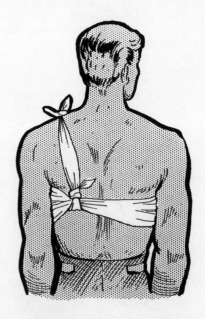

Bandaging Chest: back view.

Rules for Applying Roller Bandages:
1. Apply the outer surface to the skin.

2. Bandage from below upwards, and from within outwards.

3. Bandage the chest from below upwards; but the abdomen from above downwards.

4. When bandaging to retain a dressing or splint, leave the tips of fingers or toes exposed. The color of the nails indicates the state of the circulation of the blood in the limb. If congested, numb, or swollen, the bandage is too tight, and the splint or dressings need to be readjusted.

5. Each fresh layer of the bandage should cover two-thirds of the preceding layer.

6. Fix the finished bandage securely.

7. Whenever possible place a layer of wool under the bandage. This permits the bandage to be drawn tighter, without constricting the veins.

8. Use a bandage of appropriate size.

Methods of Applying Bandages. The four principal methods of applying roller bandages are:

1. The Simple Spiral. Adopt this method when the part to be bandaged is of uniform thickness, e.g., the finger or wrist.

2. The Reverse Spiral. The bandage is twisted upon itself at each circuit of the injured part. Adopt this method for parts of varying thickness, e.g., the fore-arm or leg.

3. The Figure of Eight. This is used for a joint or its vicinity. It is made by passing the bandage obliquely round the limb upwards and downwards, so that the loops look like the figure 8.

4. The Spica. This is a modified figure of 8, and is so called because when completed the crossings of the bandage resemble in their relative positions the grains in a head or "spike" of barley.

It is described in detail under the appropriate headings.

Bandages for various parts of the body. *To Bandage a Finger* (½- or 1-in. bandage). Turn the hand palm downwards and separate the injured finger. To dress the right hand, hold the bandage in your left, and vice versa. Make two or three fixing turns by passing the bandage round the wrist from within outwards. Lead the bandage from the root of the thumb to the injured finger and up to its tip in a long spiral. Cover the finger in a series of spirals down to its root. Then lead the bandage across the back of the hand to the wrist, on the little-finger side. Fix with a couple of turns round the wrist.

Any or all of the fingers may be bandaged thus, but between each two a fixing turn must be taken round the wrist.

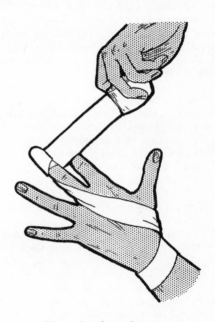

Finger Bandage: first stage.

To Bandage the Fingertip. Proceed as above, but pass the bandage over the center of the fingertip down the upper aspect of the finger to its middle joint. Fold the bandage back upon itself and carry it over the tip again to the under side of the middle finger joint. Make three such folds, the second and third overlapping the first on either side. Fix these folds in place by

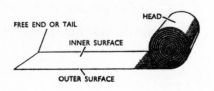

Roller Bandage.

bandaging from tip to root of the finger in a simple spiral and finish off as above.

To Bandage the Thumb (1-in. bandage). Lay the tail of the bandage across the front of the wrist. Pass the head across the back of the thumb between the thumb and forefinger. Make a simple turn round the top of the thumb and come down diagonally across the back of the hand to the wrist. Carry on across the palm, round the thumb again and so on until the thumb is covered. Finally take a turn round the wrist and secure. This is a "spica" bandage.

To Bandage the Hand (2-in. bandage). Stand opposite the injured hand, which should be extended palm downwards. Place cotton-wool pads between the fingers. Lay the tail of the bandage on the inner surface of the wrist and bring the roll obliquely over the back of the hand. Bandage the left hand in a clockwise, and the right in a counterclockwise direction. Pass the roll round the little finger edge of the hand, across the palm, round the forefinger side of the hand and horizontally across the back of the fingers, so that the little finger-nail is just exposed. The bandage circles the fingers again and passes obliquely over the back of the hand and round the wrist and obliquely up over the back of the hand again. Continue this process three or four times until the figure of 8 loops quite cover the hand and wrist.

To Bandage the Closed Fist (2-in. bandage). Place a pad in the palm of the hand and cotton-wool between the fingers. Start with two fixing turns round the wrist from within outwards. Carry the bandage over the back of the hand, round over the little finger and on to the front of the wrist at the root of the thumb. Circle the wrist and pass again over the back of the hand, the third finger, the front of the wrist, and so on five or six times. The last loop will project 1 in. beyond the margin of the fore-finger. Now pass the bandage two or three times round the bent fingers enclosed in the loops and finish off at the wrist.

To Bandage the Forearm (2½-in. bandage). Make a few fixing turns at the wrist, from within outwards. Bandage the lower forearm with a simple spiral. When the muscular part is reached, the bandage will no longer fit snugly; the lower edge will be loose. To overcome this difficulty, make a reverse spiral for the upper part of the limb. Support the forearm with your free hand and bring the bandage round the back of the limb in such a way that it lies flat. While in this position place your free thumb on the bandage and bring the head downwards. Turn it over in such a way that its upper edge folds over the thumb. A "reverse" has now been made and the *inner* surface of the roll is next the skin. Pass the bandage round the forearm again and make another reverse. (The outer surface of the bandage will now be next to the skin again.) Continue in this manner, When the bandage nears the elbow, bend the forearm at right angles to the arm, the palm facing inwards. Carry the bandage over the elbow by four figure of 8 turns. Of each, one loop encircles the top of the forearm, the other the lower part of the arm. The four crossings are in front of the elbow.

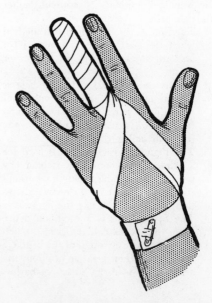

Finger Bandage: final stage.

To Bandage the Tip of the Elbow (2½-in. bandage). Lay the tail of the bandage on the inner side of the bent elbow, and pass the roll round the limb over the elbow tip. Circle the arm with a second turn and the fore-arm with a third, so that each overlaps the margin of the first turn.

Continue these figure of 8 turns round the arm and fore-arm alternately until half a dozen or so are made.

To Bandage the Arm (2½-in. bandage). Make two fixing turns just above the bent elbow. Continue with simple spirals. If the limb is exceptionally muscular, reverses may be needed. If so, make them high up on the outer aspect of the arm.

Recapitulation. To bandage the whole arm: Begin with a simple spiral at the wrist and change to reversed spiral over the forearm. Use a figure of 8 to negotiate the elbow. Complete the upper-arm with a simple spiral, with perhaps a few reverses.

To Bandage the Shoulder (4-in. bandage). Place a pad of cotton-wool in the *uninjured* armpit to prevent chafing. Make two fixing turns, with reverses if necessary, round the upper arm. Carry the bandage across the back to the opposite armpit, across the chest, and round the shoulder. Continue these figure of 8 turns four or five times until the whole of the shoulder is covered.

over the patient's head so that one end reaches to the small of the back, the other to well below the navel. Now take a 4-in. bandage and make two fixing turns round the lower chest and on top of the first piece of bandage. Proceed with reversed spirals well up the chest. Finish off with two fixing turns and pin the bandage in front. Turn up the free ends of the brace over the bandage and fix with safety-pins in front and behind.

If preferred, use two suspenders one passing over each shoulder and finish off in the same way.

The Many-tailed Bandage. After surgical treatment, a many-tailed bandage is used to retain dressings on the chest and abdomen. It has the merit of enabling the wound to be examined and the dressings changed without moving the patient. It can be made by laying several strips of roller bandage of the right length parallel to and overlapping each other. The strips are then sewn to another strip laid across their centers.

A many-tailed bandage should be long enough to go one and a quarter times round the part and deep enough amply to

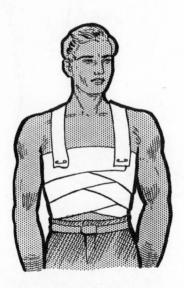

Chest Bandage.

To Bandage the Chest (4-in. bandage). A spiral bandage on the chest tends to slip down. To overcome this split a 1½-yd. length of 4-in. bandage along its center so as to make a hole 2½ ft. long. Pass this

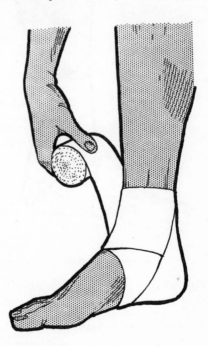

Figure of 8 Bandage for Heel: first stage.

cover the area involved. For the chest and abdomen, the tails are 3½ to 4 in. in width.

To apply a many-tailed bandage to the chest spread the bandage underneath the patient. Then cross the right and left lower ends over each other in front. Then the second lowest pair, the third lowest and so on, each successive pair securing the preceding pair. Fix the last tail with a safety pin.

To Bandage the Breast (3-in. bandage). To support one breast. Make two fixing turns round the body below the breasts from the sound to the affected side. Carry the third turn under the affected breast, up and over the shoulder, down the back, and round the body again. Continue until five or six turns have been made. Safety pins may be used at intervals to fix the crossing loops in position.

Support the leg so that the foot projects. Stand opposite the injured foot and place the tail of the bandage on the front of the ankle. Pass the roll round the tip of the heel from within outwards. Make a second round, passing the bandage slightly above the first turn. Make a third round just below the first turn on the sole of the foot. Continue like this, the fourth round passing just above the second and the fifth just below the third. But when the fifth turn reaches the inner side of the foot, do not pass it over the instep. Bring it back diagonally over the inner side of the heel across the previous turns and pass it round the back of the ankle and down over the top of the foot from without inwards. Take the sixth turn under the foot and back diagonally across the *outer* side of the heel and round the back of the ankle. It is the same as the fifth turn, but in the opposite direction. Finish off the bandage with a turn or two round the ankle.

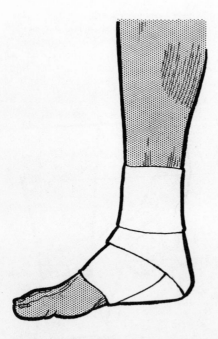

Figure of 8 Bandage for Heel: final stage.

To support both breasts. Proceed as for one breast, but take the bandage up and over the right and left shoulders alternately until each breast is covered by four or five turns.

To Bandage the Heel (3-in. bandage).

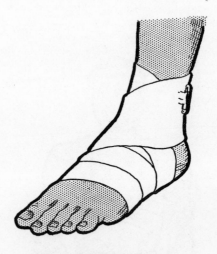

Figure of 8 Bandage for Foot.

To Bandage the Foot (Leaving the heel exposed, 3-in. bandage). Place the tail of the bandage beneath the sole of the foot. Make a figure of 8 by bringing the roll from within outwards over the top of the foot, round the ankle, across the top of the foot to the root of the little toe, and round under the foot to the starting point. Now bandage up the foot in spiral turns, with reverses, if necesary, over the instep.

Finish off with two figure of 8 turns round the ankle and foot, pinning behind the ankle.

To Bandage the Knee (3-in. bandage). There are two methods:

(*a*) *Permits movement of the joint.* Slightly bend the knee and make a fixing turn from within outwards over the kneecap. Make a second turn *below* and half overlapping the first, and a third *above* and half overlapping it. The fourth turn overlaps the upper two-thirds of the third turn. Continue in this way until the knee is covered. Finish with a turn or two round the upper leg.

(*b*) *Restricts movement of the joint.* Raise the knee so that the roll can be passed beneath it. Make a fixing turn just below the kneecap. Bring the bandage round the back of the knee and out to the front on the inner surface of the bottom of the thigh. Encircle the thigh and carry the bandage down over the kneecap. Pass it round the leg just below the knee and then upwards round the lower thigh just above the knee. Carry it round the thigh then down in a descending loop, overlapping the last one. Continue until the knee is covered.

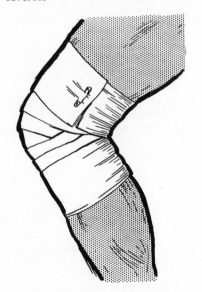

Figure of 8 *Bandage for Knee.*

To Bandage the Leg (3-in. bandage). Fix the bandage with a figure of 8 turn round the foot and ankle. Carry on up the leg with simple spirals until the bulge of the calf muscles call for reverses. Make them on the outside of the leg. Finish off with two simple spirals just below the knee.

To Bandage the Thigh (3-in. bandage). Apply the bandage to the thigh in an ascending spiral with reverses. Sometimes a many-tailed bandage is used.

To Bandage the Groin (3-in. bandage). If the patient cannot stand, the pelvis must be firmly supported. Make two fixing turns round the waist from left to right. Pass the bandage down the left groin and up behind the right buttock. Come round the waist from left to right and down the right groin; up behind the left buttock, round the waist from left to right and down the left groin again. Continue until the desired support is achieved.

To cover one groin, take a long 4-in. bandage and stand on the side to be bandaged. Make a fixing turn round the upper thigh, from within outwards. Carry the bandage up along the groin and round the back. Bring it forwards and downwards to cross the first turn directly over the dressing in the groin. Pass it round the thigh and up over the groin again, making a figure of 8. Continue these turns until the dressing is covered and secure. This is known as the Single Spica.

To cover both groins, stand on the patient's right side, or facing him if he is on his feet. Begin as for a single spica on the right side, but bring the bandage forwards and downwards over the *left* groin and round the *left* thigh. Then take it up across the abdomen to the right groin and over the first turn of the bandage. Carry it round the right thigh, behind the waist and down to the inner side of the left thigh. This completes one turn. Continue a series of turns.

To Keep a Dressing Between the Legs. Make a T bandage by stitching a piece of 4-in. bandage 1 yd. long at right angles to the center of another piece 1½ yd. long. Tear the first piece up its center for half its length. To apply, tie the second piece round the waist like a girdle with the knot in front. Pass the first piece between the legs from behind and tie the tails to the girdle on either side of the knot.

To Bandage the Chin (four-tailed band-

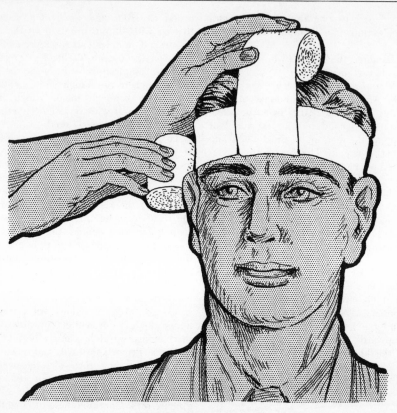

Head Bandage: first stage.

age). Cut off a yard from the widest bandage available. Tear from both ends down the middle. Stop when 3 in. from the center. This will leave an undivided central portion 6 in. long.

To apply. Place the center of the bandage on the patient's chin. Carry the lower tails upwards in front of the ears and tie them on top of the head. Bring the upper pair of tails along the line of the jaw and tie behind the neck. As the bandage is 1 yd. long, four ends are left over. Tie the two right ends and the two left ends together.

To Bandage the Head. The triangular bandage is undoubtedly the most useful, but a modified roller bandage is sometimes used.

Roll up a 2-in. bandage from each end, or stitch the tails of two bandages together so as to form one long, double-headed, or capeline bandage.

To apply. Stand behind the seated pati-

ent with one roll in either hand. Place the center of the bandage on the forehead, just above the eyebrows. Bring round the two ends and cross them well down at the base of the skull. Carry the upper end round to the front again. Turn up the other end, which lies underneath, and bring it over the crown of the head and down to the center of the forehead. Let the horizontal portion pass over it and round to the back of the head again. Turn up the hanging portion and take it back over the crown, so that it overlaps one-third of the first strip. Cross the two portions at the back and bring the hanging portion forwards again, so that it overlaps the *other* side of the center strip. Carry the horizontal portion on round the head as before. In front, secure the hanging portion once again and carry on backwards and forwards on alternate sides until the whole scalp is covered. Pin both ends round the head.

To Bandage the Eye (2-in. bandage).

72

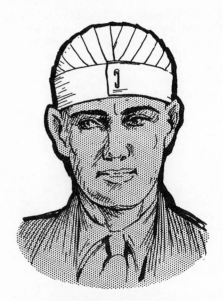

Head Bandage: final stage.

Make a fixing turn round the head, starting on the uninjured side just above the ear. When the starting-point is reached, bring the bandage over the affected eye, below the ear on that side, round the back of the head to the forehead again. Make as many turns as may be necessary and fix with a safety-pin. Both eyes can be bandaged by passing every other turn of the bandage below the other ear and up over the other eye to form a crossed bandage.

BARBER'S ITCH. Barber's itch or "foul shave" is the popular name for a skin disease, the medical names of which are *sycosis, tinea sycosis,* or *tinea barbae.* In this disease the glands at the roots of the hair in the neighborhood of the beard are inflamed. Many little yellow pimples are to be seen, each surrounding a hair, and the skin between is swollen and red. In bad cases, the upper lip and eyebrows may be affected. The cause of barber's itch is mainly a germ of the staphylococcus group, but other germs have been found to be present. Barber's itch must not be confused with other diseases which at first sight look like it, such as impetigo, ringworm of the beard, and dermatitis.

Treatment. The hair of the beard should be clipped as short as possible. Shaving, though painful, is well worth while, as it

enables treatment to reach the roots of the hairs. The sound parts of the beard should be shaved first, followed by the affected areas. A brushless cream is preferable to shaving-soap, and should be followed by swabbing the whole of the affected area with methylated spirit.

If possible the hair in the center of each pimple should be pulled out before shaving. This may, however, be too painful and may tear the skin, in which case it should not be attempted in case further inflammation arises. An antiseptic ointment must then be applied (white mercurial ointment is useful), and it is very important to rub this thoroughly into the skin. Even a weak ointment, throughly rubbed in, is better than a strong preparation if it is only smeared on. Rub in twice a day for ten minutes at a time. This treatment, if continued long enough, should cure simple cases.

Vaccines may be tried for more severe cases, and are often very useful—especially if they can be made of the patient's own germs (autogenous vaccines). X-ray treatment is also used and is generally very successful.

When they are nearly well, patients sometimes get slack and begin to neglect their treatment. This is a great mistake. The treatment must be continued until the

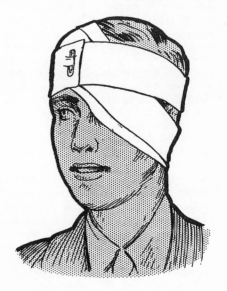

Eye Bandage.

73

disease is absolutely cured, and even then it is wise not to begin to grow the beard again (if one is worn) for at least a year afterwards. Barber's itch is usually found in delicate or temporarily run-down men, so the general health must be carefully looked after. A daily dose of salts will be found useful and frequent baths should be taken to keep the skin in healthy working order. Tonics, good food and exercise are all helpful.

BARBITURATES. The organic salts of barbituric acid form a group of powerful sedative and hypnotic drugs widely used in medicine today. Hundreds of derivatives of barbituric acid are known, but they form only a small fraction of the possible variations. The most important difference between the actions of the drugs of this series lies in the difference in intensity and duration of their action. Some, such as pentothal, when given by injection into a vein produce immediate loss of consciousness, and are used as an anesthetic for short operations. They are quickly destroyed by the body and recovery of consciousness is rapid. Others, such as phenobarbital, are slowly absorbed and slowly excreted, and produce only slight drowsiness. In between these is a wide range of drugs of which amytal and nembutal are well-known members. All are able to induce sleep rapidly when taken by mouth, and in small doses their effect will wear off in eight hours. Enormous amounts of these drugs are consumed throughout the civilized world and in the usual doses are practically harmless. Accidental and suicidal poisoning does occur from time to time and should be treated by washing out the stomach with warm water and giving hot strong coffee. (*See also* PHENOBARBITOLE.)

BARIUM MEAL TEST. Barium sulphate is a heavy, white, odorless powder which is insoluble in water. It will not allow X-rays to pass through it, and is therefore used to obtain photographs of the working of the digestive system. A bowl of barium powder is made into a porridge and is swallowed by the patient, who is then photographed under the X-rays at intervals of a few hours during the next twenty-four hours. By this means a series of photographs of the solid stream of barium is obtained in its complete journey through the stomach and bowels until it reaches the rectum and is expelled from the body. The radiologist can thus see the various organs at work and can tell whether they are functioning properly.

BARRENNESS. *See* STERILITY.

BATHS AND BATHING. The custom of bathing, both for cleansing and for medicinal purposes, dates from very early times. Bathrooms have been found among the ruins of ancient Egypt, and in Greece there are well-preserved examples dating from about 1500 B.C. Later on, when Greece and Rome were at the height of their power, bathing played a great part in the life of the people. The Romans, especially, made their baths into great social centers, and used them not only for bathing but also as meeting places in which to transact ·business, meet one's friends, and listen to lectures and concerts.

Baths promote good health by encouraging cleanliness, improving the action of the skin, stimulating the flow of blood to and from the skin, and by producing a feeling of well-being.

Kinds of Baths. Baths may be taken in fresh water, which may be cold, tepid, warm or hot; they may be taken in sea or other salt water, either hot or cold. The waters of many mineral springs all over the world are used for baths at various temperatures. These contain chemicals in large quantities which are useful in treating different diseases. There are also solid baths, such as sand baths; semisolid baths like mud or peat baths; vapor, hot-air and sun baths. For medical purposes, cold baths are given in acute diseases with great fever, to reduce the temeprature. In chronic diseases, like Bright's disease, they are given to increase the action of the skin and promote sweating, thus resting the kidneys as far as possible. In rheumatism and neuritis they help to relieve pain, and in various nervous conditions they are used to calm or stimulate the patient. Certain baths are of the greatest use in skin troubles. To discuss all the varieties of baths in detail would require a book rather than an article, but a short description will be given of the more common and important baths, with their uses. Different people feel the heat differently, so in cases of illness where absolute accuracy is desirable, a thermometer should always be used.

Cold Baths. A cold bath is one between 35 and 65 deg. F. Its daily use (in health) is a great aid to vigor and natural resistance to such infections as the common cold.

Tepid baths are those between 80 and 90 deg. F., i.e., slightly below body temperature, which is 98.4 deg. F.

Warm baths are those from 90 deg. F. to 100 deg. F. Water at 115 deg. F. can be borne by the hand, but not by the whole body. The warm bath reaction is quickening of the pulse and an increased flow of perspiration.

Salt Baths. Sodium chloride (common salt) may be added to the water—3 oz. to the gallon—and has proved valuable in the treatment of extensive burns.

BAZIN'S DISEASE or "SHOP-GIRL'S DISEASE." This occurs in girls and young women whose occupation involves a great deal of standing. The girl is frequently delicate and anemic, and may sometimes show evidence of tuberculosis. The condition begins by the formation in the skin and soft tissues beneath the skin of livid, bluish, hard lumps or nodules, as they are called. These nodules grow larger, then soften and turn into ulcers. The skin over them "sloughs" or comes away, leaving a small open sore with ragged edges. Fresh crops appear near-by, and they in turn become ulcers. In the nodular or lumpy stage of the disease there is pain, but not in the ulcerated stage.

Treatment. If it is left untreated, the disease may spread widely over the calves and may last for months and even years. If seen early, the condition will improve rapidly under treatment, though relapses are common unless the general condition of the patient is improved. The treatment consists chiefly of rest in bed and generous diet. The legs should be raised on pillows. Artificial sunlight often promotes healing, and, if this fails, short exposure to X-rays may produce the desired effect. For the tuberculous type, cod liver oil and tonics are advised; where varicose veins are the real cause of the trouble, these may be suitably treated. The use of strapping, with or without ichthyol paste, often promotes healing of the ulcers. (*See also* TUBERCULOSIS; VARICOSE VEIN.)

BEDBUGS. These insects may develop into a source of great danger and annoyance if measures are not promptly taken to destroy the eggs as well as the insects themselves. The full-grown insect is of a brownish color, very flat, and may vary in size from about a twelfth of an inch to a sixth of an inch in length. The bedbug gives forth a disagreeable smell which seems to fill the whole room, and is quite characteristic. In common with other trouble-some insects, the bite may or may not cause annoyance to persons who come in contact with it. Some people, it is true, are able to live in the most bug-infested areas without showing the least sign of having been bitten; while other individuals suffer intense agony from irritation and spots. In order to relieve the irritation the parts may be bathed with dilute ammonia or toilet water.

Not only is the bedbug an unpleasant visitor to have in one's house, but as a carrier of disease it must be looked upon as possibly dangerous. After it has been feeding on the blood of a person suffering from fever or any other infectious disease, it will spread the germs in the most indiscriminate way to other persons whom it may bite.

Drastic measures may have to be taken in order to rid a house of this pest. Mere simple cleaning will not be found sufficient, as these little creatures lurk in the baseboards and flooring. The premises which are to be cleaned must be thoroughly dismantled and all possible breeding-places must be treated with crude creosote of tar. All furniture, especially if made of wood, should be washed with soap and, after it is thoroughly dry, turpentine should be applied to all holes and cracks. Sulphur fumigation is also an excellent way of disposing of bedbugs, or kerosene may be used. Should clothing require treatment this may be carried out by soaking the garments in a carbolic solution. (*See also* BITES.)

BEDCRADLE. In certain cases, such as fracture of the limbs or painful abdominal conditions, it is necessary that the bedclothes should be raised off the affected parts. A bed cradle is used for this purpose. It is a cage-like structure, made of wooden or metal struts. In cases of emergency, an ordinary footstool can be used for this purpose.

BEDMAKING. The proper way to make up a bed for an invalid is described in the article on SICKROOM NURSING.

BEDPAN. In cases where it would be harmful for the patient to get out of bed, a bedpan should be used. It should be slightly warmed with hot, not boiling, water, and for greater comfort the margin should be covered with flannel. After use, it should be emptied as soon as possible and well rinsed out with a disinfectant fluid. (*See also* DISINFECTANT.)

BED-REST. An improvised bed-rest can be made my placing a chair upside down at the top of the bed and laying pillows along its back. This is only recommended in cases of emergency. For longer use, a properly fitted bed-rest would be more satisfactory for the patient.

BEDSORE. Bedsores can be very seri-out, especially in a patient who requires all his strength to resist the illness which confined him to bed. Any sign of redness on the skin of a person who has to stay in bed for some time should be attended to immediately, because once a bedsore commences it is very difficult to cure.

The prevention of bedsores depends very largely on good and efficient nursing, but there are certain conditions, such as complete paralysis, in which they may make their appearance in spite of careful nursing. When the circulation becomes poor and the vitality of the patient is low, bedsores will undoubtedly make their appearance unless precautions are taken.

All prominent parts, such as the spine, shoulder blades, hips, heels, elbows, etc., are especially likely to become sore, and these parts should be given attention. The patient should be washed, and before the skin is dried, the nurse should soap her hands well and gently massage the back and hips. The movement should be round and round in order to encourage the circulation of the blood where it has been hindered by constant pressure on the bed. In order to harden the patient's skin, the soap should be left on unless it creates irritation. It will be found better to dry the skin by dabbing it with a towel instead of rubbing, as the rough towel is apt to crack the skin, and a bedsore may be the result. When the skin is thoroughly dried, it should again be thoroughly rubbed with methylated spirits, or eau-de-Cologne. Finally, the body should be dusted with some fine powder, such as zinc or talc.

In very old people or patients in a feeble state of health, bedsores may appear in spite of all precautions. They should be looked upon as a serious sign and reported to the doctor immediately.

If in spite of all precautions a bedsore appears, the slough should be removed by warm boric acid dressings until the surface is clean. After this a return should be made to dry dressings, with a large cotton-wool pad over the sore.

In cases where a patient is likely to be kept in bed for some length of time, it may be necessary to use a water-bed in order to relieve any pressure on the body, but much can be done by judiciously moving the patient from time to time and by placing air-cushions underneath various parts.

As moisture on the skin will quickly lead to the formation of bedsores, it is important to see that proper care is taken in cases where there is incontinence of the bladder. In such cases absorbent pads should be placed between the patient's legs, and a

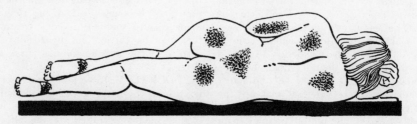

Bedsores.

soothing ointment such as zinc should be used in place of the methylated spirits.

It cannot be too deeply impressed on the nurse that above all things prevention is better than cure, and in this way only can she save herself and her patient endless worry, work, and pain.

BED-WETTING. Bed-wetting appears to be more common among boys than girls. In some cases it is difficult to cure and the greatest care and tact are necessary in the handling of the child. It is extremely unwise to punish when bed-wetting occurs, as it is very often a matter beyond the child's control. Most children learn clean habits before they are two years old. When bed-wetting persists after this age, or when as a result of illness or fright control of the bladder is lost, the condition is described as Enuresis.

Treatment. Proper attention to the bowels during the day and regular emptying of the bladder is the first important step in treatment. The diet should be nourishing but not irritating, and nothing should be given to drink after four P. M. The child should be made to empty the bladder before going to bed and should be awakened to do so after a few hours' sleep. It is a mistake to make the child feel that it is doing something wrong, as this often increases his nervousness and makes the complaint worse. The cooperation of the little patient may be gained by kindliness, and his own eagerness to obey his mother's wishes will do much to bring about a cure. Many drugs are used to try to cure children of bed-wetting. Among those generally used are belladonna, hexamine, alkalis, and thyroid extract. Treatment by suggestion and hypnotism have been tried with quite good results. All cases of persistent bed-wetting need to be examined by a doctor to exclude diseases. If the child is a boy with a tight foreskin, circumcision may cure him of the habit. (*See also* BLADDER, DISEASES OF.)

BEER. Apart from its alcoholic content, malt, liquor contains varying proportions of energy foods, chiefly in the form of carbohydrates. The quantity of protein present is negligible. Beer is usually taken as an appetizer and to quench thirst; but, at all times, it should be taken in moderation. Persons with a tendency to stoutness should not drink beer and malt liquors, for this tendency is increased. The light lager and pale ales contain the least amount of alcohol; while the old ales and heavy stouts contain the most. For invalids, only the lighter forms should be used, but never in any great quantity.

Beer is made from malt and hops, but often the brewer substitutes a proportion of raw grain, cane sugar, and glucose.

BELLADONNA. This powerful drug is obtained from the belladonna plant, which is more popularly known as the deadly nightshade. It can be readily recognized by its clusters of small purple flowers with orange centers, rather like lilac in appearance, which climb about among a tangle of other plants in the hedges. Later on, the flowers turn into bunches of black shining berries, and as they ripen about the same time as the blackberries and often grow among them, a summer seldom passes without some children being poisoned by eating them in mistake.

Belladonna is one of the most useful drugs we have, and atropine— the alkaloid which comes from the same plant—is also of the greatest use. Its chief use is in treating diseases where there are painful "spasms." A spasm is a tightening of the muscles in any part of the body so that that part cannot continue its work and the tightened muscles cause great pain. Such spasms occur in a large variety of diseases, such as asthma, bronchitis, stomach troubles, gallstones, and inflammation of the bladder. Belladonna or atropine will usually cause the muscles to relax, thus relieving the spasm. It cannot be taken for more than a few weeks at a time, however, or the effect will wear off and the patient may have too much in the system and be poisoned. Children can usually take it for a longer time than adults without harmful effects, and it is sometimes prescribed for troublesome cases of bed-wetting. In whooping cough it is of the greatest use, and will often be successful where other remedies fail.

Belladonna plasters are still very comforting remedies in lumbago, phlebitis, and painful rheumatic conditions.

Belladonna liniment is useful to rub in in order to ease the pain of such conditions as rhematism and neuralgia and lumbago. Care must be taken, however, that poisoning is not caused by too much being absorbed through the skin, as sometimes happens.

Poisoning by Belladonna. If the berries have been eaten or too much of the drug taken and there is poisoning, an emetic should be given at once and, after the vomiting has stopped, large drinks of water with sal volatile or alcohol as a stimulant. Artificial respiration may have to be performed if the breathing becomes very feeble.

The symptoms of belladonna poisoning are great dryness of the mouth and throat, enlarged pupils or dark centers of the eyes, rapid beating of the heart, sickness, excitement, and delirium with great bodily weakness.

BELL'S PALSY. This is paralysis of the facial nerve. It is called after a famous Scottish physician, Sir Charles Bell, 1774–1842. It is described under the heading FACIAL PARALYSIS.

BENIGN. This term is applied to certain illnesses and tumors which do not threaten life. The common wart is an example of a benign tumor. If tumors are dangerous to life they are called "malignant." Benign tumors may grow for years and cause no harm to the patient, but in some cases they have to be removed surgically when they have grown so large that they interfere with the working of other parts of the body. The term benign also is used in connection with the milder forms of malaria.

BENZOL. Benzol or benzene is a light, colorless fluid obtained from coaltar oil. It has a very strong characteristic odor. Applied externally, one liberal application will destroy lice. It is a highly inflammable substance and should never be used near an open flame. Benzene is a powerful poison and acts by depressing the activity of the blood-forming bone marrow. Industrial poisoning from long continued inhalation of the vapor occurs from time to time.

BERI-BERI. Beri-beri is a disease caused by the absence from the diet of Vitamin B_1, (which is described in the article on VITAMINS), and is therefore known as a "deficiency" disease. The disease is usually found in countries where rice is the chief article of food (Japan, China, India, Malay Peninsula). It is due to the eating of rice which has been polished in order to remove the husk. The vitamin is in the husk. This vitamin is found in various other foods, such as eggs, vegetables, cereals, meat, and milk, and although the disease is more common in rice-eating countries, it has been known to break out in ships, jails, and institutions, wherever the diet has a deficiency in this vitamin. The disease occurs sometimes among topers and old-age pensioners living alone. The cause is the same and is selective starvation of foods containing Vitamin B_1 brought about by poverty, apathy, and ignorance.

Symptoms. Symptoms usually begin to develop after there has been a shortage of Vitamin B_1 for about three months. There are two main types of beri-beri: "dry" and "wet." In the "dry" type there is much weakness and wasting of the leg muscles, loss of feeling in various parts of the skin, and pain in the limbs and joints. Tender swellings may appear in the calf of the leg, and the skin may feel dry. In the "wet" variety, there may be acute dropsy commencing in the legs and spreading upwards to the belly and lungs. The heart is usually affected and becomes very much enlarged, also the veins become too full, and there is enlargement of the liver. The temperature remains normal, but the mind is often affected. There are various degrees of the disease, but it usually gets steadily worse unless the diet is corrected by taking more eggs, milk, vegetables, meat, etc. The "wet" and the "dry" types are closely allied; one may follow the other, or they may both be present. In the later stages of the disease, death may occur from heart failure, but recovery is generally certain if the proper treatment is carried out.

Treatment consists of an ordinary mixed diet with the addition of the substances which contain Vitamin B_1. This can be quickly supplied in the form of yeast, vegetable extract, rice husks, wholewheat bread, and milk. If the disease has become serious the patient must be kept in bed. Bleeding may be carried out to give relief in cases where the veins have become swollen, and massage may be useful for the legs. Heart stimulants do not have much effect since the main treatment lies in correcting the diet. In an urgently ill case, Vitamin B₁ is given in the pure form by injection into a muscle.

BEVERAGES. By the word beverage is meant anything that is used for drinking purposes. Milk and cocoa, are nourishing beverages. Gingerale, lemonade, and so forth are refreshing aromatic beverages. Tea and coffee are the chief stimulating beverages.

BICARBONATE OF SODA. This is a white powder, which is alkaline. It is used in the treatment of acid dyspepsia, for nasal douches, and for soothing irritable skin troubles.

BICEPS. Biceps, which means two-headed, is commonly used to denote the well-known muscle in the upper arm, but is also the name of another muscle in the upper leg. The two muscles are alike in that they each begin in two different places and joint together to form one muscle, thus earning their name. The biceps in the arm is the muscle responsible for bending the forearm on the upper arm and is thus used in weightlifting. It comes into play in rowing, boxing, swimming, etc. The biceps in the leg is a muscle at the back of the thigh.

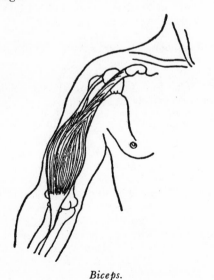

Biceps.

BIDET. A bidet is a small hip-bath used for administering douches and enemas. It may be raised on legs and be fixed in a special chair.

BILE. Bile or gall is the substance which is produced by the liver. It plays an important part in the process of the digestion of food. In appearance bile is a slightly sticky fluid, varying in color from deep golden-yellow to greenish-yellow, according to whether it is collected from the liver itself or from the gall-bladder, and how concentrated it is. It has a very bitter taste and is composed of a mixture of substances known as *mucin* and *cholesterol,* together with certain salts and two coloring matters, one of which is green and the other red. These coloring agents are formed from the dead blood cells which it is part of the work of the liver to break up and get rid of. The liver also extracts certain poisons, or toxins as they are called, from the blood for the purpose of turning them out of the body by way of the stream of bile which carries them to the intestines. It will be seen, therefore, that if the liver is sluggish and the bile not flowing properly, these poisons get taken back into the system and cause the toxic state known as "liverishness" or "biliousness." Calomel and Epsom salts are the two remedies which are specially useful in increasing the flow of bile and relieving this state of sluggishness.

The yellow substance called cholesterol is the chief ingredient of gall-stones when they are present in the gall-bladder. The bile, besides being the means by which the body rids itself of waste materials from the tissues, is also an important factor in the process of digestion. With the aid of the juice from the pancreas, which it meets in the duodenum, it plays a part in the digestion of fats. Its salts also have a strong antiseptic action and help to prevent too-rapid decay of materials in the intestines before they can be eliminated.

The amount of bile produced varies from one to two pints a day. A large part of the bile flows directly from the liver into the tube called the common bile duct and from there into the duodenum. Some trickles slowly into the gall bladder, where it is stored and concentrated. From the gall bladder it enters the common bile duct and flows thence to the duodenum. The duodenum is the passage between the stomach and the intestines. It works by means of a valve at each end, and the entrance of food into the duodenum from the stomach is the signal for the bile to flow out of the common bile duct. Active bodily exercise increases the flow of bile and will often relieve liverishness at once. Alkalis such as bicarbonate of soda in large doses are given in order to make the bile more liquid and enable it to flow more easily. Drugs which increase the flow or manufacture of bile are known as *chola-gogues*. Salicylate of soda and aloes are frequently used for this purpose.

Indirect cholagogues which act by hastening the passage of the bile through the duodenum are calomel, magnesium sulphate, podophyllin, etc. The action of olive oil on the bile is being studied. It undoubtedly has a beneficial action in some cases of gall bladder disease, but it is doubtful whether there is any foundation for the claim made that its action will cause gallstones to melt away. It is more probable that by hastening the flow of the bile it drains the gall bladder, and thus disposes more quickly of the evil results of a too-rich meal or of overindulgence in alcohol.

BILE DUCTS. The fluid produced in the liver is called bile. It is collected in numerous small vessels in the liver, called the bile capillaries, and flows into two large ducts or tubes called the right and left *hepatic ducts.* These two ducts join together to form the *hepatic duct,* and about ¾ in. farther on the hepatic duct is joined by the *cystic duct,* which is the duct leading from the gall bladder. The joint hepatic ducts and cystic duct form the *common bile duct,* and as such carry the bile into the duodenum. They enter this together with the first part of the duct from the pancreas at a point about 4 in. below the lower opening of the stomach.

As these ducts are narrow tubes less than a ¼ in. wide, it will be seen that they can be easily blocked by stones from the gall bladder or by bands and adhesions outside. Obstruction of the common bile duct by a stone or stricture makes it impossible for the liver to excrete the products of the breakdown of red blood cells, and these are retained in the circu-

lation, giving rise to jaundice. (*See also* BILIARY COLIC; GALLSTONES.)

BILHARZIASIS or LIVER-FLUKE DISEASE. Bilharziasis is a disease which is very common in Africa, especially Egypt, the West Indies, South America, China, and Japan. It is caused by the entrance into the body of certain parasites known as fluke-worms. There are three types of these worms which invade man and they seek different parts of the body. One prefers the urinary system, one the large intestine or bowel and sometimes the bladder, while the other is never found anywhere except in the large intestine. They all behave, however, in the same way. Human beings become infected by the young forms of fluke-worm which swim about in water and pierce their way through the skin of people who are bathing, or the infection may be picked up in infected food or drinking water. The young worms pass into the veins of the person they attack and in about six weeks develop into full-grown worms. When they are full-grown they find their way into the liver, hence their common name of liver-flukes, and there they pair and find their way to the bladder and large intestine, where they deposit their eggs. The eggs pass through the bowel and are passed out in the urine and the stools. They hatch and start life as young fluke worms in some other person or animal.

Symptoms. The first stage of the disease begins by a pricking and smarting sensation and redness at the spot where the worm has forced its way into the skin. This sensation usually wears off in a day or two, and nothing more is noticed for about a month or later, when symptoms of infection begin to appear, such as headache, chilliness, pains in the belly, skin rashes; then swellings of the face, trunk, limbs, private parts, etc., occur. The eggs may not be deposited in the urine until anything from two months to two years after the infection has been contracted. At that time blood begins to appear in the urine, and signs of severe bladder and intestinal trouble are observed. In the early stages of the disease the general health does not suffer much, but loss of blood at a later stage brings on a state of anemia and ill health. Persons living in infected areas who have been infected usually become safe from further attacks. If they do not and are being constantly reinfected, their condition will become serious.

Treatment. Bilharziasis is best treated by injections into the veins of antimony tartrate. It can usually be cured by this treatment unless there are very severe complications. (*See also* WORM.)

BILIARY COLIC. Biliary colic is the intense pain caused by the contractions of the bile ducts in their effort to expel a stone or gravel which has entered the duct and is blocking it. The onset of the pain is usually sudden and it is so severe that it is usually termed "excruciating." It is felt usually above and to the right of the navel and sometimes it may shoot up to the right shoulder region. A pain at the point of the right shoulder is often described, but in practice it is generally not so localized. It comes on in sharp paroxysms and the patient rolls about in great pain and doubles up to obtain relief. There may be vomiting and sweating.

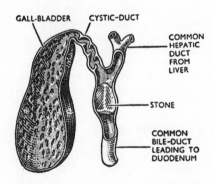

GALL-BLADDER   CYSTIC-DUCT

COMMON HEPATIC DUCT FROM LIVER

STONE

COMMON BILE-DUCT LEADING TO DUODENUM

Biliary Colic.

Treatment. During the attack morphia must be given to ease the pain and if this is not successful it may be necessary to give whiffs of chloroform. In less severe attacks a hot bath and tincture of belladonna or atropine given by mouth may be sufficient. After the pain has been dealt with the condition which caused it must be attended to.

BILIOUSNESS. The word biliousness is popularly applied to states where there is a feeling of nausea or an inclination to sickness, dirty tongue, headache, discomfort in the stomach and constipation. The term "liverish" is also used. In children, an attack of "biliousness" follows very often after eating too much rich food at a party. In adults, too, such symptoms usually follow injudicious eating or drinking. This type of bilious attack is really acute gastritis or upset of the stomach and is easily dealt with by a couple of days on starvation diet and some simple alkaline medicine such as magnesia. Should the condition continue, however, or return from time to time, especially in middle-aged or older people, a thorough examination by the family doctor or at a hospital should be arranged for, as it may be the beginning of more serious trouble.

BINET-SIMON TEST FOR INTELLIGENCE. This is a test used to gain an idea of the level of intelligence of a person. It is necessary sometimes to use some test of intelligence in the case of backward children in order to find out whether they are only backward or are really incapable of being taught at a general school among normal children. (*See also* INTELLIGENCE, TESTS for.)

BINOCULAR. This means the ability to use both eyes at once. Each eye has its own power of vision, which is obvious if one closes one eye at a time and looks at an object. The object will be seen by each eye separately, and the slight differences of impression received enable us to see things in perspective and to estimate distance. (*See also* EYE; VISION.)

BIOCHEMISTRY. Biochemistry is the name for the science dealing with the chemistry of the body. It is physiological chemistry, or the chemistry of living tissues and organs, and is a science in which a great deal of research work is now being done. Discoveries such as insulin come into the sphere of the biochemist.

BIOLOGY. This term is applied to the science of life and living things. The structure and function of all living things, plants and animals, are the concern of this science.

BIRTH. The birth of a child normally takes place nine months after the date at which the mother had her last menstrual period or "courses." If the child arrives after only seven months it is said to be *premature*. It may still live and in time become strong, but will require very careful attention in its early years. Birth earlier than six and a half months but later than three months, is called a *miscarriage*. Before three months it is an *abortion*. A *stillborn* child is one that is born dead. (*See also* CHILDBIRTH; LABOR; PREGNANCY.)

BIRTH CONTROL. Simple methods of birth control have been employed since early in the history of the human race, and nowadays there is much interest in the possibility of a contraceptive "pill," especially with the problem of overpopulation by the teeming millions in the less-developed countries of the world. There is no doubt that such a pill, consisting of the combination of a gestagen and an estrogen, can effectively prevent conception, and that taking it does not affect subsequent fertility. But it is not yet certain whether or not they also have harmful effects, and they should be taken only under the supervision of a doctor, a nurse, or a trained social worker. Gastrointestinal effects and "break-through" bleeding account for 25 per cent of women abandoning this method of contraception. The usual methods of birth control employed are still the condom or sheath, usually used along with a spermicidal jelly cream, suppository or foaming tablet; and the diaphragm, also used in combination with a spermicidal preparation. But there is still a good deal to be said for the "safe-period" and for "coitus interruptus" as old-fashioned but well-proven methods. (*See also* FAMILY PLANNING; SEX HYGIENE.)

BIRTHMARKS. Birthmarks or naevi (which is the plural of the word naevus, meaning present at birth) are inborn blemishes on the skin. They are of many different sorts, and the term should, strictly speaking, include moles and warts as well.

A birthmark is really a tumor of the very tiny blood vessels of the skin. In one area on the skin these tiny blood vessels, or capillaries as they are called, are swollen and overgrown, and there may be here and there among them a dilated larger vein or artery. It is a very common superstition that if a woman is frightened by some such small animal as a mouse or beetle while she is carrying a child, the child may have a birthmark the shape of the animal in some prominent place. There is no foundation for this theory at all.

The two most usual sorts of birthmarks are the "spider" and the "portwine stain." In the case of the spider, or arachnoid naevus, the dilated blood vessels spread out from a center with a spider's-web appearance. These birthmarks may be very small or may grow to a large size. The portwine stain is the birthmark most commonly found on the face. It is called portwine stain from its dark purple color, and it is unfortunately very disfiguring. In some cases the whole of one cheek may be covered, or the stain may be no larger than the size of a small coin. Often moles are present as well, and there may be a heavy growth of hair to add to the disfigurement.

Many birthmarks shrink or disappear without treatment before the age of three, and except in rare cases it is unnecessary to intervene before this age.

Treatment. In the treatment of all varieties, the chief aim is to remove the birthmark with as little scarring as possible. Of course, if the birthmarks are on the covered parts of the body, where the presence of a scar does not matter, by far the most useful method of treating such cases is that of removal by surgery. A single operation is sufficient, and the cure is speedy and certain. Skin may be brought from another part of the body and be grafted on if this is found to be necessary.

Spider naevi are treated by applying an electric needle to the central point, or by using a cauterizing needle. Small birthmarks are effectively treated by freezing with carbon dioxide snow.

The very extensive portwine stains are so difficult to treat satisfactorily that many authorities advise leaving them alone entirely. The blood vessels of this type are, unlike the other varieties, embedded in firm, solid tissue, and cannot be destroyed without running the risk of damaging the surrounding tissues as well. X-rays may sometimes cure such naevi, and a paint containing the radioactive substance thorium X has recently been used to good effect, but both these methods need to be used with great care.

BISMUTH. Bismuth and its preparations are included in the class of heavy metals used in medicine. Used externally, salts of bismuth may be dusted on sores and wounds as a protective and mild drying agent, but the antiseptic action is very slight. A bismuth, iodoform, and paraffin preparation popularly known as B.I.P.P. or "Bipp," invented by Professor Rutherford Morrison of Newcastle, was used with excellent results during the first World War in the treatment of wounds, and is still used, chiefly in infections of bone. One form of bismuth may be used for X-ray diagnosis of conditions of the throat and stomach, but latterly barium meals have been used instead of bismuth meals for this purpose.

In the treatment of peptic ulcers, either gastric or duodenal, bismuth oxycarbonate, a weak alkali, is effective in relieving pain. In cases of diarrhea, large doses can be given without any ill effects. In cases of dyspepsia, nausea, vomiting, or diarrhea, the following prescription will help to relieve discomfort:

Bismuth carbonate	—	30 grains
Magnesium carbonate	—	20 ,,
Sodium bicarbonate	—	30 ,,

The powder should be taken in a little milk about twenty minutes before meals whenever an attack of dyspepsia is threatened. Injections of bismuth salicylate into the muscular tissues still have their place in the treatment of syphilis.

Poisoning by bismuth may occur as a result of overdosage; but, as a rule, any symptoms of stomach or intestinal irritation caused by bismuth are due to the arsenic with which bismuth salts, especially the subnitrate, may be contaminated. Poisoning symptoms include swelling of the gums and soft palate, with a characteristic black line along the gums at the roots of the teeth. All bismuth dressings should be removed from the patient as soon as signs of poisoning appear, and no bismuth should be given internally. Owing to chemical changes which take place, bismuth is black when it leaves the bowel, and for this reason the stools of a patient who has been taking bismuth may have a grey-black appearance, but this fact need cause no alarm.

BITES AND STINGS. Insect Bites. It is sometimes difficult to distinguish between a rash and a crop of insect bites, especially when the offending insect cannot be found. An insect bite has always a small red puncture in the middle of each spot where the sting of the insect broke through the skin, and the spots due to a rash have no such central point.

The insects which most often bite human beings are fleas, bedbugs, lice mosquitoes, harvest-bugs, sandflies (also called jiggers), and wood ticks. Ticks generally remain under the skin at the point where they made the wound; so do sandflies.

Treatment. Insect bites are always very itchy, and dilute ammonia water, or a strong solution of bicarbonate of soda or baking powder, dabbed on to the bites at intervals or bound over them on a pad of cotton-wool, will ease the irritation. These are easily obtained domestic remedies, but they are often as useful as the more expensive preparations sold for the purpose. If the skin is very much irritated, however, simple calamine lotion may be spread on and allowed to dry on the skin.

Sandflies and ticks must be killed before they are removed. Kerosene, turpentine, or tobacco juice will all kill the insects if the wound is bathed in them. The dead insects must then be picked out with a blunt needle which has been put into a flame for a moment to sterilize it, and afterwards calamine lotion may be put on.

Some substances evolved during the second World War, when applied thinly to the skin, were found to repel insects for up to six hours and were instrumental in protecting troops from typhus and other insect-borne diseases. Of these insect repellants, dimethyl phthallate and dibutyl phthallate were found to be the best.

Dog Bites, etc. Mad dogs, fortunately, are rare nowadays, so that unless there is any evidence to the contrary, a dog bite should be treated as an ordinary torn wound. That is to say, wash the wound thoroughly, pour in some iodine or methylated spirits, and apply a dressing of clean lint. However, all dogbite cases should be given rabies vaccine unless the dog is found, impounded and found free of rabies. The bites of other large animals should be treated in the same way as those of dogs. A cat more often scratches than bites, but cat bites are not unknown. A pig can give a very nasty bite, and any other animal is liable to snap at a human being, especially if it is alarmed, or if it is accompanied by its young.

But if there is any reason for suspecting that the dog was mad, there is a danger of hydrophobia and prompt treatment in the form of rabies vaccine is of the utmost importance. The poison in this case comes from the dog's saliva and passes rapidly from the wound into the system of the bitten person.

Treatment. Emergency treatment must be given with the object of removing as much as possible of the poison from the wound, and of stopping it from getting into the bloodstream. (*See* HYDROPHOBIA.)

Poisonous Snake Bites. The poison in all these cases acts quickly, so immediately suck the bite hard, spitting out at once and being careful not to swallow any of the matter sucked out. Apply a tight bandage above the wound and try to make the wound bleed freely, opening it with a knife if necessary. Hold it under a tap if there happens to be one handy. If any crystals of potassium permanganate are available, rub a few well into the wound; otherwise use iodine or methylated spirits freely. Get the bitten person to the doctor as soon as possible.

Wasp and Bee Stings. Wasp and bee stings are extremely painful and happen to everybody some time during their life. A bee which has once stung becomes harmless because it leaves its sting in the wound and cannot sting again; but a wasp keeps its sting and may return to the attack again and again. If the sting has been caused by a bee, therefore, the first thing to do is to find the sting and gently pull it out. Dab on dilute ammonia, methylated spirits, iodine, or any specially prepared remedy for insect bites. If a person gets stung by a bee, wasp, or mosquito about the mouth or throat or on the upper lip, he must be taken at once to a doctor or hospital, as stings on these parts swell rapidly and occasionally prove fatal.

BITTER ALMOND POISONING. *See* ALMOND; PRUSSIC ACID.

BITTERS. In medical language the group of "bitters" contains substances which possess the common property of a bitter taste. These bitter drugs are usually given to whet the appetite and thus aid digestion. In popular language, the word bitters usually means alcoholic beverages which contain bitter or aromatic substances.

A few of the bitters used in medicine include calumba, gentian, quassia, cascarilla, serpentary, and orange peel. These all act very similarly. Calumba and quassia are known as simple bitters. Another group of bitters contains an oil in addition to the bitter substance; orange peel is the most popular of this group. Powerful drugs such as quinine and strychnine, although they do not come under the "bitters" group, may be used in medicine only for their bitter taste.

BLACK DEATH. This awesome term used to be applied to the plague which at one time was the scourge of Europe. In 1664–65 the greatest epidemic occurred in London. Modern methods of sanitation and public health have now checked epidemics, and although isolated cases may occur, prompt measures are taken to prevent the spread of the disease. (*See also* EPIDEMIC.)

BLACK EYE. A black eye is generally the result of an injury in the neighborhood of the eye. The condition is too well known to need description. Owing to the fact that the skin of the eyelids and that about the eyes is very loose, blood gathers readily in these parts, so that the bruise may often look as if the blow had been much more violent than it was. A curious effect is sometimes seen when some of the blood flows under the conjunctiva (the thin membrane covering the eye); this may remain bright red, while the blood in the eyelids is nearly black.

After operations on the nose and the hollow cavities round the nose, there are very often black eyes caused by blood which has come from the point of the operation. This disappears in a few days of its own accord.

When a black eye follows an injury to the head which has not directly involved

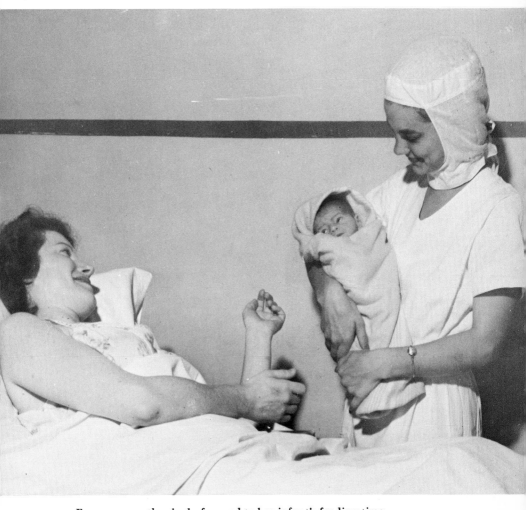

Every new mother looks forward to her infant's feeding time.
*(Children's Bureau, U.S. Department of Public Health,
Education and Welfare)*

Frequent eye examinations can help retain our most valuable sense through an entire lifetime.

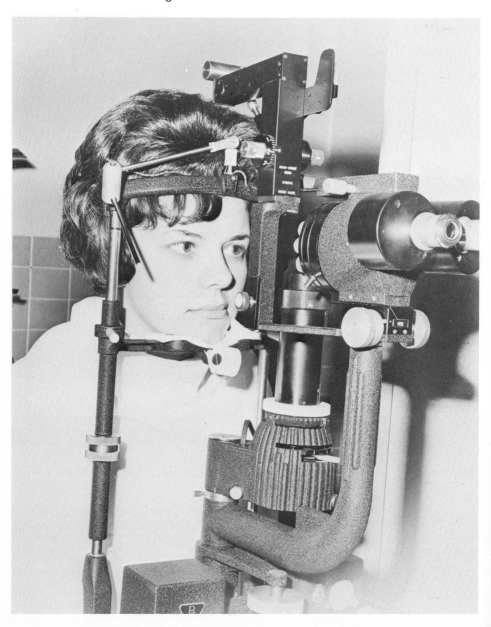

the eye, it usually means that the skull is fractured.

Treatment. If the black eye is seen immediately after the blow has been struck, cold, wet cloths should be applied to the eye, or pads of cotton-wool wet with lead lotion. Later on, when the black eye has become quite evident, hot compresses may be used, as well as gentle pressure and massage with pure olive oil. If the eye continues to be painful, however, this should be discontinued and a doctor should be consulted, as there may be some other injury to the eye itself.

The discoloration may be concealed during the day by means of a flesh-colored (water color) paint, which is quite harmless to the skin, or by a little theatrical greasepaint.

BLACKHEAD. A blackhead is a dark plug about the size of a pinhead, which appears in the sweat glands in the skin. They are found usually on the face, back of the neck, chest, and back, and are a symptom of acne. They are found, as a rule, in young people. (*See also* ACNE.)

BLACK MOVEMENTS. Dark-colored, almost black movements are passed sometimes when there is severe constipation and the stools have been delayed for several days in the bowel. Iron and bismuth taken as medicines make the stools black. The most usual cause, however, in cases where these drugs are not being taken, is the presence of blood in the stool, due to ulceration of the stomach or bowel. This condition is serious and is known as *melena*. (*See also* MELENA.)

BLACK VOMIT. Black or dark-colored vomit is usually due to the presence of blood in the stomach. It is vomited up as a dark sediment, usually described as resembling coffee grounds. (*See also* GASTRIC ULCER.)

BLACKWATER FEVER. This disease is a complication of malaria. Its chief symptom is *hemoglobinuria* or the presence of hemoglobin—the coloring matter of the red blood cells—in the urine. The disease is especially prevalent in Africa, certain parts of Spain, Italy, Greece, Russia, the Near East and Palestine; it is also found in some parts of the United States, South America, the West Indies, and in Asia, India, and the Far East.

The patient has usually lived in a malarial country for over six months, and, as a rule, there is a history of repeated attacks of malaria which have not been properly treated. It usually comes on very suddenly and may be started by a chill or a dose of quinine, although quinine is not its actual cause.

Symptoms. These vary greatly in order and severity. Usually there is a feeling of tiredness for a day or two, with loss of appetite and chilliness. This is followed with dramatic suddenness by severe shivering fits or rigors. There may be severe pains in the back and limbs, with dizziness, weakness, nausea, and the vomiting of bilestained fluid. The urine is then noticed to be red and there may be a desire to pass water frequently. The skin becomes hot, itchy, and dry and may develop a deep yellow tinge, and the spleen and liver generally become enlarged and tender. As the disease progresses the patient may become drowsy and irritable, and delirium and unconsciousness may set in. Hiccough is a symptom in very severe cases. The patient at this stage may recover; the temperature, which often rises as high as 103 deg. F., may drop after three or four days to normal and remain there. On the other hand, the temperature may remain high and death may follow, owing to suppression of urine, and other complications.

Treatment. Blackwater fever is a disease which should never be treated lightly. There are many mild cases which recover, but the outlook in severe cases is very grave. In order to ward off this disease in districts where blackwater fever is frequent, every attack of malaria should be actively treated, not with quinine, but with the newer Atabrine.

As soon as symptoms of the disease appear, the patient should be put to bed and kept lying down. He should be given fluids containing glucose, and an alkaline mixture to render and keep the urine alkaline. Cortisone or prednisone is sometimes useful Blood transfusion may be necessary, and prove helpful.

Quinine may aggravate the disease and must therefore be given very cautiously and only under medical supervision.

Convalescence is generally lengthy and

slow, and complications are frequent. After recovery it is best for the patient to leave a malarial country, as dangerous relapses are to be feared. (*See also* MALARIA.)

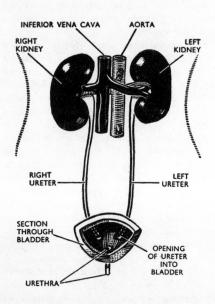

INFERIOR VENA CAVA   AORTA

RIGHT KIDNEY   LEFT KIDNEY

RIGHT URETER   LEFT URETER

SECTION THROUGH BLADDER

OPENING OF URETER INTO BLADDER

URETHRA

Bladder.

BLADDER. The bladder is a reservoir for the waste fluid of the body. It stores up the water and salts passed on by the kidneys until it is convenient to pass them out of the body in the urine. Each kidney is connected with the bladder by a long narrow tube of muscular tissue known as a *ureter,* and the bladder is connected with the exterior by a passage called the *urethra.*

The shape of the bladder varies a great deal according to whether there is little or much fluid inside. It is situated in the front portion of the bony girdle known as the true pelvis, where it is kept in place by means of rather lax ligaments so that when empty it is so contracted that there is practically no cavity, whereas when filled it expands until it holds from 8–12 oz. of urine. In abnormal conditions it will hold well over 40 oz.

When the urine has collected in the bladder sufficiently to raise the pressure above a certain point, slow rhythmical contractions take place in the muscle walls. These get stronger and stronger until they become powerful enough to overcome the circular muscle fibers which guard the exit of the bladder into the urethra. The urine is then expelled. This action is known as a "reflex" action, and occurs in the lower animals and in man until it comes under the control of the will, which has the power of regulating the reflex mechanism.

The bladder is lined on the inside by mucous membrane which is loosely attached to the muscular coat so that it is thrown into folds when the cavity is small, and smoothed out when it is distended.

Examination of the Bladder. A catheter is a hollow tube which is passed along the urethra passage into the bladder to withdraw the urine in cases where the muscle of the bladder is unable to contract sufficiently strongly to force urine out, or where there is some obstruction in the passage itself. Blocking of the passage may be due to the presence of a stone in it, or to enlargement of a gland (prostate) which surrounds the neck of the bladder in the male.

Cystoscope. This is a hollow tube with a beak at an angle which carries a small electric lamp at its end. One end has a valve which prevents the escape of fluid from the bladder until required. A telescope fits the interior of the tube and is slipped in after the bladder is washed and distended. The openings of the ureters and the entire lining of the bladder can be inspected.

Diseases of the Bladder. The commonest disease of the bladder is *cystitis* or inflammation of the bladder. This is discussed under its own heading. The two commonest disabilities of the bladder may be due to disease of the bladder itself or to disease in some other part such as the nervous system which affects the working of the bladder. They are incontinence of urine and retention of urine. Besides these the bladder is subject to rupture due to accidental crushing, foreign bodies inserted into it, tumors, stone or calculus, and such conditions as fistula and diverticulum. These conditions are discussed below.

Incontinence of Urine. Incontinence of urine is present when a person is unable to hold back the contents of the bladder until he wishes to evacuate them. The urine may escape in a sudden rush without his having the power to stop it, or it may continually dribble away. In both these cases incontinence is present. In the case where a full flow of urine is suddenly passed without the will of the individual, the condition is more likely to be due to trouble in the nervous system than to actual disease in the bladder. This condition is known as *emuresis* and is very well known in its most common form as "bed-wetting" amongst children.

The dribbling away of urine is known as *true incontinence* if the dribbling is from a bladder which is not distended, to distinguish it from *false incontinence* in which the bladder remains full owing to some obstruction such as that due to an enlarged prostate gland pressing on it, and the dribbling is only the overflow which is under such strong pressure that it is able to push its way past the obstruction.

Incontinence due to mechanical causes. Incontinence due to mechanical causes such as outside pressure on the bladder is more frequent in women than in men. In the later stages of pregnancy the pressure of the enlarged womb almost always causes a certain amount of dribbling, and some women have the same experience in the last few days of each month just before the period begins; here, again, the swollen womb is the cause. The condition called prolapse which sometimes occurs in women who have had children is also a cause of incontinence. In these cases the incontinence is usually slight and may follow on some sudden exertion. In men this form of incontinence is usually found in connection with an enlarged prostate gland, and is in fact the most obvious symptom of that condition. Even after the enlarged gland has been removed there is often a degree of incontinence for some time, but it will subside.

Incontinence due to nervous disease. The involuntary passage of urine may occur in some diseases of the spinal cord. In the early stages of the disease known as tabes dorsalis there is often a false incontinence, that is, a chronic distension of the bladder with overflow. It may be first noticed by bed-wetting at night. In the disease called disseminated sclerosis there is usually imperfect control of the bladder due to its contracted condition.

Incontinence due to nerve injuries. Injuries to the back in which the spinal cord is damaged, such as fractures, dislocations, crushing accidents, or gunshot injuries are usually followed by a period during which the urine is retained in the bladder and only escapes by overflowing. This may last for as long as two months, and may be followed by ordinary incontinence in which the bladder works as it does in a child before the age of voluntary control and it will have to be re-educated until full control returns.

Incontinence in childhood. Before the child is two years old he should have good mental control over the voiding of urine, except for an occasional lapse due to unusual excitement or some such reason. If not, he is described as having "functional enuresis," and this problem is dealt with in the section on bed-wetting.

Retention of Urine. By retention of urine is meant that a person is unable for some reason to pass urine in spite of a full bladder. There are many causes of this inability to void water. It may be due to obstruction, such as the increase in size of the prostate gland, or swelling in the region of the bladder due to inflammation, or to some sort of tumor or growth. Any of these will cause obstruction to the flow of urine by pressing on the passage by which the urine escapes from the bladder. Again, there may be an obstruction in the passage or urethra itself, such as a foreign body or a stone. The passage may be ruptured or narrowed by previous disease (stricture) or swollen by acute inflammation. Retention of the urine may be due to lack of tone in the muscle walls, a condition which is generally due to nervous disease, but in this case there will be other symptoms to show what the disease is.

There may be also an inability to pass urine due to spasm of the muscle guarding the exit from the bladder. Here the muscle which is in spasm is holding itself tightly contracted instead of opening and closing as it normally does. This may happen after an operation round the entrance to the bowel or in the region of the bladder itself.

Diverticula. These are pouches in the wall of the bladder. They are usually only discovered after examination by the cysto-

scope, already described. (*See also* DIVERTI-
CULITIS.)

Rupture of the Bladder. This is usually
met with in adult males. A *full* bladder is
easily ruptured by any form of violence
applied to the lower part of the belly,
such as a blow, kick, a crush by the wheel
of a vehicle, or a fall on a projecting
object. In fractures of the pelvis the bladder is often torn or penetrated.

Cystitis. This is inflammation of the
lining membrane of the bladder, and is
due to germs or to the action of irritating
solutions. It is known that germs can pass
through a healthy bladder without producing any changes in the walls, unless some
other factor is also present. The most common of these other factors are pregnancy,
stricture, foreign bodies, growths, operations on the bladder, and loss of tone in
the muscular walls due to nervous disease.
It is very often due to the bacillus coli,
a germ which grows normally in the large
bowel. The subject of cystitis is fully discussed under that heading.

Tumors of the Bladder. These usually
occur between the ages of forty and sixty.
Like all tumors, they are divided into two
main classes: simple or innocent tumors
and malignant or life-destroying growths.
Of tumors the most common is the *papilloma,* which is an innocent wart-like growth
of the lining membrane of the bladder. It
is quite painless and gives rise to blood-
staining of the urine. It is cured by burning with an electric needle through a
cystoscope.

Stone or Calculus. Most of the stones
found in the bladder started in the kidney
and increased in size after entering the
bladder. Some stones, however, start in the
bladder as a collection of phosphates resulting from alkaline decomposition of the
urine. A stone will also form round a
foreign body, such as the end of a broken
catheter. The same varieties of stone are
met with in the bladder as in the kidney;
those composed of uric acid, urates, or
oxalate of lime all form in the presence of
acid urine. Stones in the bladder are
usually freely movable, but may be fixed
in the opening of the passages leading from
the kidneys to the bladder or from the
bladder to the external world, or in
"diverticula" in the bladder wall.

Fistula. A fistula is a communicating
passage between the interior of the bladder
and some other organ. It is the result of
injury or disease. Fistulae in the bladder
are of three sorts. First, there is the fistula
which occurs after an operation for removal of the prostate and which may be
made intentionally when the passage
through the urethra is permanently obstructed and cannot be opened up again.
This fistula allows the urine to escape
through the skin of the abdominal wall to
the outside. Secondly, there may be a
fistula between the bladder and some part
of the intestines. This is usually due to
injury or to inflammation which has led
to the rupture of the wall of the bladder.
There may be a fistula communicating
between the bladder and the vagina in
women. This may follow an operation or
be due to a growth. (*See also* URETHRA.)

BLANCMANGE. This is a particularly
appetizing and nourishing form of food for
invalids. Peptonized milk may be added
instead of ordinary milk in cases where the
digestive organs are not working well.

BLAND. This term is generally applied
to foods of a mild and soothing nature,
such as milk and arrowroot, etc. Invalids
are usually given bland substances while
they are ill or recovering from a severe
illness.

BLAUD'S PILLS. These pills are a
very useful and popular way of taking iron
in anemic conditions. They leave no bitter
taste in the mouth, can be bought anywhere and are easy to swallow. The active
constituent of Blaud's pill is iron carbonate and it has been calculated that 45
grains daily are needed to cure iron-
deficiency anemia. This compares badly
with ferrous sulphate, which is effective in
a daily dose of 9 grains.

BLEACHING POWDER. *See* CHLORIDE
OF LIME.

BLEB. A bleb is a small blister or swelling. (*See* BLISTER.)

BLEEDERS. There are certain unfortunate families where the male members
have a peculiar state of the blood which
causes them to bleed excessively from the
smallest scratch or wound. In popular
language these people are called "bleeders," and in medical terms, *hemophilics.* It
has been generally considered that only the

men in hemophilic families were "bleeders," but it seems likely that the women may in some cases bleed more easily than is usual, without their bleeding being definitely uncontrollable as it is in the case of the men. A member of a hemophilic family should not marry and beget children without first seeking the advice of a doctor. The transmission of this disorder from generation to generation is governed by Mendelian laws and is said to be sex-linked. That is to say, an affected man will have healthy sons who will not transmit the disease. His daughters will be unaffected but will "carry" the defect which will be inherited by half her children. Half her daughters will "carry" the disease like herself, and half her sons will be "bleeders." (*See also* MENDEL'S LAW.)

Notable examples of families where there are "bleeders" are certain royal families of Europe who are no longer on their thrones. It was a matter of common knowledge that the little Tsarevitch, the heir to the Russian throne, who was killed in 1916, was afflicted in this way and would almost certainly not have grown to manhood. In another case it seemed likely that the heir to the throne would be passed over for the succession because of this unfortunate failing.

Treatment. It goes without saying that "bleeders" should be protected in every way possible from anything that might cause bleeding, since once bleeding starts it may be found impossible to stop it. No teeth should ever be extracted, and of course no surgical operation should be allowed except after special preparation by transfusion of normal blood. It sometimes happens that the condition is not very well understood, and the relations will allow a boy to have a tooth pulled out, or some little operation like circumcision or the removal of tonsils to be performed, without telling the doctor that the child comes from a bleeding family, and the truth is only discovered when it is too late to save the child.

Once the bleeding has started, the usual methods for stopping it must be tried, e.g., pressure by tight bandages. The application of adrenalin solution $\left(\frac{1}{1000}\right)$ on cotton-wool may arrest the bleeding. The patient should be taken to a doctor or hospital at once, as a transfusion of blood from a healthy person may have to be given together with injections of calcium into the veins.

If a "bleeder" is not lost in childhood and reaches the early twenties, the condition will usually improve, and it is likely that before long science will be able to discover something to cure, or at least assist, this unfortunate group of people along the lines of other diseases, in which there is something missing from the blood. (*See also* HEMORRHAGE.)

BLEEDING. All forms of bleeding are described under the heading HEMORRHAGE, and the first-aid treatment of bleeding in the SUPPLEMENT ON FIRST AID.

BLEEDING or BLOOD LETTING. Bleeding a patient is a procedure which is not often resorted to nowadays in the treatment of disease. It is done in certain cases of heart and lung disease when there is more blood in the veins than can conveniently be circulated, and it is done in healthy subjects to obtain blood for transfusion. In order to carry out this operation, the surgeon would tie a piece of rubber tubing around the patient's arm, about two inches above the elbow, thus preventing the return of venous blood to the heart and causing the veins in the arm to swell up and become prominent. A needle is pushed through into the vein and the blood allowed to run into a special bottle containing citrate to prevent clotting.

The application of leeches in order to draw off blood is a method which has fallen into disuse.

BLEPHARITIS. This is a disease characterized by inflammation of the edge of the eyelids as shown by redness, crusting, swelling, and falling out of eyelashes. A persistent blepharitis is fairly common in children. The treatment consists partly in applying suitable paints and ointments, partly in attention to diet and environment, which are often faulty, and to any other cause of ill health. Crusts on the eyelids must always be gently but completely removed by thorough wiping with cotton-wool swabs. Bicarbonate of soda, a teaspoonful to a pint, makes a good lotion for this purpose.

BLINDNESS. By blindness is meant a complete, or nearly complete, loss of the power of seeing. It is one of the worst afflictions from which a human being can suffer. The saddest part of blindness, however, is that the majority of cases could have been prevented if care had been taken at the proper time. The causes of blindness are numerous, beginning with being born blind, and going on to all the various diseases of the eye itself, either local or occurring as a complication of some general disease, and finally the cases that are due to accident or injury. (*See also* EYE; VISION.)

Born Blind. The first cause, that of being born blind, owing to complete absence of the eyes, or to some developmental defect of the eyes, is fortunately very rare, as it is naturally incurable. But it is frequently said that many children are born blind. This is quite a mistaken idea, and the sooner it is discredited the better, for a great number of babies who are condemned to lifelong blindness are blind only because of ignorance or carelessness on the part of their mother or attendant. The cause is a disease known as *ophthalmia neonatorum* which is due to the child's eyes becoming infected at birth by a discharge from the passages of the mother due to the disease called gonorrhea. "It has been calculated that this disease accounted for one-third to one-half of all the persons in blind asylums, so destructive of sight it is: but now that it is more vigorously dealt with and is notifiable by doctors and midwives its incidence has been kept down." This was written in 1930. In a general report written recently it is said that "Ophthalmia neonatorum remains the most frequent and the most distressing cause of blindness, seeing that these cases must be regarded as *almost entirely preventable.*"

Diseases of the Eye. The various eye-diseases are discussed under their own headings. In injuries to the eye, the treatment naturally depends on the extent of the injury. Briefly, the other chief causes of blindness are *trachoma, glaucoma,* and *conjunctivitis. Syphilis,* both inherited and acquired, is a very important cause.

During the last fifty years, the proportion of blind people has been slowly but steadily declining. This is due to various causes: improvement in hygiene, both at home and at work, better education, leading those suffering from eye trouble to seek skilled assistance early, and the great decrease of such diseases as smallpox, which, before the days of vaccination, accounted for so many cases of blindness, and still do in some countries. Still, there is room for a good deal of improvement. Blindness from infections should not occur; smallpox is preventable (except in a very few individuals); gonorrhea and syphilis, if treated early and thoroughly, will not affect the eyes. Trachoma, glaucoma, and conjunctivitis cause blindness which in a great number of cases might be prevented by early treatment.

Education of the Blind. No matter at what age blindness comes on, special education should be begun as early as possible. Too many people are mistakenly "kind" in trying to shield a blind person, especially a child, not only from the risk of accidents, but from all contact with the world. Even quite a small child should be encouraged to help himself in every way, by washing, dressing, and feeding himself, by examining everything with his hands, and by taking regular outdoor exercise, to grow accustomed to his limited existence as early as possible. Many children not only feel safe in their own home, or when taking guided walks, but learn to run and to swim or skate quite readily.

If blindness comes on in later childhood, the child, in a good many cases, is happier at a special school, where he is educated by specially trained teachers, and has, too, the companionship of other blind pupils. An adult who becomes blind, or who is likely to do so from disease, should be encouraged to re-educate himself as soon as possible.

It is not uncommon to find blind children developing bad habits, chiefly the making of extraordinary movements and grimaces. Parents should check this tendency kindly but firmly, as such habits are most difficult to eradicate if once formed, and are highly objectionable both to the family and to outsiders.

The ordinary education of the blind was first started by Valentin Häuy, in 1784, in Paris. At the present time, schools for the blind have been established in most U.S. cities, and societies have been started for teaching the blind at home. Various methods have been tried, but the Braille system of raised-up letters for reading is considered the best. It is very simple to learn to read by this method: writing is also easily learned, so that a blind man can not only read, but can take notes and keep accounts. Books can be printed in small bulk, and at a comparatively low cost. The system is well adapted for musical purposes, and even a Braille typewriter has been invented.

A very large number of trades have been learned and carried on successfully by blind people. There are, of course, outstanding examples of blind people who have done brilliantly in music, or at the university, or have done splendid social work, especially to benefit others similarly afflicted, but these are comparatively rare. Lack of means stands in the way of many blind people receiving more than a training for such work as the coarser kind of handwork—basket-weaving, netting, rug-making and so on. Many blind people, however, develop an extraordinarily fine sense of touch which helps them in many ways. They are also able to do such things as fine knitting and weaving, and to make artificial flowers. Music offers very good prospects for piano-tuners, teachers, organists; and many blind people earn a good living as masseurs.

Tobacco Blindness. Tobacco blindness is found chiefly among working men, and is caused either by smoking or chewing tobacco in a quantity of not less than three ounces a week. Other factors that seem to influence the ease with which tobacco affects the sight are age, sleeplessness, prolonged anxiety, and the abuse of alcohol. Some people also seem to be more easily upset by tobacco than others; that is, they are more susceptible to the effects of tobacco.

This disease very rarely deteriorates into complete blindness. It occurs always in both eyes. The patient complains that objects are imperfectly seen; they are "misty;" and that he "can see better in the dark." These symptoms are due to the fact that light-, color-, and form-sense are all diminished.

Treatment. The treatment is obvious— the use of tobacco in any form must be

stopped. It will be a month or more before any improvement takes place, but after that improvement is rapid, except in very long-standing cases, which may not entirely recover.

Hysterical Blindness. Where blindness comes on suddenly for no apparent reason in a person who has shown other signs of being of a hysterical nature, it may be found that the blindness too is hysterical. Hysteria of any sort is always a delicate and difficult subject. In the hysterical person blindness may be due to varying causes, mostly associated with nervous shock of some sort. It may be genuinely impossible for the person to see, although there is no real damage to the eye, or, on the other hand, the blindness may be "put on," since in hysteria deceptions are practiced which would not be the case if the patient were in perfect health. It is sometimes almost impossible for even the most skilled observer to distinguish between "genuine" hysterical blindness and "pretended" blindness.

Hysterical blindness occurs most commonly in women, in one or both eyes, and the symptoms may be of varying severity and character. The diagnosis of hysterial blindness is usually quite easy, because if the person is watched she is found to be doing things that would be impossible to a blind person.

The treatment is the same as that for other forms of hysteria.

Blinding from Lightning or Bright Lights. The ill effects of ultraviolet light are seen in arc-welders and electricians who have to adjust strong arclights. If they incautiously expose the eyes, the first result is "dazzling" of objects looked at, and a dimness of sight, in which everything looks yellowish in color. In about 6–9 hours the eyes begin to smart intensely; they feel as if "grit" were in them, and water profusely; the eyelids swell up and become very red, as also does the fine membrane covering the eyeball, called the conjunctiva. The iris is reddened and perhaps inflamed, and this damages the lens of the eye.

The treatment is to apply cold to the eye as soon as the first symptoms come on; this is best done by compresses of ice. When the pain begins, drops of cocaine and atropine are used; the cocaine deadens the pain, and the atropine helps to prevent inflammation in the iris. These cases always recover.

The effects of lightning on the eyes are very numerous. Small burns may be caused on the eyelids and the cornea (the transparent membrane in front of the eye). The most frequent and therefore the most important effect is opacity of the cornea and the lens, the latter forming a cataract. Both eyes are usually affected, and the cataract may be complete or incomplete; in the latter case, in a few instances, improvement may take place.

The treatment, if any is considered advisable, is the same as in the ordinary forms of cataract. This is followed by satisfactory healing in itself, but in a good many cases sight remains very poor, owing to damage in other parts of the eye—such as the optic nerve. (*See also* AMBLYOPIA; CATARACT; DEFECTIVE VISION; EYE; VISION.)

BLISTERING. Blistering is sometimes carried out as a remedy in the treatment of cases such as lumbago, rheumatism, neuritis and other painful conditions. Irritating substances such as mustard and cantharides are applied to the skin and raise a blister. This practice, however, is not recommended.

BLISTERS. A blister is a collection of fluid derived from the blood which forms beneath the surface layers of the skin. Blisters may be caused by burns and scalds, from friction, from some kinds of infection, and they sometimes occur spontaneously, generally on the legs, without any apparent cause.

Most blisters result from carelessness or negligence: the wrinkled or undarned heel of a sock will cause them through constant rubbing. Cigarettes are often the cause of blisters between the fingers, or they may be the result of picking up a very hot article or upsetting a saucepan of boiling water.

Most of the blisters encountered are the result of hurry or carelessness, and can therefore be prevented, but after a blister-provoking injury has occurred nothing can be done to prevent a blister forming or make a formed blister subside. The skin over a blister is dead and must sooner or later peel off. No general rule can be given as to puncturing or opening blisters to let the fluid escape. Site, size, cause and duration must all be considered, but large blisters are usually best opened.

Blisters on the Feet. Some people's feet are inclined to blister easily, but certain precautions can be taken to reduce the likelihood of them forming. Such people should see that their shoes are a good fit, with soft uppers and soles that are not too hard. Hard leather may be softened by soaking it in castor oil. Thick socks are always necessary when heavy boots or shoes are to be worn. These socks should be a good easy fit, and it is important to see that they have no seam in the sole of the foot if they are to be worn for long walks. Knots and lumps in the wool should be teased out before wearing, and of course large darns will almost certainly cause the delicate foot to blister if they are in a part of the sock that will be pressed on by the shoe. To keep the feet fit, bathe them night and morning, dry very carefully—especially between the toes—and powder with some good toilet powder. It is a good plan to rub the feet with methylated spirits, which dries and hardens the skin. An old army routemarch tip is to soap the socks. To do this, turn them inside out and rub the feet of them hard with a just moistened cake of soap. Scales of soap stick to the sock and oil the skin, thus preventing friction and blisters.

If blisters form in spite of these precautions, wash the feet well and dry carefully. Rub over with methylated spirits, and then puncture the blister with a needle which has been sterilized by holding it in a flame. Using a clean handkerchief or piece of linen, gently press out the fluid while taking care not to break the blister. Cover with a piece of lint or clean linen. If the blister occurs at the beginning of a walk, be very careful to keep a good wad of cotton-wool or lint or a corn pad over the place, or the skin of the blister will be rubbed off and an open sore will result with the most painful consequences. Many walkers find that it well pays them to carry a second pair of walking shoes into which to change during the walk, when the first pair has become hot and sticky.

BLOOD. Blood is the fluid which circulates through the heart, the arteries and the veins, and supplies nourishing material to every part of the body. In the veins it is dark red, and in the arteries bright red; but when exposed to air it becomes thickened and divides into a red clot and a yellowish watery fluid caled *serum.* The amount of blood in the body is now considered to be roughly one-twentieth of the total weight of the body, and in a healthy person the blood consists of 78 per cent of water and 22 per cent solids. In the body, the blood vessels form a completely closed channel through which the blood ceaselessly circulates, and never escapes except in an accidental escape which we call bleeding or hemorrhage. It is, however, always collecting new substances and discarding others.

The first duty of the blood is to feed the body, which requires a large number of different substances to keep it in health, each one of which must be present in the blood and must be carried to the part of the body where it is required. In addition, the materials for all the secretions or juices which the body forms through its various organs are obtained from the blood. Some of these secretions are used for special purposes, but in some cases, notably that of the secretions of the thyroid and suprarenal glands, they are poured back into the blood where they carry out their normal functions.

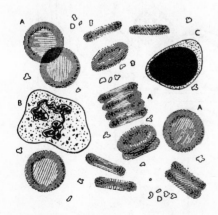

Blood Cells.
A. *Red blood cell;* B. *Polymorphonuclear leucocyte (a white blood cell);* C. *Lymphocyte (also a white blood cell);* D. *Platelets.*

Again, the blood acts as a carrier of oxygen to the tissues from the lungs. The red coloring matter, or *hemoglobin,* of the blood is the agent by which this carrying of oxygen, or *oxidation,* is performed. Heat is also distributed throughout the body by the blood, which receives heat at various points in its route and thus helps to keep the whole body at an even temperature. For instance, in passing through the muscles and glands, which are heart-producing bodies, the blood picks up heat, which is cooled off in the capillaries or little blood vessels near the surface of the body.

Blood, as well as feeding the body and providing the materials with which the various organs carry on their own specialized work, has also the very important function of ridding the body of waste matter, and is therefore an important part of the drainage and scavenging system of the body. Carbon dioxide formed in the tissues is not wanted and is carried to the lungs and there is breathed out; other waste materials are changed into urine, sweat, urea, etc.

In appearance, the blood is a red, sticky, nontransparent fluid. It is composed of a pale yellowish fluid called *plasma* in which float enormous numbers of minute bodies called *corpuscles* and *platelets.* The blood corpuscles are red and white in color. A method of estimating the numbers of these corpuscles has been invented by means of which the number of red and white corpuscles in a cubic millimeter (roughly a pinhead) of blood is calculated. The average number of red cells is about 5,000,000, and of white cells is 7,000. The red corpuscles are called *erythrocytes* and the white ones are *leucocytes.*

The red blood corpuscles are circular disks which contain hemoglobin, a compound of iron which has the power of attracting and combining with oxygen, the part of the air which is absolutely necessary to keep us alive. By means of this power, the red cells act as carriers of oxygen from the lungs to the tissues. These red cells are always being renewed, and the old dead ones are destroyed by the liver or spleen and are got rid of by means of the bile.

The white blood corpuscles are larger and very much fewer in number than the red ones. They possess the power of moving about in the bloodstream and are often described as the scavengers of the body, as they are able to eat up and destroy invading foreign bodies, such as germs. An invasion of germs into the blood causes a great increase in the number of these white blood corpuscles. They make their way to the point of invasion and wage war on the intruders; this process is called *phagocytosis* and it is by means of it that the body is continually protected from infection by germs.

The blood platelets are disk-shaped bodies, which are fewer and smaller than the red corpuscles, and play a part in the clotting of the blood.

The blood plasma is the watery fluid which contains corpuscles and platelets. It is the nourishing substance which feeds the tissue cells of the body.

Blood Examination. A method of diagnosis of disease which is used a great deal in modern medical treatment is the examination of the blood. A large drop of blood is obtained by pricking the patient's fingertip or lobe of the ear, and drawing off the blood with a pipette. To obtain a blood count or calculation of the number of the red and white corpuscles in the blood, a smear of blood is placed on a microscope slide and is placed under a high-powered lens. Then the number of cells in a given small unit can be counted and the total number roughly obtained by multiplication. In anemia the total amount of corpuscles is considerably diminished, and the diagnosis of the serious disease called pernicious anemia is made certain by the very small number found in the blood. The proportion of white to red corpuscles, the amount of hemoglobin, the shape and size of the corpuscles—all are important in the diagnosis of disease. The rapidity with which the blood clots (or coagulates) is also of great importance, as for instance the clotting is slower in jaundice, purpura, dropsy, etc. Malaria para-

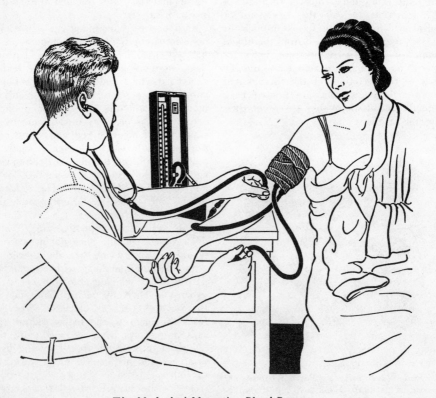

The Method of Measuring Blood Pressure.

sites are also found in the blood of malarial subjects.

Blood Groups. When an individual requires a transfusion of blood it is very important that the blood of the donor, or person who gives the blood to be transfused, should be of the same type as that of the recipient or there may be a serious reaction and collapse. For this reason the different types of blood are divided into groups. The blood in these groups has special reactions to the blood of the other groups, and although finer classifications have been worked out, individuals can in the main be divided into four groups. Group I (or AB in the newer classification) can receive safely the blood of all groups. Its members are therefore spoken of as *universal recipients*. Group II (A) can receive the blood of Groups II and IV, but against Groups I and III produces antibodies which cause clumping and destruction of the injected corpuscles. If this takes place in some of the smaller blood vessels of vital organs, the consequences are liable to be grave. Group III (B) can receive the blood from Groups III and IV. Group IV (O) can receive blood only from its own group, but can give blood to all groups, and its members are therefore spoken of as *universal donors*.

Another substance, known as the Rh (or Rhesus) Factor, has been discovered about the blood, which is responsible for certain diseases of the foetus and new-born infant. The condition is discussed under the heading RHESUS FACTOR.

Another interesting factor about blood is the "rate of sedimentation." When blood drawn from the body is left in a long tube, the cells slowly settle to the bottom. The time taken for the cells to settle is increased in many forms of disease and is used as an index of progress, as, for example, in tuberculosis.

BLOOD HEAT. The normal temperature of the blood is about 100 deg. F. When taking the temperature with a thermometer, however, the heat is judged to be about 98.4 deg. F. It is the constant circulation of the blood which keeps the body at the same temperature. (*See also* TRANSFUSION OF BLOOD.)

BLOOD POISONING. This is a condition of poisoning of the blood, due to the presence of germs or the poisons or toxins they produce. Blood-poisoning may arise from a wound or any other sources of infection. (*See also* SEPTICEMIA.)

BLOOD PRESSURE. By blood pressure is meant the force with which the blood is pumped along the arteries by the heart's beating. The strength of the heart's muscle, the elasticity of the walls of the arteries, and the volume of blood in the arteries, are all important factors in determining the blood pressure. In diseases which are accompanied by great weakness, such as anemia and heart-failure, the blood pressure is *lower* than usual, while in many other diseases it is *higher*.

The blood pressure is measured by an instrument called a *sphygmomanometer*. The usual pressure varies at different ages and for any individual is 100 m.m. plus half his age in years. A pressure of 155 or over is high blood pressure or *hyperpiesia*. This condition may be constitutional, caused by disease, or due to overeating or overdrinking. There may be temporary high blood pressure from strong emotion, pain, or exercise.

The symptoms associated with high blood pressure are breathlessness on exertion, palpitations and a feeling of discomfort in the region of the heart, headaches, giddiness, noises in the ear, irritability, and loss of the power of concentration. In most cases, a raised blood pressure causes no symptoms at all and is then an incidental finding. It is commonly found in later life and does not then usually lessen the expectation of life. It is a disorder of civilization and is in some way related to the tempo of life, selecting the bustling, overactive, stocky type of person. It is often accompanied by arteriosclerosis (q.v.), and many of its so-called symptoms are due to this.

Where high blood pressure is accompanied by symptoms, the patient should moderate his manner of living to avoid mental and physical strain, and he should obtain a sufficient amount of rest. The diet should be cut down. Meat and alcohol are best avoided, and smoking should be reduced to a minimum. Fish, poultry, eggs, fruit, and vegetables are the best foods.

It is a mistake to try to lower the blood pressure too much, as often a particular individual may require a somewhat higher blood pressure than usual to ensure good health.

Low blood pressure or *hypopiesia* may be merely an individual peculiarity, for one person may have a blood pressure lower or higher than the average. But in a severe type it may be due to disease of the suprarenal glands, such as Addison's disease. It may be the result of severe loss of blood, some forms of heart disease, and conditions like myxoedema. It is also frequently present in states of anaphylaxis and intestinal obstruction. The condition often comes on suddenly as in shock or fainting and is then only temporary, or it may be long continued.

In an acute attack, such as shock after an accident, a quick means of raising the pressure for a short time is to give an injection of adrenalin solution. Ephedrine sulphate tablets taken by mouth thrice daily are very useful, and in Addison's disease the treatment by a gland preparation called eucortone should be tried. Where the low blood pressure is due to bleeding, the lost blood may need to be replaced by transfusion, as the body will not survive a sustained low blood pressure for long.

BLOOD-SPITTING. Blood - spitting should always be taken seriously and the cause ascertained by a doctor. Streaks of blood in the sputum may be only from soft gums (due to pyorrhea) or from blood from a varicose vein in the nose or the upper part of the throat running down into the mouth. When it is more than just a streak it should be carefully noted whether the blood is coughed up or vomited up; even a slight cough may bring up a large quantity of bright and frothy blood, and this is practically always from the lungs and is often a sign of tuberculosis of the lungs, though in some cases it may be due to heart disease causing congestion in the lung. Vomited blood is usually dark in color, owing to the action of the digestive juices; this blood is usually due to bleeding from an ulcer in the stomach, and the affected person often feels faint before the blood comes up. As a general rule, dark blood will also be passed from the bowel in such cases.

BLOOD TRANSFUSION. *See* TRANSFUSION OF BLOOD.

BLOOD VESSELS. The blood vessels are the arteries and veins which carry the blood to and from the heart. The *arteries* lead from the heart and carry a supply of good blood containing oxygen to every part of the body. The *veins* lead to the heart and carry to it the waste products of the blood and the carbon dioxide. They are stronger and tougher than the arteries and the blood in them is dark-bluish red, whereas in the arteries it is bright red. The blood vessels are liable to disease from poisons present in the blood. Their walls may become thickened and lose their elasticity. They are liable to breakage or obstruction by clots. (*See also* ARTERIOSCLEROSIS; ARTERY; BLOOD; BLOOD PRESSURE; CIRCULATION OF THE BLOOD; *etc.*)

BLUE BABIES. The developing fetus normally has communications between the chambers of the heart and between the great arteries that lead from it. Since the fetus is unable to use its lungs to oxygenate its blood, it makes use of these communications to distribute the flow of oxygenated blood from the placenta to all the tissues of the body. These communications normally close soon after birth, when they are no longer needed. Sometimes, however, they persist and result in a mixing of the bad venous blood with the fresh blood from the lungs which is needed to supply the tissues with oxygen. This mixed blood is bluer in color than healthy arterial blood and imparts to the lips and skin a blue tinge. This is the reason why such cases of congenital deformity of the heart are described as "blue babies."

The pattern of heart deformity varies from case to case; from the tiniest communication which gives rise to no symptoms to the malformation so great that life can not be supported for more than a few minutes. Most cases fall in the range between these two extremes and many only become blue occasionally when the heart is working temporarily under an added load.

The heart with a congenital deformity has more work to do to maintain the circulation than a healthy heart. Many such hearts are able to carry this additional load through a long and useful life, but a large number will fail at some time. These communications are also liable to become the seat of an infection by germs known as *bacterial endocarditis.* Because of these dangers which beset the lives of such cases, successful attempts have been made to restore a normal anatomy at surgical operation. The *ductus arteriosus* is a communication between the aorta and the pulmonary artery and was first successfully tied in 1938. It has been done many hundreds of times since then with excellent results. Many other operations have been devised for the surgical correction of malformations of the heart, and this branch of surgery is advancing rapidly. Not all cases are suitable, and the selection of those most likely to benefit is a highly specialized science. By and large, most patients with a congenital heart disorder are able to lead fairly normal lives. Babies born blue and surviving into childhood the same color will usually require some form of surgery.

BLUE OINTMENT. Mercury or blue ointment is used in the treatment of syphilis and many other conditions, and rubbing on the skin is one of the ways of making sure that it is absorbed. The ointment may be put inside the sock, for then it is rubbed into the foot while walking.

BLUSHING. This is a symptom usually arising from general nervousness. The circulation of the blood is greatly influenced by the nervous system, and when an emotion, sometimes pleasurable, sometimes painful, is experienced, the blood vessels and the small arteries suddenly become dilated, thus causing a hot flush to be felt on the skin. Blushing occurs more frequently during the adolescent stage and also during the change of life in women. In shy and nervous persons this embarrassing habit often causes a great deal of distress. The only remedy is to force oneself to take an active interest in other people in order to break away from the habit of shyness.

BODY. The study of the make-up or structure of the body is called *Anatomy,* and of its working or functions, *Physiology.* The entire bony structure of the body is the skeleton, consisting of the *skull,* which includes all the bones of the head, the *spinal column* or backbone, to which are attached the *shoulder girdle* with the ribs below, and, at the lower end, the *pelvic girdle.* The legs are attached to the pelvic

girdle and the arms to the shoulder. The backbone supports the body in the upright position, the ribs form a protective cage in which the beathing apparatus and the heart are found, together with the upper parts of the abdominal organs. The pelvic girdle similarly protects the lower abdominal and reproductive organs. The backbone also serves as a protective channel for the spinal cord. The skull contains and protects the exceedingly delicate substance of the brain and the organs of sight, hearing, smell and taste. The bones of the body are covered with muscular tissue or flesh. The main part of the body between the head and the lower limbs is called the trunk. It has been seen that its walls are formed of bony and muscular tissue and it contains two large cavities, the chest or thorax, and the abdomen, which contain the organs, or viscera as they are called. The limbs, or appendages, are attached to the trunk. The whole body is protected by an outer covering called the skin or epidermis, which in turn is protected at points of friction by a growth of hair or nail. (*See also* ANATOMY.)

BOILS. A boil is a fester which may appear on any part of the body, usually at the entry of a hair follicle. It is due to a microbe which has found its way under the skin. Boils may be found in healthy as well as unhealthy persons. Certain diseases may be the original cause of boils appearing on the skin, or continuous irritation such as occurs in the wearing of a collar. When a boil occurs in persons who are otherwise quite healthy, the patient should be given some opening medicine. An adequate dose of penicillin should be given at once. Dry heat or a fomentation must be applied to the boil until it comes to a head and breaks. Yeast is a well-tried remedy for boils.

One of the most painful sites for an attack of boils is the ear, and it would be advisable to call in the aid of the doctor, who will probably pack the ear passage with glycerine or glycerine and magnesium sulphate. Warm fomentations of kaolin should be applied daily to the inflamed part, and care should be taken not to spread any infection to other parts of the body. (*See also* ABSCESS; CARBUNCLE.)

BONES. There are 206 bones in the

human body, and these, together with cartilage, or gristle, form the general framework of the body, which is called the skeleton. In appearance, fresh bone is pinkish-white in color, with a deep red center. If a bone is broken across, it is seen to consist of two kinds of tissue. One sort is dense and compact in texture, and is called *substantia compacta;* the other sort is a network of spongy fibrous tissue, and is called *substantia spongiosa* or cancellous tissue, owing to its resemblance to latticework. The outer part of the bone is always formed of the hard, dense tissue, while the inner portion is of the spongy material. On examination under a microscope it will be seen that the two sorts of tissues are really composed of the same porous material.

In the living body, the bones have blood vessels running through them and are coated with a fibrous membrane called the *periosteum.* Through the spongy bone in the middle of the long bones of the body runs a cavity which is filled with a material called the *medulla ossium,* or marrow. In the long bones the marrow is yellow in color, whereas in the other bones, and in the ends of the long bones, it is red. The periosteum is full of small blood vessels which run into numerous tiny channels in the outer bone substance called *Haversian canals,* and thus carry nourishment to the bone. If a bone is broken it will be seen to bleed from these minute vessels. A large artery runs through the marrow and is called its nutrient artery. It is accompanied by one or more veins. There is also a nerve supply.

Classification of Bones. The bones of the body are divided into four classes: long, short, flat, and irregular. The *long* bones are the bones of the limbs and are employed in movement. They are levers consisting of a body, or shaft, and two ends, which fit into joints and are movable in these joints. At each end they are covered with cartilage or gristle, while the joint is lubricated with a fluid called *synovial fluid* and is thus able to glide without friction over the cartilage-covered end of the other bone with which it connects in the joint. The long bones of the body are the humerus, in the upper arm, the ulna and radius in the fore arm, the femur (or

thighbone), tibia and fibula in the leg, the bones of the fingers and toes, and the collarbone or clavicle.

The *short* bones occur in the parts of the skeleton where strength is required, and they are compact and strong bones with a limited range of movement. The bones of the wrist, ankle and instep are short bones. The *flat* bones are bones which are meant to protect delicate structures or provide broad, flat surfaces suitable for the attachment of muscles. They are the skull-bones, the shoulder blades or scapulae, the pelvic bones, the breastbone or sternum, and the ribs. The *irregular* bones are so called from their shape, which makes it difficult to describe them with any of the other groups. The jawbone, the spine, and some of the bones of the skull are irregular bones.

Composition of Bones. Bones are composed of both animal and mineral matter in a proportion of about 33 per cent animal or organic matter to 66 per cent mineral or inorganic matter. The inorganic matter is chiefly calcium phosphate.

In young children the amount of mineral matter in the bones is nearly the same as the amount of animal matter, and their bones are, therefore, soft and flexible rather

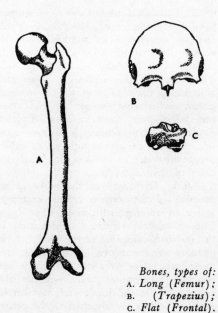

Bones, types of:
A. *Long (Femur);*
B. *(Trapezius);*
C. *Flat (Frontal).*

than brittle. These young bones are not liable to break like fully grown bones, but they bend easily. They are like young green shoots of trees which are very easily bent but almost impossible to snap in two with a clean break like old wood. Fractures of such bones are therefore called "greenstick" fractures. In the condition known as RICKETS (q.v.), the bones are very soft also.

Bone Diseases. It sometimes happens that a child is born without one or other of the usual bones, and such absence may be found in generation after generation, or only in isolated cases. The bones most often absent are leg or arm bones.

The best-known disease of bone is *rickets,* which is a chronic disease seen in young children and due to faulty feeding and bad hygienic conditions. It leads to deformities in the long bones in the arms and legs, the vault of the skull, the ribs and the pelvic bones. It is preventable by a well-balanced diet with adequate Vitamin D. Fortunately, it is becoming rare.

Acute inflammation of bone, which is called *osteomyelitis,* is a serious condition in which the bone is very tender and the patient has a high temperature and becomes very ill. *Chronic inflammation* of a bone may be due to tuberculosis. Various tumors arise in bones and are usually serious. *Periostitis,* or inflammation of the covering of the bone, may be acute or chronic. All cases of bone disease require a doctor. (*See also* OSTEOMYELITIS; PERIOSTITIS.)

BONE MARROW. Marrow is the soft substance found in the middle of bones and it is here that the red and white cells or corpuscles of the blood are formed.

BOOTS AND SHOES. A person who wears uncomfortable footwear is never in perfect health. No one can walk well—or think well—whose feet are uncomfortable. The ill-fitting shoe causes local discomfort, such as corns, callouses, blisters, and bunions; if too tight, it causes misshapen feet and affects their circulation; high heels cause the spine to be overcurved.

Shoemakers recognize these facts, and boots and shoes of correct shape and smart appearance are now obtainable in a wide variety of size. Time and care should always be given to the fitting of footwear,

as feet vary quite as much as do faces, and their individualities should be considered. The height of the heel should, for ordinary purposes, be from 1–1½ in. Serious trouble often arises from the heels being habitually worn down on one side, and the balance of the body thrown out. A rubber tip or pad on the heels will correct this; or, for casual wear, the rubber crêpe shoes now so much used. A rubber heel is recommended by most doctors, as the jar on the nervous system through the spine, unavoidable in walking upright, is much diminished thereby.

The soles and heels should be sufficiently broad to give stability and comfort in walking. One should stand up to be fitted, as the pressure on the sole increases the length of the foot by one-third of an inch, and the breadth by one-fifth. New shoes should be gradually "broken in." For adults, a good supply of shoes is a real economy, both for health, as a change of shoes is excellent for the feet, and for the pocket. If the feet tend to sweat excessively, cork soles should be used.

Children especially should have wellfitting footwear, with neither ventilation nor circulation impeded. Babies should have first woolen, then soft kid shoes. Sandals are splendid footwear for children, as they are both light and well-ventilated.

When fitting a child's shoe, the great toe should be allowed to lie straight inside the shoe, i.e., the inner line of the sole should be straight, and plenty of width allowed for the toes.

Goloshes and rubber boots generally are suitable in wet weather, but should be removed as soon as possible, as they are unsuitable for prolonged wear. What keeps out the wet keeps in the perspiration. This also applies to the rubber sneakers used in school gymnasiums; after the lesson is over, they should be changed at once.

BORACIC ACID. Boracic acid or boric acid may be obtained as white crystals or as a white powder. It is used largely to keep wounds, ulcers and sores from becoming infected. A solution of boracic acid may be employed as an antiseptic wash. Boracic lint is used a great deal for dressing wounds. Boracic powder when mixed with starch forms a useful dusting powder for infants. For sweaty feet that smell, a solution of boracic acid should be used; a little of the powder dusted into the socks or stockings may do much to prevent this condition. An ointment may be made up of 1 dram of boracic acid with petroleum jelly to make an ounce.

BORAX. Borax, or sodium borate, consists of transparent colorless crystals, with a sweetish taste. It is an excellent antiseptic and is one of the chief ingredients of many of the popular mouthwashes. As a lotion for the eyes, 10 grains are dissolved in a fluid ounce of warm water. It has been given in cases of epilepsy as a substitute for bromide in order to lessen excitability. Glycerine of borax is a very good application as an emollient for sore nipples.

BORBORYGMUS. Borborygmus is the medical name for the rumbling noises often made by the bowels.

BOTULISM. Botulism is a rare form of food poisoning due to an extremely powerful poison formed in the food by a microbe called *Bacillus botulinus.* The poison attacks the nervous system, causing paralysis.

The onset of symptoms usually occurs a few hours after the infected food has been eaten. The patient may complain of headache, and usually the vision becomes blurred or even double. There may be dizziness, and, sometimes, vomiting. There is a considerable weakness in the arms and legs, but there is usually no pain and the mind is quite clear. The voice may become very weak; the tongue is furred and the temperature is usually lower than normal. The acute stage of the disease usually lasts for about three or four days.

Treatment. This disease, of course, requires prompt medical attention, and a doctor should be called immediately symptoms appear. The patient should be kept in bed and the stomach washed out with warm normal saline. The doctor will probably give an injection of morphine, as this delays the action of the toxin. A botulinus antitoxin should be given as soon as possible.

Convalescence is generally slow, and disturbances of vision may persist for weeks after the other symptoms have disappeared. Attacks of botulism very often prove fatal, and usually several people are affected who have partaken of the same food. Foods, when being prepared or canned should be heated to an adequate temperature as the bacilli and spores are killed by heat.

BOUGIE. A bougie is a slender, rod-like surgical instrument which can be introduced into any of the external passages of the body such as the urethra, for the purposes of examining them. Medicated bougies are used in the treatment of vaginal discharges, etc.

BOVINE TUBERCULOSIS. The form of consumption which attacks cows is known as bovine tuberculosis. It can be transferred to human beings, especially babies and delicate people, by their drinking unpasteurized milk from infected cows. The dairy farmers now have their cows tested periodically for tuberculosis, and are therefore able to assure their customers that they are obtaining milk from cows which are entirely free from the disease. (*See also* TUBERCULOSIS.)

BOWEL. The bowel is now more often called the intestine, or intestines, and is described under that heading.

BOWLEG. Bowlegs or bandy legs are nearly always the result of forcing a weakly or rickety child to walk at too early an age. The upper part of the leg or thigh may be entirely in the shin part of the leg. In many cases there may be bow-knee, which is just as much the result of rickets as bowlegs are. It very often happens, too, that one leg may be bow, and the other leg may develop symptons of knock-knee, so that the curve of one leg fits with the curve of the other. This condition is due to the weight of the body pressing on the soft unformed bones of the child. As soon as the slightest tendency to bowlegs or knock-knee appears in a young infant, the mother should keep him off his feet as much as possible and the legs should be bound with well-padded splints. The general diet should be attended to and plenty of fresh foods with boneforming properties should be given, as well as plenty of fresh air and sunshine. (*See also* RICKETS.)

BRACHIAL. The term brachial means anything to do with the arm. The brachial artery is a continuation of the axillary artery along the inner side of the arm. The network of nerves in the arm is called the *brachial plexus.* (*See also* ARM.)

BRADYCARDIA. This term is derived from two Greek words and means slowness of the heart. In certain diseases the heart-beat is abnormally slow, and it is always very marked in the condition known as heartblock. It is not an uncommon finding in health and then has no serious signi-ficance. (*See also* HEAT; PULSE.)

BRAIN. The brain includes all that part of the great nervous system of the body which is enclosed in the skull. The normal weight of the brain is from 40 to 50 oz.; it is slightly heavier in men than in women, the average weight in men being from 49 to 50 oz., and in women from 44 to 45 oz.

Divisions of the Brain. The largest part of the brain consists of the "big brain" or "cerebrum," which occupies about two-thirds of the total area of the skull and is made up a mass of nervous tissue thrown into many folds. The "little brain" or "cerebellum" lies at the back of the skull and is also thrown into folds, but these are very fine and delicate as compared with those of the big brain and resemble in appearance the fine leaves of a fern. Uniting the two halves of the little brain is a wide band of nervous tissue, called the "bridge" or "pons," and this "bridge" is continuous below with the enlarged upper end of the spinal cord which is called the "bulb" or "medulla." These are the four chief struc-tural divisions of the brain: the "big brain," the "little brain," the "bridge," and the "bulb."

Nerve Centers in the Brain. Attached to the under surface of the brain, mainly to the "bridge" and to the "bulb," are twelve pairs of nerves, by means of which we are able to use our special senses of smell, sight, taste and hearing. These nerves also control the movements of the face muscles, the movements of the eyes, the movements of chewing, and the movements of the head and neck. They are numbered in order from one to twelve; but each has, in addi-tion, a Latin or Greek name. Although each nerve has its own independent sphere of action, yet the combined action of two or more nerves may be necessary to produce one particular effect. For instance, in order to obey the doctor's command to "Put out your tongue," the twelfth nerves (one on each side), which control the muscles of the tongue, must be working properly. But to experience the sensation of taste on the tongue, as, for example, when we say

that sugar "tastes" sweet, a complicated arrangement of the action of at least three, if not four, nerves is required. The act of swallowing is a very complicated one and needs the control of three nerves, the ninth, tenth, and eleventh, for its perfect performance. Similarly, when we look from one side to the other we are performing a very complicated movement which is con-trolled by three other nerves, the third, the fourth, and the sixth.

The seventh nerve is of special interest: it controls the movements of the muscles of the face, and so our facial expression. Sometimes, when people sit in a draft with the air blowing strongly on one side of their face, this nerve, which on the face lies very close to the surface of the skin of the cheek, "catches cold," as it were, or, more correctly, becomes inflamed. Then for a time it ceases to be able to control the movements of that side of the face, with the result that that side of the face be-comes partly, or completely, paralyzed. The unfortunate person who has so ac-quired what is called a "Bell's palsy" (after Sir Charles Bell, who first described it) is unable to close his eye on the side of the inflamed nerve, and so may get a sore eye from the lids not being able to brush away small particles of dust as they nor-mally do. In addition, his face looks "one-sided" because the usual creases on that side of the face are smoothed out. He can-not whistle or smile properly because he cannot use the muscles of both sides of the lips, and very often he is unable to taste on the side of the tongue corres-ponding to the affected side of the face. The condition, though very unpleasant and unsightly, is not dangerous and ultimately recovers completely, although it may, in older people, take months, rather than weeks. (*See also* FACIAL PARALYSIS.)

The complicated paths by which each part the brain is linked up with every other part, and the means by which all parts of the body are brought into com-munication with the brain, cannot be des-cribed here. But, in a few words, the brain taken as a whole consists of a countless number of nervous elements, consisting of nerve cells and their two types of processes. One type of process carries messages or impulses towards the cells; the other type carries impulses away from the cells. By means of these two sets of processes the different parts of the brain and spinal nervous system are brought into relation with each other and with every other part of the body.

The nerve cells in the brain form what is called the gray matter; their processes form the various strands of the white matter. In the "big brain" the gray matter lies on the outside of the brain, covering the surface; the white matter lies deeply. Through much painstaking experimental work, it has been made possible to map out certain parts of the gray matter of the "big brain" into various areas and to predict what will happen if one or other of these areas is injured or diseased. One such area is called the "motor" area, because when we wish to move our limbs or any part of our bodies it is this area of the brain which enables that movement to be carried out, i.e., the message is sent from this area down through the brain to the spinal cord, then is transmitted along a nerve and finally reaches the muscles, which obey the message they have received by contracting, thus causing the required movement to take place. If this area is damaged, the side of the body on the opposite side to that damaged is paralysed, because the path taken by messages from the motor area crosses to the opposite side of the brain at the level of the "bulb." Other well-defined areas of the gray matter are those concerned with the appreciation of sensation. By "sensation" we mean any experience which reaches us from our surroundings and of which we become conscious. The area for sight, for example, is situated at the back of the brain, so that we really see with the back of our heads, for if this part of the brain is injured or destroyed by disease, no matter how perfect our eyes may be, we become blind. There is a special and very important area of the brain which enables us to recognize the position of our limbs in space, without the aid of sight; and the same area tells us the position, size and shape of objects with which our limbs may come into contact. The ease with which we are able to distinguish the various objects in a pocket, for example, without using our eyes, is entirely dependent on this area of the brain.

If it becomes damaged in any way we lose this power. But the greater part of the "big brain" is composed of what are known as "silent areas," because nothing is known about them. They are presumed to be concerned with thought and memory. These "silent areas" are situated in the foremost part of the "big brain," and it has been noticed by many that in disease of this part of the brain the intelligence suffers first.

The "litttle brain" controls our balance and so enables us to alter our position in space as the need arises. It is also concerned with keeping the muscles in good tone, that is to say, in that state in which they will be ready to contract or relax to the best advantage. If there is disease of one side of the "little brain," this state of tone is lost on the whole of the side of the body corresponding to the side of the "little brain" affected, and the limbs on that side feel "floppy," and are clumsy and awkward in their movements. Balance is badly maintained and in walking the person tends to fall to the side of the damaged "little brain." The "little brain" is also concerned with the performance of complicated automatic movements and its activities are always outside our consciousness. Thus we learn to ride a bicycle with our "big brain," but after a little practice our cerebellum is able to do it for us. We can then ride our bicycle while thinking what we will have for lunch, and only realize what we are doing when something unusual crops up.

Diseases of the Brain. The brain is liable to suffer from the same types of disease, broadly speaking, as any other organ of the body, but owing to the special nature of the tissue of which it is composed, the results of such disease processes are of a peculiar character. In order to understand this, it is necessary to appreciate that the brain is enclosed in a box—the skull—which cannot expand. Therefore, anything which increases the size or weight of the brain or its coverings will cause a certain amount of extra pressure inside the skull, and this pressure not only produces pain, but many other symptoms, as well as destroying the delicate nervous tissue. Another important point is that the essential elements of the nervous system, the nerve cells and their processes, once destroyed, never re-form; their place is taken by scar tissue, which is incapable of receiving, conducting, or transmitting messages or impulses. So if a nerve cell dies, or is killed by some disease process, that unit of the nervous system can never be replaced. It has not yet been discovered whether each unit is at work all the time, but a loss of only a few nerve cells can often be shown under the microscope when there have been many symptoms of diminished nervous activity during life. Because of these two facts, the enclosure of the brain by a rigid box and the failure of the nerve cells to re-form once they have been destroyed, it should be easy to understand that in the brain the symptoms which arise from any particular disease depend not so much on the nature of the disease as on the position in the brain in which the disease is operating. For example, a slowly progressive cutting off of the blood supply such as occurs in some diseases of the arteries will produce exactly the same effects as a tumor pressing on, or growing in, a particular situation, as far as symptoms are concerned. The expert has then two problems to solve in dealing with disorders of the brain; firstly, where is the disease and, secondly, what is its nature.

To say where a disease is present in the brain may be almost impossible, or, on the other hand, may be very simple. If there is some disorder of the "little brain," for example, the signs are so definite and unmistakable, that it is only a question of determining the nature of the malady. Similarly, if one of the areas of the brain whose special action is known, such as the "motor" area, becomes diseased or injured, certain signs (in this case, signs of paralysis of the opposite side of the body) occur, which enable the nerve specialist to say with certainty that something is amiss with this particular region of the brain. In the "bridge" of the brain or the "bulb," where many of the nerves coming out of or entering the brain are attached, and where many conducting paths are crowded together, destruction of these will cause interference with the normal action of the movements controlled by these nerves and conducted along these paths, so that it is a comparatively simple matter for one who knows the structure of the brain to say when this region is damaged. But in the "big brain,"

where so many "silent" areas exist, of whose action and conducting paths we know nothing, it may be almost or quite impossible to decide where the disease is until it reaches an area whose action gives us some information. In some cases it may not, for the same reason, be possible even to say on which side of the brain the disease is, but if the disease lasts a sufficiently long time it is rare for the expert not to be able to determine the position of the disease.

Treatment of Brain Diseases. From the point of view of treatment it is of the greatest importance to establish not only the position of the disorder, but its nature. The various misfortunes that may befall us may be summarized as follows: there may be some failure in development; our disorders may be the result of injury, or of infection by a microbe which causes a reaction known as inflammation; animal parasites may make our bodies their temporary refuge; our tissues may wear out before the normal span of life is over, a process which we call degeneration; finally, tumor growth may take place and destroy or replace normal tissues. The brain is not exempt from any one of these misfortunes, but from the practical standpoint some are vastly more important than others. For failures in development, which may be of any degree from such slight ones as cause only weakness of one side of the body and limbs up to those in which the child has so little brain developed that it is a complete idiot, we can do nothing except to ensure that the most is made of such intelligence as is present, and of such movements as are possible. Very often it is advisable in the interests of the mother and other members of the family that such unfortunate children should be placed in institutions. It is always difficult to persuade the mother that where the brain is so badly developed that the child can never be normal mentally, the child will never miss that maternal care which the mother, naturally enough, wants to lavish upon the weakling. For the sake of all concerned, children who are mentally unfit should be looked after in special homes.

Injuries to the Brain. Brain injuries are always serious and should never be treated lightly. They usually follow blows or falls on the skull, and nearly always are accompanied by some period of unconsciousness. If the brain has been only slightly damaged, the injured person recovers from this unconsciousness and is then said to have had *concussion*. If there has been extensive damage to the brain tissues, on the other hand, unconsciousness deepens into what is called a coma, a state in which the breathing becomes noisy and hurried and from which it is impossible to rouse the person. It is rare for people to recover from such extensive damage to their brain as results in coma, for this state means that there has been a tearing of some of the blood vessels of the brain and that bleeding has taken place into the brain substance, an almost invariably fatal accident. In cases of only slight damage to the surface of the brain, what is called concussion, the danger is that if the patient does not take care to remain in bed until such time as his doctor permits him to get up, he will develop a severe headache, which may persist for months. A period of rest in bed, after even a few minutes complete loss of consciousness from head injuries, is essential if this headache is to be avoided.

The infections of the brain which give rise to inflammation are so many and varied that it is impossible to consider them here, except to say that because the majority of these infections do not attack the essential elements of the brain, the nerve cells, but rather the tissues supporting them and their fatty coverings, the diseases produced by these infections, though they may be disabling, are in many cases consistent with long life. (*See also* CEREBROSPINAL FEVER; MENINGITIS.)

The wearing out or premature death of nerve cells before the rest of the body cells is one of the characteristic features of old age. The failure of memory for recent events, with constant repetition of stories of "When I was a boy," is a well-recognized picture of the elderly. But sometimes this wearing out of the nerve cells occurs at an earlier age, and then the picture is a sad one. In association with the failure of memory, weakness of the will develops and all the patient's mental activities become lessened. In some cases, mental deterioration takes place so rapidly

and so completely that the patient is unable to carry on his life in a normal way and it is necessary to have him cared for in a mental hospital, if sufficient attention cannot be given at home. These patients become as children and are as easily led, and it is in these cases that unscrupulous relatives or attendants find their opportunity to influence the unfortunate victim to alter a will so that they may benefit. (*See also* MENTAL DISEASE.)

Tumors of the Brain. The brain is one of the commonest positions in the body in which tumors may develop. During the last twenty years surgery has made such wonderful strides that if the signs of tumor formation are detected early enough there is every chance that an operation on the brain can be undertaken and the tumor—if not situated too deeply in the substance of the brain—removed, at least in part. The main, and most disastrous, effects of tumor formation in the brain are those which depend on the increase in bulk of the contents of the skull, which cannot expand. These effects show themselves to the patient by an increasingly severe headache, accompanied in the late stages of tumor formation by vomiting, which is not associated with the taking of food. The headache is nearly always worse in the morning when the patient first gets up, and during the day it improves somewhat. The increase of pressure inside the skull leads eventually to destruction of the nerves behind the eye, so that failure of vision is noticed. But long before the patient notices that he cannot see so well, a doctor can, by means of an instrument with which he looks at the back of the eye, tell at once in a very large proportion of cases whether a tumor of the brain is present. In many cases also it is possible for the specialist in brain diseases to say exactly where the tumor is lying, from the signs he is able to observe. The important thing is that the early recognition of the presence of a tumor is absolutely essential if any hope of a complete cure can be promised or even attempted. A number of tumors which lie so deeply in the substance of the brain that their removal is impossible do occur, but a far larger number begin to grow from near the surface of the brain, and it is in the interests of patients suffering from surface growths that early diagnosis of their condition should be made. (*See also* CONCUSSION; MENINGITIS.)

Brain Fatigue. Any excess of mental strain or worry may cause the brain to feel fatigued. Overindulgence in alcohol, sexual excesses, or the abuse of such drugs, as morphia or cocaine may be the exciting cause. The symptoms are generally restlessness, insomnia, and the inability to concentrate on any intellectual form of work or reading. Treatment consists of rest, nourishing foods, and plenty of open-air exercise with a sufficiency of sleep. Situations liable to produce worry and anxiety should be avoided as far as possible.

Brain Fever. This is an old-fashioned term for meningitis (q.v.).

BRAN. Bran is the outer covering or husk of any cereal. It is taken to provide "roughage" in a diet which would otherwise be too thoroughly digested without leaving enough residue to give sufficient bulk to the stools. (*See also* BERI-BERI.)

BRANDY. Brandy contains 40 to 50 per cent of alcohol, and good cognac may contain as much as 60 per cent. This spirit is largely used in medicine as a stimulant, and may be given to revive a fainting patient. Brandy is considered to be very rich in energy-giving and restorative properties. (*See also* ALCOHOL.)

BREAD. The chief bread-making cereals are wheat, rye, and, corn. Wheat is specially suitable for bread-making because of the large amount of gluten which its flour forms when mixed with water. Carbon dioxide is produced by the yeast fermentation which spreads through the dough while in the oven, thus forming the texture of the loaf. During the baking process, bread undergoes many important changes. The water and alcohol (caused by fermentation) are evaporated, proteins are solidified, and the starch becomes gelatinized.

White bread is lacking in protein and fat, but is very rich in carbohydrates. The deficiency of fat is usually made up by the habit of eating butter, margarine, or other fatty substances with the bread. The mineral phosphates lacking are usually replaced in the diet by milk.

The percentage of vitamins is very small and should be supplemented by such foods as eggs, fruit, fresh vegetables, and nuts.

White bread should not be regarded as a staple food, especially for children, as it is deficient in many vital and essential elements. When bread was "the staff of life," white bread had not been invented, and all bread was wholegrain. Nowadays most white bread is enriched by adding vitamins.

Wholegrain bread. This contains more protein, fat, salts, and roughage than white bread, and also contains many vitamins derived from the germ and bran. The presence of the wholegrain, which acts as roughage, is an excellent remedy for constipation. Wholegrain bread is especially good for growing children, and there is less danger of ill-health and disease arising through vitamin deficiency when wholegrain bread forms a part of the staple food of the diet. For growing children, cod liver oil, milk, and milk-fat products should be added to the diet to ensure the proper formation of bone and teeth and prevent the occurrence of rickets.

Starch-reduced bread. This is used a great deal in special diets. It is a valuable addition to the diet of those who suffer from carbohydrate dyspepsia, and while its tissue-building properties are nearly four times that of ordinary white bread, its fattening properties due to surplus starch are entirely absent.

Malted bread. This is usually much more moist than the ordinary white breads and the percentage of starch is considerably lower. It has a characteristic sweet flavor with a slightly "gummy" crust and is easily digested.

Milk bread. Milk bread is made by substituting a portion of milk for the water used in mixing the dough. It is particularly beneficial to children because of its added nutritive value.

BREAST. The term breast is commonly used for the front part of the chest, including the two *mammae* (breasts) and the breast-bone, but in medical language the term means one or other of the mammae or glands which furnish milk. The breasts exist in the male as well as the female, but as they are not used in the male they are present only in an elementary state of development. In the female the breasts are two large hemispherical prominences which lie to the right and left of the breastbone on the front of the chest. They differ greatly in size in various individuals and at different times in the life of the same individual. In childhood there is little difference to be seen between the breasts of girls and boys, but at the age of puberty they enlarge very considerably in the female. When the body has attained its full growth the breasts remain stationary, too, until pregnancy takes place, when they begin to swell. During the period of lactation or nursing, the breasts reach their largest size. After weaning they return to a smaller size, but will usually remain larger than they were before childbearing. Other changes taking place at this time are more fully described under the heading of PREGNANCY. The female breasts shrink after the menopause or change of life, and in old age become completely atrophied.

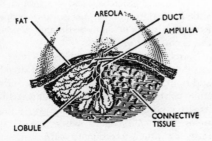

Section Through Female Breast.

The breasts are composed of glands and vessels imbedded in fatty tissue. In the center of each breast is a small eminence called the nipple. It is a deep rose color, and is surrounded by a circle of pink called the areola. This areola remains a delicate pink color until pregnancy has become established, when it changes to brown and remains brownish for the rest of life. The nipple is perforated in fifteen to twenty places by the openings of the milk-bearing ducts. On the areola are various small prominences which are really sebaceous glands, and contain a fatty substance that acts as a protection to the skin of the nipple during suckling.

The mammary gland is a complicated arrangement which filters off the materials found in milk from the blood. In the depths of the breast the milk is gathered in very tiny vessels. Several of these unite together to form little bundles no larger than a pinhead. These bundles unite again into bigger vessels called *lobules,* and the lobules converge together in groups to form *ampullae,* or reservoirs which store the milk and which lie under the areola and have direct connection with the nipple by way of tubules or ducts. The arrangement has been compared to a bunch of grapes of which the stalks are hollow. The ducts from the various ampullae do not unite, but discharge their milk from the nipple by means of small ducts.

Abscess of the Breast. If pus-forming organisms find their way into the breast, suppuration begins and an abscess forms. Infection usually enters the breast during lactation through a cracked nipple, and can often be prevented. These abscesses occur in one of three situations. They may be just under the skin or nipple and the pus may not burrow far inwards, in which case the abscess will quickly come to the surface, causing little pain or discomfort. If, however, the pus forms deep in the substance of the breast, it may track in every direction and involve the whole breast. The typical signs of suppuration are present and the patient is in great pain and becomes very ill. A third sort of abscess may have nothing to do with lactation, but may start in the region behind or below the breast. When it is called a *submammary or retromammary* abscess, and may be due to disease spreading from the lungs to the breast. The treatment of breast abscess is the same as for other abscesses. An early breast abscess can often be aborted by injections of penicillin. Hot fomentations may be applied until the abscess points, then the breast should be opened by a surgeon and drained. If the abscess is of large extent, drainage may have to be effected by means of tubes. Usually the breast heals quickly and cleanly, but occasionally small sinuses may arise and continue to discharge. These will have to be opened and packed with gauze. (*See also* ABSCESS; MASTITIS; TUBERCULOSIS.)

Cancer of the Breast. In women, the commonest sites of cancer are the womb and the breast. It frequently follows chronic mastitis, but may arise in a breast that has never given any trouble. It may be the result of chronic irritation by ill-fitting corsets, brassieres, etc., or from a blow in the breast.

The earliest symptom noticed is usually a lump attached to the skin, swollen glands in the armpit, or just a retracted or pulled-in nipple. Pain is not troublesome until the disease is well established. Eczema round the nipple which does not clear up at once with simple treatment should also be regarded as suspicious of cancer. Many women suffer from periodic attacks of pain in the breast called *mastodymia;* at first they may be afraid that their pain is the beginning of cancer, but an examination by the doctor will reassure them. In early cases of cancer of the breast, operative treatment which involves removal of the breast on the affected side is very successful, and a complete cure is frequently obtained. Many cases have been cured by modern radiotherapy, by X-rays, radium bomb, or cobalt bomb. It is the duty of every woman who has any suspicious symptom, even though it causes her no inconvenience and she has not time to be ill, to have herself examined. Delay will only make matters worse if the condition is malignant, for it is curable if recognized early.

Diseases of the Breast. The female breast is subject to various diseases, many of which are painful. Most of these diseases happen at times when there is extra activity in the breast, e.g., at puberty when the breast begins to develop, during suckling and about the time of the change of life. Acute inflammation or *mastitis* occurs most often in the early days of the nursing period, although it is not rare to find it in the breasts of babies in their first few days of life. This condition in the infant readily yields to treatment and all that is necessary in most cases is to cover the part with a pad of sterile dressing. Mastitis occurring after childbirth is a prelude to breast abscess. Cysts and glandular tumors may arise in the breast. Cysts may be due to chronic mastitis or may be caused by the retention of milk in women who are or have recently been nursing. Adenomata or glandular tumours may occur in the breasts of younger women whether they have borne children or not. They may be perfectly painless, small, not very hard lumps, or they may be exceedingly painful. In every case of trouble in the breast, especially if there is a lump of any description, a doctor should be consulted. Only if the patient comes early to the doctor can she be sure that the condition is not cancer, and, if it is cancer, early removal will give a very good chance of permanent cure. (*See also* CANCER; MASTITIS; PAGET'S DISEASE.)

BREAST FEEDING. Breast feeding is the natural method of nourishing the infant, and the normal mother's milk contains in proper quantity and proportions all the food materials necessary to keep the infant healthy. It also has the advantage of being in most cases germ free. Suckling her child also aids the mother's system to return in a natural way to the normal. It is therefore the duty of the mother both to her child and to herself to feed the child as nature intended. Only in cases of grave necessity should the infant be put off breast feeding. Full details of both breast feeding and artificial feeding are given under the heading BABY, FEEDING OF, in the SUPPLEMENT ON THE CARE OF BABY.

BREATH, OFFENSIVE. *See* HALITOSIS.

BREATHLESSNESS. Breathlessness, or shortness of breath (dyspnoea), indicates that the body is not being supplied with sufficient oxygen for its needs. It occurs after exertion in health. When it happens at rest or after only slight exertion it is abnormal, and may be due to disease of the lungs, or air-passages, or of the heart. Croup, which is also seen chiefly in children, often causes alarming breathlessness. Asthma is a condition in which this complaint is one of the chief symptoms.

In almost every disease of the lungs, such as pneumonia, consumption, bronchitis, etc., shortness of breath is present, and in pleurisy the patient makes the breathing quick and short in order to avoid the pain of deep inspirations. Practically all affections of the heart, including the fatty heart of corpulent persons, cause breathlessness; and anemia is also a common cause, especially in young women.

The treatment naturally depends largely on the immediate cause of the complaint, but in order to relieve the patient of the distressing symptom of breathlessness complete rest in bed is advisable, and propping up with pillows may be beneficial.

BRIGHT'S DISEASE. Medically termed nephritis, this disease derives its name from Dr. Bright of Guy's Hospital, who in 1827 published a paper describing its symptoms. Bright's disease includes inflammatory and degenerative changes of the kidneys. There are many varieties which include the acute, subacute, and chronic stages. It is described under the heading NEPHRITIS. (*See also* AMYLOID DISEASE.)

BROMETHOL. *See* AVERTIN.

BROMIDES. The bromides of potassium, sodium, ammonium, calcium, and iron were formerly used a great deal in medicine. Externally they have no action whatever, but internally they act by powerfully depressing the nervous system. Bromides are rapidly absorbed after administration, and are widely distributed throughout the body. They are got rid of by the kidneys quickly at first, but afterwards more slowly, so that bromides may accumulate in the body for quite a long period after they have been taken. They are of considerable value in the treatment of epilepsy. In some cases the symptoms disappear altogether and, as a rule, the severity and frequency of the fits are greatly diminished. The bromides are used extensively as hypnotics in cases where sleeplessness is caused by mental strain or any nervous disorder, but are of little use when sleeplessness is due to pain. The sleep produced is quiet and refreshing and generally without dreams. These drugs are of great value in nightmares, or in the night-screaming of children. The usual dose for such purposes is from 5 grains for a child and up to 30 grains for an adult. They very often bring relief in migraine, and cases of nervous headache. Bromide of potassium is used to diminish sexual desire, but if bromides are taken for a long period a failure of sexual vigour is produced. In whooping-cough, bromides are given in order to diminish the severity and number of the paroxysms, and many kinds of neuralgia are frequently relieved by these drugs. Concentrated solutions have the same action as any other salt in that they cause nausea and vomiting. Liquid preparations should be well diluted, and salts should be dissolved in at least half a glass of water.

Poisoning by Bromides. If bromides are taken over too long a period, symptoms of poisoning may appear, the condition being known as bromism. The patient complains of feeling depressed, easily fatigued and unfit for work. The sexual power becomes greatly diminished and the skin develops a rash exactly resembling some forms of acne. The symptoms may be removed by stopping all bromides.

BRONCHI. This is the plural form of bronchus. The bronchi are the air passages in the lungs. After the air has been breathed in through the nose it travels to the lungs by way of the *trachea* or windpipe. The windpipe divides into two smaller tubes, one of which leads to each lung. These are the right and left main *bronchi* or bronchial tubes. When the bronchial tubes reach the lung they in turn divide into numerous smaller tubes, which again divide, branching like a tree until the substance of the lung is permeated with these little air-vessels. The very smallest bronchi are called *bronchioles*. Inflammation of the lining of the bronchial tubes is the well-known disease called *bronchitis*. Bronchitis becomes serious when the walls of the smaller bronchioles are affected, since the air is hindered in its passage through them to the air cells, or *alveoli*. Spasm of the muscular tissue of the bron-

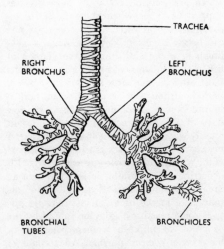

Bronchi.

chioles with swelling of the mucous membrane of the bronchial tubes is the cause of the breathlessness, which is the characteristic symptom of asthma.

BRONCHIECTASIS. Bronchiectasis is

a condition in which one or more of the bronchi becomes enlarged and dilated. The condition is usually due to a previous attack of pneumonia or bronchopneumonia, or to the inhaling at some previous time of a foreign body such as a pea or a bean, a tooth, or a bit of bone.

The patient with bronchiectasis has cough with phlegm nearly all the year round. The cough occurs characteristically first thing in the morning and with change of posture. The diseased area of lung is subject to repeated attacks of infection by germs, each attack leaving the bronchi weaker and more liable to further infection. The infection frequently spreads to the surrounding lung producing a type of pneumonia. When the symptoms are slight, no special treatment is required. When the disease is confined to one or two lobes of the lungs, these lobes are usually removed by surgical operation and a complete cure is often possible. There are many cases of successful removal of one lung in this condition. Cases unsuitable for surgery are treated by "Postural Drainage." The patient is taught to adopt a position which allows the diseased areas to drain pus and mucus into healthy bronchi whence it can be coughed up. Inhalations of penicillin in the form of a mist often enable such cases to remain free from infection.

BRONCHITIS. Bronchitis means inflammation of the bronchi and is well known to everyone.

Acute Bronchitis. Bronchitis in its acute form is a feverish cold with cough and sore chest. It is contagious and can be caught by others who come in contact with the sufferer. It is an acute catarrhal inflammation of the windpipe and larger bronchial tubes and is very common in wet climates. In healthy adult people it is rarely serious, but in very young children and aged people acute bronchitis is always a serious disease and is often fatal, chiefly because of the lung complications which so often accompany it.

Acute bronchitis usually starts as a common cold and then extends down the air passages. Very often it follows an attack of influenza or infectious diseases like measles and typhoid fever. Many people are very prone to it and the slightest exposure to cold and damp or the germs of other people's colds will bring on an attack. Great care must therefore be exercised in these cases.

Various sorts of germs are found in bronchitis as they are found in influenza, the common cold and other such diseases. The germ which is the cause of pneumonia, the *pneumococcus*, is often found in bronchitis. Many other germs have been discovered in cases of bronchitis and they are of the type often found in the healthy nose and throat. They must be regarded as secondary invaders which follow in the wake of infection by the viruses of influenza and the common cold, or which will attack bronchi already weakened by bronchiectasis or some other cause.

Symptoms. An attack of acute bronchitis starts as an ordinary cold, and then gradually extends, first to the larynx, where the vocal cords are affected, causing huskiness on speaking. There may be pain on swallowing and on talking and the throat will feel "raw." This feeling of "rawness" extends with the inflammation to the windpipe and larger bronchial tubes and produces a characteristic dry cough which is very painful.

General symptoms are fairly well marked: there is a feeling of illness, heaviness and tiredness with pains in the back and an aching feeling in all the joints. Bronchial signs begin with a feeling of tightness and rawness in the upper part of the front of the chest. At first the cough is very dry and the expectoration is scanty, but after a few days the material coughed up becomes yellowish and abundant. With the loosening of the cough the pain grows less.

Physical Signs. The breathing is definitely of a "wheezing" character. As the discharge becomes more profuse the noises in the chest become more moist and "bubbly." After about a week the light fever present usually disappears and the cough becomes loose.

In children the risk of the disease spreading is much greater, and it then spreads downwards to the smaller portions of the bronchial tubes. These fine tubes become dilated and packed with matter, and bronchopneumonia usually follows.

The lower parts of the lungs should be carefully examined every day in case there are small patches of this bronchopneumonia forming. Blowing breathing, together with a change in the general condition of the patient for the worse, such as a higher temperature, a more rapid pulse, dirty tongue, a change of color—possibly a slight degree of blueness—especially marked round the lips, a severer and more continuous cough, and difficulty in breathing, all indicate the change to bronchopneumonia.

Treatment. To lessen the risk of other people catching the cold, the patient should sleep alone and, when possible, there should be an abundance of sunlight and fresh air. A "bronchitis kettle," e.g., a kettle containing a solution of eucalyptus or menthol, should be kept near the heat so that the air is constantly moistened with water vapor. The room should be kept at a constant temperature of about 65 deg. F., but must be well ventilated. Drinks of hot lemonade and a hot-water bottle on the chest are helpful. The patient must remain in bed, and drink as much bland fluid as possible. The dry cough is usually very tiring, and for this the kettle will be found most useful. A syrup of codeine, or some other sedative are the medicines usually prescribed to quiet the cough.

Inhalations, such as a teaspoonful of compound tincture of benzoin in a jug of hot water, may alleviate the dry cough. The water should not be too hot, and in practice the best way to be sure of a suitable temperature is to pour boiling water in the jug and to wait for five minutes by the clock before adding the benzoin and inhaling. Care must be taken not to inhale before the end of the five minutes as, if the vapor is too hot, the larynx may be badly scalded and the inflammation rendered worse than before.

After one or two days the expectoration becomes more free, and then the various expectorant mixtures which aid the production of phlegm are very useful.

In children the amount of the discharge is sometimes so great that it is difficult to bring it up. If there should be any difficulty in breathing, or should the color become dusky, an emetic such as salt and water, or a tablespoonful of ipecacuanha wine, should be given and repeated if necessary. This procedure will bring up quantities of phlegm, and greatly relieve the condition.

Severe bronchitis or threatening bronchopneumonia requires treatment directed against the invading germs. Fortunately they are usually sensitive to antibiotics in adequate dosage, penicillin (often combined with streptomycin), or else tetracycline.

Chronic Bronchitis. Chronic bronchitis is often associated with the condition known as emphysema. It may also follow repeated attacks of acute bronchitis. It occurs most frequently in the aged and in males. It is the cause of "winter cough" in the aged, and returns with the utmost regularity as soon as the weather gets cold and changeable.

Symptoms. In old men, shortness of breath, especially on exercise, is the most noticeable symptom. They "puff and blow" on going up hill or up a flight of stairs. There is no pain except that due to the cough which comes every autumn and remains all winter. During the summer months there is little cough, and the patient may be quite free from the condition.

In children, chronic bronchitis with cough, usually at night, is a common accompaniment of enlarged tonsils and adenoids.

In the young the condition may persist for years without impairment of health and without apparently damaging the lungs.

Putrid bronchitis is sometimes met with, though, as a rule, evil-smelling expectoration is a sign of bronchiectasis, gangrene, abscess, or tuberculosis.

Dry catarrh is fairly often seen. It is characterized by paroxysms of coughing of great intensity with little or no expectoration.

Treatment. A change to a milder climate will often prevent the attack. California, Arizona and New Mexico, are winter resorts in which the subjects of chronic bronchitis can live with the greatest comfort. With care chronic bronchitis may prove to be only a trivial ailment.

For many years vaccines have been used in the treatment of bronchitis, but they have often proved disappointing. Fortunately bronchitis responds well to the antibiotics, the best one for long-term use being tetracycline (terramycin).

Great care should be taken in the early part of the winter to have clothes of sufficient warmth to give ample protection.

BRONCHITIS KETTLE. In the treatment of bronchitis as well as some other diseases it is necessary to keep the air at a constant moist temperature. To do this a special kettle with a very long spout which expands at the end is used. If one is not obtainable any large domestic kettle may be used with an improvised funnel of brown paper, cardboard or several thicknesses of newspaper. An electric vaporizer may also be used.

BRONCHOPNEUMONIA. Pneumonia which affects the bronchial tubes as well as the lungs is called bronchopneumonia. Pneumonia proper usually starts in the lungs, whereas bronchopneumonia affects more particularly the smaller *bronchioles*. It is more often found in children and the elderly. The condition when it arises in young children is easily recognized and is of a serious nature. The child has the symptoms of a severe cold, but is obviously much more ill than it would be with an uncomplicated cold. It may be very flushed and restless or, in some cases where the toxemia is severe, may be very drowsy. The temperature is high, 103 deg. to 105 deg. F., and the pulse rapid, while the breathing is quickened and noisy and there is a dry cough. Bronchopneumonia is often a complication of infectious diseases, especially of measles, for which reason measles should always be treated seriously. Bronchopneumonia in infants is liable to be fatal; and in older children, though not so dangerous to life, is still a very serious illness and one which may cause future ill health.

Treatment. In the case of an infant or young child, treatment will be on the following lines: the child is kept in bed but may be lifted in the arms occasionally to change its position. The head and shoulders should be slightly raised with an extra pillow to help the breathing. The temperature of the room must be kept the same day and night, and should be about 65 deg. F. A vaporizor should be kept going in order to moisten the air. As the chest must be easily reached without disturbing a very sick child, the night dress must be slit up or open in the front. If the temperature is as high as 105 deg. the child must be sponged from time to time all over in tepid water of a temperature between 85 deg. and 90 deg. The diet should be of milk and water in equal parts with the addition of a couple of teaspoonfuls of sugar of milk, and a teacupful should be given by spoon or bottle every three hours. Water should be given in sips between the feeds. Penicillin, usually given along with streptomycin, has proved very effective in treatment, given in suitable doses and under the careful supervision of a doctor. The bowels should be opened daily by a dose of syrup of figs. Oxygen is life-saving in many cases, and is administered to an adult through a mask which fits over the nose. Infants and children are enclosed in a tent through which a steady flow of the gas is maintained.

BRONCHOSCOPE. This is an instrument for examining the interior of the larger bronchial tubes. It is a tube which is passed down the back of the throat through the larynx and the windpipe. The science of bronchoscopy deals with the use of bronchoscopic tubes and instruments for the purpose of extracting foreign bodies that have been inhaled into the lung, or treating other affections of the lung.

BRONZING. In certain diseases, especially in Addison's disease, the skin becomes pigmented and has a decidedly bronzed appearance. It is also a symptom in exophthalmic goitre, diabetes, and chronic arsenical poisoning.

BRUISES. A bruise is caused by damaging the soft tissues under the unbroken skin. It may be of any severity, from a very slight injury to an extensive, deep-seated, and intensely painful one. In extreme cases, dangerous or even fatal bleeding may occur from damage to an important organ. People who suffer from scurvy, hemophilia ("bleeders"), and fat and anemic females are liable to be bruised from very trivial causes.

In bruising with rupture of a blood-vessel, the blood spreads quickly through the underlying soft tissues. A bluish-black patch results, with pain, tenderness, and swelling. In severe bruises, where there is much stretching of the skin, blisters may form. When the bruise is deep, the extravasated blood takes some time to reach the surface, and the bruise may not show until some days after the injury. Serious bruises may give rise to shock, and if nerves or muscles are damaged, slight paralysis may develop. This is often seen after shoulder injuries.

Most bruises heal readily, during which time the well-known alterations in their color take place, owing to changes in the blood-pigment. If the patient is seen immediately after the accident, the part should be elevated and firm pressure applied by means of an elastic bandage. If, however, a bruise has already formed, rubbing several times daily is the best and most speedy means of dispersing the blood. If the skin is injured, e.g., if blisters have formed, an antiseptic dressing should be put on, and massage only employed after healing takes place.

Cold applications, such as icebags and evaporating lotions, were formerly much advocated, and are certainly soothing. In severe cases of bruising, however, they should be used cautiously, as they are apt to lower vitality of the part, causing it to take longer to heal. (*See also* BLACK EYE.)

BUBO. Bubo describes inflammation or swelling in a lymphatic gland. The term is usually employed in connection with swellings in the groin due to venereal diseases or plague. It may, however, be allied to swelling in other lymphatic glands.

BUBONIC PLAGUE. This is an acute infectious fever caused by the germ called *pasteurella pestis,* which is conveyed by fleas from rats to man. It is more prevalent in the East than in any part of the world. The incubation period may vary between two to ten days, but in the average case symptoms generally appear about three days after invasion of the germ. Onset is generally quite abrupt, marked by a feeling of chilliness, and the temperature may rise to 103 deg. F. or higher. The pulse becomes rapid, and there is severe headache and aching of the limbs. Giddiness is complained of, and the patient usually experiences a loss of muscular control, causing the gait to become staggering. There may be great general weakness and marked mental apathy. In the majority of cases of bubonic plague the glands in the groin become affected, and less frequently other lymphatic glands. The bubo or swelling, which may appear on the groin, is as a rule very painful and may vary from the size of a walnut to the size of a small

orange. The urine generally becomes scanty and there may be traces of albumin present.

Death may occur at any stage of the disease; but in cases which improve, convalescence may be very prolonged. Plague is a disease with a very wide range of symptoms and which is therefore divided into various types. The most effective treatment is with streptomycin by injection.

BUNION. Inflammation of a bursa of the foot, usually in the neighborhood of the big toe, is a very common complaint and can be very painful and crippling. It may be due simply to the pressure of badly fitting footwear, such as boots or shoes that are too narrow or too short, but very often the big toe is deformed by arthritis and the bursa which forms to protect the joint becomes inflamed. Bunions must be treated like other forms of bursitis. (*See also* BURSITIS.)

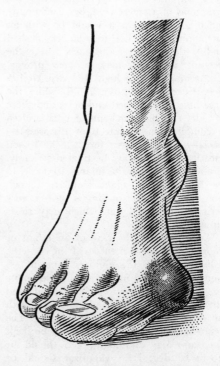

Bunion.

BURNS AND SCALDS. A burn may be caused by dry heat, such as fire or hot metal; by lightning or an electric current; by corrosive acids, such as nitric acid or vitriol; or by corrosive alkalis, such as caustic potash, caustic soda or quicklime.

A scald is caused by moist heat, such as boiling liquids, steam, hot oil or tar. The extent of the damage varies from mere reddening of the surface of the skin to charring of the deep tissues. The amount of damage done depends upon the intensity of the heat and the length of exposure. The chief dangers from burning or scalding are shock and blood poisoning. Even the smallest burn is very painful. The best dressing for a small scald or burn is gauze wrung out in a solution of salt in water, one teaspoonful to the pint. All but minor burns require expert treatment and should be taken to the doctor. The subject is dealt with more fully in the SUPPLEMENT ON FIRST-AID TREATMENT.

BURSA. A small enclosed sac containing clear stricky fluid. These little bags of fluid are found in various parts of the body where two parts would rub on each other. They are placed between the parts to minimize friction. The most usual situation in which they are found is therefore round joints. Bursae are liable to injury and inflammation.

BURSITIS. Inflammation of a bursa is known as bursitis. In acute inflammation the bursa becomes distended with fluid, and the tissues in the neighbourhood become swollen, hot and red. The treatment is similar to that of an acute abscess, hot fomentations and rest being necessary. If pus forms in the bursa it must be let out. In certain occupations the bursa in a particular region may be subject to repeated irritation and a condition of bursitis may become chronic. The commonest forms of chronic bursitis are "housemaid's knee," "miner's elbow" and "weaver's bottom." In these chronic forms of bursitis the movement which causes the irritation to the bursa must be avoided and the part rested. Iodine painted on over the region of the bursa will help to reduce the swelling, and an elastic bandage for support may be very useful.

Persons who habitually carry weights in the same way, like porters, are subject to bursitis in various parts of the back and shoulders.

BUTTER. Butter is a very valuable part of the daily diet and has been in use since very early days. Nowadays the manufacture of butter is a highly skilled proceeding undertaken usually under the supervision of expert chemists and bacteriologists, and butter offered for sale must conform to certain standards laid down by law, and usually reaches the public in as pure a form and as clean a manner as is possible with a foodstuff produced in such large quantities. A good standard of milk is required. The cream is separated from the milk and is pasteurized to kill undesirable germs. It then has the proper organisms added to it in order to acidify it, and when they have ripened it suitably the churning process takes place. After churning the salt is added and it is packaged.

As a food, butter contains a large proportion of the fat soluble Vitamins A and D, and is therefore especially valuable for children who are still growing, since Vitamin A influences the general growth of the tissues and Vitamin D the growth of the bones and teeth.

BUTYRIC ACID. This is an acid with a sharp taste which is present in rancid butter. This acid may form in the stomach owing to indigestion, and its presence generally imparts a very unpleasant odor to the patient's breath.

BYSSINOSIS. Byssinosis is a chronic lung condition, with bronchitis, caused by working in the card-room of a woolen mill and inhaling the tiny particles of wool over a long period.

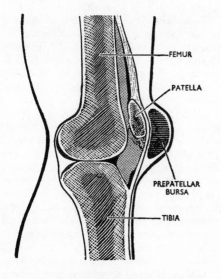

Bursitis.

FEMUR

PATELLA

PREPATELLAR BURSA

TIBIA

CACHEXIA. This term comes from two Greek words and means a bad habit. In medicine the term is applied to conditions in which there is much wasting and general loss of flesh.

CADAVER. Cadaver means a dead body, but the term is applied especially to the dead body of a human being.

CAECUM. The caecum is the first part of the large intestine or bowel. It forms a large pouch with its closed end pointing downwards and its open end communicating directly with the colon. Its average size is about 2½ in. long and 3 in. broad. The appendix is attached to the caecum. (*See also* INTESTINE.)

CAESARIAN SECTION or OPERATION. This is a method by which the child is removed from the mother's body through an opening which is made in the abdominal wall by surgical means. It is frequently necessary to perform this operation when the child cannot be born in the natural way without endangering the life of the mother; as, for example, in cases of obstruction caused by tumors, or of deformities of the pelvis. The death rate from Caesarian section is very small, and if it is properly carried out no serious complications are likely to arise. In many cases both mother and child have been saved from serious injury and even death. The operation gained its name from the fact that Julius Caesar was said to have been born in this manner.

CAFFEINE. This powerful substance is found in the leaves and beans of the coffee tree and in the leaves of tea. In character it is slightly bitter to the taste, and is composed of colorless, silky crystals which dissolve easily in cold water. It is a well-known fact that tea and coffee are stimulants and increase mental alertness, but excessive indulgence may cause excitement and insomnia.

In bronchial asthma, caffeine citrate may be given before bedtime and during the night. It is useful in dropsy due to kidney disease and in heart failure due to pneumonia.

CAISSON DISEASE. This is a condition which occurs in divers and others who work under high atmospheric pressures. Symptoms do not develop until after the diver returns to normal atmospheric pressure. They are produced by the liberation of bubbles of nitrogen gas in the tissues. Airmen flying in rarefied atmospheres over 20,000 ft. suffer in the same way.

Symptoms. In the mildest forms there are headache, giddiness, and fainting which may pass off without any ill-effects. In more severe cases there are agonizing pains in the limbs, joints, and trunk, known by workmen as "the bends," from the position in which the limbs are held. Abdominal pain and distension, with nausea and vomiting, may be due to escape of gas into the intestines. There may be complete paralysis. In severe cases there is vertigo and coma, and death is not uncommon. As a rule, the milder forms, including the "bends," generally recover without any permanent ill effects. Even cases of complete paralysis may recover in a few days, through usually improvement is more gradual.

Fat men should not be employed as caisson workers as they are more liable to be affected than others. To prevent the occurrence of this disease, the workers should pass from the atmosphere of very high pressure to the normal one by means of a series of air-locked chambers, where the pressures are gradually lowered, staying a definite time in each chamber.

Treatment. When symptoms of caisson disease do occur, the patient should be placed in a chamber and the pressure should be raised to that at which he was working. He should then be gradually brought back to the normal atmospheric pressure.

CALABAR BEAN. A powerful drug known as physostigmine or eserine salicylate is obtained from the calabar bean. Physostigmine applied locally to the eye causes the pupil to contract, and is used extensively by oculists in the treatment of certain eye disorders, especially glaucoma. It has been given internally for chronic constipation, and for chronic bronchitis when there is not enough expectoration. If it is given in large doses this drug acts as a poison, and causes death from asphyxia.

CALAMINE. The natural zinc carbonate when washed and pulverized forms a smooth powder which is known as calamine. It is an excellent treatment for skin diseases and may be made up as a lotion, or prepared with petroleum jelly as an ointment.

CALCIFEROL. The pure substance isolated as Vitamin D is the product of the action of ultraviolet rays of light on a substance, ergosterol, contained in most living cells and foodstuffs. (*See also* VITAMINS.)

CALCIUM. Calcium is best known as the carbonate limestone or chalk. Calcium chloride is used to increase the clotting power of the blood. It is employed in itching skin affections such as urticaria, pruritus and prurigo, and is said to be useful in the treatment of chilblains, small doses being taken at frequent intervals. Calcium carbonate and calcium phosphate in equal parts, a teaspoonful thrice daily, is an excellent remedy for diarrhea of gastric origin. Calcium carbonate is extensively employed in conjunction with magnesium carbonate in the treatment of gastric and duodenal ulcers. Lime water is used in the preparation of milk for infant feeding, as it reduces the size of the curds: 1 to ½ teaspoonful should be used. Lime water may be taken by adults in doses of 1 to 4 fluid ounces for acidity of the stomach or to check looseness of the bowels.

Used externally, the prepared chalk of calcium may be used as a dusting powder.

CALCULUS. Calculus is the term applied to a stone-like material found in the body, particularly in cavities of the body. These stones or *calculi* are most commonly found in the bladder, gall-bladder, kidneys, and ureters; they are sometimes present in the pancreas. The stone may be of various substances cemented together, such as uric acid, phosphates or calcium. Generally there is an original cause such as infection, a foreign body, remains of blood corpuscles, or fatty tissue. The calculi vary greatly in shape and may be sand, gravel, or stones, according to size. So long as the calculus stays in the cavity in which it has formed it may give rise to no symptoms whatever, but immediately it begins to move intense pain is felt. (*See also* BILIARY COLIC; GALLSTONE.)

CALLUS. A callus, or callosity, like a corn, is a thickening of the horny layer of the skin, but unlike a corn it has no core, and merges into the surrounding skin. Callosites appear on the feet or hands, and are due to friction and pressure.

Treatment. On the feet they occur when badly fitting shoes are worn; not only shoes that are too tight, but those that are too loose can produce callosities, following blisters due to the constant friction. The remedy here is obvious. They also occur in some deformities of the feet where one part of the foot has to take all the pressure. In these cases (unless operative treatment can relieve the situation) it is best to take the advice of an orthopedic surgeon (who is skilled in curing deformities) as to the type of footwear necessary. As a simple instance, flat foot is frequently accompanied by a troublesome callus under the head on the middle toe; this is relieved by specially made shoes. The cost is little more than that of ordinary good shoes. It will generally be found that with properly fitting shoes calluses gradually disappear, but if any further measures need to be taken the treatment described under CORNS will be found suitable. It is, naturally, far easier to remove a callus, as here there is no troublesome core. Some patients find an ordinary ring-pad, such as is used for corns, useful when the callus is small. A swelling called a bursa may form beneath a callus, and, if it becomes inflamed, may be a very troublesome complication, causing much suffering. If neglected, it discharges through the skin and an inflamed passage remains, resembling an ulcer.

Calluses are also seen very frequently on the hands, most commonly on the "pads" at the base of the fingers. They are seen in athletes, such as rowers, baseball and tennis players, or gymnasts, and are produced by various trades—carpenters', blacksmiths' and so on. Harp and other wire-stringed instrument players show some degree of callus at the ends of the fingers, where their "trade-pressure" occurs. Chemical injuries occurring frequently in the course of work, such as with acids or brine, frequently produce calluses.

As on the feet, calluses form on the hands as a kind of natural armor, to protect against irritation, and usually give no trouble except that they are unsightly. It is best to leave them alone unless the person is prepared to give up his work or his games, as more harm than good would be done by removing a protective layer and continuing to expose the skin to irritation. They have, however, the disadvantage that the sense of touch over the affected parts is diminished; and also that, in the dry and horny skin, cracks not infrequently occur, which penetrate to the true skin and become very painful. The treatment for these is mentioned under CHAPPED HANDS AND LIPS.

CALOMEL. Mercurous chloride, more commonly known as calomel, is a heavy white powder used as a purgative. It is powerful in effect, and is given in a dose of ½ to 3 grains. The milder vegetable laxatives are better for routine use. It should be given at bedtime and should be followed by a morning glass of salts. Calomel is often dusted on ulcers or sores, especially if they are of syphilitic origin.

CALORIE. Calorie is the name given to a heat unit, and is the amount of heat required to raise the temperature of 1 gram of pure water by 1 deg. C. For certain practical purposes, as, for example, in determining food values, the large Calorie is used, and this is the amount of heat required to heat 1 kilogram of water 1 deg. C. Though, correctly, a capital "C" should be used in speaking of these values, it has become customary to express them as "calories," but it must always be remembered that this food Calorie is one thousand times as large as the unit used in physical studies. (See Appendix 2: Table of Foods and their Neutrient Values.)

CAMPHOR. Camphor is a white crystalline substance obtained from the camphor laurel which grows in Formosa and Japan. Oil of camphor is of a pale yellow color, with a fragrant odor. Camphor is powdered by rubbing it with a few drops of alcohol. Its stimulating effects make camphor a favorite ingredient in many liniments. It is frequently used in the treatment of chronic rheumatism, lumbago, neuralgia and in the chest complaints of children.

Camphor Poisoning (Symptoms). Large doses of camphor may cause excitement, giddiness, staggering, and in some persons a feeling of exhilaration similar to the effect of alcohol. In severe cases the pulse generally becomes much slower; there may

be severe pains in the stomach and head, faintness, delirium, convulsions, and finally death from collapse.

Treatment. An emetic should be given, followed by strong tea or coffee. The patient should be kept as warm as possible with hot-water bottles.

CANCER. The human body is subject to tumor growths of various sorts. These are divided into two classes, benign growths and malignant growths. Benign growths are all the cysts and tumors which do not shorten life. Malignant growths are those which cause a great deal of damage to the body and when untreated lead to death. The general health is greatly impaired, and the organ, such as the stomach or liver, in which the cancer is growing becomes less and less able to carry on its work until the day comes when it can no longer function at all. They are also apt to spread to other parts of the body and to return after they have been cut out. Malignant growths are of two sorts, carcinomas and sarcomas, but for convenience they are generally referred to simply as "cancer."

Cancer is largely a disease of middle and old age, but sometimes occurs in young people. When younger people are attacked by cancer it usually runs a much quicker course than in older persons, and may be considered an acute disease. In older persons, when it is discovered too late to operate upon successfully it can still often be held at bay and alleviated for a great number of years.

It is often said that cancer is a disease of civilization. It is true that there is a larger proportion of cases in the so-called civilized countries than amongst the less civilized races, but it is by no means unknown among primitive races, and as it is so much more a disease of old age than of youth it is possible that in civilized countries more people are kept alive until the cancerous age. The same thing applies to the increase in the number of deaths from cancer. It is obvious that as fewer people are allowed to die from other causes, such as consumption, and more people are kept alive to the age of fifty, there must be an increase in the number of deaths from cancer until some means is discovered of curing cancer at a later stage in its course.

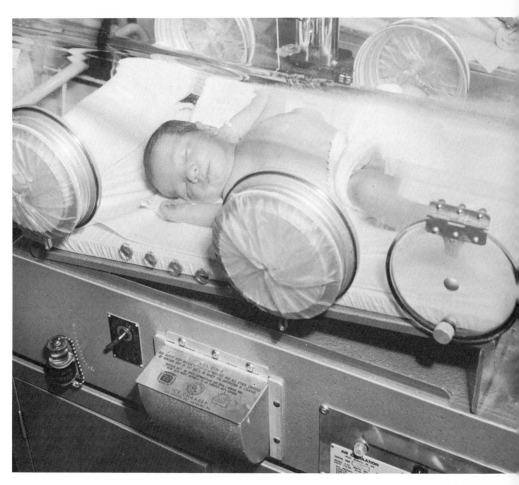

An incubator carefully protects the premature infant's
fragile health.

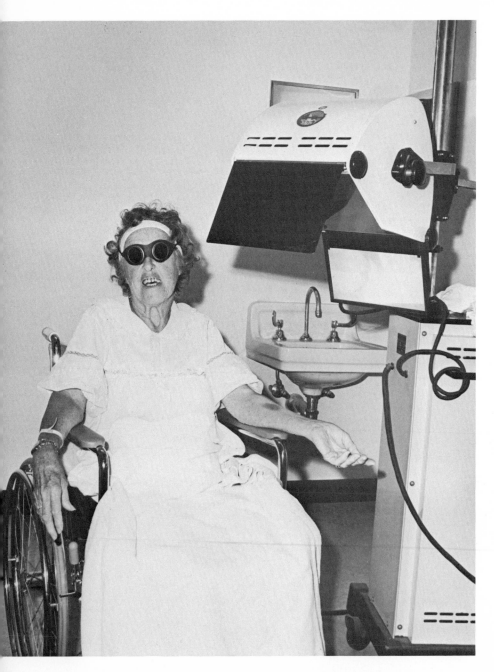

The use of X-ray therapy has proven successful in the treatment of many diseases.

It may be pointed out here, however, that cure of cancer after it has taken a good hold can only amount to getting rid of the tumor by some such means as surgically cutting it out and great damage may be done to the surrounding parts before the cancer is discovered. By far the more important thing is to prevent cancer from occurring at all, or to discover its presence at a very early stage.

Different Kinds of Cancer. The difference between carcinoma and sarcoma lies in the character of the cells of which they are composed. The whole human body is composed of millions of cells. These cells are described in a separate article and it is sufficient here to state that the life of a cell in the body is like the life of the body itself. The cell begins, grows and develops and finally dies and is succeeded by other cells. Like bodies there are normal cells and abnormal cells, that is, well and sick cells. There are also cells of different types, like people of different races. The two most important groups of cells are first the group containing the cells forming the skin, the linings of the mouth and various organs and passages of the body and the glands. The other group consists of the cells forming the connective tissue or, generally, the flesh, and the tissue composing such parts of the general framework of the body as the bones, muscles, and gristle. A malignant growth of the first group of cells is called a *carcinoma* and of the second group a *sarcoma*. Both sorts of growth are popularly grouped together and called *cancer*.

Of carcinomas and sarcomas, the carcinomas are by far the more numerous. Sarcomas develop in the tissue surrounding bones, muscles, etc., while carcinomas attack glands, organs such as the stomach, and soft parts like the lip, and the skin itself. Skin cancers are described later in this section.

As well as the breast, womb, stomach, lung, which are the most frequent sites, cancer is found frequently in the intestines and rectum, gall bladder, liver, larynx, tongue, esophagus (the passage from the mouth to the stomach), and bones.

Occupational Cancers. People engaged in certain occupations run a greater risk of contracting cancer than others, and in these cases the cancer is almost certainly due to constant irritation of a part either directly, or as the result of a frequently used chemical substance. For example, in cotton-mills, mule-spinner's cancer is a form which occurs in male workers. This cancer arises in the scrotum and is due to constant irritation of the part by the continued saturation of the clothes with the lubricating oil used. Precautions are now taken to prevent this trouble. Workers with rubber may get cancerous growths on the skin, and all workers with tar products, such as creosote, benzine and paraffin are liable to cancer.

What Cancer Is. It is not known what causes cancer, but the effect of whatever causes it is to make groups of the cells grow in an irregular fashion. The tissues of the body, which include everything except bone, fluids, and oddments like nails and hair, are made up of living cells which grow in a definite manner, and are destroyed and repaired in an orderly fashion. In the normal person, when cancer invades the body from its unknown source, certain of these cells begin to grow in an unusual manner. They grow more quickly, are imperfect in form and are arranged differently. The become more powerful than the normal cells around them and begin to destroy them, feed upon them and eat them up, as it were. From a small lump the tumor grows until the whole cavity of the organ it has attacked is filled up and the organ is of no further use.

There is no evidence that cancer is infectious, though it often happens that several members of the same family die of this complaint. Nor has it been proved to be hereditary, though frequently children of cancerous parents may die of cancer. It is much more likely that it is the same faulty hygiene, diet, and manner of living, together perhaps with some similar weakness of constitution which is shared by different members of the family, which is responsible for their suffering from the same disease.

Causes of Cancer. The causes of cancer are as yet unknown, except that constant irritation of a part seems to be directly responsible for a certain number of cancers, such as the trade cancers. There is no doubt whatever that excess smoking, especially of cigarettes, is the chief factor in the cause of cancer of the lung, as was clearly shown in the Royal College of Physicians Report in 1962 and in the U.S. Surgeon General's report in 1964. It is thought by some workers carrying out research on the subject that there may be a definite cancer virus or germ, which like other germs gains admittance to the body and settles in a weak spot, but this theory has never been proved. It has been shown that the sex hormones have some relation to certain types of cancer, and cancer of the prostate may be controlled by the administration of stilbestrol. Chemists, physicists, microbiologists are continuing researches into the causes of cancer together with a great band of skilled medical research workers all over the world. Much work also is being done in the great hospitals and in research laboratories. It would seem that it is only a question of time until the cause of cancer becomes known and then its prevention and cure by medical means may well become comparatively simple.

Early Diagnosis of Cancer. It is very important that cancer should be diagnosed as soon as possible so that treatment can be undertaken at the earliest possible moment. This is unfortunately often a difficult matter, as there is very little to attract the victim's attention to the condition in its early stages. Pain is not an early symptom in most forms, and quite a large cancer may grow without causing any noticeable pain whatsoever. A lump may be noticed in the breast, but in the deep organs of the body the tumor has usually reached a large size before it is felt. In the majority of cases the first thing that draws attention to the cancer is that it has begun to interfere with the working of some organ, and the patient goes to the doctor complaining of some trouble such as indigestion, difficulty in breathing, difficulty in swallowing, or irregular discharges and bleeding from the womb, or increasing weakness and loss of weight. It will be seen, therefore, that it must necessarily be difficult to recognise cancer patients at an early enough stage, unless people are encouraged to have periodical medical examinations, and are brought to see the folly of neglecting even small symptoms of ill health. Even more difficult is the case of

persons who have been accustomed for years to a slight degree of ill health, such as chronic nervous dyspepsia or irregular actions of the bowels. These people frequently do not notice themselves at what point their chronic discomfort turns into permanent and definite disease, at which time it is perhaps too late.

Cancer in Women. It is generally known that more women are attacked by cancer than men. This is because the reproductive organs play so much larger a part in women than in men, and the womb and breasts are very liable to cancerous growths.

The cares of a house and family mean, for many women, that for their childbearing period, and until the family grows up, their own health and comfort must take a secondary place. Hence the great frequency of the tragedy in which the mother, having seen her family grow up successfully, begins to take notice of her own vague pains and discomforts only to find that it is too late.

Treatment of Cancer. The most successful treatment for cancer known at present is complete removal by operation at an early stage, and as so much depends upon the earliness of the operation, not a day should be wasted unnecessarily after the diagnosis has been made. Some authorities prefer treatment by "deep" X-rays or radium, as a means not only of slowing the growth and rendering the patient more comfortable, but actually of cure, though operation has the most advocates. Radium treatment is better than operation, however, in some cases such as cancer of the tongue. The truth is that both radium and X-ray treatment give good results in early cases of cancer, but it is not known yet how long such cures last and operation is more certain—at any rate, up to the present. In late cases of cancer, where little can be done but perform "palliative" operations to make the patient more comfortable, a great deal can be done by X-rays and radium to give relief. Mention has already been made of the encouraging results in cancer of the prostate which have followed the administration by mouth of stilbestrol, a synthetic sex hormone. More recently a chemical known as nitrogen mustard, when injected into a vein, has been found to produce shrinkage of certain cancers in parts remote from the site of infection. These heartening discoveries lead us to believe that the solution to the puzzle of cancer lies not far away. (*See also* BREAST, CANCER OF.)

Secondary Cancer. This is a cancer that arises from cancer of some other organ by direct growth or by means of the lymph channels. Both these processes are very well seen in long-standing cancer of the breast, where not only the substance of the breast, but also the overlying skin, shows firm nodules of growth, and the lymph glands under the arm and about the collar-bone become enlarged and firm, showing that they, too, are affected. Cancer cells may be borne by the bloodstream to a distant tissue, forming another type of "secondary growth."

Cancer of the skin. The skin, like every other part of the body, is afflicted with tumors or "new growths." These may be divided, for convenience of description, into the harmless or *benign* growths such as warts and moles which cause no risk to life, but may be disfiguring or troublesome from their size or position on the body; and the harmful or *malignant* growth, which, if unchecked, will inevitably cause the death of the patient, just as does a malignant growth in any other part. They are all familiarly called "cancer of the skin," though there are several varieties which begin in different ways.

Cancer of the skin arises from an overgrowth of a group of the cells making up the skin tissue. For some reason, these begin to grow rapidly, using the neighboring healthy cells for food, and often spread to other parts: in short, they behave like an invading army of lawless marauders—an army that is too often, alas, victorious over the law-abiding body cells! (*See also* EPITHELIOMA.)

CANCRUM ORIS or CANKER OF THE MOUTH. This is a disease of the mouth which generally appears in childhood between the ages of one and five. The patient is usually in a very debilitated state owing to some disease such as measles, diphtheria, scarlet fever or whooping cough. Deep, foul ulcers appear on the inner side of the cheek and may spread rapidly and pierce through the cheek. The gums and lips may be similarly affected. The tem-perature is usually very high, and in cases where there is general blood poisoning or bronchopneumonia, the patient may even die. The disease is due to germs and unhygienic surroundings.

CANITES. This is a term applied to blanching or whitening of the hair. (*See also* HAIR.)

CANNABIS INDICA. Cannabis indica is an Indian hemp from which a powerful drug is obtained, which is also known as *hashish* or *bhang*. It acts as an antispasmodic and a narcotic or sleep-producing drug. The patient may have a sensation of mild intoxication, feeling very gay and pleased with everything, but when taken to excess it leads to loss of appetite, trembling of the limbs, and insanity. Very large doses have been recovered from, however, and no death from cannabis indica is on record.

It is used in medicine in the form of a tincture or of an extract, and may be administered in cases of neuralgia and migraine. It is also useful in the treatment of colics, whooping cough, and painful menstruation.

CANNULA. A cannula is a tube used for withdrawing fluids from the body. A double cannula is used to wash out a cavity of the body: one tube being used for the inflow of a fluid and the other tube for the outflow.

CAPILLARIES. The tiny blood-vessels of the body are called *capillaries.*
They continue the circulation of the blood between the smallest arteries and the smallest veins, called the *arterioles* and the *venules,* and are so small that they cannot be seen with the naked eye. The capillaries form dense networks throughout the tissues of the body. They are thickest in size just under the skin, and smallest in the linings of the organs deep in the body, and in the brain. The number of capillaries in any given organ depends upon the need of that organ for blood. The denser the network of capillaries the greater is the supply of blood.

The structure of the capillaries is interesting. They consist of walls made up of a single layer of cells whose margins are joined together with a cementing substance. The capillaries branch out from the walls of the arteries and veins, and from the arteries they obtain blood rich with oxygen and nutritive materials. The walls of the capillaries are able to pass oxygen, carbonic acid and nourishing materials from the blood through their walls into the tissues for the purpose of feeding the tissues. Similarly the capillaries collect waste materials out of the tissues, which they return to the veins for destruction and excretion from the body. The white blood-corpuscles or leucocytes, which protect the body by attacking disease germs which have found their way into the blood-stream, are able to pass through the capillary walls, backwards and forwards between the blood and the tissues. (*See also* ARTERY; BLOOD; LEUCO-CYTES.)

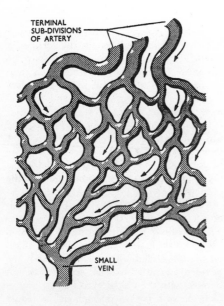

TERMINAL
SUB-DIVISIONS
OF ARTERY

SMALL
VEIN

Capillaries.

CARBOHYDRATE. One of the largest and most important groups of substances from which the body obtains its food is the group of carbohydrates, which are so called from the fact that they contain carbon, hydrogen and oxygen. Carbohydrate is the body's principal source of heat and energy. Every cell in the course of its normal working, whether this be the production of muscular energy or the secretion of some natural juice, consumes carbohydrate with the liberation of heat. Whatever the food source of carbohydrate, it is absorbed from the gut and used in the form of a simple sugar.

The principal carbohydrate foods are sugar and sweetstuffs, and the starchy foods such as bread, grain cereals, rice, and potatoes. At different times the body will require different amounts of carbohydrates. In winter more will be required than in summer, and the individual who has to perform much physical exertion will need more than the person who leads a sedentary life. (*See also* DIGESTION.)

CARBOLIC ACID. Carbolic acid or *phenol* is obtained by distilling and purifying coaltar. It may be obtained as colorless crystals with a peculiar smell and a sweetish, pungent taste. When they are treated with about 6 per cent of water these crystals become fluid and are carbolic acid as we know it. Carbolic is a powerful caustic and irritant, and when applied to the skin in concentrated form will cause burning and pain. A white spot may appear on the part, which becomes red when the acid is removed. Externally, carbolic is largely used as a deodorant and disinfectant. The raw acid may be used for disinfecting drains, bedpans, etc. A week solution is used to wash wounds to keep them antiseptic, and mosquito bites may be relieved by the application of weak carbolic. It is also useful in keeping the mosquitoes away. Carbolic cleanses, heals, disinfects, and allays pain. Carbolized gauze and carbolized lint are also prepared and used frequently for dressings for wounds.

Poisoning by Carbolic Acid. Carbolic acid may be absorbed through the skin and mucous membranes. Poisoning has often occurred as a result of the prolonged use of carbolized dressings, or if the carbolic acid has been taken internally. On swallowing, an intense burning pain may be felt in the mouth, gullet and stomach, and white ulcerated areas may appear in the mouth. The skin becomes cold and clammy, and breathing gradually becomes more and more feeble and finally stops. Treatment consists of washing out the stomach several times with 10 per cent alcohol and water. Apomorphine is a suitable emetic. White of egg and large doses of any harmless oil may be given. Chalk and limewater and caffeine are also antidotes. The patient must be kept as warm as possible by the use of hot-water bottles or electric pads. Medical aid should be called in as early as possible.

CARBON DIOXIDE. Carbon dioxide is a gas also known as carbonic-acid gas or carbonic acid. This gas must be given off by the body if health and life are to be continued. It is of great value if breathing is difficult in the newborn child, and it has been given to stimulate the breathing in cases of opium poisoning and pulmonary collapse.

Any atmosphere which is overcharged with carbonic acid may produce symptoms of headache, loss of appetite and lack of energy. When it is inhaled in a pure form, death results from asphyxia.

Carbon-dioxide Snow. This may be made from the gas which has been allowed to escape from a cylinder into some suitable receptacle. The snow can be molded so as to form a pencil, which may be applied to birth-marks, port-wine stains, lupus or rodent ulcers. The application is usually for about half a minute or a little longer. (*See also* ANESTHESIA, LOCAL.)

CARBON MONOXIDE. Carbon monoxide is a very poisonous, odorless gas. It is the dangerous gas given off in the exhaust of an automobile, and by oil burning lamps and heaters. In extreme cases death may occur very quickly and artificial respiration may prove of no avail, owing to the difficulty of separating the gas from the blood. The presence of this gas is very treacherous in coal mines, as miners may go on working in a poisoned atmosphere without being aware of it. Many people who have gone to sleep in a closed automobile or have otherwise breathed air overcharged with carbon monoxide have gradually become unconscious and died from the poisoning.

When entering a room filled with gas in order to rescue a person, the mouth and nose should be covered with a damp cloth and the windows should be thrown open immediately. On no account should an open flame be used. The person should be dragged or carried out into the fresh air, the clothing loosened as much as possible, and artificial respiration started. The doctor should be called as soon as possible and he will see that inhalation of oxygen gas is given when necessary.

CARBUNCLE. A carbuncle is an inflammatory condition of the skin and tissues under the skin, and is usually due to infection by a germ known as the staphylococcus. The carbuncle usually starts as a simple boil or group of boils, often at the root of a hair on the skin, but it spreads rapidly to the tissues around and under the original boil and may become very large. Occasionally it spreads inwards and downwards and may burrow in any direction. The carbuncle forms a hard swelling which is dark red in color, very hot and tender to the touch, and painful. Pus forms at several points, and if the carbuncle is left without proper attention the skin may become riddled with sinuses and the whole region may become a soft, boggy mass of pus and dead tissue, which will leave an unsightly hole when the carbuncle finally heals up. In cases that are at all severe, the patient becomes very ill with a high temperature, rapid pulse rate, constipation, and furred tongue. There may be severe poisoning of the system, causing restlessness and loss of sleep and perhaps delirium. The condition may rapidly become dangerous to life, especially in elderly or debilitated persons. Cases where there are two or more carbuncles at the same time, or where the carbuncle is on the lip or face or behind the ear, are especially dangerous to life.

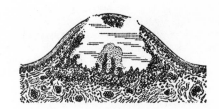

Carbuncle.

Treatment. The treatment is, in the less severe cases, the same as for a boil. Hot applications, such as kaolin or poultices, or better still, a radian-heat lamp, should be continued until the matter comes to the surface, when it may be allowed to escape through small incisions. The wound is sprayed twice daily with hydrogen peroxide to remove the dead tissues, and is dressed with clean gauze or boracic fomentations.

As soon as the condition is recognized, however, for it is apt to be serious, the doctor should give injections of penicillin, or one of the other antibiotics, such as terramycin or aureomycin, by the mouth. Surgical treatment may be necessary.

Carbuncles sometimes occur in persons who are already suffering from kidney diseases, diabetes, or chronic alcoholism, and in such cases they are apt to be especially dangerous, as the patient has not sufficient strength to throw off the infection. (*See also* ABSCESS; BOIL.)

CARCINOMA. Carcinoma is the most frequent form of cancer. It is described under the heading CANCER.

CARDIAC. This is an adjective meaning anything to do with the heart, as, for instance, cardiac weakness, cardiac murmur, or cardiac stimulant. The heart and its diseases are described under the heading HEART.

CARIES. The term caries means decay, and is usually used in connection with decay of teeth, or bones. The cause of the decay in bone may be inflammation due to invasion by septic germs, syphilis, or tuberculosis. If septic organisms are present there will be a discharge of pus or matter. Dental caries is quite different from that occurring in bone, and a description will be found under its own heading. (*See also* NECROSIS; TEETH.)

CARMINATIVE. Any drug which produces a feeling of warmth and which relieves the feeling of overfullness in the stomach is known as a carminative. These drugs act by relaxing the muscles of the stomach and intestines. The taking of liqueurs at the end of a meal is a well-known example of the carminative action. The principal drugs of this class are the volatile oils. Other examples of carminatives are aniseed, allspice, cloves, cinnamon, bitter orange and dill.

CAROTENE. A yellow pigment contained in carrots, tomatoes, spinach, and other vegetables, which when taken into the body is converted into Vitamin A by the liver, and is secreted in milk.

CAROTID ARTERY. The two great arteries down each side of the neck are called the carotids, or common carotids, and by them blood is carried to the head and neck. The right common carotid artery

rises from the *innominate artery,* where it branches off from the *aorta* just behind the junction of the breastbone and collarbone. It travels upwards until a point at the level of the larynx, or Adam's apple, is reached, when it divides into two main branches, the *external carotid* and the *internal carotid.*

The left common carotid artery rises from the uppermost part of the *arch of the aorta* and travels upwards to the same distance as the right common carotid, where it also splits into the left external and internal carotid. The external carotids supply the scalp, the face and the greater part of the neck, while the internal carotids feed parts within the skull and the cavities which contain the eyes. Aneurisms of the carotid artery are not often met with, but when they do occur they press on the wind-pipe and larynx and cause breathlessness and sometimes difficulty in swallowing. (*See also* AORTA; ARTERY.)

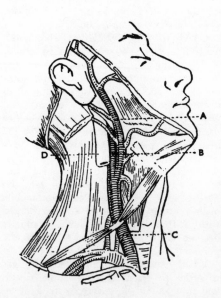

Carotid Artery: A. *External Carotid;* B. *Internal Carotid;* C. *Common Carotid;* D. *Jugular Vein.*

CARRIER. It sometimes happens that a person may harbor dangerous germs in his body and yet remain in good health. These harborers of germs are known as "carriers." In some cases they have never actually had an attack of the disease of which they carry the germs. More often they have suffered from infection and continue to excrete the germ after apparent cure or during convalescence. Germs of diphtheria or cerebrospinal fever may thus be carried in the throat for years, and germs of typhoid fever or dysentery may be present in the stools. Sometimes the germ carried is not one of any particular disease, but may be a virulent streptococcus or staphylococcus germ which will cause severe infection or inflammation if it is conveyed to a delicate person or operation case. Where the germ is carried in the nose or throat, the tonsils should be removed and measures taken to improve the health of these parts. Typhoid or dysentery carriers should be treated as they would be for the disease and all known carriers should be kept strictly away from kitchens, invalid nursing, or any means whereby they can spread infection.

CARTILAGE. Cartilage, which is commonly known as gristle, is found in various parts of the body, chiefly in joints. The walls of the chest, the wind-pipe, the bronchial tubes, and the structure of the nose and ears are of cartilage. Most of the bones of the body develop from cartilage, which is replaced by bone as the infant grows older. This type of cartilage is called *temporary*. The cartilage in joints is called *articular* and it is of great importance in the structure of movable joints. If two bones were to rub continually against each other they would in time wear their surfaces away and thus would no longer fit tightly enough to make a useful joint. To prevent this rubbing, the end of each bone in a joint is coated with articular cartilage, which is a pearly bluish-white colour, smooth and elastic, and serves to break the force of concussions and enables the bones to glide smoothly one against the other.

The cartilages which form the ends of the ribs where they join on to the breast-bone and the cartilage in the nose, larynx, etc., are of a stronger and tougher variety, and are liable in old age to *calcify*, that is, grow hard and bony owing to becoming pickled, as it were, in calcium salts. The cartilage of joints is subject to tuberculous disease. The cartilages become very sensi-

tive and when the joints are completely relaxed, as at the moment of going to sleep, the cartilages lie on each other and their pressure causes sharp pain and abrupt awakening, which is one of the most distressing symptoms of this condition.

Certain joints of the hinge variety have small separate pads of cartilage, each of which is called a *meniscus*. These menisci are easily dislocated and cause pain and loss of power in the joint until they are replaced. The commonest of these dislocations are those of the semilunar cartilage of the knee and the cartilage of the jaw.

CASCARA SAGRADA. Cascara sagrada, or sacred bark, is the dried bark of the Californian buckthorn, collected at least one year before being used. It is a very serviceable drug for the treatment of constipation. Its great advantage is that gradually increasing doses are not required. The liquid extract is very bitter, but this can be circumvented by taking the drug in capsule form, or the taste may be concealed by various aromatic substances, a well-known palatable preparation being cascara evacuant. Cascara sagrada acts as a tonic to the bowel and does not purge or cause unnecessary pains. The drug should be taken on retiring at night and continued for about ten days, gradually lessening the dose until finally the medicine may be stopped altogether. For constipation in a child, try one to three drops in syrup, one to three times a day.

CASEIN. The chief protein constituent of milk is known as casein; it is much the same thing as white of egg, but contains more nitrogen and a greater amount of phosphorus. Casein is converted into an insoluble protein, the curd, by the action of acids and rennet. First the rennet converts it into a substance known as paracasein. Then the paracasein mixes with the calcium salts of the milk and forms the curd. In human milk the curd is much less firm than in cow's milk. The value of this curdling action is not apparent, but it is believed that casein in the solid form may stay longer in the stomach and thus be submitted to gastric digestion, instead of passing promptly into the duodenum, as happens with liquid material. The action of rennet goes no further than the curdling; the digestion of the curd is carried on by pepsin, a digestive substance found in the gastric juice.

In order to obtain a light, easily-digested curd, milk may be diluted with soda water, and for a baby's bottle may be diluted by adding lime-water.

CASTOR OIL. One of the most useful drugs we possess is castor oil, which is obtained from a plant that grows freely in India. The oil is abstracted from the seeds of the castor oil plant (*Ricinus communis*) and is colorless or pale yellow. It is exceedingly disagreeable to take in an undisguised form, but since it is so very valuable as a medicine the patient would be well advised to make up his mind both to swallow it and to keep it down when it is swallowed.

Castor oil is so useful because it is almost the only purge which will clear the bowel thoroughly with one dose of medicine, and it does not cause unpleasant griping pains. For this reason it is used when some doubtful article of food has been eaten and it is desired to get it thoroughly cleared out, or in cases where the intestine is being irritated by something which has not been removed by other aperients.

The action of castor oil is lubricating as well as aperient, so that a smooth and effortless movement of the bowels is obtained without any of the violent muscular contractions that are caused by doses of other aperients such as aloes. For this reason castor oil is a useful opening medicine for pregnant women. Young children, too, take it very well. It is most useful in the single dose method, because if taken continuously it has a binding effect on the bowels.

The chief tip to help the squeamish to get it down is to avoid getting the smell and taste of it. One method is to hold the nose, approach the spoon to the mouth and gulp it down. The taste, however, is almost as bad as the smell, so pour a few drops of peppermint water, brandy, lemon juice, or coffee in the bottom of the medicine glass, pour in the castor oil, and cover with more of the brandy or whatever has been used. In this way the whole quantity will slide down the throat without the oil being tasted. Castor-oil can now be obtained in capsules and there are also many preparations on the market in which the taste and smell are reduced to a mini-mum. The dose of castor oil for an adult is 2–8 teaspoonfuls, and half a teaspoonful or more can be given to an infant.

CATALEPSY. This is a condition in which there is a blind obedience to any suggestion made. People so affected will imitate any action seen; they will repeat like parrots any short sentences spoken to them; and they will allow their limbs to remain placed in any awkward position. While they are apparently quite happy, or at any rate do not seem to mind, patients with catalepsy will hold any position in which they are placed for several hours without obviously getting tired. In many cases there is also an obedience to orders, however absurd, or however dangerous their nature. This is something like the condition which is seen in people who have been deeply hypnotized, but goes beyond it. Catalepsy is more often seen in people suffering from a grave mental disorder, dementia praecox, but it may also occur occasionally in the course of some forms of hysteria. There is usually no difficulty in deciding from which trouble the patient is suffering, as in the more severe condition other signs are present. Also, it is rare for catalepsy to persist for more than a few days except in dementia praecox.

CATARACT. The lens of the eye is a crystalline substance, rounded on both sides, and placed just behind the iris or colored part of the eye. It focuses the image of an object looked at upon the retina. (*See also* EYE.)

Cataract is a disease in which vision is more or less obscured because the lens of the eye becomes opaque, or, rather, loses its transparency. The patient "sees through a glass darkly." This intransparency is caused by the formation of minute drops of albuminous fluid among the fibers of the lens. These fibers are arranged on one another like the leaves of a book. The lens grows slightly all through life, and the increase would be greater than it is but for a process known as condensation, which is always going on. In childhood the lens is soft, but from the age of about twenty-five the central parts become harder, forming what is called a nucleus, while the outer part, or cortex, remains soft. At thirty this process is readily seen when the eye is examined, and it goes on, becoming more and more marked until at about the age of seventy all is nucleus. As the nucleus hardens the pupil of a middle-aged person begins to look greyish, while that of a child is perfectly black. This smoky appearance, which is quite normal, is sometimes mistakenly taken to mean cataract.

Cataract is a very common disease; it has been estimated that it is present in 96 per cent of people over sixty, but it is usually so slight that it gives rise to no trouble. Sometimes, however, the density of the lens increases, and the patient has what is known as a *hard or senile cataract*. It begins usually at about fifty-five or sixty. It is commonly thought that senile cataract is hereditary, or occurs as a result of other diseases of the eye, both of which ideas are incorrect. Cataract is so common, as has been seen, that it is easy to imagine heredity to be a factor; and doubtless other eye disease may be present in an elderly eye, but it occurs quite independently of these.

Roughly speaking, there is only one symptom, that of increasing difficulty of sight. This is worse in a bright light, because then the pupil contracts, and the patient is only using the central portion of the lens, wherein is the worst of the opacity. He often walks with bent head, and shades his face with his hand, in order to cause enlargement of the pupils. In the great majority of cases both eyes are affected, though the cataract is not necessarily equally advanced; this point is of considerable importance when treatment is to be decided upon. When the cataract is advanced, and practically the whole lens is affected, the appearance is as if the pupil were filled with ground glass. "Black" cataract, so called, only differs from the ordinary form in the color of the lens, which in old people may gradually assume a dark brown or black discoloration.

The various treatments that have been tried to prevent or retard cataract are legion, but none of them is of the slightest use. Two palliative or "relieving" measures only need be noticed. One is a preliminary operation (iridectomy), which is favored by some surgeons; the other is the use of atropine drops in very weak strength, which assist in dilating the pupil, and so give better sight for the time being by illuminating the outer and less affected portions of the lens. Atropine must be used with very great care, and only under medical supervision, or a disease known as *glaucoma* might be caused. Indeed, some specialists entirely forbid its use in any patient over forty unless the tension (or hardness) of the eye is low.

Treatment before operation. The only cure, as is generally known, is to wait until the cataract is "ripe" and then to have it removed by operation. The ripening may take a considerable time, the usual being two to three years. An eye specialist will, of course, decide when the time has come to operate, but as a general rule the cataract is ready when the patient has lost his reading power. In other words, the lens is sufficiently hard to be removed. If "overripe," further changes take place in the lens and its capsule or covering, and an operation then is not nearly so satisfactory as one performed at the proper time.

Before operation is finally decided upon, however, several factors must be taken into account. The age of the patient, for example, will affect such a decision. A man of seventy-five or eighty has not a very long expectation of life, and also, at that age, changes in the cataract are exceedingly slow, so that it is often best to operate rather early. The state of the general health, too, is of very great importance: such complications as chronic bronchitis, with its troublesome cough; deafness, which is a most awkward extra disability; a large amount of sugar in the urine (a little does not matter, as it so often occurs in elderly people); albumen in any quantity in the urine; skin disease affecting the face; great feebleness; or excitability or unsoundness of mind—all must be considered very carefully.

The state of the eye itself should also be borne in mind. It is useless to operate on an eye in which other parts are affected. It is always advisable, therefore, to have the eyes thoroughly examined by a specialist *early,* before the cataract becomes so dense as to obscure the back of the eye and make examination difficult or impossible. Most specialists allow the patient to use his eyes as much as he likes, within reasonable limits, while awaiting operation; some, however, prefer the better eye only to be used for reading.

The operation is usually performed under a local anesthetic, and though it naturally demands great skill, it is safe and successful even in aged people.

Treatment after operation. The treatment *after* operation is simple, and a good result depends to a very great extent on the obedience and quietness of the patient. It was formerly the custom to insist on complete darkness after the operation, but this, together, with the patient's anxiety about his condition, sometimes produced a form of mental trouble—generally relieved when the room was brightened. Surgeons still vary in their after-treatment, but the modern tendency is to have few dressings and a moderate amount of light. It is considered best by some to err on the safe side: they tie up the eye for three or four days after the operation, changing the dressings and examining the eye once daily. Others prefer to use no dressings whatever on the eye, except a wire shield for safety's sake, but advise the patient to open the eyes from time to time, for short periods, after the first two hours have elapsed.

All insist on bed (except in the case of diabetic or very stout patients, who are more comfortable up), but allow the patient to sit up on the third or fourth day. At first he should be careful to lie on his back or the sound side, and should put no strain on the eye by trying to help himself in any way; his attendants must do everything for him. The room is shaded but not dark, and the bed is placed with its head to the window. At the end of a week the patient is usually up.

When the patient has recovered he will require two pairs of glasses, one for reading and the other for distant sight, the two pairs are necessary because glass lenses naturally have no power of accommodation in the same way as has the natural lens.

Cataract occurs at various periods of life, and very many causes have been suggested; some are doubtful, and some are rare, and only the more usual forms are considered below.

Soft cataract. This occurs at an earlier age than the form which has just been described. In these cases the nucleus is not yet fully formed and the cataract forms "streaks" throughout the lens, the outer portions generally being more affected. The patient not only complains of increasing defect of sight, but notices "motes" before his eyes; not floating, as are frequently seen by healthy eyes, but stationary. A bright object may be seen multiplied, especially a bright light in the dark. A moderate degree of shortsightedness may come on, which is for a varying time relieved by spectacles. This is often known as "second sight," as the patient may previously have been wearing glasses for "old" or "long" sight, and now finds that he can read better without than with them. This stage may continue for a considerable time; but, as a rule, soft cataract is far more rapid in its onset than hard cataract. It may take a few months, or weeks, or only days, and may be caused in various ways, the two most common appearing to be as a result of diabetes, and from damage.

Treatment. In soft cataract treatment, atropine is useless. The operation performed is usually a very simple one. In *diabetic cataract,* both eyes are always affected and the cataract develops remarkably quickly. In general, operation gives satisfactory results, though diabetic patients have dangers of their own. Under no circumstances are both eyes operated on at the same time, even if the cataract is equally advanced. Diabetic cataract has been known to clear up, but so rarely that it is never considered wise to wait "on the chance."

Traumatic cataract. A cataract due to injury begins to form immediately after the damage is caused to the lens. The younger the patient and the greater the damage, the more quickly will the cataract form. The trauma is not necessarily from a direct blow or wound, it may be from such a distant agent as a lightning flash, though this is rare.

Treatment. The surgeon's duty is to "stand by" until the cataract is ready, and seize the precise moment for operation. Atropine is generally administered to keep the iris dilated, and out of the way of the rapidly swelling lens. In older people the operation may be performed early; in the young it is best to wait as long as is safe.

Congenital cataract. This condition is found in children. In rare cases it may be severe enough to be noticed at a very early age; but generally it is only discovered when the child goes to school, as it is seldom severe and does not get worse. The child is seen to hold his books very near his eyes, and draw his brows down, in order to reduce the light and so enlarge the pupil. This form of cataract is always present in both eyes, and is caused by two of the leaves of the lens, one in front and one behind the central point, being laid down opaque instead of transparent. The other layers are all clear.

Treatment. If vision is fairly good, it is often better policy to correct it as far as possible with glasses, and leave well enough alone. On the other hand, if vision is seriously interfered with, the proper course is to operate.

CATARRH. Inflammation of mucous membrane in any part of the body is known as catarrh. When a mucous membrane is inflamed owing to the action of harmful bacteria or the presence of irritating material it usually gives off a slimy discharge of mucus, as in the case of acute nasal catarrh or bronchitis. Catarrhal conditions of the bowel and stomach are frequent both in temporary and chronic form.

Nasal Catarrh. Nasal catarrh or persistent discharge from the nose is often looked upon as a disease, and is popularly supposed to be incurable. It is not, however, a disease, but only a symptom that something is wrong with the nose. A great many conditions can give rise to nasal catarrh and most of them are curable. The most frequent cause of nasal catarrh is repeated attacks of the common cold, which is an infectious disease and is caused by a virus. When the virus infection has burned itself out, which normally takes place in a few days, the inflamed mucous membrane is readily attacked by the numerous germs which normally have their abode in the nose and throat. The germs often flourish and multiply in the channels and caverns (or sinuses) of the nose, and such persistent infection is the commonest cause of chronic nasal catarrh.

Treatment. One of the best methods of treating chronic nasal catarrh is by a simple nasal douche. This should not be sniffed up the nose, but allowed to run from a glass douche, or else syringed up by a rubber ball syringe. If the douche is sniffed up it may convey infection to the other parts of the nose and even to the ears. A favorite douche is made by taking equal parts of bicarbonate of soda, borax and common salt, and mixing them into a powder. A half-teaspoonful of this powder to a half-pint of warm water is douched up the nose once or twice a day. Some people prefer nasal drops of menthol in liquid paraffin, 10 grains of menthol to 1 oz. of liquid paraffin. If these simple methods do not clear up the nasal catarrh after carrying them out regularly for three or four weeks, the nose should be examined by a doctor as there may be an infection of one of the air sinuses, or polypi may be present, or the bone of the nose may be bent, preventing proper drainage.

CATARRHAL JAUNDICE. This is the popular but inaccurate name for infective hepatitis, or epidemic jaundice. This was one of the major medical problems of the second World War, malaria, venereal disease, and infective hepatitis being the three most important diseases in the Mediterranean area. It is believed to be spread by droplet infection, but flies may also be to blame. Its onset is sudden, with high fever, and sometimes bronchial catarrh; loss of appetite and digestive symptoms are common. It is difficult to differentiate from malaria and other fevers until jaundice appears. The symptoms may last from 25 to 40 days. It is rarely fatal, but is known sometimes to leave the liver in a permanently damaged condition which may later develop into cirrhosis. No effective treatment is known. (*See also* CIRRHOSIS OF THE LIVER.)

CATGUT. Catgut is a material used in surgery for tying blood-vessels or stitching together skin and tissues. It is necessary for this purpose to use a material that can be thoroughly sterilized and which will also be absorbed in time. A material that is absorbed too quickly would not serve the purpose, nor would one that could not be absorbed at all. The gut or intestine of various animals has been found to answer the purpose almost perfectly, and the prepared material, from whatever animal it comes, is collectively called *catgut*. The most usual sort of catgut is that prepared from sheeps' gut. The intestines of the sheep are soaked and scraped clean of mucous membrane until only the elastic tissue remains. This is twisted into, strands and put to harden in a mixture of sulphuric and chromic acid in order to toughen it so that it will not absorb too quickly. It is then kept for from two to three weeks in a 1 per cent solution of potassium iodide, and then sealed in sterile tubes ready for use. It cannot be boiled. Catgut remains unabsorbed in the tissues for roughly as long as the time it has been steeped in the acid preparation, so that the surgeon can use a catgut that will remain firm until the tissues are united sufficiently to hold together without it.

CATHARTIC. A medicine which is used to produce an evacuation of the bowels is known as a cathartic. This group of drugs includes many varieties, and some have a stronger action than others. Certain substances, such as Epsom salts, are used to make the stools more liquid as well as to increase *peristalsis,* which is the rhythmical tightening and loosening of the walls of the intestine whereby the contents of the intestine are passed onwards.

The milder cathartics include aperients and laxatives such as liquid paraffin, sulphur, etc., which usually produce one or two motions a day without any irritation to the bowel. The more severe cathartics include such medicines as castor oil, calomel, senna, cascara, phenolphthalein, etc., which produce more frequent and more watery stools. Drastic purgatives include jalap, podophyllum, and croton oil, and have no place in medicine.

CATHETER. Tubes of rubber, gum elastic, or metal which are used for passing into a cavity through a narrow canal, are called catheters. The most usual one is the urethral catheter, designed to pass through the urethra or canal through which the urine is discharged from the bladder. If a patient is unable for some reason to pass urine, it has to be withdrawn by a catheter. Because of the danger of infection, catheterisation of the bladder should always be regarded as a temporary measure designed to relieve acute stoppage of urine. When as a result of enlargement of the prostate difficulty in passing water is experienced over a long period, the condition will have to be dealt with by surgical operation. Long rubber catheters are used for the purpose of washing out the stomach or duodenum and for draining the gall-bladder. The eustachian catheter is of metal or vulcanite, and is used for passing by way of the nose up the *eustachian tube* into the ear for the purpose of inflating the ear. The eustachian catheter can be used only by a doctor skilled in the procedure; but it is sometimes necessary for a patient to use the rubber catheter himself, either for gastric lavage or for emptying the bladder. It is essential, therefore, that he should realize the necessity of thoroughly cleansing the catheter. The bladder especially is very easily infected, and inflammation of the bladder, or cystitis, is one of the most troublesome complaints it is possible to have. A glass or metal box should be kept ready in which the catheter can be replaced as soon as it has been used and sterilized. Before use the instrument should be boiled for five minutes in a clean pan kept for this purpose only, and the hands should be well washed before handling it. Before inserting the catheter, a little sterile petroleum jelly or glycerine of borax may be smeared on the end to act as a lubricant. After use the instrument should be well washed inside and out in running water and drawn through a little methylated spirit or surgical spirit to dry it. It must then be put immediately into the covered box which is kept for it.

CAUL. On the head of a newborn child there may be a sort of cap formed by the membranes with which it was covered in the womb. As a general rule the baby's head ruptures these membranes in passing and they are left behind, but occasionally a portion remains adhering to the baby's head. This is known as the caul. This membrane used to be considered to have magic powers and a dried caul carried by a sailor at sea was supposed to protect him from drowning.

CAUSTIC. Caustics are substances which are able to destroy tissues. They may be applied to the skin as a liquid or a solid. The best known caustic is silver nitrate or caustic lunar which is greatly used to destroy warts and to discourage "proud flesh" in healing ulcers. Caustics, on the whole, are used very little except in the treatment of warts, corns, and growths, as their action is inclined to cause much irritation and pain. Solutions of caustic potash have been used to remove the outer skin in certain chronic skin diseases and the weaker solutions may be applied to relieve itching and the irritation of insect bites.

CAUTERY. It is sometimes necessary to destroy portions of tissue, and this can be done by cautery much more efficiently than by the action of caustics. There are many kinds of cautery, but as a rule this operation is carried out by an instrument heated by an electric current or in a flame. *Actual* cautery is carried out with a white-hot iron, while *button* cautery is carried out with an iron heated in hot water. In *galvanic* cautery a platinum wire is heated by electricity and applied to the part to be destroyed. (*See also* DIATHERMY.)

CELL. Cells are the tiny units of living matter of which the human body is built just as a great building is built of bricks. In the case of any building its bricks can be seen, but in the body the cells are so minute that high-powered microscopes are required to see them. Under the microscope a single cell looks like a tiny drop of jelly with a speck in it. In the beginning our bodies start as a single cell containing this speck which is called the *nucleus*. The firmer substance of the cell is called the *protoplasm*. The nucleus contains still smaller particles called the *nucleoles*. The protoplasm of which the cell chiefly consists is able to move and to take substances into itself for feeding purposes. Its chief characteristic is that it *grows* and *multiplies,* and changes its form, so that the one cell from which we start in our mother's womb reproduces itself with great rapidity through all the stages of larger and larger embryos until a complicated human body has been built up, composed of millions of cells of different sorts and uses and the baby is born. It continues growing by cell multiplication and differentiation and finally becomes a man or a woman.

Cell reproduction and growth. Cells reproduce themselves by dividing. A change begins to take place in the nucleus which divides into two halves which are known as the daughter nuclei. Each of these daughter nuclei forms the nucleus of two new cells. These again divide, which makes four cells from the original one. Division continues in this way until masses of cells are formed. At an early stage the cells which are to form the organs, the bones, and so forth of the body are differentiated from the others, and when they reproduce themselves they form other cells in their own likeness. As well as building the body and its various organs, the cells produce the various substances which are used in the mechanism of the body, the lubricating oils, the food digesters, etc. The life of cells is naturally not as long as the life of the body; they die and are replaced many times. They can also become ill or damaged and be repaired. It will be seen, therefore, that the cells are the agents by which the body is built up, and is kept in repair. Certain diseases of the body, noticeably tumors and especially cancers, are caused by irregular growth of certain cells. For some reason which has not been determined, they cease to obey the strict rules which miraculously govern cellular growth and become a law unto themselves. They grow and multiply with a complete disregard for the host of whom they form a part and by whose death they also die.

CELLULITIS. When the cellular tissue under the skin is infected by harmful germs it becomes inflamed. The inflammation may be localized to a particular small spot, in which case a boil or abscess forms, or it may be general over a larger area but may not show any tendency to gather to a head. This condition is called cellulitis and shows that the tissues are successfully resisting the invasion of germs. There will be an area of reddened skin with no very definite edges. The skin may be shiny and the region is swollen and tender.

Treatment. To treat the condition heat should be applied locally, either in the form of hot baths or fomentations, or in a dry form such as radiant-heat lamps or hot pads. The part should be kept raised if possible and must be kept at rest. The doctor will give one or other of the antibiotics, penicillin by injection followed by a synthetic penicillin by mouth, or terramycin. The cellulitis may disappear without coming to active suppuration. But if suppuration arises it must be treated, as in the case of an abscess, by incision. (*See also* ABSCESS; BOIL.)

CEREALS. The cereals have always provided an important source of food to the human race. The varieties which we make most use of today include wheat, rye, corn, oats, barley, and rice.

In earlier times the grain from these cereals used to be eaten whole or roughly ground up, and it is only within the last hundred years that the finer processes of milling have eliminated the germ and outer covering of the seed. Owing to their deficiency of protein and fat, cereals and their food products should be supplemented with other substances such as milk, cream, nuts, butter or eggs, as, for example, bread and butter, milk puddings, etc. It is especially necessary in the case of children to see that the diet is not lacking in any of the necessary vitamins. Semolina, macaroni and vermicelli are included in the food products obtained from cereals.

CEREBELLUM. The cerebellum is the part of the brain which lies below and behind the cerebrum. (*See also* BRAIN.)

CEREBROSPINAL FEVER. This is an infectious disease caused by a tiny germ known as the meningococcus, which enters the patient's body through the nose and throat, and is conveyed by the bloodstream to the nervous system, where it causes inflammation of the coverings of the brain and spinal cord. It often occurs in epidemics, especially in the winter and spring, and very large numbers of people may be attacked, owing to the fact that others act as "carriers." They do not themselves fall victims to the disease, but they harbor in their noses and throats the microbes which can infect those with whom they come into contact. Cerebrospinal fever can occur at any age, but children are the more liable to be affected, and it is particularly dangerous in infants between the ages of six months and three years. There are many and varied forms of the disease, but the acute type is by far the most common.

Symptoms. The patient has an intense headache, usually felt at the back of the head; he feels generally out of sorts, and the temperature goes up. The earliest sign which may make one suspect the presence of cerebrospinal fever is stiffness of the muscles of the back of the neck. This soon becomes very marked, and the patient finds that any attempt to bring the head forward

gives him pain. He therefore lies in bed with the head drawn backwards and resents any attempt to make him bring the chin down towards the chest. There is very often a shivering attack at this stage, or in children, a convulsion.

Vomiting, not associated with the taking of food, may occur, but is more common in children than in adults. The physical and mental attitudes soon become typical of irritation of the brain; the patient lies huddled up in bed, unwilling to move, resenting any interference, whether this is to feed him, to examine him, or even to talk to him. He may become delirious, talking utter nonsense, or he may lie in a condition of complete apathy, taking no notice of anything, the eyes being open and staring, with a peculiar vacant look. Young children are especially liable to lie motionless, this condition being interrupted at intervals by a distinctive cry, which can never be forgotten by anyone who has once heard it, so high-pitched and anxious is it. The cry is independent of any headache the child may have and is quite purposeless though no less distressing to those who have to listen to it.

In a considerable number of cases a rash appears over the body and arms during the first week of the illness. The rash may take the form of large rose-red spots, or it may look rather like a measles rash. The patient loses flesh rapidly, and at the end of a week appears quite wasted. Loss of sleep, which is the usual accompaniment of the severe headache, adds to the patient's misery. If the illness has not been diagnosed by the end of the first week and the essential treatment has not been given, the outlook for recovery is poor, but in few other illnesses, if any, is it possible for a patient to be so ill and yet to recover completely as in cerebrospinal fever, provided that the adequate treatment is forthcoming early enough. The certain diagnosis is made by examination of the fluid which surrounds the spinal cord. Some of this is taken by puncturing the space between the spinal cord and its coverings in the lower part of the back and withdrawing the fluid with a syringe. In cerebrospinal fever the fluid looks cloudy when it is withdrawn, owing to the presence of many pus cells in it. In these pus cells there can be seen, under the highest power of the microscope, the microbes which have caused the disease. Sometimes, if very few of these are present in the fluid, it may be necessary in order to be able to see them under the microscope, to make them multiply first by feeding them for twenty-four hours on special food which they like and will thrive on. Therefore in certain cases a definite diagnosis may not be possible until the day after the fluid has been removed, though in most cases it can be made the same day.

Treatment. Until the discovery of the sulphonamide drugs the treatment of cerebrospinal fever was by a serum given into the spinal canal, and this treatment was sometimes dramatically successful, though relapses were not uncommon. Treatment by sulphonamides has, however, removed the dread with which this fever was once regarded, and has altered the whole outlook on the disease. Early diagnosis is all-important, hence puncture of the spinal canal and examination by a bacteriologist of the fluid thus obtained must be carried out whenever the disease is suspected. Sulphadiazine or sulphadimidine are the sulphonamides usually given, in full doses, for not more than a week, by mouth, or intravenously. Penicillin may also be given by injection, but the sulphonamides are more helpful.

A case of cerebrospinal fever is best treated in hospital, as the illness is not only an exhausting one, but requires skilled nursing. If the patient is nursed at home, the main trouble is to ensure that enough food is taken to maintain his strength as far as possible. In the early stages, if the patient is irritable and resentful of attention, it may be very hard to persuade him to take even a liquid diet. Raw eggs, beaten up in milk, freshly prepared meat-essences, and as much water as he can be induced to take should be given in small quantities at frequent intervals. Later in the course of the illness, if the patient is only semiconscious, the act of swallowing cannot be relied on, as some of the food may "go the wrong way" and enter the lungs. Feeding by means of a nasal tube, inserted by the doctor, three or four times a day, must then be resorted to. According to the age of the patient, from a quarter-to

a half-pint of peptonized milk, or of beef-essence, is given at each feed. A raw egg may be given with the milk. The bowels must be kept well opened. Tepid sponging often helps to soothe the restless patient when the fever is at its height. Those in attendance should pay great attention to personal cleanliness, and should come into contact with as few people as possible while they are in charge of the case, for fear of spreading the disease. They should gargle twice a day either with a weak solution of permanganate of potash (a solution which is faintly pink is the right strength), or with a half-strength solution of peroxide of hydrogen. The nose may be sprayed with a weak antiseptic solution. Those nursing a case of cerebrospinal fever rarely themselves contract the disease; the danger is that they may give it to other people. (*See also* MENINGITIS.)

CERVICAL. This word is derived from the Latin, and literally means "of the neck." It is the adjective used to describe structures lying in the neck, and is also used to denote the *cervix* or neck of the womb.

CERVIX. The cervix is the neck of the womb. It is a frequent focus of illhealth in women because it is so often torn during childbirth. If the tear is neglected and becomes infected with harmful germs, it may cause the state of poor health which many women fall victim to, in which there is a chronic discharge from the vagina and feelings of discomfort and tiredness. A doctor should always be consulted, as the condition is very amenable to skilled treatment.

CHAFING. When two surfaces of skin rub together it produces a condition of irritation known as chafing or intertrigo. (*See also* INTERTRIGO.)

CHALK. Chalk or calcium carbonate is used in medicine in many different ways. In the prepared form, which is calcium carbonate freed from most of its impurities by washing and drying, it is used as a dusting powder, and it also forms one of the ingredients of many of the tooth powders. It is used internally in cases of diarrhea and colitis, and also in chronic dyspepsia.

CHALK-STONES. Chalk-stones are often referred to as gout-stones or *tophi*, and are found under the skin of gouty people. Although these deposits are called chalk-stones they are made up of sodium-biurate. The most common site for these stone-like deposits is about the knuckles and the lobes of the ear. (*See also* GOUT.)

CHANCRE. A chancre is an ulcer which develops about four weeks after infection by one of the venereal diseases, usually syphilis. A fluid may exude from it which is found to be teeming with germs. The sore may be of the hard or soft variety, but it is generally understood that the term *hard chancre* is applied to the sore which is an early symptom of syphilis. This sore generally appears in the region of the genitals, but chancres may occur on the lip, tonsil, tongue, breast, finger, and elsewhere. The *soft sore* is a venereal disease, but not syphilitic, and may be treated and cured in a short time by the used of antiseptics; but as in the case of hard chancre, it is essential to seek the aid of a doctor as soon as the infection is discovered, to obtain proper attention and treatment. (*See also* SYPHILIS.)

CHANCROID. This term is applied to a soft sore, caused by venereal disease. (*See also* CHANCRE.)

CHANGE OF LIFE. Women have many ways of referring to the period when their childbearing life ceases, but the most common popular name for it is the change of life. Doctors talk of it as the climacteric or menopause, or sometimes even as the critical age. This last name is very suitable because the change of life is always a critical age for women. Many women pass through the change with little discomfort; some have a bad time for a couple of years, and then take a new lease of life and begin to enjoy themselves again; while others, unfortunately, settle down to a life of invalidism and misery. Many of the sufferings of these women could be avoided with proper care and consideration during the critical age.

The chief physical change that takes place at this time is that the ovaries and other organs of reproduction cease to perform their function and become atrophied and shrivelled. This change occurs at different ages in different types of women, but it is somewhere between the ages of forty and fifty-five—between forty-five and fifty

being the most usual age. As a general rule, it may be taken that the earlier the menstrual periods start, the longer they will go on, and that women in the same family are likely to have the change of life at about the same age. Certain factors affect the age at which the change may be expected. For instance, spinsters and child-less women are likely to reach the change some years before married women who have had children and have led a normal sexual life. States of health in which the vitality is lowered may also bring on the change at an earlier age.

Physical Changes. It is not always easy for a woman to know when she is approaching the change of life, and the first time a period is missed for a few days she may imagine that she has become pregnant. In most cases the periods cease gradually, either by becoming scantier until they finally cease or by missing three or four consecutive months, then appearing again in a regular fashion for some months until they again disappear for several months. The time taken from the first irregularities until the final cessation of the periods is usually between one and two years. In a few cases the periods stop suddenly and completely, and there is generally a great disturbance of the general health with this type of climacteric. In the earlier stages of the change there may be an increased flow at the periods instead of the usual diminished flow. This excessive flow, or *menorrhagia,* as it is called, should cease after a few months. If it does not, a visit should be paid to the doctor, as it may be the sign of some trouble, such as a fibroid tumor or even the beginning of cancer, and such conditions can be cured if taken in time.

The unpleasant symptoms which are very general among women at the climacteric are due to an upset of the glandular balance. This upset indirectly affects the working of the nervous system, which shows its resentment in various symptoms such as flushes nervousness, and irritability, "pins and needles," dyspepsia, and neuralgia. It is also noticeable that many women become unduly fat at this time.

Flushing. Of the symptoms of the climacteric flushing is the most distinctive. It is a rush of blood to some part of the body, such as the face, or it may be a sudden unexpected hot feeling all over the body.

These hot flushes may be followed by bouts of chilliness. Palpitations are also frequently present. The heart may suddenly be felt thumping rapidly, and the woman may feel breathless and alarmed for a short time. These flushings are very unpleasant, but are in no way dangerous, and always vanish after the change of life has become established.

Obesity. The tendency to put on flesh about the time of the climacteric is distressing to many women. There are a few cases where the increase in weight is accompanied by dryness of the skin, falling out of the hair, dulling of the intelligence and slowing of the heart's action. In these cases there is some glandular deficiency in the thyroid gland or the pancreas which should be corrected by the administration of thyroid extract, or in certain cases, insulin. These remedies should, of course, only be taken under a doctor's care. Most cases of obesity in middle-aged women, however, are due to faulty habits rather than to any disease, and the treatment is the same as for obesity at any other time. When a woman who has hitherto led an active life finds herself temporarily unable to do as much as she used to in the way of work and exercise, she is very apt to put on flesh rapidly, unless she curbs her diet and limits the amount of starchy food she eats. (*See also* OBESITY.)

Nervous symptoms. As well as the physical changes that take place at the change of life there are mental changes. The sexual desires are diminished in most cases, though in happily married couples complete loss of desire rarely, if ever, takes place as a result of the menopause.

In many other ways the general health of a woman may suffer at this time. She may have indigestion in various forms, constipation may be troublesome, etc. All these conditions should be corrected in the ordinary way, but it is a very great mistake for a woman to consider herself an invalid at this period. Her activities should be modified so that she may go slowly, avoid as much worry as possible, and have extra rest when the need is felt. A placid and easy-going existence is best, but the slowing down should be regarded as temporary,

just a well-earned rest before embarking on a new phase of life. Many women really begin thoroughly to enjoy life after the menopause; and their health improves almost as if the cessation of the reproductive functions had released more energy for the upkeep of the body.

CHAPPED HANDS AND LIPS. Normal healthy skin is rendered resistant to outside irritation, and kept in a soft, smooth condition by the fat and moisture contained in its outermost or horny layer, and poured out upon the surface of the skin by the sebaceous and sweat glands. If the horny layer of the skin is for some reason deprived of too much of its fat and moisture, it becomes dry and rough, and tends to crack or "chap." This is most commonly seen on the hands and lips; it is, indeed, rare in other parts unless actual disease is present. Some skins are naturally drier than others, and so chap more easily, but all require some external irritant before chapping occurs, such as exposure to cold and windy weather; a habit of biting the lips; too much washing with hot water and soap, particularly strongly alkaline soaps (as in washing powders), which will dissolve the fat out of the skin; and imperfect drying of the skin, especially in cold weather.

Treatment. The treatment of chapped hands and lips is fairly obvious; it lies in prevention. If the skin is properly protected, chapping will not occur. Warm or tepid water should be used for washing, not (if it can be avoided) hot or cold, and the skin should be carefully dried afterwards. If it is inclined to be dry, it should be lubricated. The time to apply lubricants is immediately after the natural fat has been removed by washing. Lanolin is perhaps the best preparation to use, as it most nearly approaches the natural fat. A very little should be applied, well rubbed in, and the excess wiped off. At night more may be used, and loose cotton or chamois gloves should be worn. Lanolin may also be applied to the lips, or a softening lipstick used, the base of which is either lanolin or cocoa butter.

If cracks have already occurred, lanolin again is the best preparation to use; a lanolin cold cream is also good; camphor-ice or ointment acts as a mild counterirritant, and is often very successful in curing chaps.

A word may be said about the very general use of cold cream or glycerine preparations as emollients. The former is an excellent cleansing cream, but as its chief components are wax, liquid paraffin, or similar substances which are not fats, the skin is only greased, not softened. Glycerine (like soap) "softens" the skin by swelling its horny layer and thus mechanically closing the cracks; but the skin is to some extent harmed by this, and loses a little more of its natural resistance to irritants. Pure glycerine should never be used for chaps, as it has a great affinity for water, and unless diluted with a watery solution such as rose-water, will take up water from the skin; this will cause the condition to become worse, and will give rise to much pain.

CHAULMOOGRA. Chaulmoogra oil is obtained from an evergreen shrub which grows in Burma and other parts. This oil is used in the treatment of leprosy, and is sometimes given for tuberculosis and rheumatism.

CHEST. Chest is the popular name for the *thorax* or upper part of the trunk of the body. It is a framework of bone and cartilage in which are found the principal organs of breathing and circulation. The lungs and heart are vital to the maintenance of life, and are of soft, easily damaged material and require room for expansion. The chest therefore takes the form of a strong bony cage in which these vital organs are protected from injury and in which they have room to contract and expand freely.

The chest extends from the shoulders to the diaphragm. Its principal bony structure is the spine. From the spine the twenty-four ribs extend, curving round to meet the breast-bone or *sternum* in front. The first five ribs on each side extend directly from the spine to the breast-bone, the second five join into one bone before being attached to the breast-bone, and the last two on each side float loose in front, and are attached only to the spine, and not to the breast-bone. The ends of the ribs, where they join the breast-bone, are formed not of bone but of cartilage, which gives them a certain amount of flexibility, and enables them to be moved by the chest muscles as they expand and contract in the process of breathing in and out.

The measurement round the chest in men is usually between 32 and 42 inches, but the girth is not so important as the difference between the measurements taken during breathing in and breathing out, which gives the range of movement of the chest. A good range of movement is found in good health. Many people are born with narrow chests which are not necessarily weak chests. They should, however, try to develop them by breathing exercises, correct posture and as much fresh air as possible, as the narrow or small chest is more liable to lung troubles than the broad chest. It is useful to accustom weak-chested children at an early age to sleeping with the window open at night.

The chest in old age or as a result of chronic bronchitis may become rounded, or, as it is called, barrel-shaped, through chronic enlargement. In this type of chest the range of movement will be very small, probably not more than one inch difference between breathing in and breathing out. Rickets in infancy is responsible for two common sorts of deformity of the chest. The condition called *pigeon-breast* is very common in rickety children, and there may also be bony swellings on the ribs where they join on to the breast-bone causing a condition popularly known as

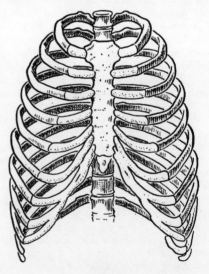

Chest.

"rickety rosary." (*See also* HEART; LUNG; RIBS, ETC.)

CHICKEN POX. Chicken pox or varicella is an acute infectious disease characterized by a rash and accompanied by fever. Infection is spread by direct contact, by a third person, or by inhalation of the virus which causes the disease. Children are chiefly affected, but adults are also liable to infection. The incubation period lasts from 11 to 21 days, but symptoms generally make their appearance about 14 days after infection. The rash may be the first symptom, but in adults especially, the eruption of the rash may be preceded by headache, backache, discomfort, and shivering.

At the beginning of the disease there may be a slight rash or flush, appearing one or two days before the true rash develops. The typical rash may appear on the second day. It attacks the front and back of the trunk of the body, then the face, and later spreads to the upper arms and the thighs; the scalp, also, may be affected. The legs, forearms, feet and hands are generally involved to a lesser degree, and in very rare cases the mucous membranes of the mouth or throat. The spots quickly become pustular and may burst in about 2 days' time. The rash comes out in crops for the first 2 to 7 days, so that spots in various stages may be seen simultaneously on the body. The vesicles or spots finally dry up into a scab which may take from 4 days to 4 weeks to drop off. Scarring does not occur unless the tissues of the skin have been destroyed, but on separation of the scab a slight redness may be present which usually fades and leaves a white spot which may last for years.

The temperature is usually only slightly raised, but in severe cases may be high for a few days. Gangrenous chicken pox, resembling smallpox, in which the tissues of the skin die, is to be met with in very debilitated children, and is sometimes fatal. In hemorrhagic chicken pox, bleeding may appear under the skin, or there may be bleeding from the mucous membranes.

Chicken pox is one of the milder diseases, and its course should be uneventful, except for the severe types. Complications do not, as a rule, arise, but cases of earache, inflammation of the kidneys, laryngitis, and various nervous complications such as encephalitis sometimes occur.

Treatment. The patient should be put to bed until the temperature has returned to normal and all spots have reached the crusting stage. Usually the only treatment required, beyond that necessary for any mild fever, is a local application to ease the irritation of the skin. The patient must never be allowed to scratch the spots. A dusting powder of equal parts of starch, zinc oxide, and borax may be applied. During the period when the crusts are beginning to form the body may be sponged with warm water containing enough potassium permanganate to color it pink. In the final stage, after the crusts have come away, zinc ointment may be applied to the tender skin which is left.

The period of quarantine generally lasts for about 20 days for those persons who have been in contact with the disease, and the patient must be isolated until the last scab has come off, which usually takes from 3 to 4 weeks.

CHILBLAINS. This complaint is only too well known. It occurs during the winter months only, and is found especially in children who are below par (though it may occur at any age). The patients are usually those who are susceptible to colds and chills, and in whom, though the heart itself may be healthy, the circulation is somewhat defective. There appears to be congestion or "crowding" of the blood at the extremities, i.e., the fingers, toes, ears, and nose, and chilblains develop as a reaction to cold. They are also seen sometimes on the cheeks in weak infants. Cold, damp weather, rather than a dry, frosty atmosphere, tends to encourage the appearance of chilblains; other factors which bring about this condition are underfeeding, dressing in thin clothes, which do not keep the body warm enough, and tight shoes and gloves, which restrict the circulation of the blood.

The trouble begins with an itching, burning sensation in the affected parts, followed by swelling which is smooth and shiny, and often soft in the middle. These swellings are caused by the tiny veins in the skin becoming greatly dilated, and pouring out *serum* (the fluid part of the blood) into the tissues. Because of the intense itching, the chilblains are invariably scratched and rubbed, blisters form, which break down, and small ulcers result which are difficult to heal. Chilblains usually recur with annoying regularity during cold weather, and many sufferers find that a remedy which gave them relief for one winter has no effect when used in following years.

Treatment. Obviously it is preferable to prevent an illness than to deal with it in a progressive stage, and the method of prevention outlined below is therefore no less important than the general and local treatments which are described first. They all work towards the same end, that of improving the circulation, both local and general. Internally, cold liver oil and tonics, are given to improve the general health. Calcium preparations have become very popular of late years. Various ways of giving this have been tried, but the most convenient method is to use calcium lactate tablets, 5 grains, 2 or 3 to be taken 3 times daily. It was thought that calcium, which has an effect on the clotting power of the blood, might be an infallible remedy in cases of chilblains; sometimes it does produce excellent results, but in other cases, the effects are disappointing; it is, however, well worth a trial.

The local applications recommended are too many even to name; only those which have been proved efficient will be mentioned. When itching is the most prominent symptom, calamine lotion, menthol, or cold water applications seem to give most relief.

Iodine, in ointment, tincture or collodion, appears to be the most generally successful routine treatment, but must not be overdone, or an "iodine itching" may occur, which may be almost as troublesome as the chilblains themselves. A convenient method is to use the weak tincture of iodine (5 per cent) as a paint for two nights, and, on the third, a mild ointment. This may be continued as long as the iodine causes no irritation. If the chilblains have broken, a mild ointment should be used, the object of treatment now being not to stimulate the circulation but to heal the ulcers. Cold cream, boric ointment, and ammoniated mercury in zinc paste are all good. Arctic explorers use an "ointment" of whisky and soap, which is said to be equally effective.

In bad cases, hot-air baths, X-rays, and local treatment with ultraviolet light have all been useful.

The preventive method has been neatly summed up: prepare in summer for the winter. In other words, preventive treatment must not be given up as soon as the winter's crop of chilblains disappears. *All* cold must be avoided. The clothes must be sufficiently warm, wool being worn both in summer and winter; cold baths or even cold water for washing the hands should be avoided, and the skin should be thoroughly dried afterwards. The patient must be warned against sitting too near the heat and using hot-water bottles on the affected areas.

General as well as local massage and vigorous exercise all help to improve the circulation. Tight boots, shoes, gloves, and collars are forbidden; also garters and goloshes, all of which tend to restrict the circulation in the extremities. In short, if the circulation can be so improved that the patient's hands and feet (and therefore the rest of his body) are always warm, chilblains will not occur.

CHILDBIRTH, PREPARATIONS FOR. In a normal case with a first baby, the birth can often be calculated to a definite date by counting nine months and one week from the first day of the last period before the pregnancy began. This should give the earliest date at which the baby may be expected. There are often variations, usually in the way of arriving too soon, but with first babies it is surprising with what punctuality most of them make their appearance in the world. The date of "quickening" is also a guide, as it occurs halfway through the pregnancy.

Before the date of the expected arrival of the child, the mother, if she is wise, should have had several medical examinations to see that all is in order. The most dreaded complication of the later stages of pregnancy and the confinement and lying-in period is the condition called eclampsia, in which convulsive fits occur. This condition can usually be avoided if examinations of the pregnant woman's urine and blood pressure are made from time to time during the pregnancy. The medical examinations may reveal other important matters as well. For instance, if the child is lying in the wrong position for birth, it may be necessary to turn it around in the womb. It will also be ascertained whether twins are present, and whether the bony ring surrounding the exit from the womb is larger than the head of the child. If it is not, and the condition is not disocvered until the birth has begun, there will be serious trouble; whereas, if it is known in time, several things can be done.

When all these preliminary examinations show that pregnancy is progressing normally, it is the duty of the expectant mother to keep in good health, and to prepare for the approaching event with a quiet mind. Nowadays most deliveries are done in hospitals but in rural districts where a hospital is not available certain preparations should be made. The nurse or midwife should be engaged well beforehand, as the best ones quickly get booked up. She will advise as to the choice of a room for the confinement, what to prepare in the way of waterproof sheets and other necessary equipment.

Equipment that will be needed. For a well-equipped confinement which is to take place at home, instead of in hospital, the following articles are required:
- 1 waterprof sheet (about 1½ yd. square).
- 2 draw-sheets (these can be made from old sheets).
- 2 accouchement sheets.
- 2 large rolls cotton-wool.
- 1 roll gauze.
- 3 binders.
- 3 dozen large sanitary napkins (a special size is made for use in confinements).
- 3 dozen small sanitary napkins.
- 2 dozen surgical safety-pins (large and small).
- 2 enamel bowls (about 1 ft. across).
- 2 hot-water bottles.
- 1 covered slop-pail.
- Bed-pan.
- Douche-can and 3 ft. rubber tubing.
- Scissors.
- Bath thermometer.
- Linen thread.
- An antiseptic.
- Surgical alcohol.
- Petroleum jelly.

- Boric powder.
- Talcum powder.
- Usual toilet articles, tooth-brush, soap, etc.

It will usually be found that some of these things, such as the waterproof sheeting, bedpan and douche, can be rented from a druggist. An accouchement set can, of course, be bought complete from a druggist, but the expectant mother may find it more convenient to buy these items separately.

In addition to the above list, a supply of clean towels, sheets and pillow cases should be available; also, an old nightgown will be needed to wear while in labor, and several should be provided for the lying-in period. These should be made to open in front, to be convenient for breast-feeding. The layette, or outfit for the baby, is described in the special supplement on the BABY. It should be ready a couple of weeks before the birth is expected.

A week or so before the date when the confinement is expected to begin, the room in which it is to take place should be thoroughly "spring-cleaned" and all unnecessary furniture and ornaments put away. A single bed should be chosen for the confinement and should not be too low, or it will mean a lot of stooping for the doctor and nurse. (*See also* ECLAMPSIA; LABOR; PREGNANCY; PUERPERIUM.)

CHILL. A person usually complains of feeling chilly when he has been exposed to a draft or when he has been out in the wet on a cold day. Shivering may be followed by symptoms of a common cold, and in more severe cases, pneumonia. Chill may be experienced in many diseases, especially in cases of malaria. The patient should be put to bed and kept warm with hotwater bottles and blankets, and hot drinks should be given. An excellent drink is made with whisky, lemon, sugar, and hot water. This should be given after the patient has been put to bed.

CHIROPODY. By chiropody we mean the surgical care of the feet, which of course includes the treatment of corns and calluses. A person who specializes in the care of the feet is called a chiropodist. (*See also* CORN.)

CHLORAMPHENICOL. *See* CHLORO-MYCETIN.

CHLORAL HYDRATE. The hydrate of chloral is a powerful hypnotic or sleep-inducing drug, and is chiefly used because of its rapid action. Soon after administration of a moderate dose, the patient will fall into a deep sleep, which generally lasts several hours, and which is indistinguishable from natural sleep. On waking, the patient feels refreshed, and there are no symptoms of headache or confusion. Its great advantage is that a dose which is sufficient to induce sleep is not large enough to cause intestinal disturbances or any other harmful effects. Children react very well to this drug.

It is particularly useful in the treatment of simple insomnia from overwork or worry, but it does not relieve pain at all, and, therefore should never be given when insomnia is due to this cause. It has been administered as a soothing drug in cases of delirium tremens and puerperal convulsions, but such large doses are required that they may have a harmful effect on the patient.

Poisoning by Chloral Hydrate. The taking of chloral hydrate becomes a vice with some people, and a "craving" for it seems to be established very quickly. In cases of chronic poisoning the chief symptoms are stomach and intestinal upsets, skin rashes, great heart and respiratory weaknesses, and general debility. The mind may be disturbed, and people have been known to become permanently weak-minded. A slightly larger dose than the patient is accustomed to taking may be very quickly fatal.

Treatment. This consists of washing out the stomach or administering an emetic. The patient must be kept warm by means of hot-water bottles, hot blankets, friction, and massage. An injection of hot coffee may be given into the bowel, and the patient should be prevented from going to sleep by flapping him with wet towels, and shouting to him. An injection of strychnine may be given.

CHLORIDE OF LIME. Chloride of lime, or chlorinated lime, as it is sometimes called, is a white powder made by exposing slaked lime to the action of chlorine gas. This lime is a powerful disinfectant and bleaching agent, especially when mixed with an acid.

In order to disinfect drains or toilets, about 1 lb. of chloride of lime should be mixed with 1 gal. of water and poured down the drain; it also acts as a deodorizer to remove bad smells.

Articles of clothing may be disinfected by soaking them in a solution of 2 oz. of chloride of lime to 1 gal. of water and allowing them to stand for about 24 hours. (*See also* DISINFECTION.)

CHLORODYNE. This is a medicine used for relieving pain. It contains chloroform, dilute hydrocyanic acid, morphia and alcohol, as well as flavoring substances. It is used to induce sleep, especially if the sleeplessness is caused by pain. The mixture should never be given to infants unless under medical supervision.

Doses repeated too frequently may lead to symptoms of opium poisoning. (*See also* OPIUM POISONING.)

CHLOROFORM. Chloroform is a colorless liquid, with a sweetish taste and a peculiar odor. It is largely used as a general anesthetic. When breathed in it causes loss of consciousness with abolition of all sense of pain, and it is a safe anesthetic to give to young children or old people if given mixed with plenty of air and by a doctor who understands its administration.

It may be used as a local anesthetic for toothache, the tooth being plugged with a piece of cotton-wool soaked in chloroform. Because of its sweet taste, it is very often used as a flavoring agent in order to disguise the nauseousness of other medicines. The compound tincture of chloroform and morphia acts as an anodyne; it is a similar preparation to chlorodyne. (*See also* ANESTHESIA.)

CHLOROMYCETIN (CHLORAMPHENICOL). This is one of the many recent antibiotics to find a place in the treatment of disease. It was originally obtained from a mold, *Streptomyces Venezuelae*, found in the soil of a field in Venezuela. Since then its chemical structure has been worked out, and it has been manufactured in the laboratory and the synthetic substance used in treatment. Chloromycetin, like aureomycin, is active when given by mouth, but has the disadvantage of upsetting side effects. It is effective in a wide range of diseases; it has been shown to be curative in typhus and active against the other rickettsial diseases, though probably superseded by aureomycin in the treatment of his group of illnesses. It is without dispute the most effective drug at our disposal in the treatment of typhoid and paratyphoid fevers. The synthesis of an antibiotic in the laboratory is an event of considerable importance, since it opens a new front in the fight against disease and provides a new stimulus to the ingenuity of the synthetic chemist.

CHLOROSIS. Chlorosis, or "green sickness," as it is sometimes called, is a form of anemia which occurs chiefly in young girls, though it has become rare in recent years, owing to the healthier lives they lead. A fuller description is given under the heading ANEMIA.

CHOKING. The treatment of choking is always a question of rendering first aid, and so is dealt with in the FIRST AID SUPPLEMENT. It is also referred to in the article on ASPHYXIA. For simple choking caused by a piece of food sticking in the throat or some such accident, an adult may be struck on the back between the shoulders, smartly but not too violently. A very young child may be lifted by the ankles and held upside down for a few seconds. If these methods are not successful, send for the doctor at once.

CHOLECYSTITIS. This is the medical name for inflammation of the gall bladder, and is described under the heading of GALL BLADDER, INFLAMMATION OF.

CHOLERA, ASIATIC. Cholera is an acute disease due to a specific organism known as the *Vibrio cholerae*. The condition is characterized by very frequent watery stools, muscular cramps, suppression of urine, and collapse. The germ is conveyed to man by means of infected water. Food and flies also convey the disease. Convalescent patients may act as "carriers," and occasionally persons in apparently good health, who show no symptoms whatever of cholera, may be carriers, and by spreading the infection in their stools may prove to be a grave danger to the community. The disease occurs most frequently in India, China, and other Far Eastern countries, but epidemics have broken out in Egypt, Europe, and very occasionally in America. The incubation period varies from a few hours to 5 or 6 days, but, on an average, symptoms appear about 3 days after the infection has taken place.

Symptoms. Cholera may start quite suddenly, or there may be a few days of diarrhea which gradually becomes more severe. The stools quickly quickly assume what is known as the "rice-water" appearance, and there is generally a marked loss of water from the body accompanied by severe cramps in the legs and abdomen. Vomiting of watery fluid and intense thirst may add considerably to the patient's misery.

The face at this time begins to develop a very pale and pinched appearance, the eyes are sunken and the expression is anxious. The skin loses its elasticity and becomes cold and clammy, the heart may become weak, and the pulse and voice feeble. Symptoms of collapse may be very marked, and the urine may be suppressed and scanty. The patient may either die quickly, or pass in a few days into the reaction stage. When the stage of collapse has passed, diarrhea gradually diminishes, and the motions begin to lose their watery appearance and become more solid. The skin becomes warmer and the patient no longer appears pinched and blue. The heart improves and the urine output begins to increase. This reaction stage may be followed by rapid recovery, but sometimes a relapse occurs during the convalescent period, with a return of the diarrhea. Severe complications may sometimes arise, chiefly during the reaction period.

Preventive Treatment. In an epidemic, precautions should be taken to prevent the spread of the disease, and a certain amount of protection may be gained by boiling all water and milk, eating only cooked foods, and by avoiding all foods liable to cause diarrhea. Vaccination will afford considerable protection for about one year.

Treatment. As soon as there are any signs of diarrhea the patient should be put to bed at once, kept as warm as possible, and given small doses of opium. The violent vomiting and the intense thirst may be relieved by iced drinks. The body temperature must be kept up by means of warm blankets and hot-water bottles. The patient should drink water, albumen, or glucose water, in small quantities frequently. In cases where there is much loss of fluid from the blood, injections of salt solution are given into the veins. This is one of the chief modern advances in the treatment of cholera, and it has reduced the death-rate in some places by about one-half. Potassium permanganate pills should be given every quarter of an hour for the first four hours, and then every half-hour until green bile appears in the stools. The administration of chalk has been highly recommended, and appears to be beneficial. A new compound of sulphathiazole and formaldehyde has recently been tried on a small scale in India, with remarkably rapid relief of symptoms and an exceptionally low death rate. During convalescence the diet must be increased very cautiously and only diluted citrated milk, jellies, and similar bland substances should be given.

CHOLESTEROL. Cholesterol, or cholesterin, is the name of a substance which is present in the bile. It is found in the yolk of egg and in the blood. Gallstones are frequently composed of cholesterol. (*See also* BILE; GALLSTONES.)

CHOREA. Chorea is more popularly known as St. Vitus's dance. It is chiefly a disease of childhood, in which there are irregular and involuntary actions of the muscles of the face and limbs. (*See also* ST. VITUS'S DANCE.)

CHOROID. The choroid is the middle of the three coats of the eyeball, and lies between the white and the retina. In the front half of the eye it forms the ciliary processes, and beyond these, the iris. It is black in color, and its use is to prevent "dazzling" and to ensure that objects are seen clearly.

Choroiditis. When the choroid becomes inflamed, the patient complains that he sees everything through a mist. Objects appear distorted and altered in size; floating specks or "sparks and balls of fire" before the eyes may be noticed. The causes of choroiditis are many: syphilis; tuberculosis; many infections, including those from nose, throat and teeth, or chronic "poisonings" of the system; acute rheumatism; gonorrhea; injury; eyestrain, increasing short sight; and changes due to old age.

Treatment. Except in syphilitic cases, where prompt measures may bring about a cure, choroiditis is very difficult to treat. In septic cases, such as those due to wounds and acute infections, the whole eye may become so diseased that it must be removed. Eyestrain should be carefully avoided, especially in those with short sight and tuberculosis, when dark glasses should be worn. In old people—rarely before seventy-five—the disease occurs as a simple "wearing out" of the choroid. The patient has a central blind spot, but always retains sufficient vision to enable him to get about. In general, treatment is directed towards any possible *cause*, and attention should be given to the general hygiene. Tonics such as cod-liver oil and iron are helpful, especially for children. (*See also* EYE.)

CHYLE. Chyle is the term applied to those ingredients of the food which, after passing through the stomach and being mixed with the gastric juices, are absorbed from the intestine, not by the blood, as is the case with the greater part of the absorbable ingredients of food, but by the *lymphatic channels.* The special lymphatics which deal with the absorption of chyle are called the *lacteals,* because of the milk-like appearance of their contents during the process of digestion. The parts of the food which are absorbed by the lacteals are the fast. The cycle is carried by way of the *thoratic duct* to the *left subclavian vein,* where it is emptied into the blood stream. (*See also* BLOOD; DIGESTION.)

CHYME. When food is swallowed into the stomach it is mixed with and acted upon by digestive juices, of which the chief is hydrochloric acid, and the process of digestion begins. When the food is well soaked with the gastric fluid and has been thoroughly mixed by the action of the stomach, the valve at the lower end of the stomach opens and the stomach contents are passed on into the duodenum in a form called chyme. In the duodenum the chyme meets other digestive juices, and the process of digestion continues. The chyme is passed on from the stomach to the duodenum in small quantities which are propelled forward by the contractions of the stomach, so that by the time it reaches the duodenum it should be well mashed up into an easily-flowing stream.

CICATRIX. Cicatrix is the technical

name for a scar. New scars are usually purplish or red, but after a time they become white and glistening. (*See also* SCAR.)

CINCHONA BARK. This name is given to the dried bark of the stem and branches of cinchona trees, of which there are several varieties. This was also known as Jesuit's bark, owing to its extensive use by the priests in the Spanish settlements of South America. It was first introduced to Europe by the Countess of Cinchon, wife of the Viceroy of Peru, in 1640. Quinine as well as other powerful drugs, is extracted from it. The red cinchona bark produces the most quinine, and it is from this variety that preparations of the drug are made. Quinidine, also, is obtained from cinchona bark, and is used for its action on the heart. (*See also* QUININE.)

CIRCULATION OF THE BLOOD. The blood is circulated throughout the body by the heart and the bloody vessels. The different parts of the circulatory system are described in separate articles under the headings ARTERY, BLOOD, CAPILLARIES, HEART, VEIN. Only a brief description of them is given here.

The *heart,* which is the central organ of the blood system, lies within the chest or thorax. It is a bag-shaped organ with a wall of muscle, and while the body is living it contracts at a regular rate, thus pumping blood throughout the body. The blood, pumped by the heart's contractions, or beats, as they are called, flows into a system of long tubular vessels called *arteries,* and is carried by them to every part of the body. These arteries are branched in every direction to supply the limbs and outlying parts of the body with blood. Their branches are again branched, and so on until the smallest arteries are reached. These end in tiny vessels called *arterioles,* and the arterioles open into a network of infinitesimally small vessels called *capillaries,* which are only visible under a microscope. The arterial bloodstream contains oxygen from the air breathed in and nutriment from the gut. When the blood reaches the capillaries, nutriment and oxygen are passed into the tissues of the body, and thus they are fed and enabled to carry on their work. The capillaries, as well as passing nutriment

into the tissues, collect from the tissues the waste materials which must be removed from the body in order to keep it in health. These waste materials pass from the capillaries to tiny vessels called *venules,* which are in the same relation to the *veins* as the arterioles are to the arteries. The venules flow into the smaller veins, and the smaller veins join on to the main veins in a similar system to that of the arteries. By the veins, therefore, the

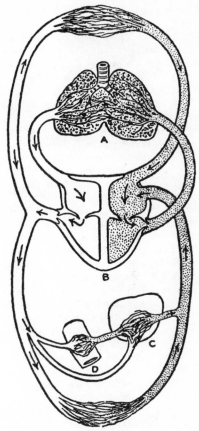

Circulation: Diagram showing circulation, Arterial blood to the left, Venous blood to the right. A. *Lungs;* B. *Heart;* C. *Liver;* D. *Intestine; Capillaries at top and bottom.*

bad blood containing the waste materials is carried to the heart. This system of blood supply by the arteries and blood collection for return to the heart by the veins is known as the systemic or greater circulation of the blood. There are, however, two minor circulations.

In the lesser, or *pulmonary circulation,* the venous blood enters the heart at the *right auricle.* From this cavity it is carried to the *right ventricle,* and from it is passed along the pulmonary arteries to the lungs, where it circulates throughout the whole tissue of the lung in the capillaries, giving off carbon dioxide and other noxious substances which are exhaled by the lung, and receiving oxygen. After circulation through the lungs the blood, which is now re-oxygenated, purified and turned into arterial blood, passes back through the *pulmonary veins* to the *left auricle* of the heart, whence it passes into the *left ventricle* and out into the systemic circulation again.

The other lesser circulation is that of the blood which circulates through the spleen, pancreas, stomach, small intestine and the greater part of the large intestine. This blood is not returned directly to the heart from these organs, but is carried by the *portal vein* to the liver, where it percolates in the small vessels of the liver, discarding toxic substances and leaving the organ by the *hepatic veins,* whence it is passed to the *inferior vena cava,* which conveys it to the *right auricle* of the heart.

The function of the circulatory system of the body is to convey to the tissues the fluid called blood, which contains the nourishment required to keep the body alive and in working order. This nourishment consists of oxygen obtained by the lungs from the air and nutritive substances obtained from the food. The way in which the nutritive substances are absorbed into the blood is described elsewhere. The second function of the circulatory system is to remove from the blood the impurities which it has absorbed from the system during its journey through the body. Two distinct sets of blood vessels are used for these purposes. The arterial system conveys the pure and nutritive blood throughout the body and the venous system returns the impure blood to the heart. The heart serves the double purpose of dispatching the arterial blood on its journey round the body and receiving back the impure blood, and also of dispatching the impure blood on its way to the lungs for purification and

receiving it back for restoration to the main circulation.

CIRCUMCISION. Circumcision is the operation of cutting off the foreskin of the penis. This is quite a simple operation in baby boys, without any danger attaching to it, and is practised as a religious rite by Jews and Mohammedans. Among Europeans circumcision is usually done only when the foreskin is abnormally tight, and cannot be retracted over the glans of the penis. In the infant the operation is so slight that the child may run about as usual immediately afterwards. In the adult the operation is more serious and 48 hours in bed will be required and restricted activity for several days thereafter.

CIRRHOSIS OF THE LIVER. This often goes by the names of "gin-drinker's liver" and "hob-nailed liver," in the former case because of the belief that it is caused by the consumption of too much alcohol, and in the latter because the liver shrinks and develops a hard, knobby surface. Although it is undoubtedly true that too much alcohol is a factor causing cirrhosis of the liver in some cases, it is no longer held to be the only or even the main cause, since cirrhosis may occur in cases in which alcohol has played no part, as in the case

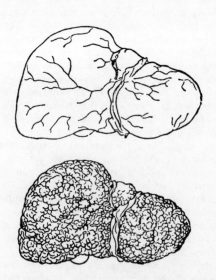

Cirrhosis of the Liver: ABOVE: *Normal Liver;* BELOW: *"Hobnailed" Liver.*

of young children and in races like the Hindus who do not take alcohol.

Cirrhosis has been produced experimentally in animals by feeding them on a diet deficient in a food derivative called cystine. There is much evidence pointing to cirrhosis being due to failure to absorb or use this and other closely related substances. The condition is known to follow an attack of infective hepatitis and other affections of the liver by microbes. The liver becomes congested with blood, at first enlarged, and later beginning to shrink and harden. In some cases, however, it does not shrink, and has much the same appearance as a liver that has undergone fatty degeneration.

Symptoms. The majority of the sufferers from cirrhosis of the liver are males over forty, and it is more common among heavy drinkers and among traveling salesmen, than in other occupations. The patient usually has a feeling of discomfort in the pit of the stomach, with nausea, indigestion, sickness, and vomiting. There may be bleeding from the stomach, the blood being either vomited or passed through the bowel. The patient usually looks thin and slightly yellow-faced, and he often develops small, dilated, spider-like veins over his nose and cheeks. Later on the belly sometimes becomes distended with fluid, and the feet and ankles may swell.

Treatment. The bowels must be kept open, and a daily dose of bicarbonate of soda in warm water will relieve the feeling of nausea. No alcohol must be taken, and the patient should take as much exercise as possible. A high-protein diet is usually prescribed. Such a diet contains much meat, fish, and milk. It is often supplemented by preparations of Vitamin B and cheese.

To avoid the complications of vomiting blood and dropsy, an operation has been devised which diverts the flow of blood from the portal circulation to the vena cava, so that it does not have to pass through the hardened liver. (*See also* EDEMA.)

CITRIC ACID AND CITRATE. This acid is found in lemons and oranges, and they owe their sharp flavor to it. The acid may be extracted from these fruits in the form of colorless crystals which are very easily dissolved in water; 35 grains to 1 fluid ounce of water will make a solution the same average strength as lemon juice. It is greatly used to provide cooling drinks, especially in cases of fever. An effervescing drink may be made by placing 20 grains of citric acid and 25 grains of bicarbonate of soda each in half a glass of water; sugar may be dissolved separately, and the three ingredients mixed together in a large tumbler just before drinking. Sodium citrate is used in medicine for three purposes: first to prevent the clotting of blood, second to make the urine alkaline in infections of the urinary tract, and third to promote a fine curd in milk.

CLAUDICATION, INTERMITENT. This is a form of intermittent lameness associated particularly with arteriosclerosis, though it may occur temporarily in other diseases which have a weakening effect on the walls of the arteries. The patient feels intense pain in the legs after walking for a short time and has to stop. As soon as he sits or lies down the pain ceases, only to return again when walking is resumed.

CLAUSTROPHOBIA. Dread of being shut up in a small or confined space, such as a room with the door shut, or in a crowd, is known as claustrophobia. (*See also* AGORAPHOBIA; PSYCHOTHERAPY.)

CLAVICLE. The collarbone, or clavicle, is a long bone lying in a horizontal position between the breastbone and the arm. With the *scapula* it forms the shoulder girdle. The collarbone gives width to the shoulders and supports the arm, which joins on to its end at the tip of the shoulder and is thus held free of the body. It is very liable to be broken, especially by falls in which the individual puts his hand out to save himself and thereby receives a severe blow on the hand. Fortunately, however, the break is usually only a crack which stays in position and is easily healed.

CLAW-FOOT. Claw-foot is a deformity of the foot in which the arch is greatly exaggerated, so that the balls of the toes are brought near to the heel. The condition is seldom present at birth, but is usually due to some form of spinal disease. The very high instep makes it difficult to obtain suitable shoes, and corns and callosities form easily. There may be severe pain in the instep. In early cases the condition may be treated by putting the foot in plaster of Paris, in a position to correct the deformity, followed by massage and exercises and the wearing of special shoes.

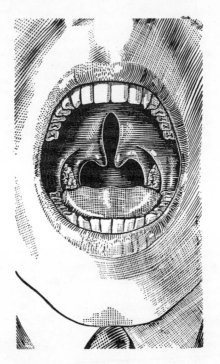

Cleft Palate.

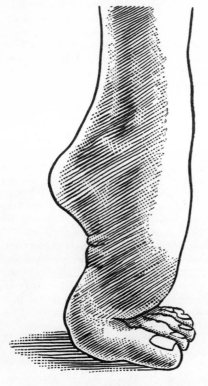

Claw-Foot.

CLEFT PALATE. The palate or roof of the mouth is formed by two plates, of bone in front and muscle behind, which normally join together in the middle line of the roof of the mouth. Occasionally, however, a child is born in whom the two sides of the roof of the mouth do not completely join up, with the result that a gap is left. This condition is called cleft palate, and if left untreated will cause great difficulty in feeding and speaking. The only way to close the gap is by operation which should be done in early childhood, preferably during the first three months of life. If the gap cannot be closed by operation a specially prepared dental plate should be worn.

CLIMACTERIC. The climacteric and menopause are medical names for what is commonly called by women the change of life. A full account is given under the heading CHANGE OF LIFE.

CLIMATE. A temperate climate—that is to say, neither very hot nor very cold—is certainly much healthier than one where the air is heavy with moisture from marsh or jungle, where dysentery, yellow fever, cholera, malaria, and other dire diseases are common. We must not forget, however, that even in those tropical countries which used to be called the "White Man's Grave" there have been vast improvements of late years. For it was found that some of these diseases were carried by mosquitoes and flies, which, as we all know, are dirt-carriers, and may easily be disease-carriers even in this country. By chasing these pests out of their haunts it has been possible to clear many parts of the world from the fevers that formerly made them impossible for white people to live in and unhealthy for any race of human beings. For example, by getting rid of the mosquitoes, Americans were able to free Cuba from the fevers which used to be such a terrible plague; and where North America joins South America, the narrow strip of land through which the Panama Canal was cut, formerly a fever-ridden district, has now as low a death rate as many average American cities.

The countries lying on or near the equator are hot. Some, like Central Mexico, are hot and damp; others, like Central India, are hot and dry. The hot, damp climates are not nearly so healthy as the hot, dry ones; but even there, liver complaints and bouts of malaria have always been a drawback to people going out to trade, explore, or fill civil or military positions, or to do medical or missionary work. Hot countries are generally unhealthy because the insect "carriers" of disease flourish in such climates. It is generally true that the standards of public and personal hygiene are lower too. Education of native races in modern methods of hygiene and insect pest control is doing much to make tropical and subtropical countries safe to live in.

Rheumatic and chest illnesses are what we have to face if we settle in a very cold country, but on the whole there are fewer illnesses to fear than in hot parts of the world. Mountain climates are not good for the aged, or for those with heart or kidney disease. The air being thinner—*rarer* is the correct word—the pulse is faster and we breathe more quickly. Also, we have that buoyant feeling which makes it easy and delightful to walk many miles on a mountain vacation when, at home, one or two miles would tire us out. The air is dry and not laden with germs. The sunshine is plentiful during the day and there may be frost at night. Sudden snowstorms are likely to come on, alternating with brilliantly hot sunshine.

Some climates, as we have seen, predispose to certain illnesses; some are good for one kind of ailment, some for another. But even more important than climate are the conditions under which we live, such as housing, diet, habits; all these influences have to be considered where illness occurs.

In one respect medical opinion has changed very much during that last half century. Whereas, formerly, tuberculous patients used to be kept in heated rooms and sent to warm climates, they are now encouraged to sleep out of doors in all weathers and given as much fresh air as possible.

CLINICAL. This term is derived from the Greek word for a bed, and is used in connection with the bedside treatment of a disease. A *clinician* is a doctor whose opinions and teachings are based upon experience gained at the bedside of his patients. The term *clinic* is used to denote a place where medical instruction is given in the presence of the patient whose symptoms are studied and whose treatment is considered. A *clinical* thermometer is one which is used when taking the temperature of a patient.

CLOT. A clot is a solidification of the blood. In normal persons the blood clots on exposure to air at a definite rate of speed and this clotting time is useful as a test of the state of the blood. An abnormal clotting of the blood while in a blood vessel is called *thrombosis*, and clots at the menstruation periods and after childbirth are common.

CLOTHING. At a very early date, man, with his scanty hair and thin skin, became envious of the natural covering of other living beings, and stole from them to clothe himself. His first clothes were doubtless fashioned from the skins of beasts he had slaughtered for food; but later he became proficient in weaving, and there is historical evidence to show that wool, camel hair, silk, and linen fabrics have been in use for many thousands of years. The history of cotton does not go back so far, but even this was known in India some time before the Christian era.

Nowadays, the majority of garments are made of cotton, linen, or rayon (frequently called "artificial silk") from the vegetable kingdom, wool and silk from the animal, and plastics from the chemist's laboratory. Furs, feathers, and leather are also used for special purposes. These materials may be used pure or as a mixture.

Cotton. This is obtained from the fluffy covering of the seeds of the cotton-plant, and can be woven into fine, smooth, and durable material. It is only very slightly shrunk by washing. It is unsuitable for undergarments in cold countries, as it soaks up the perspiration and remains moist; this moisture is rapidly evaporated with much loss of heat, so that the body soon feels chilled. Cotton is a good conductor, which signifies that the heat of the body is rapidly conducted away and dissipated. Air, on the other hand, is a bad conductor, so that cellular cotton, which contains many air-spaces, is a far warmer material.

Cotton, however, is good for outer wear, as dust, dirt, and germs in the air cling far less readily to it than to rougher materials; it is also easily washed. For these reasons it is often used as uniform wear for those in occupations which involve undue exposure to dirt and infection, such as hospital and nursery nurses, housemaids, librarians, mechanics and others.

Flannelette. A cotton material, the surface of which has been rendered fluffy so as to include more air, is known as flannel. It is much warmer than smooth-woven cotton, and because of this and its cheapness as compared with wool it has been very widely used. Unfortunately this fluffy material is also very inflammable, and has been responsible for the loss of many lives by burning. Nowadays, flannelette is often rendered noninflammable by soaking it in certain chemicals, such as a solution of alum, but it should be noted that washing gradually destroys this power, so that the flannelette in time returns to its inflammable state. There are many other similar materials, which it is impossible to name in detail, but they are all inflammable in proportion to their fluffiness. Flannelette should not be confused with *flannel,* which is made of wool.

Linen. The stalks of the flax-plant yield fibers from which linen is made. This material is finer and smoother than cotton; its properties are the same, except that it is an even better conductor of heat, so that it, also, is not very suitable for winter underclothing. Linen and muslin may be rendered noninflammable by a "fireproof starch," but this, as in the case of flannelette, is partly removed by washing.

Wool. Derived from the fleece of sheep and similar animals, wool is most valuable for clothing. It absorbs and retains the perspiration, and is a bad conductor of heat, so that it is most suitable for underclothing. It is practically noninflammable, as it only

smoulders without catching fire. Woolen materials are warm, partly because of the comparatively great amount of air contained in the spaces between the fibers, partly because the fibers themselves contain a large amount of natural oil in their substance. This, however, varies a good deal with the process of manufacture; if this is carried out carelessly, much of the oil is removed and the wool is harsh, wears badly, and is not nearly as warm as well-manufactured material. Bleaching, for instance, may remove the fat; hence a good deal of unbleached or natural wool is used for underclothing. Woolen garments should be washed carefully, or the valuable oil content will be lost. As wool readily absorbs perspiration, which consists not only of water vapor but also of materials given off by the body, woolens need frequent washing; very hot water, or strongly alkaline soaps, will dissolve out the oil and shrink the fibers, and a good-quality woolen will be rendered no better than a cheap one. Soft, warm water should be used; no soda, but a good soap and above all, the woolens should be squeezed and not rubbed. Before drying, the garment should be squeezed, or put flat through the wringer, not wrung in the usual matter, as this twists and breaks the fibers. For very dirty or greasy clothes, a strong detergent may be used. Drying out of doors is by far the best method, as sunlight and dry air kill off any germs which may be present, bleach the clothes, and prevent the removal of the oil which occurs when the garments are dried in an automatic clothes dryer.

Wool is made up in many ways, both for outer clothing, as in tweeds and flannels, and underclothing, as in flannel and woven materials. Garments are also hand knitted. The closer the weave, the warmer is the material; but woolen materials, unless they are very thick and closely woven, are not suitable for outer wear in cold, and, especially, windy weather. The popular "wooly sets," so often worn by toddlers in winter, and consisting of a cap, coat, and pull-on leggings of loosely woven or knitted wool, are unsuitable for wear out of doors, except in mild weather. They have no wind-breaking power at all. Doubtless, if "wooly sets" declined in popularity, the high death-rate of small children from bronchitis, bronchopneumonia and other such diseases would also decline. Children, as well as adults, should in cold weather wear a coat sufficiently closely woven not to allow the wind and cold air to penetrate to the skin, and in very cold weather cloth leggings may be added.

There are many materials of wool and cotton mixture which are also used for inner and outer clothing. To some people with peculiarly sensitive skins, wool causes irritation or even dermatitis; in these cases a silk or cellular cotton garment should be worn next to the skin, and the woolen garment over this.

Silk. This is obtained from the cocoon of the silkworm, and has both advantages and disadvantages for underclothing. It is a very bad conductor of heat, so that it is both warm in winter and cool in summer; it is cleaner in wear than wool, and far more easily washed, with little shrinkage. If exposed to fire, it burns very slowly. On the other hand, it is much less absorbent than wool, so cannot hold perspiration to the same extent; it is comparatively expensive, and not nearly as durable as either wool or cotton.

Nylon. Nylon is a cellulose product, obtained from wood-pulp, coal, and other sources. It is extensively manufactured under various names, and in many instances is taking the place of silk, cotton wool, and furs for fabrics. Its chief attraction is that it is easily washed and requires little or no ironing afterwards.

Fur, leather, and waterproof materials. All these materials are very valuable as outer garments when the weather is cold, windy, or rainy. Leather and oilskins are especially valuable, as they are almost entirely impermeable, and so are excellent wind-breakers. This impermeability, however, acts both ways, and so prevents ventilation of the skin by causing stagnation of the air between the skin and the coat. This is quickly realized if a waterproof garment is worn in warm weather; the discomfort soon becomes very great.

Dyes. A troublesome dermatitis is sometimes produced by the dyes which are used for coloring materials. Aniline dyes, which are commonly used, sometimes contain arsenic, which is irritating when ap-

plied to the skin. This harmful effect is perhaps most often seen on the feet and legs, when stockings colored with an aniline-arsenic dye are worn. The warmth and moisture of the feet appear to hasten the action of the arsenic. Dyed furs, also, may be the cause of irritation of the skin. Dermatitis occurs most often on the back and sides of the neck, and the chin, where the fur collar rubs the skin, and occasionally on the wrists. As in these cases the only cure is to discard the fur, it is best to get a guarantee from the furrier that the dye used is harmless.

Considering all these qualities, then, the ideal material for clothing must *protect* the body against both cold and heat, in virtue of its property as a bad conductor; it must be *noninflammable,* or as nearly so as possible; it must be *permeable,* so that the skin is well-ventilated; and it *must not irritate* the skin.

Warmth and Color of Materials. Clothing gives warmth, not in itself, but in proportion as it can retain the natural heat of the body. The warmest materials, in the following order, are wool, fur and down, silk, cotton, and linen. It must also be remembered, however, that this property does not depend only on the material itself, but also on other factors. Garments worn loosely are warmer than tight garments, because of the thicker layer of air between them. Several thin garments worn in layers are warmer than a single garment of the same weight, for the same reason. The color of the outer clothing is important, as each color has its own heat-absorbing power. These, in order, beginning with the greatest, are black, dark blue, light blue, dark green, turkey red, light green, dark yellow, pale straw, and white. Rough materials are warmer than smooth ones, as they increase the circulation in the skin by their slight constant friction.

The power of absorption is very important in determining the warmth of a material, as it allows perspiration to be absorbed from the skin, and this is evaporated from the garment, not from the skin itself, so that the chilliness produced by direct evaporation is avoided. This power is of considerable consequence from the point of view of health. After exercise, for instance, a cotton garment quickly becomes damp and cold; wool, on the other hand, remains warm and dry, and prevents chilling of the body surface, which is very dangerous.

General rules for dressing. Clothing, to be suitable and healthy, must preserve the whole of the body at a uniform temperature. As a general rule, too much clothing is worn, especially by men, and by the unfortunate children of a too-fond mother. It is even more objectionable to health than too little; the overclothed person is apt to be much affected by the cold, and to be prone to coughs and colds, and other affections of the respiratory passages. On the other hand, the dress of women and children offends chiefly against uniformity of temperature—the body is warmly clothed, but the extremities are far too thinly clad. Exception has already been taken to "wooly sets;" it is no less distressing to see small children dressed in winter weather in a thick coat, but with a lengthy expanse of cold blue leg between thin socks and short pants or skirts. These extremes are bad for both the health and the appearance. Children should always have long warm woolen stockings in cold weather, regardless of fashion. The "hardening" of children should proceed cautiously; the middle course should be taken between swaddling and over-exposure. In warm weather the clothing may be reduced to a minimum, provided chills can be avoided.

Clothing should be changed according to the weather, not the calendar. There was formerly a custom of "sewing in" the children for the winter. When the careful mother thought the season far enough advanced, she arrayed her children in all the warm underclothes they possessed, and sewed the garments firmly together. Whatever the temperature, the little unfortunates remained *sewed in* until the following spring.

The clothing should not interfere with any natural functions or movements, so as to lead to injury or maldevelopment of that part of the body which it covers. The collar should not be too tight, as the neck contains many important vessels which are liable to suffer from pressure. Garters should not be allowed to restrict the circulation of blood to the legs, and suspenders should be worn instead. The waist and the feet have probably suffered most from tight or ill-fitting coverings, and are important enough to be discussed in separate articles. (*See also* BOOTS AND SHOES; CORSETS.)

Children's Clothing. At the extremes of life, *warmth* of clothing is the great essential. Little children lose heat rapidly and are liable to take cold, because, as their circulation is more rapid than that of the adult, more blood is carried in the same length of time to the skin vessels, and so more heat is given off from the skin. Also, in children the skin surface is larger in proportion to its contents than is the case in adults. In infancy, the clothing should be warm and easily washed, but not heavy and uncomfortable. (*See also* LAYETTE in the SUPPLEMENT ON BABY.) Wool, unless irritating, or flannel should be worn next to the skin by both infants and growing children.

Clothing in Old Age. In old age, as the vital processes decline and the circulation becomes feeble, the function of heat production and regulation is impaired, and the temperature of the body tends to fall. If chill ensues, restoration to the normal temperature is slow and uncertain. Clothing should be warm and light, as heavy clothes are just as burdensome to old people as to little children. Woolen or flannel garments are again the most advisable in their case, and extremes of temperature should be avoided as far as possible.

Nightclothes and Bedclothes. Nightwear should be of woolen material in the winter, and of silk, rayon, or very fine wool in the summer. Bedclothes should be as light as possible, provided that they are reasonably warm; it is far better in cold weather to use a light *ventilated* eiderdown or feather quilt than to pile on additional blankets. Feathers, like wool, are warm, both because of their natural oil and the amount of air they contain. Cellular blankets, although they may seem expensive, approach the ideal bed-covering for warmth and lightness, and are well worth the initial cost. The mattress should be of hair, which is the most expensive, or wool, or a mixture. A few good vegetable substitutes for hair are now obtainable. Feather beds are unhealthy, as they press so closely on the body as to interfere with the ventilation of the skin and thereby produce over-heated and restless sleep. Mention may be made here of the use of hot-water bottles. While it is a mistaken policy for the young and healthy to become so accustomed to these that they cannot do without them, neither is it good for young or old, or those of a delicate constitution, to leave a warm room to go to an icy bed. Electrically heated blankets and bed-warmers, although they lack the charm of the hot-water bottle, are simple and effective methods of taking off the chill. If a hot-water bottle is used to warm a child's cot, it *must* be removed before the baby is put to bed.

CLOVE. Cloves are obtained from the dried flower-buds of a species of myrtle grown in the Indian Archipelago. Cotton-wool dipped in oil of cloves and applied to the hollow of a decayed tooth, or a clove chewed, is generally found to relieve toothache. Their main use is in cookery because of their aromatic flavor; they also impart a pleasant odor to the breath.

CLUB FOOT. Club foot, or talipes, is a deformity in which the foot is twisted. The condition may be congenital (present at birth) or it may occur later in life as a result of paralysis or injury.

There are four varieties of club-foot: (1) *talipes equinus,* in which the heel is raised from the ground, causing the patient to walk on the ball of the foot; (2) *talipes calcaneus* is the opposite condition, where the heel rests on the ground and the front of the foot is raised; (3) *talipes varus* is the condition in which the sole of the foot is turned inwards, so that the patient walks on the outer edge of the foot; and (4) in *talipes valgus* the foot is turned outwards, causing the patient to walk on the inside of his foot. These forms are usually combined, as in the condition of *talipes equina-varus,* where the heel is drawn up and the sole is turned inwards, or *talipes calcaneo-valgus,* where the heel rests on the ground and the sole is turned outwards.

Treatment. For the cases present at birth, treatment must begin in the early weeks of life while the bones are still very soft and pliable. The position of the foot must be corrected several times daily, the mother or nurse gently but firmly turning the foot

to the normal position and holding it there for a few minutes. In addition to this, the muscles of the legs should be massaged daily. A splint should be used at night to hold the foot more firmly in position, so that, as the child grows older, the bones will gradually assume a normal shape. If massage and manipulations are not carried out immediately after birth it may be necessary later on to resort to surgical operation.

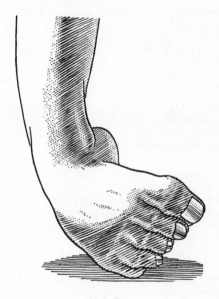

Club Foot.

When the deformity is due to paralysis, treatment by massage and electricity may be found beneficial. For cases which are due to contraction of the muscles following an injury, operation may be necessary. In most cases it will be found necessary to wear a special apparatus in order to support the ankle and keep it in the correct position for walking.

COAL-MINER'S LUNG. This is a condition which is common amongst coal miners, in which the linings of the lungs become impregnated with particles of coal-dust. It is described under ANTHRACOSIS.

COCAINE. Cocaine is obtained from the leaves of two South American plants. The dried coca leaves have been used from time immemorial by natives, who roll them up with a little lime and chew them.

Derivatives of cocaine such as procaine and novocaine are largely used in medicine to relieve pain, and a few drops of it may be injected under the skin as a local anesthetic when a very small operation has to be performed. Operations on the nose and mouth may be carried out after painting a solution of cocaine over the part. Cocaine ointment is useful when applied to the skin in cases of itching, eczema, and shingles, but it must never be used in cases where the skin is broken. A solution is used to soothe pain in the eye due to the presence of a foreign body, and operations may be carried out while the eye is thus anesthetized. Its use as a local anesthetic has largely been replaced by a number of safer synthetic drugs such a procaine, and it is now rarely used for its general action. In moderate doses the bodily and mental powers are greatly increased for a short time, and under the influence of this drug travelers and hunters have been able to perform feats of strength and endurance far beyond the normal. A feeling of happiness and excitement is induced, and all sense of bodily or mental fatigue is abolished. Unfortunately, this drug is very dangerous to take, as a habit is quickly formed. The victim of the cocaine habit soon develops symptoms of acute indigestion, insomnia, emaciation, and insanity, and an early death follows. It is almost unknown for a cocaine addict to be cured of the craving.

Poisoning by Cocaine. A single large dose may cause extreme mental excitement, delirium, and convulsions. If cocaine is taken habitually in small doses, the patient becomes a victim of sleeplessness; eventually he loses all moral sense.

Treatment. In cases of acute poisoning, the stomach should be washed out by means of a stomach tube. Anesthesia by chloroform and ether may be necessary to stop the convulsions. (*See also* ANESTHESIA.)

COCCUS. The name coccus is given to spherical-shaped germs which produce disease and is derived from the Greek word for a berry. The most commonly known are streptococci, staphylococci, and pneumococci, of which accounts are given in the article on GERM.

COCCYX. The coccyx is the name

given to the last bone of the spine which is composed of four rudimentary vertebrae, and corresponds to the tail in animals. In early life the joint between the coccyx and the *sacrum* is movable, but it becomes fixed in later life. It sometimes happens that the coccyx is slightly bent inwards, and this may be the cause of backache. A coccyx that is too long may cause discomfort after sitting for a lengthy period. The coccyx may be damaged or displaced by sitting down suddenly on something hard. A displaced coccyx can be returned to position, but is apt to slip out again. In a few cases rigidity of the coccyx may cause difficulty in childbirth. (*See also* VERTEBRA.)

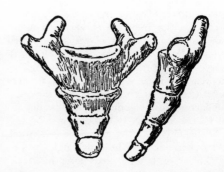

Coccyx.

COD-LIVER OIL. This is a very valuable and easily digested form of fat. Not only is it easily absorbed into the blood by itself, but it seems also to aid the absorption of other foods. It is made by extracting the oil from the livers of codfish. Scottish oils are said to contain the most vitamins, the oil obtained from Newfoundland ranking second, then the Norwegian. Owing to its richness in Vitamins A and D, cod-liver oil is invaluable in the prevention and treatment of rickets. It is a valuable fattening food in wasting diseases, and in convalescence. It appears to improve the resistance to bronchitic infection in chronic coughs and it is useful for children suffering from undernourishment. It is often given in the treatment of some chronic skin diseases.

An emulsion is more easily taken than the pure oil, and doses should be very small at first—about one teaspoonful—

gradually increasing the amount to about four or more teaspoonfuls. A mixture of cod-liver oil and malt extract may be found more palatable; it should be taken immediately after a meal or at bedtime. When it is impossible to get the patient to take the oil internally, it may be rubbed into the skin. It will often accelerate healing when applied to chronic ulcers of the skin. (*See also* FOOD; VITAMINS.)

COELIAC DISEASE. This is a troublesome disease of children due to an unexplained malabsorption of fat, and, to some extent, of starches, diagnosed by examination of the stools. It is treated by injections of Vitamin B and liver extract, and by giving bananas, which contain protein and starch in an easily absorbed form.

COLCHICUM. Various drug preparations are obtained from the root and seed of colchicum, or meadow saffron. They are used in the treatment of gout. Given during an attack, colchicine, which is the active principle, acts very rapidly and markedly relieves the pain. It is a drug which should be used with great caution, as in large doses it gives rise to great abdominal pain, vomiting, diarrhea, and prostration and collapse.

COLDS. The common cold, which is sometimes called by the technical name of *coryza*, or acute nasal catarrh, is the commonest ailment to afflict mankind. The most painstaking research has failed to solve the riddle of its cure.

Symptoms. The symptoms of a cold are well known to everyone. Sometimes an attack starts with shivering and chilly feelings down the back, sometimes with a sore throat and sometimes with headache and stuffiness in the nose. In whatever way the attack starts, however, there will soon be a "streaming" nose and perhaps watering eyes. The watery discharge from the nose may clear up in a couple of days, or it may progress to a thick yellowish discharge which will take up to a week to get rid of. Sometimes the discharge settles down to become a chronic catarrh of the nose, which may be quite difficult to deal with.

Causes. Cold in the head is an infectious disease caused by a virus, which is a germ too small to be seen by an ordinary microscope. People with colds should remember that they are infectious; they should avoid crowded places, refrain from visiting sick or delicate persons, and, if they must go about among their fellows while in the "streaming" stages, be careful to cover the mouth and nose with a handkerchief when sneezing or coughing. The cold that is only a slight inconvenience to some individuals may be a severe trouble to others who are more susceptible to germs. Immunity against the common cold is short-lived. This is thought to be due to the germ having many different but closely related types, infection with one of which will not protect against invasion by another; it is, perhaps, the reason why attempts at prevention and treatment have had such gloomy results.

Treatment. Many people have their pet precautions against colds, which they take either as a general health routine, or when there is an epidemic, or, perhaps, when they have been with someone who is suffering from a cold. Spraying the nose and gargling certainly may ward off trouble, or at any rate lessen the severity of infection, but the day will inevitably come when the most careful person will fall a victim. A healthy mode of life, and fresh air in the house, without drafts, are really the best preventives. The teeth, nose, and throat should be examined if the tendency to catch cold is very marked.

When preventive measures have failed, a cold should run its course very quickly if it is dealt with at once. An attack may be cut short if the patient takes a hot bath and retires to bed with hot drinks and a hot-water bottle to induce perspiration. A couple of aspirin or similar tablets, may relieve the discomfort. If the symptoms have subsided by the morning it is helpful to begin taking a tonic, and particular care should be taken for the next few days to avoid catching another chill. If, however, the cold is well developed, continue the same treatment or use any of the favorite cold remedies, such as ammoniated tincture of quinine, a few drops of camphor on a lump of sugar, or two aspirins every four hours (those to be taken only if the patient is in bed or confined to the house). If the throat is sore, gargle at intervals with salt and warm water or some simple gargle such as glycerine of thymol. For the sore nose and nasal discharge, inhalations are of the greatest assistance. Menthol crystals, compound tincture of Benzoin, or oil of eucalyptus may be used by pouring boiling water over the crystals or liquid in a bowl and holding the head over the bowl, while breathing in the scented steam. A large towel placed over the head and bowl forms a tent to keep the steam from escaping. Soothing substances, such as chloretone inhalant, may be sprayed in vapor form into the back of the nose with pleasant effects, by a special spray called an atomizer, or an ordinary liquid spray may be used with glycerine of thymol or some such substance.

When the cold is over, a tonic will tone up the general health. (*See also* INFLU-ENZA.)

COLIC. Colic is the term used to denote pain due to irregular or violent contractions of muscular tubes in the body. The most usual form is that due to spasmodic contractions of the bowel and is called *intestinal colic*. There may be *gastric colic* in the stomach, *biliary colic* due to irregular contractions of the bile ducts, *renal colic* in the ureters, etc. The cause of colic is usually some kind of obstruction in the bowel or duct concerned. This obstruction is often a stone, but may be due to kinking or constipation. The muscular walls of the ducts try to pass on the stone by their contractions and pain results. The pain of colic is sometimes very severe and the victim is "doubled up" and often vomits. Unlike other pains, it waxes and wanes rapidly.

Treatment. Colic may be so severe that morphia will have to be administered, as in the case of biliary colic. Atropine is the most useful drug for counteracting the tendency of muscles to go into spasms. The most common form of colic is intestinal colic due to constipation, undigested food or to a chill. Sips of hot water with peppermint or ginger in it or a dose of chlorodyne may relieve the pain. Frequently, a hot-water bottle held to the part will be all the treatment necessary to relieve the pain temporarily.

If colic does not yield to simple remedies quickly, it is always best to call in a doctor, as it is impossible for the ordinary person to be sure of the cause of the pain.

The commonest cause of colic in babies is cold, and this should be remedied by giving sips of warm water and applying heat to the abdomen; great care must be taken, however, that the fomentation or hot-water bottle is not too hot for the delicate skin of the infant. Frequent attacks in infancy are usually due to underfeeding or improper feeding and may be associated with constipation.

COLITIS. By colitis is meant inflammation of the large bowel or intestine. The condition is described according to its nature as mucous colitis, catarrhal colitis, and ulcerative colitis.

Mucous Colitis. The distinguishing feature of this condition is the passage from the bowel of quantities of membraneous-looking material which consists entirely of mucus. Mucus is the slimy material which exudes from the mucous membranes, or linings, of the various organs or passages of the body. In the case of mucous colitis the mucus is from the lining of the large intestine, and it may be due to a catarrhal condition of the bowel or to a nervous condition in which too large a quantity of mucus is being given off.

Symptoms. The mucus passed in mucous colitis is very varied in character. It is sometimes passed in long bands of a ribbon-like appearance, which may be mistaken for segments of a tapeworm. It may be of considerable thickness and bear on its surface the marks of the folds of the intestine, or it may be in the shape of a tube surrounding portions of the stool, so that people are led to believe that they have passed pieces of the bowel itself. It occurs most commonly in females. Patients who develop mucous colitis have often been subject to occasional attacks of cramp in the bowels, usually lasting a day or two, dyspepsia, flatulence, etc. The main symptom is constipation of a severe nature requiring the constant use of purgatives to overcome it. The motions are generally hard masses often covered with mucus.

The constipation may be replaced by a continuous diarrhea with frequent loose motions containing much mucus and a quantity of thin watery material. There is some dull, aching pain and a feeling of discomfort and uneasiness along the whole course of the large intestine. There may be attacks of severe pain, lasting several hours, followed by the passage of quantities of tough and stringy mucus. The pain is caused by the efforts of the bowel to rid itself of the tenacious mucus which clings to it. Most of the sufferers of this complaint are thin, anemic, pale and poorly nourished, always complaining of feeling cold and of pain in the back and in the loins. They are often very neurotic and take a morbid interest in their symptoms. Symptoms often come in attacks which can be correlated with emotional upsets and difficulties at home and at work.

The disease is never fatal, but is apt to last a long time, and be very difficult to cure.

Treatment. In this condition treatment must aim at three things: overcoming the tendency to constipation; improving the patient's nutrition; stimulating and strengthening the nervous system. The diet must be ample and nutritious, well cooked and daintily served, consisting chiefly of eggs, raw or lightly boiled; soups, meat jellies, custards, finely minced beef, calves' feet jelly, fish souffles, pounded chicken, and crisp toast or crackers. The patient must avoid green vegetables, starchy foods, fruits, pastry, and cheese.

The bowels must be made to open regularly every morning, and this can be done by suitable doses of metamucil sufficient to produce a soft motion. The antibiotics and sulphonamides have proved disappointing, but prednisone is often helpful. (*See also* IRRIGATION OF THE BOWEL.)

Convalescence. If possible, when the patient begins to improve, a vacation should be taken in order that the patient's thoughts and attention be turned away from his ailment and occupied with change of scene.

Acute Catarrhal Colitis. Acute attacks of inflammation of the bowel are usually due to the eating of some doubtful article of food or something else which "disagrees" and are part of a general stomach and intestinal upset.

Symptoms. The symptoms are well known. There is colicky pain in the lower or middle part of the abdomen, sickness, and diarrhea; there may be fluid and offensive motions, which may contain an excess of mucus; the temperature may rise and skin rashes, such as urticaria or nettle-rash, may occur.

Treatment. The patient should be put to bed, and given plenty of plain water, which must be boiled, to drink. He should not be given any food. In order to keep up the patient's strength thin liquids like chicken broth, whey, or albumen water may be given. Give a good purge of milk of magnesia. If the patient is a baby, give $\frac{1}{2}$ to 1 teaspoonful, and for an older person from 1 teaspoonful for a small child up to 2 tablespoonfuls for an adult. As soon as the diarrhea has ceased, bring the patient back gradually to normal diet, restricting the diet again immediately if there is any sign of a return of the diarrhea. Usually, cases due to contaminated food clear up entirely in a few days, but sometimes the colitis becomes chronic and may drag on for months. It is well, therefore, to treat the matter with care at the beginning in order to avoid such a complication.

Ulcerative Colitis. Colitis in which the bowel ulcerates is a not uncommon disease of middle life; it is very difficult to cure and is of serious import. It is not always known what causes it, but as it closely resembles tropical dysentery it is thought by some authorities to be due to some similar germ. Chronic ulcerative colitis occurs in persons of an unusually timid and sensitive personality. The disease is usually a chronic one. It progresses for a while and is followed by a phase of apparent cure which only too often gives way to relapse later. Relapses are found to follow periods of upset and anxiety and remission occurs when the cause is removed. It begins gradually with increasing diarrhea in which mucus, pus, and blood are passed. The number of stools increases to as many as twenty a day, and improvement then usually takes place. Sometimes it takes on a severe form and is occasionally fatal.

Treatment. The treatment is similar to that for mucous colitis. However, special medicines are required in cases due to amoeba or other known causes. Severe cases may need admission to hospital, when they are treated by rest and blood transfusion. Occasionally it is necessary to put the diseased bowel at rest by by-passing it with a surgical operation (*See also* DIARRHEA; DYSENTRY; ENTERITIS.)

COLLAPSE. This term is applied to a

condition of extreme exhaustion. It may follow some prostrating disease such as pneumonia, cholera, infantile diarrhea, etc. Any condition in which there is a great loss of fluids from the blood vessels may bring about a state of collapse. This is very similar to the condition of surgical shock. The main difference between the two lies in the onset, which is more gradual when the state is due to some disease.

Symptoms. The face is pale and haggard and the eyes are sunken and glassy. The body may be covered with cold sweat, while the temperature is generally reduced to 95 deg.–97 deg. F. The voice is very weak, and the pulse feeble. The patient may be conscious but unable to pay attention to what is going on around him, while in other cases unconsciousness may occur.

Treatment. The patient should be kept as warm as possible, by means of hot-water bottles placed at the feet and sides, and warm blankets to cover him; he should be allowed to lie on his back, with his head low. Medical advice must be sought. Stimulants should only be administered under medical supervision in those cases where collapse occurs as a result of bleeding, or when bleeding is likely to occur.

COLLARBONE. The medical name for the collarbone is the clavicle, and it is described under that title.

COLLES' FRACTURE. Colles' fracture is a break in the radius at the lower end, just above the wrist. This type of fracture is usually caused by a fall on the hand when the arm is outstretched, and the end of the bone may be impacted, or driven on to the upper part. Colles' fractures usually unite without leaving much deformity of the arm, and the arm is fit for use in three or four weeks.

COLLODION. This is a thick liquid made by dissolving gun-cotton in ether and alcohol, or with acetone. When painted on the skin the ether dries rapidly, leaving a thin protective film. This forms an excellent covering for small wounds after they have been thoroughly cleansed and dried, but it must not be used on discharging wounds. Collodium callosum, which is collodion used in conjunction with salicylic acid, is a rapid and painless solvent for corns and warts.

COLOCYNTH. Colocynth, or bitter ap-

ple, is obtained from the dried pulp or pith of the fruit of a species of cucumber, which is imported from Smyrna and Spain. It is a powerful purgative and should be used with discretion.

COLON. The large bowel, or large intestine, is called the colon. It is described under the heading INTESTINE.

COLOR BLINDNESS. Some people are unable to distinguish between colors, and are called *color blind.* The degree of color blindness varies, the commonest form being the inability to distinguish between red and green; blue-yellow color blindness is much rarer and total color blindness very rare indeed. The condition is more common in men than in women, and occurs equally in all races. It is apt to run in families, several brothers, perhaps, being affected; or it is sometimes transmitted from grandfather to grandson, the son escaping the defect. Color blindness may exist in one eye only, the other having normal color vision. The acuteness of vision is unaffected in any way, and, as a rule, the "patient" feels no inconvenience. He may even name the colors of things correctly, because he has been told that a geranium is scarlet, or that the grass is green; but he sees only a difference in shade, not in color. It is usually a friend or relative who discovers the condition. In tests among a large number of people, both men and women, it was found that 6 per cent of men were wholly color-blind, 25 per cent were partially color-blind, and 11 per cent of women were partially color-blind.

It is a curious fact that, as a class, color-blind persons are above the average in intelligence; the defect is, indeed, frequently associated with very high ability, many of the greatest men having suffered from it. Such was John Dalton, the famous chemist, who, having discovered it in himself, set to work to study it, and in 1794 published the first scientific account of color blindness.

The methods of testing for color blindness for practical purposes must show that the candidate can distinguish between colors used in his employment. Formerly, and still to some extent, "Holmgren's wools" were used. The candidate was given a certain colored skein of wool and asked to pick out, from a large number of mixed skeins, the other skeins of the same color, whether lighter or darker in shade. It was possible to discover, by this method, whether a person was color blind, and, if so, to what colors. It was not, however, accurate, and naturally produced considerable dissatisfaction among men who were rejected by what they considered to be an unfair test.

Edridge-Green, a modern investigator, does not consider the "wool" test nearly good enough for practical purposes. He has therefore devised a lantern, by means of which colored lights are shown to the candidate, who must *name* them correctly. The naming of colors was not included in the wool test; but as Edridge-Green says, quite rightly, the engine-driver (for example) must *name* the color of a signal-lamp to himself before he can decide what is his duty. Not only are the clear lights shown, but these are modified to imitate their appearance in different weathers, such as haze, fog and heavy rain. By this excellent test it is clearly seen whether the candidate is fit or unfit to have charge of a ship, an engine, and so on.

Acquired color blindness. This occurs in disease of the light-perceiving apparatus, i.e., the retina, the optic nerve, and the sight centers in the brain. It differs from the congenital or natural form in that there is an associated failure of acuteness of vision. It generally occurs in a definite order: first the green fails, then the red, and lastly the blue. This is well seen in tobacco blindness, of which a full description is given under BLINDNESS.

It is easy to see that acquired color blindness may be a source of great danger to sea-captains, engine-drivers, and others, and they are retested from time to time to ascertain that their color vision remains perfect.

COMA. Coma is a state of deep unconsciousness. It is usually a matter of serious importance. Poisoning by various poisons which take effect on the nervous system, such as alcohol, prussic acid, opium, and any of the sleep-inducing drugs such as those derived from barbituric acid (like veronal) cause coma. Certain injuries and disorders which cause pressure on the brain, such as fracture of the skull, brain tumor, and apoplexy, may bring on coma.

There may be coma in very severe attacks of influenza, malaria, sleeping sickness, and even measles. Coma is also a symptom of uncontrolled diabetes. Coma vigil is the name given to a state which occurs in severe fevers, in which the patient lies muttering to himself, often with his eyes open, but really in a state of unconsciousness.

Treatment. When a person is found lying unconscious without any obvious cause and cannot be wakened, a doctor should always be sent for, even if it is suspected that the cause is really heavy drinking. The coma of diabetes can now be dispersed almost immediately by an injection of insulin. (*See also* DIABETES.)

COMFORTER. A pacifier, or dummy nipple, is used by many mothers to soothe a crying and irritable infant, but the disadvantages attached to this method of pacifying the child are so numerous as to heavily outweigh the advantages. The pacifier is such a common method of transferring infectious germs to the child that it can only be looked upon as a constant source of danger. It may be taken for granted that the nipple falls from the baby's mouth dozens of times during the day, and there is no doubt that it is generally put back again into the mouth without being sterilized or even washed.

COMPOUND E. *See* CORTISONE.

COMPRESS. A compress may be applied firmly to a part of the body, to relieve inflammation or to prevent hemorrhage. It is most useful for treating a sprain, or for the prevention of a black eye. To make the compress, lint or flannel cloth should be folded to double thickness, and wrung out in ice-cold water. A piece of oiled silk, or similar waterproof material, is used as a protective covering, and the compress is then bandaged over the painful part.

COMPRESSION. Compression of the brain is due to a piece of bone or a clot of blood pressing on the brain. In some cases a tumor, or inflammation of the outer coverings of the brain, may be the cause of compression. It is a much more serious condition than that of concussion, and the treatment of the case will depend on the exciting cause. (*See also* BRAIN).

CONCEPTION. Conception means to become pregnant. (*See also* PREGNANCY.)

CONCUSSION. Concussion of the brain is caused by a fall or a blow on the head. Loss of consciousness follows, and on recovery the patient is unable to remember either the blow, or the events which occurred immediately before his lapse into unconsciousness. This is known as *retrograde amnesia*. If there is no such gap in his memory, he has not suffered from concussion. When the patient recovers consciousness he nearly always suffers from shock. He will probably vomit, and will almost certainly have a headache. If the concussion is slight, the patient may be able to understand what is said to him.

Treatment. The patient should be laid on his back, and the clothing should be loosened so that he can get as much fresh air as possible; no food or drink should be given, except, perhaps, sips of water. He must be kept perfectly quiet until the arrival of the doctor. Lapse of consciousness through concussion lasts only for a brief period; no attempts should be made to arouse the patient from deepening unconsciousness, or a lapse after a lucid interval, as this indicates that he is suffering from a more serious injury, such as bleeding inside the skull, or hemorrhage in some other part of the body. (*See also* BRAIN.)

CONDENSED MILK. This is cow's milk from which most of the water has been evaporated. Condensed milk which is prepared with the addition of cane sugar is a white, or rather yellowish-white, product of about the same thickness as honey. Condensed milk prepared without the addition of sugar is not boiled down to the same degree, and therefore remains more liquid. Children should not be fed wholly on condensed milk, as it is deficient in vitamins and may lead to the development of scurvy. Dried milk may be obtained, which contains the necessary vitamins, but orange juice should be added to the diet in order to eliminate any risk of scurvy.

CONDYLE. By condyle is meant any rounded eminence such as occurs in the end of a bone and takes part in the formation of a joint.

CONDYLOMA. This is a wart-like growth or tumor often found near the opening of the anus. Growths of this type can be removed by the use of caustics or by surgery.

CONFINEMENT. This term is used in connection with childbirth, usually to denote the lying-in period. (*See also* CHILDBIRTH; LABOR; PUERPERIUM.)

CONGENITAL. This term is used to describe any disease or condition which is present at birth. Conditions such as congenital dislocation of the hip may not be noticed until the child starts to walk. Some congenital deformities of the hands and feet are polydactylism, that is, the presence of extra fingers or toes; overgrowth of one or more fingers or toes; and club foot. Syphilis is one of the most common congenital diseases.

CONGESTION. This condition occurs when an abnormal amount of blood collects in any organ or part of the body, causing swelling. The passive, chronic form of congestion, as when the blood vessels are overfilled, is due to some weakness of the circulation, but more often the condition takes an active, acute form, due to inflammation. It is serious when the lungs are affected. Treatment depends so much on the part that is congested that no definite rules can be given here. Congestion of the lungs, and of the kidneys, is discussed under those headings; congestion of the brain is dealt with under the heading MENINGITIS. In certain diseases, congestion is artificially induced as a method of treatment.

CONJUNCTIVA. The conjunctiva is the thin membrane lining the eyelids and covering the white of the eye. It continually "sweeps" the eye in the act of blinking, and keeps it moist and free from friction by mucus poured out by its glands on to the surface. It is well supplied with blood vessels, and its constant exposure to the air renders it very liable to attacks of inflammation called conjunctivitis. (*See also* EYE.)

CONJUNCTIVITIS. Anything that irritates the conjunctiva causes conjunctivitis; there are many forms. The three chief symptoms are soreness, redness, and varying discharge from the eyes.

The pain is generally described as smarting, scalding, or itching. The secretion of the eye may be only slightly increased, so that the eye feels sticky, and the eyelids and eyelashes are "gummed" together in the mornings; or there may be a copious running of a watery or thick pus. The tiny vessels usually seen in the white of the eye are enlarged and scarlet.

These signs vary a good deal in different patients and in different types of the disease, and because the symptoms may appear to be chronic or mild, it does not necessarily follow that the eyes are less harmed than in the acute forms of conjunctivitis. *No eye trouble, however slight it may seem to be, should in any circumstances be treated as of no account.*

Treatment. In treatment, the cause, as far as possible, must be corrected. The eyes should be rested and protected from any irritants such as smoke, bright lights, or cold winds. Warm antiseptic washes should be used several times daily; these serve to wash away the secretion and germs, and are also very soothing. A soothing ointment is applied to the edges of the lids.

Every case should be treated as if infectious; it is impossible to be too careful. Any dressings should at once be burned. The patient should never be allowed, as sometimes happens, to use the same towel over and over again to wipe away the discharge; and, of course, no other person, especially a child, should be allowed access to towels, etc., used by the patient. These details may seem unnecessarily troublesome; but, if they were carefully attended to, a great deal of eye trouble would be avoided.

Simple Conjunctivitis. This is caused by any persistent irritation, such as dusty or fume-laden air, eyestrain, working in a too brilliant light, the misuse of alcohol, etc.

Treatment. The treatment is according to the cause, which should be removed, and the eyes should be bathed frequently with a mild alkaline lotion, such as weak bicarbonate of soda in warm water.

Angular Conjunctivitis. This is a chronic form of conjunctivitis in which the reddening of the eyes is especially noticeable in the corners. It is treated by zinc drops or ointment.

Catarrhal Conjunctivitis or Pink Eye. The disease is very contagious, and may attack several members of a family, or run through a school. In addition to the usual symptoms, a dislike of light is present, and adults generally suffer a good deal of pain.

Treatment. Catarrhal conjunctivitis is easy to treat as it usually recovers of its own accord in a week or two. Frequent washing with an antiseptic loction and the use of an antiseptic ointment are all that is necessary.

Follicular Conjunctivitis. At first sight this has a great resemblance to trachoma, which is described below. The likeness is, however, more apparent than real. This form is found to occur only in sickly or neglected children, and is due to uncleanliness and bad hygiene. Adenoids are often present.

Treatment. If the case is severe, the "sago-grain" bodies may be removed, but in most cases astringent lotions cure successfully. The general hygiene should be looked to, and tonics are useful.

Granular Conjunctivitis or Trachoma. In this chronic conjunctivitis, small nodules, aptly described as "sago-grain" bodies, form under the conjunctiva and set up a persistent irritation. As the disease progresses the inflammation gradually dies down, but the mucous membrane of the eyelids is destroyed, so that the eye is ill-nourished and sight may be affected. The scar tissue in the eyelids contracts and causes the eyelids, with the eyelashes, to turn inwards. This gives rise not only to great discomfort but to considerable injury to the eye itself.

Treatment. Treatment varies according to the stage of the disease. If the condition is acute, it is treated as purulent conjunctivities. When the "sago-grains" have formed, they are mechanically removed. When trachoma has reached the stage of overgrowth, an astringent application such as copper sulphate lotion is used. This treatment requires a great deal of patience, as it may take months or years to attain a good result. In "healed" cases, where a scar membrane replaces the conjunctiva, the best application is diluted glycerine drops.

Purulent Conjunctivitis. This is one of the most dangerous forms and is most common in infants and young adults. In the great majority of cases it is due to gonorrheal infection. When it occurs in infancy, it is generally known as *Ophthalmia neonatorum.* (*See* BLINDNESS.) In most cases the infection is conveyed to the infant's eyes at birth, from the passages of the mother. On about the third day, the baby's eyes are seen to be reddened, and a watery discharge flows from them. By the next day the condition is much worse. The eyelids are swollen, purple-red, and glazed. The discharge is now copious, and consists of thick yellow matter.

Treatment. Unless treatment is very prompt and effective, the result of *ophthalmia neonatorum* is some permanent damage to the sight, or even total blindness. Fortunately, there is a simple method of prevention, which consists in disinfection of the infant's eyes immediately after birth with a drop of 1 per cent silver nitrate into each eye. *This should be done as a routine measure in all cases, whether "suspicious" or not.* If, however, the disease occurs, the most important and difficult part of the treatment is to keep the eye free from pus. If possible, the child should be admitted to hospital with its mother, not only because it can then be fed naturally but so that both the mother and child can be treated. The baby's eyes are washed out every hour or even half-hour, as the discharge produced is extremely copious. A solution of penicillin is dropped into the eyes every few minutes until the infection is overcome. In addition, one of the antibiotic drugs, especially penicillin, or aureomycin, is given internally bringing about a quick and dramatic improvement. All dressings should be burned immediately, and towels, clothes, etc., thoroughly treated with disinfectant before being washed.

In *adults,* cases of purulent conjunctivitis are even more dangerous to sight. The patients are generally young men. The symptoms are very similar to those found in the infant, except that they are more severe and the general health is greatly disturbed. The eyelids are much discolored and very swollen.

Treatment. The treatment is as before with a few modifications. In adult cases it is not uncommon to find only one eye affected, and every effort should be made to protect the "good" eye, both by means of antiseptics and by covering it. The patient is told to sleep on the diseased side, so that no pus will trickle over into the other eye.

CONSTIPATION OR COSTIVENESS.

Constipation is a very common condition in which the bowels do not move often enough or are not completely emptied when they do move. The number of motions required for health varies for different people. The majority of people have the bowels opened once a day, but two motions a day are quite usual; some other people have a motion only every other day without apparently feeling any bad effects. Constipation may be temporary, and due to some passing illness or lack of tone, but in many people it tends to be chronic, and some means of correcting it has to be carried out continuously, or a state of health continually below par will arise.

The stool of a normal healthy person is light brown in color, 4 to 5 in. long, and about 1 in. thick, and should be passed in not more than two or three pieces. It should be light enough in weight to float in water. There are great differences, however, in the color and amount of the stools in perfectly healthy people, due to what and how much they eat and drink.

Probably too much attention is paid nowadays to the working of the bowels, for most people can miss an occasional day without any harm being done; instead, they worry unnecessarily and purge themselves with an aperient, when, in all probability, the function would resume its normal operation the next day. It is thought by some authorities that there is very little absorption of poisonous materials or toxins from the bowel into the bloodstream if the contents of the intestines are solid, and that unhealthy absorption of toxins takes place much more easily from fluid contents of the bowel. The action of aperients on the bowel is to hasten the contents of the stomach into the bowel in a liquid state. It seems therefore sensible to think that as long as there is no disease in the stomach or intestine a slight degree of constipation is preferable to making the contents of the bowel fluid by aperients. Any state of ill-health in the alimentary tract will, however, be made worse by constipation, so where definite symptoms arise the constipation should be treated.

Symptoms. The symptoms that are attributed to constipation are numerous. The complexion becomes sallow and "muddy," the tongue is furred and the breath may be offensive. The appetite will not be good. There may be sick headache, mental depression, and sleeplessness. In fact, almost any symptom of ill health may be present in a mild form. As a general rule pain is not present with constipation unless aperients have been taken, when the pain is due to the contractions of the bowel which they cause. Any sudden or violent pain, especially with sickness and collapse or a rise in temperature, should be attended to at once by a doctor, as it may mean ulceration or obstruction in the bowel. Pain at the actual moment of passing the motion may be due to piles, a condition described under its own heading.

Treatment. The treatment of chronic constipation, where there is no definite disease causing it, is the treatment of the general state of health and the regulation of the diet and daily habits. The most important thing will probably be daily exercise. A certain amount of exercise is absolutely necessary for everyone who does not obtain sufficient muscular exertion in the course of his day's work, and in this respect it may be remarked that housework in a small house, except on days when washing or strenuous cleaning is done, is not enough exercise for healthy women. They need a brisk walk as well. The object of the exercise is to stimulate the working of the liver so that it will produce and send into the intestine enough bile to secure proper digestion of the food. It goes without saying that the call to stool should be answered as soon as it occurs. In most persons' lives it is convenient to so train the bowel that the call comes at the same time every day, and it should be at a time that is likely to be a convenient one. This training can be begun in the very earliest days of babyhood.

The question of diet is, of course, of the greatest importance in the treatment of constipation. As a general rule it will be found that the diet of the constipated person is too solid, too concentrated, and too easily digested. A certain amount of irritating matter or roughage is required to give the bowel something to bite on. This roughage is best obtained from cereal, brown bread, green vegetables, and certain fruits like figs, or prunes, which are not entirely digested. Also, few people drink

enough fluid. Three or four pints of water should be the normal consumption per day.

If attention to the diet, exercise, and daily hygiene do not cure the constipation, it will then be necessary to take a simple aperient. This is fully discussed in a special article on aperients.

CONSTITUTION. It is usual to speak of people as being of different constitutions, meaning just the general condition of their bodies, especially with regard to the way they resist various diseases. It is well known that certain people are more liable than others to some forms of disease. The disease is said to "run in the family," or in medical terms they have a "diathesis" for that disease. Gout, rheumatism, diabetes, and tuberculosis are examples of diseases which are supposed to run in families and which some people are constitutionally more liable to contract than others. A "sound constitution" is probably the very best thing that a child can inherit from its parents; a body in which every organ is sound in structure and in perfect working order, the nervous system is steady and reliable, and what may be called the "plumbing" of the body, the complicated system of piping and pumping which carries on the circulation of the blood, is in good trim.

Although certain sorts of constitutions are inherited, that does not mean that the disease to which the person is constitutionally liable must inevitably overtake him. On the contrary, by knowing that he is liable to contract the disease he is enabled to take precautions, and if he can live in suitable surroundings and avoid things which would undermine his constitution, he need not fear that the illness will occur. For example, the children of consumptive parents, if placed in surroundings where they are no longer exposed to infection and where they can get lots of fresh air and good plain food, will be no more likely to grow up consumptive than any other children; but if they continue the faults of living which led to the illness of the parents, notably living in houses of which the windows are never opened, they will take the disease, while their neighbors who have no constitutional tendency will go free.

A doctor when he first examines a patient will ask questions about all his family and parents—at what ages and from what causes they died. This is because he is trying to gain some idea of what the constitution of his new patient is likely to be, and this knowledge will be of the greatest importance in his treatment of the patient in the future.

CONSUMPTION. Consumption is the old name for the disease which is now called tuberculosis. Consumption of the lungs is called phthisis; consumption of the skin is called lupus. All forms except LUPUS are discussed under the heading TUBERCULOSIS.

CONTACT LENS. A thin shell of glass or plastic, made to fit over the cornea, used instead of spectacles to correct refractive errors, especially by actors and athletes. It is used with a thin film of saline, and takes some time to get accustomed to.

CONTAGION. The word contagion means the process by which certain diseases are communicated from one person to another. This may be done by direct contact with the patient who is harboring infectious germs, or by handling the clothes of such a patient. The term infectious is generally used when the disease is communicated to another in a more indirect way; but on the whole, the borderline between the two terms is a very narrow one.

CONTRACEPTION. This term is derived from two words: contra, against, and conception, to conceive. It is applied to the prevention of conception, or birth control. (*See also* SEX HYGIENE.)

CONTRACTED FINGERS. The condition in which the fingers become contracted is known as Dupuytren's contraction, after a famous French surgeon of that name. It is often hereditary and is found in succeeding generations of the same family, usually among the males. The skin and tissues beneath it in the ring and little fingers of one or both hands become thickened and drawn together, so that the fingers become folded over into the palm of the hand. It is thought by some authorities that a glandular deficiency may cause the condition, and some cases have done very well on treatment by extract of thyroid gland.

Treatment. In early cases, massage may give relief and even stop the condition from getting worse, but when the fingers become

really deformed the tissues beneath the skin may have to be operated on, and in the case of a manual worker it may be advantageous to remove the little finger entirely. (*See also* FINGERS.)

CONTRACTURE. Contracture means the *permanent* shortening, distortion or deformity of a muscle, or group of muscles.

CONVALESCENCE. When one refers to the convalescent period it is generally implied that although the patient is no longer ill, he is still far from his normal healthy self. The convalescent period is a very important one, and it is at this time that good nursing is so necessary. The building up of the wasted tissues should be gradual, and is carried out by means of nourishing food and plenty of fresh air.

The Surroundings. The room in which the patient lies should be as bright and airy as possible. The bed must placed in the way of a draft, or in such a position as to allow the sun to stream on to the patient's face. In winter, the room should not be allowed to become overheated, and this can be avoided by keeping the windows open whenever possible. Visitors should not be allowed to stay more than a few minutes at first, but the time and the number of visitors may be increased gradually as the patient becomes stronger. It is difficult for a normal, healthy person to realize how tiring it is for an invalid to talk and appear cheerful when the strength is very much below par. On the other hand, a patient must never be allowed to become bored, so the nurse will have to use her own judgment. It will be found that visitors are quite willing to be turned out of the convalescent room if the nurse considers her patient is becoming tired and strained.

Diet. As regards food for the invalid, this must be light and digestible, and, of course, the individual taste must be considered. Nourishing soups such as beef tea and chicken soup are as a rule appreciated by most invalids. Milk, either alone or with sodawater, and egg-nogs or thin arrowroot, should be given. Another point to bear in mind is that the patient may be able to eat only very little at a time, so he must be tempted to eat or drink at least every three hours. Breakfast should consist of either half a grapefruit, or the juice of an orange, a small pot of tea and some toast or thin bread and butter. It is a mistake to send too much at first unless the patient's appetite is normal; the sight of too much food often causes an invalid to shudder and turn away from it, whereas a tray daintily set out with just enough to tempt the appetite may encourage him to ask for more. An egg-nog with a little sherry or brandy mixed with it may be given about eleven o'clock, and one or two plain cookies should be sent in with it. The midday meal at first may consist of chicken jelly or soup, broth, or any such light nourishing substance. Milk puddings and custards should be made with fresh milk. As the appetite increases, more solid foods such as steamed or boiled fish, roast lamb or grilled lamb chop, sweetbreads or tripe, and vegetables may be added to the diet. It is a mistake to ask the patient what he would like to eat; as a rule the answer is "nothing," but a request for any particular form of food should not be ignored if it is at all advisable for the patient to have it.

Care of the Patient. If the patient is in a very weak and debilitated state, everything possible should be done for him until he regains his strength. He should be sponged over at least once during the day, and the hands and face sponged morning and evening. The back and limbs should be massaged daily with methylated spirit or eau-de-Cologne in order to prevent bedsores forming. Absolute cleanliness should be maintained and care must be taken to see that the skin is properly dried. Dry skins should be rubbed with equal parts of methylated spirit and oil, as this prevents cracking. After massage has been carried out the body should be powdered over; equal quantities of oxide of zinc, boracic, and starch powder make an excellent and reliable dusting powder.

Tonics. In most cases a tonic is necessary to give tone to the system and to stimulate the appetite. There are many iron preparations which may prove very helpful to the patient such as Blaud's Pills. Children should be given cod-liver oil and malt. Often a change of air to a bracing climate will tone the patient up and do much to bring him back to a normal state of health. Very old people, or delicate or very young children, should not be taken to too bracing a climate, as this may do more harm than good. A mildly bracing place should be chosen at first; and not less important are the possibilities of securing suitable diet and cooking and cheerful surroundings.

CONVULSION. A convulsion, commonly called a fit, is a violent irregular motion of the whole body or of part of the body, due to involuntary contractions and relaxations of the muscles, and may be likened to an earthquake in the system. The most common convulsions are those which occur in infancy and are called infantile convulsions; those occurring during attacks of St. Vitus's dance called choreiform from its other name of chorea; those due to epilepsy; to lockjaw (tetanus); or advanced kidney disease (uremic convulsions). Women also suffer from convulsive fits in a disease of the later stages of pregnancy (eclampsia). All these are described under the diseases which cause them.

COPPER. Copper sulphate, more commonly known as blue vitriol or blue stone, is of considerable value in medicine. Used externally, the sulphate is applied as a caustic to reduce growths on the skin and an ointment of copper citrate is useful in the treatment of ulceration of the eyelids. Sulphate of copper is often used to kill germs found in reservoirs and to act as a disinfectant, but this procedure is not unattended by danger, as, owing to the amount required to be really effective, there is a risk that symptoms of poisoning may arise from consumption of the water. Very dilute solutions of copper sulphate have been used for chronic forms of inflammation of the eye. It is particularly useful in phosphorus poisoning; three or four grains of the sulphate in water should be given every few minutes until vomiting occurs.

Poisoning by Copper. Large doses of salts of copper violently irritate the stomach and intestines, but as a rule acute poisoning is rare. Copper may be taken in very small quantities over a long period without producing any ill effects, but on the other hand symptoms of poisoning may arise causing severe colic.

Treatment. Treatment consists of washing out the stomach by giving large quantities of warm water followed by white of egg or milk. If the pain is very severe, opium may be prescribed to allay the irritation.

CORD. There are several structures in the body referred to as cords. The most important is the *spinal cord* which is about 18 in. in length, extending from the top of the spine to the upper border of the second lumbar vertebra; it is continuous with the brain. The *umbilical cord* is the cord by which the child is attached to the mother at birth. The *spermatic cord* extends from the internal abdominal ring to the posterior border of the testis and is composed of arteries, veins, nerves, lymph glands and the *vas deferens*. There are also *vocal cords* in the larynx.

CORN. A corn or clavus is too well known by the majority of people to require a detailed description. It is a circumscribed overgrowth of the horny layer of the skin, occurring as the result of prolonged pressure due, of course, to the use of improperly fitting footwear. The corn has a deep core or "eye," while the surrounding parts are over-grown, and there may be a varying degree of inflammation.

The troubles which corns produce are often out of proportion to their apparently small size. As walking becomes very painful, the sufferer alters the normal position of the foot to gain relief, and may in time become flat-footed. Apart from local disabilities, the radiating or "shooting" pains of the corn may extend to the knee, and many people have been credited with "gout of the knee-joint" which disappears entirely with the removal of the corn, especially if flat-foot has been corrected at the same time by suitably "built" shoes.

Treatment. The true remedy for corns, then, is correctly fitting shoes. Without them all other measures are temporary and palliative only. Much may be done to stop the formation of corns by having several pairs of shoes and wearing them in turn. Each pair presses a little differently, and so lessens the chance of damaging one particular part. When a corn has formed, relief from pressure and consequently from pain is given by the well-known corn-plaster, which consists of an adhesive ring of cotton-wool which surrounds the corn. Strict attention to cleanliness of the feet,

by daily bathing, also relieves the pain to some extent.

To remove the corn, it should first be softened by a thorough soaking in hot soapy water, to which sodium carbonate (washing soda) is added in the proportion of two tablespoonfuls to a basin of water. Soakings on several successive days may be necessary before the corn will soften. It should then be rubbed down as briskly as possible with pumice-stone or a friction cloth.

The central core and the surrounding callosity can also be softened by various medicaments. A rapid method, which is best used only by a medical man, is to place a drop of *liquor potassae,* 15 per cent, or strong acetic acid on the corn, and rub in as vigorously as can be borne. The horny layer is rapidly dissolved into a greasy pulp. Both, especially the strong acetic acid must be used cautiously, and not on any account allowed to touch the healthy skin. The acetic acid method is, in any case, somewhat painful. A milder, but still rapid, method is to apply *liquor potassae,* 5 per cent, rub in, and immediately neutralize by a drop of dilute acetic acid or white vinegar.

Slower, but painless, methods consist in the use of milder horn-dissolving agents, the chief of which is salicylic acid, used either as a "medicated plaster" or as a paint in combination with collodion. The plaster consists of a small center of salicylic plaster, surrounded by an ordinary corn plaster. The medicated part should be placed over the corn, and the whole kept in place by a narrow strip of surgical plaster. It should remain in place for three days, when it will be found that the superficial part of the core and the surrounding horny part will have softened and may be removed easily.

In obstinate cases, ionization with zinc, or treatment by X-rays, have been used. Surgical removal is sometimes resorted to as when the central core is very deep it cannot easily be removed by medication. This is a matter for the doctor, and should in no circumstances be undertaken by the patient, absolute surgical cleanliness being a necessity in this, as in every operation. Many a person has lost, if not his life, at least his foot, through a carelessly cut corn.

If, however, infection occurs at the site of a corn, treatment should be that of an acute abscess. The most sensible procedure is for the patient to consult his doctor as soon as possible.

"Soft" corns belie their name by being very troublesome. They occur in any position between the toes, and even after what seems to be a complete removal are exceedingly apt to recur. Cleanliness of the feet is here even more important than in the case of hard corns, especially if there is much sweating of the feet. The most suitable application is spirits of camphor, which should be painted on at night; during the day zinc oxide or talc powder should be used, and wool placed between the affected toes. A powder containing starch (as do many toilet powders) should not be used, as it is apt to irritate a damp skin. These are, naturally, only palliatives; the most satisfactory method is surgical removal which, however, may need to be repeated if the corn recurs.

CORNEA. The cornea is really the window of the eye. It is a transparent membrane covering the iris and the pupil. At the side of the eye it joins the white. It is well supplied with nerves, and so is extremely sensitive. (*See also* Eye.)

Ulceration of the Cornea. The cornea is readily damaged when the eye is exposed to an irritant. This destructive process is called ulceration. An ulcer may occur at any point on the cornea, and, when it heals, an opaque scar is left. Sometimes the ulcer eats through the cornea and damages other structures in the eye. This may cause any degree of damage to the sight, from a mere cloudiness of vision to complete blindness.

The *cause* may be a wound of any sort, from a slight scratch to the most extensive damage. Many varieties of conjunctivitis may lead to ulceration. Often ulcers arise without any cause being determined.

Septic Ulcer. This is one of the most important and serious forms, as it is the most frequent cause of loss of sight among active workers with the hands. Some of the worst cases occur among farm laborers and miners. Two or three days after the injury a severe gnawing pain in the temple begins, so bad that the patient "walks the floor" at night and soon becomes worn

out through sleeplessness. Unless treated, the ulcer tends to wander over the cornea and may attack neighboring parts.

Treatment. To prevent this, it is necessary to destroy the active margins from which the spread goes on. This is done by "touching" the ulcer with carbolic acid or the cautery. Another very important part of the treatment is to attend to any accompanying disease of the eye. When the condition begins to improve, the healing process is hastened, and the scar tissue cleared up as far as possible, by the daily application of weak cortisone ointment and massage, a most valuable combined treatment.

Keratitis. The term keratitis is used to denote inflammation of the cornea without ulceration. The most important form of keratitis affects children at about the age of puberty, sometimes several members of the same family, and girls rather than boys. The cause in the great majority of cases is congenital syphilis, other signs of which may be present. Injury is frequently the exciting cause which lights up the disease.

Symptoms. Two common forms of the disease are seen. In the *mild* form the eyes easily tire, and vision is blurred. Greyish spots are seen on the cornea. The patient recovers in a few weeks. In the *severe* form the symptoms are much more acute; pain, especially, may be very distressing. The cornea becomes obscured by closely packed blood vessels which from their appearance are called "salmon patches." In the course of a few weeks the patient is practically blind, but recovery takes place in 6–12 months. The outlook is generally good, unless complications occur.

Treatment. The eye is treated by atropine drops. Antisyphilitic treatment is given, and the general hygiene is carefully regulated. A difficulty in many cases is that the patient loses interest in everything but his own "hopeless" condition. Both he and his family should be made to realize that this despairing frame of mind is quite unnecessary, as his blindness is only temporary.

Conical Cornea. In this condition the cornea, instead of being a flattened curve, rises up into a cone-shaped prominence. It is corrected by glasses or by an operation.

CORONARY THROMBOSIS. The coronary arteries carry blood to the muscle of the heart. They are commonly involved in the widespread disorder of arteries called *arteriosclerosis*. This disorder produces a thickening and hardening of the arterial wall with consequent narrowing of the blood channel. When the bore of the coronary arteries is so narrowed that it is insufficient to supply the heart with enough blood to carry out its work efficiently, then the heart "complains" by means of a special symptom known as *angina of effort*. Angina of effort is a type of pain in the chest which is constantly brought on by exertion and relieved by rest; it is dealt with in a special section. When a coronary artery is so narrowed that the blood inside it clots, there arises the condition known as coronary thrombosis. The blood supply to a part of the heart is completely cut off and the affected area of heart muscle dies and ceases to function. The blood supply is normally so good that when this occurs a degree of repair to the dead or "infarcted" area of heart very often takes place. It will never be what it was before, though, and some degree of impairment of heart function is the rule after coronary thrombosis. This will often take the form of anginal pain, or shortness of breath on exertion, and it is usual to advise such patients to curtail their activities.

Symptoms. The symptom of coronary thrombosis is severe pain lasting several hours or days and felt deep in the chest under the breastbone. It is often accompanied by sickness and shock. Unlike angina, it persists in spite of rest, and, indeed, often occurs when the patient is at rest. There is no known way of preventing this accident, but once it has happened its effects can be minimized by enforcing a period of rest in bed for at least a month. Preparations which delay the clotting of blood, like heparin and dicoumarol, are often given to prevent extension of the clot. After recovery, life should be conducted at a slower tempo both physically, and mentally, and it is usual to advise retirement from competitive business and manual work. It is fortunate that this disorder happens at a time of life when this is usually possible.

CORPUSCLE. This word literally means a little body. The blood cells are called corpuscles. (*See also* BLOOD.)

CORROSIVE. A corrosive substance is one which destroys tissues or any part with which it comes in contact. There are a large number of substances of a corrosive nature, and many fatal accidents have occurred through drinking them. These poisons include the strong acids, strong alkalis, and caustics. The more important acids include oil of vitriol or sulphuric acid, hydrochloric acid, nitric acid, oxalic acid, acetic acid, and carbolic acid.

The more common alkalis which act as corrosive poisons include caustic soda, caustic potash, washing soda in strong solution, and ammonia. Among the caustic salts are zinc chloride, silver nitrate, and chromic acid.

Symptoms come on very quickly after such a poison has been taken by mouth. There is intense pain in the mouth, throat, and stomach, followed by vomiting, which is usually bloodstained. There is generally great difficulty in breathing and the patient may die of collapse in a short time. Even if the symptoms pass off, the patient may succumb from destruction of the tissues and perforation of the stomach.

Treatment. The doctor must be sent for at once, and, if possible, the nature of the poison should be stated; this may be ascertained from the label on the bottle from which the poison was taken. *In the case of corrosive acids and alkalis, it is generally considered to be wrong to give an emetic; in any case it is unlikely that the patient will be able to swallow at all, but if he can be made to vomit immediately, the good will be greater than any possible harm.* Soothing liquids such as milk and white of egg, or a wine-glassful of olive oil in the same amount of warm water, or gruel may be given. The antidotes for the common types of poisoning are set out under POISONS.

Shock must be guarded against by keeping the patient as warm as possible. Hot-water bottles should be placed at the feet, sides and chest and warm blankets placed over him. The clothing should be loosened and the room well ventilated. Artificial respiration should be carried out if necessary. If these instructions are fulfilled promptly there is every chance of keeping the patient alive until expert medical attention can be given; in fact, the doctor may not find it necessary to do anything further. Strong tea or coffee, warm but not hot, may be given later as a stimulant.

CORROSIVE SUBLIMATE. This is a salt of mercury known also as perchloride of mercury, mercuric chloride, or bichloride of mercury. The chief use of this substance is as a disinfectant or antiseptic. It is one of the most powerful of all the antiseptics and even in very dilute solutions will kill virulent germs, but it must not be used on metal instruments because it corrodes them. Corrosive sublimate solutions are generally tinted blue in order that the distinctive color may help to guard against accidents, as it is extremely poisonous. Mercury was the first substance found to be effective in the treatment of syphilis and the perchloride is still sometimes used to this day. It may be applied locally to syphilitic ulcerations and treatment should be begun as early as possible.

Cases of poisoning by this substance should be treated promptly by giving white of egg. An emetic should be given in this case as, in spite of its name, it does not act as a corrosive but as an irritant. (*See also* MERCURY POISONING.)

CORSETS. Fortunately for the health and comfort of women, the days of injurious "tight-lacing" are past. The modern corset is cut to fit, and acts as a comfortable control for the over-exuberant figure.

Special corsets are sometimes ordered. For instance, though as a rule an expectant mother needs no support, some have very slack abdominal muscles, which allow an uncomfortable tilting forward of the heavy womb. These patients are much benefited by wearing a maternity corset, which supports the abdomen without interfering with health by compression. A corset should not be worn during pregnancy; if the breasts become uncomfortably heavy, they should be supported by a specially cut brassiere.

Surgical belts and corsets are prescribed both for men and women in a variety of disorders. Sometimes, for instance, in rupture; after operation; in curvature of the spine due to faulty position; in curvature due to disease, and so on. As each is individual to the patient, they cannot be described in detail. (*See also* ABDOMINAL BELTS.)

CORTEX. The outer layer of an organ is called the cortex. The *cerebral cortex* is the thin layer of gray matter on the surface of the *cerebrum*. (*See also* BRAIN.)

CORTISONE. A steroid hormone isolated from the adrenal cortex by Dr E. C. Kendall of the Mayo Clinic and his co-workers in 1935. The adrenal or suprarenal glands consist of an inner medulla, which secretes adrenaline, and an outer cortex from which some thirty steroid hormones have been isolated, the most important being cortisone and hydrocortisone (the natural hormone secreted by the adrenal cortex, slightly more potent than cortisone). The secretion of these cortex steroids is controlled by a pituitary hormone, corticotrophin or ACTH, and when this is no longer being produced the secretion of the adrenalin cortex steroids stops.

In 1949, Dr. P. S. Hench and his colleagues of the Mayo Clinic discovered that cortisone had a most favorable effect upon the serious, painful, and disabling disease, rheumatoid arthritis, and cortisone was at once hailed as a miracle-worker, equally effective when taken by the mouth as when given by intramuscular injection. As time went on, however, it was found that about half the patients treated developed upsetting side effects, mainly due to salt and water retention: hypertension, glycosuria, obesity, as well as mental depression. Patients who needed large doses developed even more serious conditions, such as bleeding gastric ulcers, collapse or fractures of bones, severe mental disturbances, and activation of quiescent tuberculosis.

Controlled trials were carried out in Britain under the direction of the Medical Research Council and other interested bodies, and it was found that, over a number of years, in rheumatoid arthritis cortisone was no more effective than aspirin, so that it is no longer recommended for its treatment. Fortunately, synthetic steroids were developed in the laboratory that were found to be even more potent than cortisone, though they may still give troublesome gastric side effects. In the laboratory, an alteration in the steroid molecule of cortisone produced the synthetic prednisone, and a similar alteration in hydrocortisone produced prednisolone. It has been found that these new synthetic steroids give good results in the treatment of rheumatoid arthritis, and side-effects are only likely to occur in patients who are getting large doses. To avoid gastric upsets, the tablets are crushed and given with meals, and they now have a coating that dissolves only when it reaches the intestine.

The injection actually into an affected joint of hydrocortisone brings about a reduction of pain and swelling, which usually lasts for about two or three weeks, but repeated injections at short intervals are to be avoided, as it may harm the joint. A 1 per cent solution of hydrocortisone as drops has been found to be useful in the treatment of inflammation of the eyes.

Selye, working in Montreal, has produced evidence to suggest that cortisone acts by protecting us against the harmful effects of "damaging agents" such as chemical and bacterial poisons by silent adjustments taking place in our adrenal glands.

CORYZA. The medical name for nasal catarrh. (*See also* COLDS.)

COTTON WOOL. Cotton wool or absorbent cotton, is made of the hairs of the seed of the cotton plant. It becomes absorbent after the fatty and oily substances have been removed; this is termed "absorbent cotton wool," and it is used extensively in medicine. To mop out small cavities such as the ear or nose, cotton wool should be wrapped round the end of a match or an orange-stick. The proper way to do this is to take a small piece of cotton wool and place the end of the stick in the middle, and twirl the cotton wool well round with the tips of the fingers. When mopping out the nose or ear of an infant it is better not to use a match as this may cause damage to the delicate organs; the cotton wool twisted by itself will be found adequate. Cotton wool when purchased from the druggist is in a highly compressed state and if it is warmed a little in front of a fire it will fluff out and be much more economical to use, but this should only be done by a responsible person and never by a child. It should be remembered that cotton wool is very inflammable and many accidents have been caused by its use on fancy-dress costumes.

COUGH. Cough is an important symptom of disease of the lungs and air passages.

Act of Coughing. Coughing is an action by which air is driven from the chest and throat in an explosive fashion. The impulse to cough is usually the result of some irritation of the various branches of a nerve called the "wanderer" or *vagus* nerve. This nerve gains its name from the way its branches wander over the body. It supplies the heart, the chest, the stomach, the intestines, and other parts.

Varieties of Cough. In diseases of the larynx, or voice-box, the cough is usually hoarse, barking and "croupy." In ulceration or thickening of the mucous membrane of the throat, the cough may be husky.

Cough in Diseases of the Lungs. In *bronchitis* the cough is at first short and dry and may be painful. As the secretion is increased it becomes moist, and may also be paroxysmal; there may be bouts of coughing and fairly long free intervals.

In *tuberculosis* cough is an early symptom. At first it is dry and hacking, later it becomes loose and is accompanied by expectoration mixed with slime and matter. It is often most severe in the morning. In some patients advanced tuberculosis may be present without any cough.

In *pneumonia* the cough is infrequent, short, dry, restrained, and associated with severe pain in the side. In acute *pleurisy* the cough, although it is usually present, is seldom so noticeable as in acute pneumonia.

The paroxysmal cough of *whooping cough* is characteristic; a series of coughs follow each other so rapidly that there is no time to draw in the breath between them. The patient becomes blue in the face, the veins of the forehead and scalp stand out, the eyes become prominent, and the tongue is often protruded. Bleeding from the nose may occur. At last a sudden inspiration takes place with a loud whoop. This may be followed immediately by a second or several series of coughs and whoops before the paroxysm is over. At the end of the paroxysm a quantity of mucus is generally expelled with some violence, and in young children vomiting is usual. During the attack the child may seize some piece of furniture for support.

Enlarged glands at the root of the lung may give rise to very severe and persistent coughing.

Diseases of the Heart. Inflammation of the membrane lining the heart (pericarditis) is sometimes accompanied by a painful cough. Aneurism of the aorta is usually associated with a dry and brassy cough, either by direct pressure on the windpipe, or by irritation of the nerve which leads to the muscles of the throat. Any condition in which the heart's action is feeble, and where consequently the circulation through the lungs is carried on imperfectly, may give rise to a troublesome cough.

Nervous Cough. This term is applied to all forms of cough in which no definite cause can be discovered. It is often a mere habit, and it may be associated with emotion, especially that caused by speaking in public.

Hysterical Cough. Cough is fairly common in cases of hysteria. It may be very severe and persistent and give rise to anxiety as to the condition of the lungs.

Diagnosis. Some forms of cough are characteristic, e.g., that of whooping cough, and the brassy cough of the sufferer from aneurism. The greatest difficulties arise when there are no obvious diseases of the throat, chest, or heart.

Treatment. The treatment of cough due to the diseases of the chest or of the heart will be found under the various headings concerned. Where the throat is the seat of the irritation, gargles, sprays, pigments, and pastilles are all useful; these include such remedies as medicated glycerine jujubes, or licorice pastilles. If the cough is due to a relaxed throat, the back of the throat should be painted two or three times a day with an astringent such as glycerine and tannic acid, or with a weak solution of iodine, or the more specialized preparations such as Mandl's solution, etc. Removal of enlarged tonsils and adenoids, or of a uvula which is too long, may also be necessary.

Inhalations are of great value when the irritation proceeds from the larynx. Nothing is more effective in soothing laryngeal irritability, and the persistent cough which attends it, than the inhalation of the vapor from compound tincture of Benzoin or menthol crystals.

Children who suffer from a cold on the chest may be relieved by rubbing the chest with liniment containing camphor. Food and fresh air should be supplied in liberal quantity. A soothing cough mixture should also be given.

When the cough is loose and the expectoration is free, a stimulating mixture should be given.

COUNTER IRRITANT. Irritation of the skin in order to relieve pain of some part of the body is known as counter irritation. Counter irritation is often applied to the chest in cases of bronchial catarrh by rubbing camphorated oil well into the skin.

There are several groups of counterirritants varying in the degree of severity of their action. Mild counterirritants such as mustard, turpentine, camphor, or iodine, which produce a feeling of warmth to the skin, are called *rubefacients*. Rubefaction is the medical term for the redness which appears on the skin after the application of such drugs. The more severe type of counterirritant when applied to the skin produces small vesicles or blisters which run together, forming one large bleb full of clear fluid.

COURSES. This is a popular term for the menstrual periods which occur in women (*See also* MENSTRUATION.)

COWPOX. This is believed to be a form of smallpox among cattle, but which may be communicated to human beings who come in contact with it. It is a relatively mild disease showing none of the severe symptoms of smallpox. There is usually a slight rise in temperature, and a sore generally appears on whichever part of the body has come in contact with the diseased cow; generally it is on the hand, through the process of milking. It was noticed that persons who had suffered from cowpox did not develop smallpox, and it was this observation which led Jenner in 1796 to carry out, for the first time, vaccination of man with cowpox lymph obtained from the hand of a dairymaid. The lymph which is used nowadays to confer immunity against smallpox is taken from the sores on a tuberculin-tested calf and, after being mixed with glycerine and water, is stored in a cool dak room before being used. (*See also* VACCINATION.)

CRACKS. Cracks may occur in several parts of the body and where they are present should always be healed as soon as possible, not only because they are usually painful, but also because they make an open doorway for the entrance of germs into the blood. The most common cracks are those on the hands and lips. Cracks on the skin of the hands are called chaps, and are described in a separate article.

Cracked Lips. Cracks on the lips are usually at the corners, which are apt to be moist from the saliva from the mouth, or in the fullness of the lip where the cold winds catch it. The habit some people have of constantly moistening their lips with their tongue is very apt to cause cracks in the lips in cold, dry, windy weather. These may be very painful and are also very ugly.

Treatment. The best way to prevent them, and to cure them when they have occurred, is to keep the lips moist in cold weather with a good cold cream, or plain lanolin, which is simply the purified oil obtained from sheep's wool and cannot harm the most delicate skin. It is interesting to notice that chapped lips are far less common than they used to be and the explanation is certainly that most women now use lipsticks, even if they are only colorless ones, and these lipsticks are made of some simple harmless greasing material, generally lanolin, white paraffin, or cocoa butter. Thus the lips are protected from both frost and cold winds and also in summer from excessive heat.

Cracked Nipples. Another crack, that is common amongst mothers and can cause a great deal of trouble and excessive suffering is the crack in the nipple. This crack comes a few days after the mother has begun to nurse the baby if she has not taken care to harden the nipples before her confinement. The pain when the baby suckles is very great, and when cracks develop, feeding from the affected breast should be stopped for 24 hours. Compound tincture of benzoin should be applied and a nipple-shield used for the first day after suckling is resumed. In many cases an abscess forms, and the baby may have to be weaned. Great care should therefore be taken to prepare the breasts before childbirth by the methods described in the article on PREGNANCY.

Cracked Fingers. Cracks on the thumb or fingers are caused by the same things as chaps on the backs of the hands: generally the hands have been exposed to cold and dry winds, or have been wet in the cold. These small but deep cracks can be very painful and a great nuisance, especially to a woman who has sewing or knitting to do.

Treatment. They are difficult to heal unless they are covered with a bandage to keep them from being continually torn open again. The hard edges of the crack should be rubbed off with pumice stone and the crack filled with an ointment containing salicylic acid and kept covered up until it is completely healed. To prevent chaps and cracks on the hands there is nothing so useful as glycerine in some form or other. It may be used in a diluted form mixed with rosewater and rubbed into the hands at night during the cold weather.

Cracked Tongue. Cracks in the tongue happen sometimes where there is a tooth with a rough edge, which constantly irritates the tongue, and sometimes when the stomach is upset and out of order. Excessive smoking may also cause this condition.

Treatment. When they are the cause the teeth will have to be put in order and rough edges filed down. Any digestive trouble will have to be attended to and smoking cut down or given up. The mouth may be washed out frequently with glycerine of thymol. If the crack does not heal quickly a doctor should be consulted at once, as it may be the beginning of an ulcer, which may lead to more serious trouble.

Anal Fissure. This is a painful and troublesome crack in the skin of the anus, which is the lower opening from the bowel. As the stools are continually passing over the crack and infecting it as well as irritating it, these cracks are very difficult to heal completely.

Treatment. The part should be kept scrupulously clean and nupercainal ointment may be rubbed over the crack before and after each motion of the bowels; the motions should be kept soft, but not moving more than once or twice a day. If the crack does not heal it should be seen by a doctor.

CRAMP. Cramp is a painful spasm of any muscle. The muscles which are most often subject to cramp are those of the legs and feet. The attack may be due to lying or sitting too long in a strained position. Exposure to cold, general debility, fatigue, or diabetes are some of the conditions which may produce cramp. Cramp is also used loosely to describe any colicky attack in the abdomen. Cases of drowning from cramp are usually due to heart failure. In cramp in a limb, the best way to relieve the pain during an attack is to stretch the affected limb. This may be very difficult and extremely painful, but it is well worth the effort. If the victim is unable to do this, the affected part should be rubbed energetically until the spasm gradually gives way. (*See also* COLIC and CRAMP in the FIRST AID SUPPLEMENT.)

CRANIAL NERVES. These consist of twelve pairs of nerves which come from the brain itself. They control the senses of sight, smell, hearing, speech, etc., also all movement and sensation about the head and neck.

CRANIUM. The cranium is that part of the skull which contains the brain, though the whole skull is often wrongly referred to as the cranium. The bones that form the skull are divided into two classes, the cranial and the facial. (*See also* SKULL.)

CREAM OF TARTAR. Acid potassium tartrate is also known as bitartrate of potash or cream of tartar. In doses of ½ to 1 teaspoonful in ½ pint of warm water, it acts as a mild purgative. A very pleasant drink for feverish patients is imperial drink, which is made by adding a teaspoonful of cream of tartar to a pint of home-made lemonade.

CREOSOTE. Creosote is obtained by the distillation of wood, the best kind being made from beech wood. Creosote has the same action on the body as carbolic acid, and has been used externally as an antiseptic. It is used as an inhalation in bronchitis and lung complaints, and may be inhaled either from boiling water or by means of some form of inhaler, so that the vapor can be conveniently drawn into the chest through the nose and mouth.

Creosote is also taken internally. It should be taken in capsule form, diluted with a quantity of almond oil or cod-liver oil; dose, 1 to 5 minims taken immediately after meals.

The ointment of creosote is made up with creosote, hard paraffin and white soft paraffin. It is used in various skin diseases such as dermatitis and inflammations of the skin.

CRESOL. Cresol, or cresylic acid, is a straw-colored liquid obtained from coal tar by distillation. It becomes brown on keeping or on exposure to light, so should be preserved in stoppered amber-colored bottles.

It is a powerful disinfectant and Lysol is made from it. A tablespoonful to 1½ pints of water is a convenient strength for disinfecting instruments, linen, drains, etc. For the hands, one tablespoonful to 2½ pints will be found strong enough.

Cresol has a reputation in the treatment of whooping cough, when the substance is vaporized by heat. This may be carried out by pouring a teaspoonful of cresol on to a heated metal plate, or a special vaporizer can be obtained for the purpose.

Cresol and its various preparations, being so common, have led to many cases of poisoning. The symptoms are very similar to those of carbolic acid poisoning and the treatment is the same.

CRETINISM. A cretin is a child who suffers from a peculiar form of idiocy, owing to the absence or deficiency of the juices of the thyroid gland. This gland lies in the front of the neck and it plays a very important part in the physical and mental well-being of human beings. The thyroid gland is one of the ductless glands of the body whose juices are carried directly into the bloodstream. (*See also* DUCTLESS GLANDS.)

Cretinism seems to be more prevalent in certain parts of the world than in others and in such cases is due to deficiency of iodine in the drinking water. The condition is very common in Switzerland, Northern Italy, and France. Cretinism occurs also from time to time in the U.S. and Great Britain, when it is due to an inborn arrest of development in the thyroid gland.

Symptoms. If a child is born with the thyroid gland undeveloped, nothing unusual is noticed until the child reaches the age of about 6 months. It will be noticed then that the child is backward, and physical as well as mental signs begin to develop. The head appears to be large and flat, and the tongue is unusually large and tends to protrude. The hair becomes thin, and the skin appears to be very dry. The abdomen is seen to be very prominent and the back is curved in. Speech, if it develops at all, is very late and defective. Quite a number of these children die young, but there are many who grow up. Without treatment they are idiots, and they remain dwarfed, rarely attaining the height of four feet.

Treatment. Treatment should commence immediately the condition is discovered. Continuous administration of thyroid gland extract is necessary to make up for the deficiency in the patient. The child will, under this treatment, begin to react very quickly, and so long as the treatment is kept up will continue to develop normally, both mentally and physically.

CRISIS. The word crisis as used in regard to illness means a turning point, and is used to mark the moment in severe illness when the patient suddenly takes a turn for the better and the high temperature drops quickly. As a general rule, the more quickly the temperature rises in the first place the more quickly it will fall when the crisis is past. The most marked crisis is that which occurs in untreated pneumonia. The patient has been getting steadily worse and the fever and breathing are very bad. The crisis arrives almost always on the ninth day, though occasionally there is a rapid crisis which occurs on the fifth day. The patient at the height of pneumonia is desperately ill and it does not seem that he can hang on to life much longer. Then the observers notice that his skin has become moist and cooler, he may pass a large quantity of urine and will drop into the first quiet sleep he has had for days. From that moment recovery should begin and go on steadily. Other severe fevers, such as measles, influenza, etc., have a minor crisis when the fever has reached its height. This is often as soon as twenty-four hours after the first rise of temperature.

The word crisis is sometimes used to denote an attack of pain in the illness called tabes dorsalis.

Some diseases, such as Addison's disease and Graves' disease, proceed naturally with periods of improvement and periods of replase. These episodes when symptoms are of unusual severity are referred to as crises.

It has been explained that crisis means the rapid drop of temperature in severe illness, but it happens in some diseases that the drop of temperature is slow but sure, and the patient recovers very gradually. This sort of ending to an illness is described as an ending by lysis, not crisis. (*See also* LYSIS.)

CROUP. This is a condition of difficulty in breathing accompanied by a harsh cough. It is due to a spasm of the muscles which guard and control the entrance to the lungs.

Causes. In young children the portion of the voice-box containing the vocal cords, which is known as the glottis, is so small that the slightest swelling which narrows the opening, or the presence even of a little mucus causing a blocking of the passage, will give rise during the night to attacks of suffocation which may be frightening.

Symptoms. The child is usually between the ages of 2 and 5 years, and seems perfectly well during the day, though he may possibly have a slight cold. He wakes up suddenly about 11 p.m. with intense difficulty in breathing. His breathing is jerky, air is drawn into the lungs noisily and it makes a whistling sound. There is also a hoarse cough. After a period of time varying from a few minutes to an hour or more, the attack ends and the child falls asleep again as though nothing had happened. These attacks may be repeated night after night.

Although it is very alarming, croup is rarely fatal, and simple treatment is all that is usually necessary to stop the attack.

Treatment. The attack of difficulty in breathing, which naturally inspires so much alarm, is treated by applying to the front of the neck a sponge or handkerchief soaked in water as hot as possible and wrung nearly dry. Care should be taken not to burn the skin. The water should be changed and the sponge or handkerchief kept hot until the suffocation has disappeared. Between the attacks the child should be kept in a warm room, and a vaporizer should be used. The bowels should be kept open regularly. The child must be kept as quiet as possible and all excitement and irritation should be avoided. If the condition of rickets is present this must of course be treated.

Other Conditions which resemble Croup are:

Congenital Laryngeal Stridor. This is a condition which is present at birth or just after. The difficulty in breathing is continuous and ceases after a few months. It does not cause any distress and is never fatal.

Catarrhal Spasm of the Larynx. In these cases there is some degree of cough or hoarseness present. The onset of the attack is fairly rapid, but not sudden as in false croup. The breathing is not jerky. It is never fatal.

Catarrhal Laryngitis (Acute Laryngitis). In this case there is a history of a previous cold, difficulty in breathing and some degree of fever. The difficulty in breathing becomes steadily worse and lasts longer each time. The condition may be a simple sore throat or it may be due to diphtheria, and in such cases medical advice should be sought early.

Whooping Cough. In this case there will be the characteristic "whoop."

Enlarged Tonsils and Adenoids. These may cause some obstruction to breathing and produce a noise very similar to that of croup. The treatment is to remove the tonsils and adenoids.

CROWING. This is also called *laryngismus stridulus,* laryngospasm or croup, and is a form of convulsion affecting the muscles of the throat, causing the patient to make a crowing noise rather like the whoop in whooping cough. It is a condition which affects children between the ages of 6 months and 2 years and occurs in children who have rickets; adenoids are frequently found to be present. (*See also* CROUP.)

CRUSH SYNDROME. Severe crushing of a limb by injury (such as fallen masonry) gives rise to toxic symptoms at present thought to be due to absorption of an injurious substance resulting from the crushing. It causes suppression of urine and other serious symptoms, and treatment is still experimental.

CRUTCH. A crutch is an appliance which is used to support the weight of a body when a patient is suffering from a diseased or injured limb. The head of the crutch, which consists, in the simplest form of crutch, of a cross-piece at the top of a wooden pole, should be well padded to prevent undue pressure on the armpit, otherwise the nerves of the arm may become paralyzed.

CURARE. This substance has been known to medicine for many years as an extremely powerful poison, acting by paralyzing the nerve ends at their point of action in muscles. Certain tribes of South American Indians used this poison to coat their arrowheads and probably knew something of its practical pharmacology thousands of years ago. Purified extracts, standardized so that the effect of dosage can be predicted with some certainty, have recently been introduced to obtain muscular relaxation during surgical operation. The outstanding advantage of the drug is that it permits the anesthetist to maintain a lighter level of anesthesia throughout operation except at those moments when complete relaxation is required. Curare does not replace the usual methods of producing anesthesia, but enhances them and makes them safer. It has been used as well to relax the spasms of tetanus, and in strychnine poisoning. The use of this drug in practical medicine has been a great stimulus to the synthetic chemists and there are now a fair number of laboratory-made substitutes available.

CURD. *See* CASEIN.

CURETTAGE. This term is applied to an operation in which the interior of the womb is scraped with a *curette.* A curette is an instrument shaped rather like a spoon with a long handle.

One of the commonest reasons for this operation is the removal of fragments of the products of conception, which if left in the womb would result in infection and bleeding. It frequently has to be performed after a miscarriage.

CURVATURE OF THE SPINE. The normal movements of the spine are forward, backward, and sideways, but if any exaggeration of the these movements appears, curvature of the spine may result. (*See also* SPINAL CURVATURE.)

CUTICLE. The cuticle is popularly

used to refer to the layer of skin which grows round the base of the nails, but it is really the outer covering protecting the whole skin of the body. (*See also* SKIN.)

CUTIS. The cutis is the true skin. (*See also* SKIN.)

CUTS. A cut, however small, should be thoroughly cleansed before one tries to stop the bleeding, in order to avoid a septic (poisoned) wound. The simplest way is to hold the injured part under a running cold water tap for a few minutes. The surrounding parts should be washed away from, never towards, the wound. Broken glass, etc., should be removed if seen; the cut should not be probed.

After washing, mild tincture of iodine should be dabbed (not rubbed) freely over the cut and the surrounding skin, and a clean dry bandage put on. A perfectly clean handkerchief is suitable. Adhesive tape or ointment should not be applied.

Even fairly profuse bleeding may often be stopped by a firmly applied bandage; boric powder is sometimes useful. For more serious cuts, where the bleeding cannot be stopped, a tourniquet should be put on above the wound, and medical aid summoned at once. (*See also* FIRST AID SUPPLEMENT.)

CYANOSIS. This term is applied to a bluish discoloration of the skin which is due to the blood not being properly mixed with oxygen. It occurs in health in the tips of the fingers, nose, and ears during cold weather. In such cases it is due to slowing of the circulation in the skin. Blueness of the lips does not occur in health and is due either to slowing of the circulation in the heart or to inadequate mixing with oxygen in the lungs. More rarely, it may be the result of mixing of venous and arterial blood, such as happens in congenital malformation of the heart. More rarely still, it is due to drugs like phenacetin and some sulphonamides.

CYSTITIS. This means inflammation of the bladder. It is usually due to infection by a germ, together with a lowered state of health. Some types of germs are so powerful that they alone will cause inflammation of the bladder, but these are not common.

The causes are injury or congestion of the bladder wall and stagnation of the urine. Stagnation of the urine may be due to a variety of causes in the passage from the bladder to the exterior (the urethra), such as stricture (narrowing of the passage), enlargement of the prostate gland which surrounds the neck of the bladder, the presence of stone or other foreign body; and also to various conditions affecting the nerve supply to the bladder.

Congestion of the bladder may be due to inflammation of the neighboring structures such as the womb, to tumors of the bladder, etc. Damage during pregnancy or after childbirth is also quite a common cause.

Virulent germs may reach the bladder from the urethra, or the germs may descend from the kidneys down the ureters. Germs are more liable to enter the female than the male bladder from below, because the female urethra is much shorter. The passage of a catheter may cause inflammation of the bladder.

Symptoms of Acute Cystitis. Pain in the lower part of the belly, also agonizing pain in the bladder and at the end of the penis in the male, after passing water. Water has to be passed frequently and urgently. The water contains an abundant deposit of slime and pus with perhaps blood in varying quantities.

Treatment. Rest in bed and food consisting of a milk diet, with plenty of fluids, are necessary. The pain is much relieved by hot hip-baths, of which two or three a day may be taken lasting for 20 minutes. The bowels must be kept open with suitable aperients. The catheter should not be passed while the condition is acute, nor should any attempt be made to wash out the bladder. Aureomycin and chloromycetin are very effective.

Chronic Cystitis. In this condition there is some pain, but usually much less than in the acute stage. There is more a feeling of weight in the lower part of the belly. There may still be a desire to pass water frequently and to evacuate the bowel. Damp and cold, sexual and alcoholic excesses will make the discomfort worse.

The water is cloudy, smells offensive and may be difficult to pass. It often contains pus and blood and is frequently alkaline. Of the complications the most serious is infection of the kidneys.

Treatment. This depends on whether the germ causing the cystitis makes the urine acid or alkaline. When the water is acid the germ is usually the bacillus coli, a germ which normally lives in the large intestine. Drugs are given which tend to make the water alkaline. Citrate of potassium and bicarbonate of soda in large doses are given. A course of sulphadimidine or one of the antibiotic drugs will usually destroy infection by bacillus coli. When it fails to do so there may be some abnormality in the urinary tract, such as an enlarged prostate or a stone in the bladder, which will require special treatment. If infection persists in spite of this, the water must be made acid by giving sodium acid phosphate, and urotropine is given in fairly large doses. There may be a temporary aggravation of symptoms such as some discomfort and frequency in passing the water, so the patient should be warned of this in order to prevent disappointment. The hexamine is usually effective in clearing up the infection.

Local treatment may be carried out by washing out the bladder.

An antiseptic fluid is introduced by way of the urethra into the bladder two or three times a day. The bladder is washed out again and again until the returning fluid is quite clear. The fluid usually used is weak silver nitrate.

Further Points. The drinking of large quantities of water is very important. At least a tumblerful of fluid should be drunk hourly in the early stages. A large quantity of fluid acts mechanically and helps to clear the membrane of the bladder from its germs; it also keeps the urine dilute. (*See also* BACILLURIA; BLADDER.)

CYSTS. Cysts of one sort or another are tumors or swellings filled with fluid or semisolid substance. They grow in almost any part of the body, and vary in size from little pea-sized lumps to great un-

sightly growths, which are very disfiguring. Most cysts are harmless, though ugly and uncomfortable. A few varieties are mentioned below. The commonest variety of cyst is the *sebaceous cyst* or *wen,* which is formed by the blocking of the sebaceous or fat-glands of the skin. These wens may grow in any part of the body, but are most common on the face, neck, and head. A curious variety of cyst is the *dermoid cyst* which is present at birth, but usually does not develop until later in life. It is usually found on the face and contains such sub-

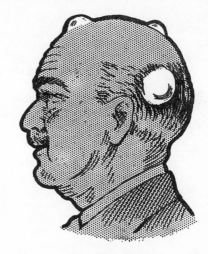

Cysts, Sebaceous.

stances as skin, hair and even teeth. *Hydatid cysts* are dangerous cysts which are caused by a worm resembling the tapeworm. This worm inhabits the intestines of sheep and dogs and is conveyed to human beings by these animals. They usually occur in the liver or lungs. *Ovarian cysts* of various sizes are fairly common in women, and in some cases grow to astonishing sizes. Further information about these varieties of cyst and their treatment is given under their own headings.

DACTYLITIS. Inflammation of the the finger is known as dactylitis. It is a condition which starts in one of the small bones of the finger and is nearly always tuberculous in origin. It may

be a sign that tuberculosis is present in some other part of the body, so it is necessary that the general health should receive attention. Dactylitis may also occur in children owing to inherited syphilis. The diseased finger usually requires to be operated upon, and if the condition is due to tuberculosis, the treatment will take the form of plenty of fresh air, good food, and sunlight.

D.D.T. The discovery of D.D.T. (technically dichlorodiphenyl-trichlorethane) as an insecticide was one of the notable advances in medicine during the second World War. It was first synthesized in 1874, but the discovery of its insecticidal properties was the result of methodical research by Paul Muller, a Swiss working at Basle.

D.D.T. fulfils the requirements of an ideal insecticide. It is lethal to insects, while being relatively harmless to animals and plants. It is stable so that its effects persist in the areas in which it is deposited and it does not lose potency under the effect of sunlight. It does not injure fabrics or corrode metals and it is cheap to produce. Perhaps its only serious rival in this field is benzene hexachloride, which is in the process of development.

During the second World War, D.D.T. was widely used in the control of mosquitoes. By spraying the interior walls of houses with a 5 per cent solution in kerosene using 1 qt. for every 1,000 sq. ft., it was found possible almost completely to eradicate mosquitoes and houseflies. Respraying only needed to be carried out every month. This spray was also found to destroy bedbugs.

A 5 per cent powder should be found useful in the home. Weaker concentrations may well be found ineffective. Such a powder is a good treatment for fleas on dogs and is effective against the common clothesmoth. D.D.T. can be incorporated in an oil-bound waterpaint to eradicate bugs from the walls of infested houses.

A single application of an emulsion containing 2 per cent D.D.T. to the hair when left without washing for fourteen days will cure headlice (pediculosis capitis.) A dust containing 10 per cent D.D.T. has been widely used in refugee camps to combat pediculosis of all types. About 1½ oz. are needed to disinfest the body and clothes of a person with body lice.

DAMP. Damp plays a very important part in many illnesses. If the air is saturated with moisture, the skin is unable to get rid of the normal amount of sweat which is necessary to perfect health. Wherever there is dampness there is always a feeling of chilliness, even in spite of a fire. A hot, moist atmosphere is very harmful because this also interferes with the proper evaporation of perspiration and a feeling of heaviness is the result. Workers in cotton mills suffer a great deal from lung troubles such as bronchitis and pneumonia through getting their clothes soaked with sweat and omitting to dry them properly before going out into the air.

Cold, damp air is most harmful to people who suffer from rheumatism and arthritis as it seems to make their pains worse. It is a very common thing for people to say that they know when it is going to rain because they feel it in their bones. Sometimes corns have jumping pains, or an old scar may feel unusually tender.

Many diseases appear to occur more frequently in damp climates. Bronchitis and pneumonia are among the more common. (*See also* CLIMATE.)

DANDRUFF. Dandruff, or scurf, is due to a mild chronic inflammation of the skin of the scalp. The inflammation may be present for many years, the only disturbance being a slight itching. The head is "scurfy," i.e., the horny cells of the scalp are shed in large numbers and form scales; and there is a tendency for the hair to come out. Each fallen hair is replaced by one thinner and weaker, until the hair is seriously thinned. Finally, the hair roots become atrophied, and baldness results.

This is one of the commonest of skin diseases; it has been estimated that one in every three people is affected. It is due to infection of the surface layers of the scalp with a mold and is conveyed from person to person by hairbrushes and combs. It is aggravated by neglect of washing, brushing, and combing, with the consequent accumulation of cells and dried perspiration upon the scalp. The use of harsh drying shampoos and lotions, the excessive use of oils, and anything which hinders the natural perspiration of the scalp (tight hats or headdresses, wigs, etc.), all aggravate the condition. Some people, such as those with tender skins, which turn red and are irritable on very slight provocation, are especially liable to dandruff. Acne or rosacea, oily skins, and defective digestion are frequently accompanied by dandruff.

Treatment. This long list of causes shows that the treatment must be general and preventive as well as local. The *preventive* treatment consists of avoiding anything harmful to the scalp, and due attention to the hair. The *general* treatment consists of regulating the diet and attending to the ordinary rules of hygiene.

The milder cases of dandruff should be cured by regular care of the hair. If possible, it should be washed daily, and the juice of half a lemon mixed with the final rinsing water.

The cure of a well-established case requires endless patience and care, as the condition is very obstinate. Women with long hair would be well advised to have it cut, as the application of medicaments to a scalp covered by long hair is not only very tedious and difficult, but the resulting appearance is far from attractive.

Many substances have been used, such as sulphur, salicylic acid, resorcin, iodine, pyrogallol, etc. (Fair-haired people should only use the first two, as the others darken the hair.) The most valuable of these is sulphur, which may be applied as an ointment or emulsion, the latter being the cleaner method. The preparation is applied at night and well rubbed in, and a linen cap worn. A bathing cap, so often advised, should *not* be worn; it is most unhealthful for the scalp. The sulphur is allowed to remain on for ten days and then washed off; after which the treatment is repeated until the cure is complete.

Since light treatment and X-rays produce such wonderful results in other cases of chronic inflammation, it was hoped that they would be equally successful in cases of dandruff, but the results have so far been disappointing. Improvement may occur at first, but the condition soon relapses, and may even be aggravated.

DAY BLINDNESS. This is a disorder of the sight in which objects cannot be well or comfortably seen either by daylight or by strong artificial light, but are seen more clearly and comfortably by a half-light, as in shadow or twilight.

It is not a disease in itself, but a sign of disease, and may be caused by various conditions. There may be a cataract or "blind spot" in the lens of the eye, with the result that the vision is obscured when the pupil of the eye is small, as it is in bright light, but becomes clearer when the pupil grows large, as it does in poor light. If there is irritation or inflammation of the lids, or eye, or if the eye is dilated from the use of atropine or any other cause, there is always some degree of discomfort in the light, so that the patient can only open his eyes (if at all) in the shade. It occurs naturally, but only for a short time, when one passes suddenly from darkness into light.

The disease causing the symptoms should be treated. A central "blind spot" can be to some extent relieved by giving drugs which enlarge the pupil of the eye, or by making a new pupil. Inflamed eyes are relieved by a shade or by tinted glasses, until the disease which caused the condition has cleared up.

DEAD FINGERS. There are people who suffer from what is popularly called dead fingers. The fingers, and sometimes the toes, may suddenly go white and cold and remain so for a short period and then rapidly regain their normal color. The disease is considered to be due to a disturbance of the nervous system. Particulars are given under its medical name, RAYNAUD'S DISEASE.

DEADLY NIGHTSHADE. *See* ATROPINE and BELLADONNA.

DEAF MUTISM. This means that a person can neither hear nor speak. It may date from birth or be acquired at an early age, and in nearly every case the deaf mutism exists because the child cannot hear and so has never learned to speak, as speech comes from the imitation of sounds heard. The most usual cause of deaf mutism dating from birth (*congenital deaf mutism*) is a defect in the development of the internal ear; this may be hereditary and is said to be comparatively common in children who are the result of marriages between near blood relations, such as first cousins. Deaf mutism acquired at an early age may be due to a variety of diseases, such as meningitis, scarlet fever, mumps, and inflammation of the internal ear.

Treatment. The first thing to do in the treatment of deaf mutism is to make sure that the condition is not due to some disease of the ear which ought to be treated. If the deaf mutism is due to a defect of development of the ear no treatment will be of any avail, and the child should be sent to a special school for deaf mutes. Teaching speech by signs is now out of date, as it restricts conversation to those who are acquainted with the deaf and dumb alphabet. Nowadays deaf mutes are taught by lip-reading and by the sense of touch: the pupil watches the movements of the teacher's lips and at the same time places his hand over the teacher's throat to feel the movements of the larynx. Although the education of deaf mutes is a long and tedious business, the results usually obtained make it well worth while. (*See also* DEAFNESS; DUMBNESS.)

DEAFNESS. This may be due to blocking of the outer passage (external meatus) of the ear by wax, to blocking of the middle ear (the little space behind the drum) by catarrh or inflammation, or to disease of the internal ear (nerve deafness.) Many persons, when they become deaf, say that there is deafness in their family, and make little or no effort to get cured; but an extremely small percentage of cases of deafness is due to any family influence. Deafness is common, much more common than most people imagine, and it is much more easily treated in its early stages than in its late stages, when it is almost always incurable. Wax can be removed easily by syringing the ear with a solution of bicarbonate of soda in warm water; this dissolves the wax, which the stream of water washes out. Catarrh of the middle ear is usually an extension of a cold in the nose up the little tube that leads from the ear to the middle ear itself. It is often brought on by violent blowing of the nose when one has a cold or by using a nasal douche and sniffing it up the nose too hard. Catarrh of the middle ear is best treated by inhalations of menthol or compound tincture of benzoin (1 teaspoonful to a pint of boiling water); a specialist can clear the ear by blowing the catarrh away with a little silver eustachian catheter; but this is a difficult procedure that needs much practice. Inflammation of the ear and chronic discharge from the ear cause deafness, but require treatment by a doctor to get them well. Otosclerosis is a kind of bilateral progressive deafness, especially for low tones, which develops usually in early adult life. It is sometimes hereditary and is due to changes in the bone surrounding the internal ear. It can often be helped by a delicate surgical operation, stapedectomy.

Internal ear deafness (nerve deafness) is usually due either to old age, or to a poisoning of the nerve of hearing by tobacco or quinine, or by the poisons of such diseases as mumps or syphilis. This last type of deafness is the most difficult to cure, and the cause must be found and treated.

DEATH. Death is represented in art by a skeleton with scythe and hour-glass, or as a reaper, cutting down bearded grain and innocent flower alike. But however he is painted or written about, we cannot escape him; and death, in one form or another, is witnessed by most of us before we have gone far on life's journey. The child sees its kittens or rabbits die; it watches the autumn leaves flutter to the ground, brown and apparently lifeless; perhaps someone in the family dies.

There are ten thousand doors, says the English poet, Webster, that may open "for man to take his exit." Death, that is to say, may be natural, owing to the natural decay of old age; or it may be violent, as by drowning, a street accident, a snakebite; or it may be the result of disease; and under each of these headings there are many forms it can take.

In a sense, we begin to die as soon as we are born. Our bodies are built up of millions of tiny cells; these are called tissue. Each time we exert ourselves, whether bodily or mentally, as in walking, scrubbing a floor, talking, or merely thinking, we use up some of this tissue, and it is destroyed and replaced by fresh matter. This is going on all our lives, so that we are continually dying and continually being reborn until death.

How do we recognize death? When death takes place two things occur: (1) the circulation of the blood through the body and (2) the act of breathing stop. Changes take place in the cell tissue and, consequently, in the appearance of the dead person.

That the circulation has really stopped may be ascertained by listening carefully for the heartbeats. For the breathing, a mirror may be held before the face and note taken of whether it becomes misty, or a feather may be placed on the upper lip and we may watch for the faintest fluttering.

Those in attendance should close the eyes and mouth, bandage the jaw and straighten the limbs.

A few hours after death the body is cold. Bruise-like marks on the back show that blood no longer actively circulating is collecting there. During the next few hours the muscles stiffen, to relax again in about four days. A greenness on the abdomen two or three days after death shows that decay has begun.

Duties of Relatives. It is the duty of the relatives personally to report the death to the local office of Medical Examiner or Coroner. If a doctor was in attendance during the last illness, written notice must be accompanied by the doctor's certificate of the cause of death. Failing any relative who was with the dead person when death took place, or attending on him, the duty of informing the registrar falls on some other relative. Failing any relatives, it falls on someone present at the death, then on the occupier of the house, then on someone living in it, or the person arranging for the funeral. The body must not be buried until the coroner has given a certificate; this is handed to the clergyman at the funeral.

Sudden or violent death and deaths in prison are matters for the coroner. It would be the duty of anyone witnessing a sudden or violent death or finding a dead body to inform the police.

Cremation. Anyone wishing his body to be cremated after death should leave written instructions to this effect. If he forbids this form of burial, it cannot take place.

DEATH RATE. As in death itself the two great events are the stoppage of the circulatory system and the stoppage of the breathing, so in the figures showing the death rate over the country year by year and quarter by quarter it is disease of these two systems that stands at the head of the list of causes of death: first the heart and circulatory system; then influenza, pneumonia, and other diseases of our breathing apparatus. So it is the stoppage of these two essential things, things that work automatically, as it were, all our lives, without calling attention to themselves so long as they are healthy, that accounts for most deaths.

High in the list of causes of death is the disease, cancer. Nowadays, people are less nervous than they were of going to see the doctor if they are worried about a lump, or have any other symptom that brings to their minds the fear of this disease. They know that the dread disease is curable so long as it is recognized early enough.

Next in the list of causes of death come diseases of the nervous system, and then come various diseases of the circulatory system.

The above are the main causes; but there are others that make us think. For instance, there are still far too many deaths of infants from diseases peculiar to early infancy. Research into the causes of this loss of life is being organized, and it is to be hoped that the reasons will be recognized soon and the number of deaths greatly diminished.

There are far too many deaths resulting from various types of accidents. There is a gradual increase in the number of such fatalities, a number far too great for a modern civilized community.

DEBILITY. Debility is a term used to describe a state of health which is very much below normal yet without being due to actual disease. The term is not used unless a search for organic disease has failed to reveal its presence.

General debility may be caused by insufficient or improper food, lack of exercise, unhealthy surroundings, or as a sequel to exhausting illness. Nervous debility usually owes its origin to some long-continued anxiety in persons of nervous temperament. Financial or business worries or unsatisfactory love affairs will often cause nervous debility.

Any form of debility should be treated with adequate rest, plenty of fresh air, good and nourishing food, and a proper amount of exercise and tonics.

DEBRIDEMENT. Debridement describes the opening up and clearing of a contaminated wound, with removal of blood clot, dirt, and foreign material, and excision of damaged tissues.

DECOMPOSITION. In science, decomposition means the splitting up of chemical compounds into simpler substances. This chemical change is taking place all the time in our bodies and is a necessary part of the body's normal working. Complex food substances are broken down in the process of digestion so that they can be readily absorbed and utilized by the tissues. The cells of the body, by decomposition of absorbed materials, provide themselves with the means of growth, and energy to carry out their work.

Decomposition of foodstuffs is very important in regard to the health of the human being. Decomposition takes place owing to the presence of germs which generate poisons. Ptomaine poisoning is due to the presence of germs in food and in some cases death has occurred after eating such food. Age alone is not responsible for decomposition, because if food is kept under proper conditions it will not decompose as rapidly as food which is exposed to the action of germs. Foods when properly canned or bottled may keep for years, also meat if it has been kept in a refrigerator where bacteria cannot survive. All decomposed food should be avoided, and care should be taken to prevent unnecessary decomposition taking place by storing food in a cool, dry place and providing suitable covering to keep out dust and flies which carry germs.

DEFECTIVE VISION. There are two sorts of blindness and defective sight: in the first there is an easily recognizable defect in the eye; in the second, however, there is no obvious cause in any part of the eye. The term *amblyopia* is used to mean this latter form of defective sight.

Amblyopia due to defective development is frequently found along with other defects of the eye. The most common is long sight (hypermetropia), where one eye is affected, and the other is nearly normal. In these cases squint frequently occurs. The child's habit of using the "good" eye and resting the squinting one undoubtedly aggravates the condition; but it is of no use, as was formerly done, to occlude the good eye with a ground-glass lens so as to make the squinting eye do its proper work. The power is lost as soon as the good eye is allowed to resume its rôle of fixation.

The treatment of this form of amblyopia should be on preventive lines as far as possible: if a child is noticed to use one eye more than the other, for instance, or if there is any other peculiarity in his sight, he should be treated as soon as possible by an oculist. If this is not the case, some impairment of vision will occur even if the adverse conditions are removed later in life.

In lead poisoning, various retinal changes are met with, with corresponding symptoms. The prognosis in these cases is very bad. Further deterioration of vision, with changes in the optic nerve, is sure to follow, even when the source of poisoning has been removed.

In functional amblyopia, sometimes called amblyopia fugax, from its transitory character, the loss of sight may be complete or partial. It comes on in the course of a few minutes, and may last from half a minute to an hour. It is sometimes preceded by "flashes of light before the eyes," and may be followed by an attack of migraine. It may occur quite frequently; no changes are seen in the eyes. There is another similar form in which, however, the attacks are longer and edema (or swelling) of the retina will be found. This is due to spasm of the retinal arteries. The attacks are infrequent, and unless very severe, no permanent harm is done. (*See also* AMBLYOPIA; BLINDNESS; VISION.)

DEFICIENCY DISEASES. Deficiency diseases are a group of diseases due to lack of an essential element in the food called a vitamin. Disease may be due to deficiency of vitamins in the diet or failure to absorb them from the gut.

The first disease that was recognized to be due to vitamin deficiency was scurvy, which is caused by lack of Vitamin C, the vitamin present in fresh vegetables or meat. Scurvy formerly used to break out in ships on long voyages, and it was found that it could be prevented by taking daily a small amount of lime juice, as it was called. (In reality it was lemon juice from Mediterranean lemons, which were called limes by mistake; lemon juice, it has been found, contains much more Vitamin C than does lime juice.) Vitamin B, when lacking, causes a disease known in the East as beri-beri, in which the affected person has severe neuritis and eventually various forms of paralysis. At the siege of Kut, in the first World War, it was observed that the soldiers who had hand-milled (unpolished) rice escaped beri-beri, but those who fed on white (polished) rice contracted it; the reason for this was that the "germ" of the wheat contains something that prevents beri-beri. Rickets, the third deficiency disease to be recognized, is due to an absence of Vitamin D, the existence of which was made known only after Vitamins B and C were discovered. It has been found that rickets can be prevented by sun-light and by taking animal fats. Slight deficiencies in vitamins cause comparatively minor ailments such as constipation and night-blindness, mental depression, and lethargy. An ordinary good mixed dietary is the best assurance of an intake of vitamins sufficient to maintain good health. (*See also* VITAMINS.)

DEFORMITY. Any abnormal condition of the body whether congenital (present at birth) or acquired later in life may be termed a deformity. Deformity may be due to faulty development of the child or the result of injury or disease.

Certain deformities such as extra toes or fingers seem to run in families, but such deformities are very easily got rid of if attended to at birth, and no discomfort or unhappiness is caused when the child grows up. Those which are most common are club foot, dislocation of the hip, cleft palate, harelip, and wry neck. Other congenital deformities may not be so easily treated and may even be so bad as to prevent a normal life being led.

Deformities due to injuries are very common and are the result of scarring of the skin, shortening of the muscles, and damage to bones. Many people are so badly scarred by burns that the tissues are destroyed, leaving very disfiguring marks. Skin grafting has done much to prevent ugly deformities, especially on the face; this is carried out by taking skin from a healthy part of the body and causing it to grow over the disfigured parts. When muscles have been damaged they usually shorten during the process of healing. This condi-

tion may be treated by massage; but, as a rule, a surgical operation is required to put matters right. Unless broken bones are properly reset, a considerable amount of deformity will result. It is usual to have X-ray photographs taken after a fracture has been reset in order to make sure that the bones are in the correct position.

Various diseases are responsible for deformities of the bones and by far the most common is tuberculosis. It attacks the growing bones of young children and may even destroy part of the bone; the ligaments also become diseased, thus causing the bones to assume abnormal positions. Most of the cases of humpback are due to tuberculosis of the spine and many displaced hips are due to the same cause.

Rheumatoid arthritis is a disease which affects many of the joints in the body. Serious deformities are caused by this inflammatory condition and many people become altogether bedridden by it. However, the chief general disease which leads to deformity is rickets. This condition causes the bones to become soft and, as soon as any pressure is put on them—for instance, when the child begins to walk—the bones become distorted and many deformities are thus produced. Humpback, curvature of the spine, bowlegs, knock-knee, and deformity of the pelvis are a few of the conditions which may arise through rickets. Many women have a difficult and dangerous time at childbirth because of the damage done to the pelvis by rickets in early childhood.

Paralysis due to nervous disorders may cause serious shortenings of the muscles. Infantile paralysis, especially, is the cause of many permanent deformities. The limbs gradually waste away through not being moved or used, and a withered arm or leg is often one of the results of this condition. Surgeons who deal with cases of deformity are known as *orthopedic* surgeons, and surgeons who build up parts of the face or body are known as *plastic* surgeons. During both World Wars, when terrible injuries were inflicted and very often parts of the face were blown away, burned, or otherwise destroyed, the plastic surgeon was able to work wonders by building up and repairing the features. It was no uncommon thing for a man to have a new nose built on to his face, or for a great gap in the jaw to be filled in so that the face presented a normal appearance. This type of work has now become very advanced and there is no longer any need for people to lead unhappy lives owing to ugly facial disfigurements or deformities.

DEGENERATION. By degeneration is meant a gradual change for the worse in the tissues of our bodies. It may be the natural process of growing old, when all our organs are wearing out and the stocks of energy of one sort or another that keep our bodies in working order are getting less; or it may be due to causes that are not inevitable, such as illness or poisoning of the tissues by substances which are taken into the body from without or are manufactured in the body itself.

With regard to the degeneration of old age, everyone knows that they cannot expect to be as strong and stand as much strain in their old age as in their youth and prime. In a machine which is made up of many parts, it is to be expected that one part after another will wear thin or wear out entirely; for the machine we can go out and buy another part to replace the worn one and the machine becomes as good as new; but in the machinery of our bodies, a part once worn out cannot be replaced. We cannot buy ourselves a new stomach or a new pair of kidneys or eyes; all that we can do is to take as good care as possible of our machinery while it is in good working order, and when it is wearing thin, treat it with a much consideration as possible and make it last as long as possible. The normal healthy person should expect to be doing and enjoying a full day's work until at least sixty years of age. Then the time arrives when notice must be taken of a downhill trend of our bodies and mental faculties. The nervous system is not what it was, various glands do not function as well as formerly, the heart is not so strong as it once was. In fact, the changes of old age are setting in and the time has come to slow down.

It happens very often, unfortunately, that these signs of degeneration are observed not at the time of normal old age, but when most people think they are only approaching middle-age, about forty or fifty. The degeneration in this case is due to the poisoning of the tissues from various causes that might have been prevented if proper care of the body had been taken in the journey through life, and the habit of worrying and overworking, overindulgence in alcohol or smoking, or habitual overeating and underexercising had been avoided. The early degenerating due to definite diseases such as Bright's disease, pernicious anemia, etc., is not dealt with here, since it is obvious that the sufferer from a chronic disease must take special measures to keep himself going if he is to reach old age at all. But, apart from disease, far too many people carelessly allow themselves to start on the downward journey at far too early an age. The man who becomes plump from self-indulgence in his thirties will have a sixty year old body when he is fifty, unless he mends his ways. This is an artificial degeneration. The machine has been badly used and will not, of course, last as long and as well as the machine which has been well treated and properly cared for.

DELIRIUM. This is a mental disturbance which is marked by excitement, bodily restlessness and flights of the imagination, and accompanied by senseless chattering. Delirium occurs in many disorders, but is a particularly distressing accompaniment of any high fever. To the onlooker it is a terrifying thing to hear a relative talking utter nonsense, or "wandering" as it is often called, and to see him or her tossing about from side to side in a vain endeavor to obtain rest. Fortunately, this disturbance lasts for a comparatively short time. In most fevers like scarlet fever, or diphtheria or in pneumonia, delirium does not necessarily mean that the patient is very gravely ill; it is only the height of the fever which is causing the delirium. But in certain diseases it is a very bad sign if the patient develops delirium. Typhoid fever is one of these diseases. In this disorder, the delirium is rather different in type; instead of being noisy and restless the patient sinks down into bed and mutters nonsense.

Delirium is one of the features of the attack in that form of insanity known as acute confusional insanity, which very often is associated with such physical conditions as poisoning by alcohol, belladonna, food poisoning; or which occurs in some cases after childbirth or after severe hemorrhages. Acute confusional insanity is a common type of mental disorder and, happily, the patients, on recovery, nearly all forget their illness and have little or no recollection of anything that happened during their sad experience. In the attack, the signs of delirium are all present, but they are all exaggerated. The patients are lost in time and space, and do not recognize those about them. They are noisy and restless; they may roll about the floor and it is consequently difficult to keep them in bed. Hallucinations are nearly always present. That is to say, the patient may hear voices, see visions, or smell odors which do not in fact exist. In some cases, rather quaint visions are seen; the patient describes small, brightly dressed people, one to two inches in height, who amuse and interest him by their antics. More often the visions are unpleasant—weird animals or devils are seen. According to the degree of restlessness and confusion, it is for the medical practitioner to decide whether a patient who has the delirium of acute confusional insanity should be nursed at home or temporarily be removed to an institution. It is comforting to know that when the latter alternative is decided on, the period of residence is likely to be short and recovery from the attack almost certain.

DELIRIUM TREMENS. This is not the result of a very large single dose of alcohol; it occurs in those people who are steady drinkers, never drunk, but never completely sober. It comes on very often if, owing to such unforeseen circumstances as an injury, or attack of pneumonia, all alcohol is suddenly stopped. Delirium tremens is really a variety of acute insanity which is marked by delirium with trembling and excitement, and in which there is great anxiety, mental distress, and confusion. It lasts only a few days and with proper treatment, recovery is the rule; but any further indulgence in alcohol renders the patient liable to another, and possibly fatal, attack. The mental signs of an attack are mainly those of confusion and anxiety or states of intense terror. Terrifying visions, well described by many novelists, are seen. These visions commonly take the form of animals crawling over the bed and up the walls, or of terrible enemies who

threaten the patient with immediate death. Restlessness may be extreme, the patient throwing himself all over the room in an attempt to escape from his horrible visions, and it is not surprising, therefore, that he is completely unable to sleep. The patient looks, and is, physically ill; his face is an unnatural reddish color, his breath is offensive, and he cannot take food. There is a trembling of the limbs which may be limited to the arms or may also be seen in the legs. The temperature is often slightly raised.

Treatment. It is difficult to treat a patient in his own home because he is likely to be very noisy and violent, and it may take two or three attendants to prevent his hurting himself. On the other hand, the disorder is likely to last only a few days, and the patient on recovery, though weak, is perfectly clear in his mind, and may resent having been moved. This problem has to be settled for each individual case according to circumstances. The great point about the treatment, wherever it is given, is to ensure that the patient obtains sufficient sleep, and for this reason paraldehyde or one of the barbiturate drugs is usually given. Next to sleep, sufficient food is the main requirement of a patient with delirium tremens, as it is notorious that alcoholics do not take enough food. In an attack of delirium tremens, milk is the best diet in the worst stages. Thiamin and Vitamin B complex are also useful. On recovery, the patient must be warned that for the rest of his life he must be a total abstainer.

DELIVERY. By delivery is meant the stage of childbirth during which the child actually passes from the womb of the mother. In a normal delivery the head of the child comes first, and the rest of the body usually comes away within the space of a few seconds. After delivery has taken place, the mother should rest in bed for at least a week but if this is not possible, daily rests should be taken and all heavy work should be avoided. Falling of the womb and its complications very often occur because the mother has neglected to take sufficient rest after her child has been delivered. (*See also* CHILDBIRTH; LABOR.)

DELTOID. This is the name given to a thick muscle of the shoulder. It derives its name from its likeness to the Greek letter delta.

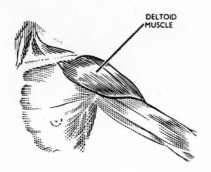

DELTOID
MUSCLE

Deltoid Muscle.

DELUSIONS. Delusions are false beliefs or judgments which cannot be accepted by persons of the same race, class, age, and education as the person who expresses them. This rather lengthy definition of delusions is necessary, because what is a delusion for an intelligent American might well be accepted as a natural belief for a savage in the wilds of Africa, or for a child of five years old. For example, if such a child drapes a tablecloth round his shoulders, puts his father's hat on his head, and proclaims himself a king, we are amused and say that he has a vivid imagination. The same conduct in an educated man would result in measures being rapidly taken to secure his detention as a person of unsound mind. The most important feature of any delusion is the intense conviction with which the deluded person persists in his belief or judgment.

No amount of argument, or what a normal person would call "proof to the contrary," will shake an insane delusion, and time so spent is only wasted. So long as a delusion lasts, that person is definitely insane, inasmuch as he has lost insight into his true condition.

Delusions are many and varied, but they mainly reflect the mood of the patient. A depressed patient has delusions of misery and woe; he has committed unpardonable crimes; brought ruin on his family; his brain is rotten; or his limbs are made of glass and will break if he moves them. An excited patient tends to have delusions that express his sense of wellbeing; he possesses vast estates, can break every athletic record, and go for weeks without sleep.

Some patients have what are called systematized delusions, because not only are these delusions supported by argument, but they govern the patient's conduct. It is in patients with systematized delusions that we find cunning, but insane, criminals. A patient with such a delusion hears voices, for example; these voices tell him that certain people are plotting against his life; in order to save his own life it is necessary that these other people should be killed. It must always be remembered that a delusion is a sign of grave mental disorder. In every other respect a patient may appear well and mentally normal; but if he is the victim of a delusion, careful observation is essential lest the delusion should influence his conduct and place him within reach of the law.

DEMENTIA. This is a permanent loss of mind which results from destruction of certain nerve cells in the brain. It must be distinguished from *amentia,* a condition in which the mental powers have never developed. Dementia may be the last stage in some other mental disorder, or it may occur as the result of the wearing out and breaking down of the nervous system in old age, or the specialized cells of the nervous system may be starved of blood through disease of the arteries of the brain and so perish. The chief causes of disease of the brain arteries are excessive consumption of alcohol, chronic disease of the kidneys, and syphilis.

Dementia Praecox. This term was formerly used to describe the mental illness known as schizophrenia and is described under that heading.

Senile Dementia. This is a condition of old age in which the mind gives way before the body. The memory fails and the patient lives in the past. He becomes irritable and hard to please, and laughs and cries more easily than would be expected of an adult. He often loses things because he forgets where he has put them and then accuses others of stealing them. If not treated tactfully and sympathetically such people often develop ideas of persecution or imagine that their relatives wish to rob them. Finally, there is the "second childhood" in which everything has to be done for them as they are incapable of even feeding themselves. Only kindly and tactful attention can make the last few years of these unfortunate folk anything but a burden to them.

DEMULCENT. A demulcent is the name given to any substance which has a soothing effect on the skin or mucous membrane. In cases of poisoning white of egg acts as a demulcent on the lining of the stomach; and any soothing ointment is a demulcent to the skin.

DENGUE FEVER. This is a type of fever which is very common in most tropical countries, and which usually commences with great suddenness. It is a disease which is practically never fatal and it must not be mistaken for other conditions, such as measles, malaria or influenza.

Symptoms. As a rule a feeling of chilliness with rheumatic pains in the joints may be felt a little time before the fever actually begins. As the temperature rises, there is severe headache and aching pain at the back of the eyeballs. The joints all over the body seem to ache, and the pain is more severe on movement. The tongue is at first moist and furred, but soon becomes dry and coated, and the throat may be sore. Vomiting is not uncommon, and there may be diarrhea, though oftener there is constipation. In severe cases the temperature may rise as high as 104 degrees F., and delirium is not unusual. The crisis occurs about the third day, accompanied by sweating and diarrhea. The headache is relieved and the temperature may fall, and what is known as "the stage of calm" is reached. At this time the patient may feel extremely weak, but be well enough to get up for a short period.

On the fourth day, or sometimes as late as the seventh, from the date the illness began, the rheumatic pains return, the temperature rises slightly, and a rash resembling scarlet fever or measles appears. The rash begins on the hands and the backs of the wrists, and spreads to the arms, body and legs. In the meantime the temperature returns to normal and the spots may take two or three weeks to clear up completely. The rheumatic pains may be felt for a little time after the fever has gone and the patient may suffer from insomnia.

Treatment. The patient should be kept in bed until the rash has disappeared. Aspirin, in doses of 10 grains every 6 hours, may be given in order to relieve the rheumatic pains. Doses of health salts should be given as soon as the fever begins. The convalescent period is straightforward and rapid, but there may be a persistent feeling of weakness for a long time after. A change of climate is usually necessary if this weakness does not wear off.

DENTAL CARIES. This term means decay of the teeth, and is caused by bacterial activity involving the dentine. Damage to the enamel which protects the tooth leads to weakening of the dentine by the chemical action of fermenting food and by bacteria. Once the protection given to the pulp by its dentine surround has been destroyed, inflammation of the pulp results.

Chief causes of dental caries, other than any constitutional weakness, are poor diet and inattention to dental hygiene. Vitamin D is of particular importance in the diet, and this deficiency can be avoided by the consumption of milk, eggs, butter (or margarine), fat fish (herrings, particularly), and cod-liver oil. Green vegetables, fresh fruit and fruit juices are valuable for their additional property of Vitamin C, and extra calcium is supplied by cheese and bread.

From every point of view it is wise to take care of the teeth, and it is obviously better to prevent trouble occurring than to find that neglect has brought about a condition which can cause pain and ill health, and which may require much time and patience to cure. Regular visits to the dentist, regular brushing of the teeth—certainly twice a day, and preferably after meals as well—gentle massage of the gums, and sufficient hard foods to give the jaws exercise in biting and chewing, will all contribute to good health. (*See also* CARIES; NECROSIS; TEETH.)

DENTAL CARE. Like everything else, there is a right and a wrong way of cleaning teeth. To begin with, the proper toothbrush must be used and the best kinds are made with bristles which are not too soft and which do not come out with use. Some people, it is true, have very tender and soft gums, and the slightest rubbing may cause bleeding, and for them a softer brush will be best; but for the average person, a medium-hard brush will be right.

The choice of dentifrice is also a matter of individual taste, and any which is made by a reliable firm is sure to give satisfaction. Some people cannot use those which are made up in the form of a soap, as the foamy lather in the mouth causes them to feel nauseated. Most dental pastes are very pleasant to use, and as a rule they contain an antiseptic substance which leaves the mouth fresh and clean. A gritty tooth paste or powder should never be used for more than an occasional clean-up.

How to Use a Toothbrush. The whole point of cleaning the teeth is not merely to polish the outer surfaces, but to clean between and behind the teeth as much as possible. In order to do this the brush should not be drawn across the teeth, but an up-and-down movement should be used. This enables the bristles of the brush to work themselves into the spaces between the teeth, and in this way any particles of food are removed. The dentifrice should be applied to a dry brush, and each side of the mouth, behind as well as in front of the teeth, should be brushed for a few minutes. After the dentifrice has been worked well into the teeth the mouth should be rinsed out with water. If an additional antiseptic rinse is desired, a few drops of hydrogen peroxide, or some other antiseptic mouth wash may be added to the water.

After the teeth have been thoroughly brushed, the toothbrush should be rinsed under the tap and dried. This is an important point, otherwise the brush will soon become soft and the bristles will tend to break off or come out. It is better to hang the toothbrush up on a rack or small nail for the purpose, as this allows it to drain properly. At least two toothbrushes should be kept for the purpose of cleaning the teeth; this ensures the use of a dry brush night and morning. In most books on dentistry it is advised to clean the teeth after every meal, but for the average person who is busy and away from home most of the day this is not practical, and a brush night and morning should be sufficient to keep the mouth clean.

Discolored Teeth. The color of the teeth varies a great deal with different people,

and it is not everyone's good fortune to be blessed with teeth like pearls, but much can be done to whiten them, especially if they become discolored by too much smoking. A few drops of hydrogen peroxide sprinkled on the toothbrush and used about twice a week will tend to remove yellow stains. Again, the hydrogen peroxide can be used as a mouthwash, but it should be kept in the mouth for a few minutes and not rinsed out, otherwise the cleansing effect will be largely lost.

Care of the Gums. If the gums feel unduly tender and are inclined to bleed, a visit to the dentist may be indicated. If there are any signs of pyorrhea, it will be necessary to have the matter attended to immediately. It is unwise to put off paying a visit to the dentist whenever there are signs of bleeding gums, because very often teeth which may later on have to be extracted could be saved by a little early attention.

To improve the health of the gums, and thereby improve the health of the teeth, the gums should be brushed at least once a day for a few minutes. Ordinary kitchen salt in half a glass of water is a very good thing to use for hardening the gums. The brush should be frequently dipped into the salt water and every square inch of the gums should be gone over.

Dental Care for Children. Children after about the age of four are, as a rule, quite capable of starting to use a toothbrush themselves. They should be given an attractively colored one in order to encourage them to use it. In this way the habit of cleaning the teeth daily will be formed. Mothers should remember that a thorough brushing of the teeth at night, and certainly after the last meal is eaten, has more effect in preserving the teeth than brushing at any other time, but the morning brushing is also important. The effect of diet on the teeth is an important question which does not come into this article, but the eating of fresh, firm fruits after a meal is an excellent way of keeping the teeth clean. Giving a child an apple to chew after a meal is just as good as sending him to clean his teeth, and the exercise necessary to chew the apple will help to strengthen the jaws and teeth.

Care of Dentures. Artificial teeth, just

like natural ones, require to be kept clean and in good condition. They should be taken out night and morning and scrubbed thoroughly with soap and water. At one time it was considered undesirable to leave them in overnight, but most people nowadays prefer to sleep with them in and provided due attention is paid to their cleanliness, there is nothing against this procedure.

Dentures, like one's own teeth, are liable to have scale form on them, and if this is allowed to accumulate, the teeth will become dirty and even offensive. It is wise, therefore, to soak the dentures periodically overnight in one of the many proprietary cleaning agents which are obtainable. These will not only remove the tartar, but will cleanse and sweeten the plates and make them more comfortable to wear. It is not possible to say how often this should be done, as different people's teeth form scale at very different speeds, but one cannot go far wrong if the teeth are cleansed in this way at least once every two weeks.

Dental Floss. This is used for cleaning between the teeth and for dislodging matter which may be clinging to the surfaces and necks of the teeth. The floss consists of strands of nylon or similar material suitable for being drawn or slipped between the teeth.

Dentifrice. Any substance used for cleaning the teeth is termed a dentifrice. There are many preparations to be had in liquid, paste, or powder form.

A tooth powder should not be too gritty or the continual rubbing may cause the enamel on the teeth to become chipped. Each person should use a dentifrice suitable to the individual needs. For example, if the mouth is acid, causing tartar to form behind the teeth, an alkaline dentifrice containing magnesia should be used to neutralize the acid. Most preparations contain an antiseptic in some form or another, and the flavoring substances used are generally agreeable to the taste.

Dentine. The hard substance which forms the greater part of a tooth is known as dentine. It resembles bone, but it is made up of different structures which vary somewhat in different teeth. Ivory, which is obtained from elephants' tusks, is an example of dentine. (*See also* TEETH.)

DEODORANT. This name is given to any substance that deordrizes or destroys offensive smells. It is important when dealing with this matter to remember that the mere fact of covering up a smell is not removing the cause. Many deodorant substances also act as disinfectants; carbolic acid, for instance, is a powerful disinfectant, but it is only mildly deordorant and will not be of much use in covering up a very foul smell. On the other hand, chloride of lime is capable of acting both as a strong deodorant and as a disinfectant.

There are many preparations on the market which are sold for personal use in order to do away with offensive body odors. Perfumes are used by many people for this purpose, but their use should be limited to small quantities otherwise their use may become objectionable.

In the sickroom the air can be deodorized by a solution of a pleasant-smelling disinfectant. The windows should be thrown open top and bottom to allow fresh air to come in. Buckets of water placed in a room will remove the smell of paint. (*See also* DISINFECTANT.)

DEPILATORY. This is the name given to any drug or method by which hair is removed from the body. Many depilatories are composed of sulphide of barium, but the effect produced by the use of this substance is temporary and hair will grow again in the course of a week or two. It is necessary to mix barium sulphide with water to make it into a paste. The paste is spread over the part of the skin to be treated and left on for about five minutes, then scraped off with a very blunt knife.

Shaving is a popular method but tends to coarsen the hair and increase its growth. Plucking the hair with small forceps is a method which has become popular within recent years. The eyebrows, especially, are trimmed in this way. It is, however, a painful process unless the skin is slightly deadened by an application of ether or some such substance. Rubbing the skin with pumice-stone is sometimes carried out in order to remove hair from the arms and legs.

All these methods only remove the hair for the time being, because in order to destroy the hair for ever it is necessary to remove the root. Electrolysis is a method by which permanent removal of the root may be carried out. This is done by treating each hair separately with a fine needle through which an electric current is passed. It is a task which requires a very skilful operator as there is great danger of damaging the tissues of the skin and thereby causing disfigurement. Diathermy is another electrical method of removing hair and it is claimed to be more satisfactory than electrolysis. X-rays are the most effective depilatory known and are used to produce loss of the scalp hair in the treatment of ring-worm.

DEPRESSANT. This is the name given to a group of drugs which have a depressing effect on various organs of the human body. These drugs act either through the brain center or through the nerve supply. For example, when chloroform is given, it depresses the brain and eventually causes the patient to become unconscious. Many drugs are given to depress the action of the heart, and they act by slowing the conduction of the impulses in the nervous tissues of the heart.

DEPRESSION. This is a mental state in which there is a feeling of ill-being and sadness, slow thinking, and a general sense of inactivity. The outlook on life is gloomy, all movements are slow, the expression is dull. Everything becomes a burden, and work almost an impossibility. The patient who is suffering from depression feels worst in the early morning when the vitality is at its lowest. At this time he is usually overcome by a feeling of despair at the thought of having to face another day. Frequently these patients neither seek nor will take medical advice. They declare that "nothing can be done," "their case is hopeless." It is in such a frame of mind that suicide is attempted. In almost every case of depression this thought of suicide enters the patient's mind. He is so wretched that he feels he cannot go on. Very often there is little warning before the attempt is made; the patient conceals his misery and may even pretend to those around to be better. It is fortunate that this state of depression occurs in attacks, and provided that during these attacks the patient is watched and prevented from attempting to take his life, the outlook for recovery from any one

attack is good; but other attacks may occur.

Treatment. The bodily health must be well looked after both during and in between the attacks. Very often it is found that physical ill health or an emotional shock is the precipitating factor, and cure will follow the removal of the appropriate cause. Severe cases require admission to a mental hospital both to protect them from injury and to give them treatment. Convulsions are induced electrically and are often followed by remarkable improvement. During an attack of depression, however mild, it is wise to stop work, as mental stress and worry only make the condition worse. Complete mental rest, with very light exercise in the open air is the best treatment.

DERMATITIS or INFLAMMATION OF THE SKIN. When the skin is irritated in any way, whether from outside or inside, it behaves like all the other parts of the body in like circumstances: it makes a protest. To this is given the name dermatitis, or inflammation of the skin. The greater the amount of the irritation, and the more sensitive the skin, the more severe is the resulting inflammation.

The first stage is that of *erythema* or redness, due to the wall of the blood-vessels dilating or relaxing. The next is that the relaxed vessel walls allow fluid to be poured out into the tissues of the skin; this means that the cells of the horny or topmost layer of the skin, instead of being shed as invisible single cells when their work is done, stick together and come off as noticeable *scales*. If the amount of fluid is greater, it flows out between the cells on to the surface and dries there, forming what are called *crusts*.

If the fluid is poured out more rapidly than it can make its way to the surface, it makes little pools in the epidermis, or upper layer of the skin. These form tiny blisters, and are called *vesicles*. Larger blisters soemtimes occur, which are called *blebs* or *bullae*. In some cases the fluid produced is actually so great as to wash off the outer layer of the skin, leaving an inflamed red surface from which drops of fluid are continually seen oozing. This is known as *moist* or *weeping* dermatitis.

In very chronic inflammation, the whole

skin layer and the tissues underneath become thicker and harder. This process is called *keratosis*.

In view of these different results which may be brought about by irritation of the skin, and remembering that one or another, or two or three together, may be seen at the same time, it is easy to understand the great variety of skin "pictures" that may be found, the difficulty of treating them, and the patience that must in many cases be exercised by both doctor and patient if a good result is to be obtained. There is, at present, no one-day cure for dermatitis.

Sometimes dermatitis occurs in which one form of reaction predominates and it is convenient to recognize and treat this. It must always be remembered, however, that it is the *cause* of the dermatitis that is of importance, not the *form* it takes.

Red or Erythematous Dermatitis. This is generally found on the face, and may be produced by the sun, or by such irritants as poisonous plants. If it occurs where two surfaces rub together, as between the thighs, it is apt to become moist. It is treated by lotions containing such powders as zinc oxide or zinc carbonate, or by simple dusting powders. Liniment exsiccans, which is composed of tragacanth, glycerine, and water, is excellent for slight cases, and "black wash" or weak tar lotions in chronic cases. Ointments and other greasy applications are unsuitable.

Swollen or Edematous Dermatitis. This generally occurs along with some other variety. It is generally seen on the upper part of the arms, and the body, where small, swollen areas, about the size of a dime, are seen. Sometimes crusts occur. It is treated in the same way as the erythematous variety.

Pimple or Papular Dermatitis. This occurs in two forms. There may be pimples on the inner surfaces of the arms and the back of the neck, which are burning and very itchy, or there may be a chronic crop of pimples, generally on the limbs, which are due to a too-great growth of the skin tissue. The surface of the pimples may be flattened or pointed, and pale pink to dark red; as there is always itching, many pimples may be scratched off and crusts of dried blood are seen on the top. This form of dermatitis so closely resembles the skin disease called lichen planus that for a long time it was thought to be a variety of this disease and called lichen simplex; it may also be confused with prurigo, if the itching is unusually severe.

In the acute forms the treatment is by lead and tar lotion, or by dusting powder, and if this is done early it may prevent the formation of vesicles. The chronic form is very difficult to treat. It is generally best to "make haste slowly," and use weak tar lotion or "black wash," which produces a slow but steady improvement. Zinc gelatine is useful in cases where there is much itching. Argyrol and other silver compounds, and salicylic acid or salol, in a paste, may be tried cautiously; at first only on a small area of skin.

Vesicular Dermatitis. The main sign of this fairly common type is little blisters. It usually occurs on the face, or to a lesser degree on the hands, and is the result of exposure to some strong irritant, especially a plant of some poisonous kind. It develops very rapidly from the red to the pimply, and then to the blistering stage. The blisters break on the surface of the skin, and a mild case may end in this way. In a more severe case more and more blisters are formed, which burst on the surface and form crusts. These act as nurseries and breeding grounds for germs, and so the fluid that is poured out becomes changed into pus or "matter." If the discharge becomes still more profuse, weeping dermatitis results. If the blood vessels are much dilated, as sometimes happens, the affected parts are of a bright scarlet color; this was formerly called red eczema.

It is treated by lotions or mildly antiseptic powders. The discharge and crusts should be removed from time to time by spreading the part with strips of lint or old washed linen soaked in oil, or by a starch poultice. As the condition improves, a paste may be used. This may be made of equal parts of magnesia and petroleum jelly; or Lassar's paste, which is made of equal parts of zinc oxide, starch powder, lanolin and petroleum jelly, may be preferred. In weeping dermatitis, an astringent or drying lotion, such as black wash, or lead or aluminium acetate in a weak solution, should be applied by placing strips of lint soaked in the lotion over the part.

Sometimes in this, and the red eczema variety, the patient is much relieved by the use of ointments such as Hebra's, which is composed of equal parts of lead plaster and petroleum jelly. This should be applied by spreading on lint and placing over the skin, then bandaging. It should be changed twice daily. If the hands are affected, and the patient is carrying out treatment at home, the application of strips and bandage may be a matter of some difficulty. In these cases is it more convenient if he has several pairs of washable cotton gloves, a clean pair to be used each time the dressings are changed. If his "dresser" turns the gloves inside out, puts them on, and "washes" them all over with the ointment, then re-turns them for the patient, the dressing will be easily and satisfactorily performed. If liked, he can wear a second pair of gloves over the first. Sometimes it is necessary to try one or two ointments before one is found to suit the patient.

Blistering dermatitis may be taken as a good example of how to dress an inflamed skin. It will be noticed that the lotions, pastes, and so on are not applied directly to the skin by "dabbing" on, or rubbing in, but are first applied to lint, and this gently laid over the inflamed parts. The object in treatment is to assist the skin in its work of healing, not to rub off the tender new skin as soon as it forms.

Scaly Dermatitis. This is usually the last stage of the other varieties. It may occur on any part, but is especially noticeable on the legs.

The treatment is directed to soften and remove the scales. Ointment and pastes are therefore used, and very well rubbed in. Tar or salicylic acid, both of which help to dissolve the horny scales, may be added to the ointment in small proportions. Old people sometimes suffer from a very chronic scaly dermatitis on the legs. They are greatly benefited by an application consisting of oil of cade (prepared from tar) and cod-liver oil. As the condition improves, the proportion of the oil of cade should be increased, and "by the time the codliver oil has disappeared from the prescription, the leg is usually well!"

In obstinate cases, where the deeper tissues have become thickened, the upper hard skin must have a more severe treatment. It may be scrubbed with soap spirit or soft soap, and dressed with soap plaster, containing 2–3 per cent of salicylic acid, spread on linen. This treatment, together with massage, should be employed until the skin is quite soft and supple and all thickening has disappeared, or the condition may return. In still worse cases, the upper layers of the skin are dissolved off with caustic potash before a dressing is applied. This is very painful, but exceedingly useful when other means fail.

Sometimes, in very thickened skin, fissures or cracks occur, owing to the stiffness and hardness of the skin. They are treated by tar and salicylic acid in ointment, varnish, or plaster.

As has been said, anything which irritates the skin will cause inflammation in some degree. Irritants are of very varying kinds. They may be *physical,* such as light, heat, or cold; *chemical,* such as many drugs, poisonous plants or woods, soaps, dyes, and so on. Irritation may be due to *infection,* using the word in the widest sense, and including infection by insects, such as in scabies ("the itch"); fungi, such as in ring-worm; and germs, as in lupus or tuberculosis of the skin.

Treatment. The treatment of dermatitis or inflammation of the skin has already been discussed from the local point of view; that is, as far as regards applications to the skin itself. The aim in treatment is to take away what the skin has in excess, and to supply what it has not; for instance, to remove discharge, scales, or thickened skin; to supply fat to a dry skin; to relieve itching and heat. It is hoped by these means that the skin will be put at rest sufficiently to cure itself.

Diet. It is known that some articles of food produce a rash in some people. Sometimes a patient knows quite well that a certain article of food increases his skin trouble; but in doubtful cases a skin test may be used. The patient may then have a reasonably plentiful and varied diet, and be quite certain that he is safe from aggravating his skin trouble.

There are, however, a few special cases that need mention. In very acute inflammations of the skin the temperature may be raised (though this is rare except in children), and in these cases the diet should be as for a feverish condition. In any case where the trouble is severe, the diet should be light and readily digested. If other diseases are present, such as any form of indigestion, diabetes, or pernicious anemia, in which a special diet is part of the treatment, they should have preference in treatment; but, if possible, any food *proved* to increase the skin rash in a particular case should be avoided.

Foods that warm and flush the skin, such as very hot drinks, spiced dishes, curries, pickles, condiments, and salted meats, should be avoided. These stimulate the circulation in the skin, and thus tend to increase dermatitis; they also increase any itching that may be present. Very hot, strong, "stewed" tea is certainly harmful, as it tends to flush the skin. Coffee, especially when strong, has rather a special effect in increasing itching; this is chiefly noticed if there is dermatitis about the anus.

A special word must be said about alcohol. It is sometimes said that alcohol "goes to the head," or "goes to the legs," according to how an individual is affected by its use; but it certainly "goes to the skin" in all cases. It has a greater power than any other food of increasing the circulation in the skin, and so flushing and warming it. Any form of dermatitis is rendered worse by alcohol, especially the more acute forms, and those in which itching is found.

Soap and Water. Soap and water should be used sparingly on areas affected by dermatitis. If it is absolutely necessary to use soap in a case, the patient should choose a pure, superfatted, unscented kind; he may make experiments to decide which variety suits his skin best; and should use it as little as possible. When it is necessary to clean ointment or paste from an acutely inflamed skin, it is best done by using medicinal liquid paraffin.

The above advice refers to the more acute types of eczema; in the chronic, dry, hard, and scaly forms it is not necessary to employ such tender measures. On the contrary, household "soft soap" and a stiff nailbrush are often very helpful in breaking down the hard skin; or still more severe methods may be devised.

In very hot regions an acute moist dermatitis is often rendered worse by the increase in the discharge made by the pouring out of the sweat, while a "dry eczema" is improved thereby.

Drugs. To allay itching and anxiety and to promote restful sleep, phenobarbitone is often given. A group of drugs, of which benadryl is one example have been found to diminish the sensitivity of the skin to damaging agents, and they are often used to good effect in dermatitis.

Persons who develop dermatitis after exposure to an irritating chemical or natural product will usually have to change their jobs, as their idiosyncrasy is likely to remain with them for the rest of their lives.

DERMOGRAPHIA (Skin-writing). Dermographia is a peculiar condition in which one is able to write or draw a pattern on the skin, and the result is immediately shown in vivid red, raised marks. The patterns usually remain quite visible for several minutes, then gradually fade.

This peculiar condition often accompanies urticaria or hives, but the patterns usually itch, while in true dermographia the patterns do not itch. Nothing can be done for this condition; it is one of those medical curiosities which is due perhaps to some disorder of nervous control.

DERMOID CYSTS. This is the name applied to growths found in the body which contain structures that really belong to the skin. For instance, skin itself may be found growing inside, or hair, etc. (*See also* CYSTS.)

DESCENDING COLON. Part of the large intestine is known as the descending colon. (*See also* INTESTINE.)

DESQUAMATION. Derived from a Latin word meaning to scale, the term desquamation is used to describe the peeling of the skin which follows certain diseases. In scarlet fever, peeling of the skin occurs after the rash has faded; in severe cases, considerable loss of hair may accompany peeling. Desquamation of a branny appearance follows the fading of the spots in measles.

DETERGENT. This name is given to any drug or substance which is used for cleansing or purifying. Soap, for example, is a detergent. Many alcoholic preparations will clean greasy skins effectively.

DHOBIE ITCH. This is a Hindu name for ringworm of the body. It is a disease which is very common in the tropics, and it derives its name from the belief that clothes become infected while being washed. The washerman in India is known as the dhobie. Full description of the disease is given under RINGWORM.

DIABETES (DIABETES MELLITUS.) Diabetes mellitus is the medical name for the disease which is commonly known simply as diabetes, or sugar diabetes. It is, unfortunately, a fairly common disease after middle age and used to come sooner or later to a fatal ending; but with treatment by *insulin,* diabetic people can now lead useful lives.

Throughout literature from the earliest times there are references to a mysterious disease, which was accompanied by the passage of large amounts of urine, but it was left to an English physician, Thomas Willis, to make the discovery that the urine in this disease was sweet. This was done by the obvious method of tasting the urine, when it was discovered to be "wonderful sweet," as if it contained honey or sugar! It was another hundred years, however, before another English doctor, Dobson, carried out various experiments with the urine of diabetic people and noticed that such urines fermented like alcohol; and therefore he came to the conclusion that the sweetness observed by Willis was due to sugar, a fact which he was later able to prove. This sugar, which is known as dextrose, glucose, or grape sugar, is obtained from the carbohydrate or starchy materials which are taken as food, but a certain amount comes from the protein parts of the diet as well.

Symptoms. A typical case of diabetes is a wasting disease, with the well-recognized symptoms of passing large quantities of urine (polyuria), thirst and hunger, together with sugar in the urine (glycosuria). If the malady is left untreated it will continue to get worse, until the patient falls into a fatal coma or state of unconsciousness. There are, however, all degrees of severity of the disease, from a condition in which there is merely a trace of sugar in the urine, to one in which the symptoms are so pronounced as to make the patient seriously ill.

It is usual to regard everyone who continually has sugar in the urine as diabetic; but it must be emphasized that sugar in the urine, especially when it is only temporary, is not of such great importance. It is really quite a frequent occurrence. Some cases are due to leakage of sugar from a faulty kidney, and many untreated cases of persistent and fairly well-marked sugar in the urine never develop into true diabetes. The exact amount of sugar present can only be measured after a meal of carbohydrate has been eaten, and, where diabetes is suspected, this examination is well worth doing, because in many cases it will save the person, who is merely suffering from the simple condition, an unnecessary amount of bodily and mental anguish. The onset of the disease is gradual, and either the frequent passing of urine or a marked thirst may be the first things to direct attention to the condition. The digestion remains good and the appetite may be enormous. The tongue is usually dry, red, and glazed, and the saliva is scanty. The gums become swollen. In spite of the enormous amounts of food consumed, the patient usually becomes very thin and wasted, the skin is irritable and there is constipation.

Complications. *Coma:* The most serious complication of severe diabetes is coma or unconsciousness, which is caused by poisoning of the blood, or *acidosis,* caused by the faulty chemistry of the body. In a typical case of coma there is increased depth of breathing, the pulse grows weak, and the patient gradually loses consciousness, sinks into a deep coma, and dies, sometimes within twenty-four hours. The coma may come on without any warning, or there may be headache, confusion, and a staggering gait before the coma comes on. In other cases there may be weakness, giddiness, and livid hands and feet.

Skin Eruptions: In diabetes, boils and carbuncles are very common. Eczema and intolerable itching are very often present. Profuse sweats may occur, and in certain cases there may be "bronzing" of the skin.

Other Complications: Diabetic persons are very liable to consumption and are often carried off with an attack of pneumonia. There may be some degree of kidney trouble causing swelling of the feet and ankles, but general waterlogging of the tissues is rare owing to the amount of urine that is passed. Neuritis, neuralgia, numbness, and tingling in the limbs are common. A diabetic person is often morose, and some become restless and anxious to a degree. In diabetes the sexual function is impaired and impotence is common, and is usually an early symptom. It is rare for an untreated diabetic women to conceive, and if she does she generally has an abortion, but a diabetic mother if properly treated will usually bear a healthy child. There is, in fact, no known instance of a diabetic mother having a diabetic child.

Treatment by Diet. Diabetes is due to a change in the organ called the pancreas, and from the nature of things this change is progressive if left untreated. This progressive tendency may be checked by dieting, but may unfortunately be made worse where the diet is unsuitable. In some cases the tendency to become worse is very marked and even suitable dieting will fail to check it. These are the cases where the preparation called *insulin* is necessary. About 40 per cent of diabetics can be treated by dieting alone.

The three main articles of diet are protein, fats, and carbohydrate, and any of these may produce some sugar during the course of digestion, or cause acidosis if not given in the right proportions. This especially applies to the type of diet which contains too high a proportion of fat and too little carbohydrate.

The value of each type of food is measured by the amount of energy it can give when it is digested. According to the amount of energy which is necessary for a person of a certain weight, so the total amount of food can be regulated to correspond. This total has to be made up of the three main food substances in their correct proportions. It is mainly the carbohydrate foods which cause an increase in the level of sugar in the blood, which in diabetes "spills" over into the urine. Thus the essential feature of a diabetic diet is that it contains little carbohydrate (bread, potatoes, etc.), and such a diet is clearly unsuitable for a patient already wasted by the severe form of the disease. Such cases always need insulin. In each particular case the diet must be worked out by giving small amounts of food to begin with, and then slowly increasing the amount to the quantity which suits the individual. The patient is first starved till there is no sugar in the urine: increasing amounts of food are then given day by day until there is sugar in the urine. This gives the tolerance limit for that article of food, and on this knowledge the final diet is worked out.

Discovery of Insulin. The part of the body which is not working properly in diabetes is the little organ lying near the stomach, which is called the pancreas in human beings. In animals it is called the sweetbread. For a long time it was thought that the pancreas as a whole was out of order in diabetes, and attempts were made to treat diabetes with extracts from the pancreas, but these were not successful. It was only in 1922 that it was realized that it was the substance produced by a small group of cells situated in the material of the pancreas and called the *insulae,* or Islands of Langerhans, that was responsible for seeing that the sugar taken into the blood was burnt up into energy and made use of by the body. For such a small part of the body the responsibility of these little cells is great. It is now known that only when these cells in the pancreas are out of order does the condition called diabetes arise.

After this discovery, the obvious thing was to try to obtain the particular juice that the Islands of Langerhans manufacture, in order to feed it to patients who were dying for lack of it. This was at last accomplished by the efforts of a young Canadian doctor, Frederick Banting. His preparation was given the name of *insulin,* and will remain one of the great discoveries of all time. Many people who were condemned to a miserable and inevitable death from diabetes were after his discovery able to carry on their work in comfort. A young American doctor, Minot, was enabled by Banting's discovery to regain his health and carry on with his research work, which led to the almost equally great life-saving discovery of the use of liver in the treatment of pernicious anemia, a disease which, like diabetes, had meant an inevitable and lingering death.

Insulin Treatment. As has been stated above, the first hope of the diabetic patient

191

is in diet, but if this fails, insulin must be resorted to. It must be remembered, however, that it may take some months to find a suitable diet on which the patient does not lose weight and on which his general condition does not get worse. The strength of insulin preparations is measured in "units" according to its effect on the sugar in the blood. Unfortunately, patients vary in their response to insulin, so that the present "unit" of measurement is not very accurate, but it is the most satisfactory way of measuring the strength of insulin that has yet been discovered. Most preparations of insulin are such that a cubic centimeter of the liquid contains 10 or 20 units of insulin.

The introduction of the long-acting zinc protamine and globin insulins has been a great advantage to patients, by avoiding the frequent injections previously necessary.

Insulin Poisoning. Insulin poisoning may appear when insulin is being given in too large doses. The face usually flushes and is accompanied by profuse sweating; the patient feels giddy and has a sense of physical coldness about the limbs, and there may be blanching of the face. Sometimes the first symptom is a feeling of nervousness or tremulousness, so that the patient finds it impossible to coordinate his movements, e.g., if he tries to write he scrawls on the paper. There may be vague feelings of apprehension—a fear of some disaster about to take place. Later, confusion and delirium appear, with finally collapse and unconsciousness. Convulsions are rare.

These symptoms usually come on from one to three hours after an injection of insulin, but not infrequently may be seen from four to six hours, or even twelve hours after injection.

Sugar given by mouth will quickly relieve all the symptoms, so that there is little or no danger associated with the use of insulin if the patient is carefully warned to take sugar whenever any symptoms, such as those described, follow an injection. The patient should carry with him some glucose, or even a candy bar. He soon begins to recognize the symptoms, and by taking the sugar can prevent their further development.

Should the patient be unconscious, the sugar must be given by injection into the veins and the collapse treated on the usual lines by stimulation with suitable drugs (strychnine, camphor, hot coffee, etc.)

Effect of Insulin. Insulin acts by restoring the diabetic patient to a normal individual. The food must be regulated and the necessary insulin dosage discovered and given *by injection* with the utmost regularity. When this is done, the blood sugar can be kept at a normal value. Many patients with long-standing diabetes are able to resume work, and appear to be as fit as the average person.

Insulin is required in cases in which diet does not control the disease and in patients where the diabetic condition is associated with symptoms such as: eye changes, which often end in blindness; neuritis of various degrees; intense local and general irritation; weakness of the limbs, and pains in the back and sides; diabetic gangrene.

It is important, of course, to be certain that the case is one of sugar in the urine due to diabetes, and not a case of *renal glycosuria,* where the sugar leaks through into the urine from the kidney. In this case the insulin will only lower the blood sugar still further and may eventually give rise to signs of insulin poisoning.

In young people, and those in whom the disease is fairly acute, it is advisable to give insulin, as this gives the best chance for the diseased pancreatic cells to regain some of their activity.

Sulphonylurea Treatment. Tolbutamide and Chlorpropamide, given by mouth, have been found to lower the blood glucose. They are best suited to elderly or infirm patients with mild diabetes, who do not respond to diet alone.

Treatment by Diet. Insulin does not cure diabetes: it merely replaces a deficiency. In the young, however, there is definite evidence that recovery of the cells of the pancreas may take place when the disease is controlled by insulin, though no cases of a cure have yet been recorded.

The aim is to arrange a satisfactory diet which will give the patient the necessary amount of insulin to keep his urine sugar-free.

As a rule, the best results are obtained by placing the patient on a fixed diet which is calculated to be sufficient in all respects, and then to give increasing doses of insulin until satisfactory results are obtained.

The protein should be in the neighborhood of ½ gram or less per pound weight, while the carbohydrate should be small.

SAMPLE DIET FOR MODERATELY SEVERE CASES OF DIABETES

Breakfast (9:30 a.m.).
  2 oz. bacon.
  1 egg.
  1 oz. white bread.
  ½ oz. butter.
  ½ oz. thick cream.
  4 oz. vegetables.
Lunch (1 p.m.).
  Beef tea.
  4 oz. whitefish.
  ½ oz. starch-free bread.
  ½ oz. butter.
  ½ oz. cheese.
  1 oz. thin cream.
  2 oz. vegetables.
Tea (4 p.m.).
  Tea.
  ½ oz. thin cream.
  ½ oz. arrowroot biscuit.
  ½ oz. butter.
Dinner (6:30 p.m.).
  Clear soup.
  4 oz. meat.
  1 oz. bread.
  ½ oz. thick cream.
  ½ oz. cheese.
  ½ oz. butter.
  4 oz. vegetables.
  Coffee.

This diet is given as an indication of the line to be adopted, and may require modification according to circumstances. Experience shows that, provided sufficient insulin is taken, there are fair limits of diet between which the patient can live and thrive. Weighing every article should not be necessary. Once the diet is settled, it is only necessary to teach the patient how much food is represented by a given weight, and he soon learns to eat approximately the same amount of food each day without weighing it. Soluble insulin is given twice a day, by injection about thirty minutes or so before the morning and evening meals.

Very often it is possible to keep the urine sugar-free by a single morning injection of the slower-acting zinc protamine insulin, either alone or combined with soluble insulin. Mild cases may be controlled by an injection of globin insulin, which is intermediate between the other forms in its duration of action.

Any illness, such as an ordinary cold, an attack of influenza, or practically any deviation from normal health, may give rise to marked increase of sugar in the urine, even when the patient has remained on a constant diet and the dose of insulin which is normally sufficient to keep him sugar-free. Such patients may even pass into diabetic coma as a result of some trifling ailment. Greatly increased doses of insulin must then be used for a time, and the same increase should be given before a surgical operation. Before insulin was available the surgeon hesitated to incur the grave risk associated with an operation on a diabetic person. In desperate cases, when an operation had to be attempted, coma often supervened and the patient died. Since the advent of insulin it is safe to say that the diabetic person has as good a chance as anybody else.

Insulin in Pregnancy. It was the common experience in the days before insulin that in diabetes the menstrual periods disappeared sooner or later. Even when this function persisted, pregnancy was very rare, and, if it did occur, the strain on the mother was so great that it seldom ended satisfactorily. Nowadays it is fairly common to meet with diabetic patients on insulin treatment who become pregnant and bear children without ill effects. The average diabetic patient who becomes pregnant runs no greater risk than does a normal woman, provided she is carefully treated on modern lines.

DIABETES INSIPIDUS. This is a chronic disease in which there is a great increase in the amount of urine passed, but it does not contain sugar as does the water in ordinary diabetes. It is a rare disease and is sometimes popularly called "drinking diabetes." It is so described because one of the chief features of this form of diabetes is a terrible and unquenchable thirst, so that the victims drink quarts of water or other liquids which seem to pass straight through them without appeasing their thirst.

Symptoms. The two most noticeable symptoms which are also present are the increase in the amount of pale-colored urine passed and the evident and distressing thirst. The beginning of the disease may be very slow and practically unnoticed or it may come on very suddenly. The frequency with which the patient has to make water causes distress and discomfort during the day and loss of sleep during the night.

The mouth, tongue, and throat are dry and parched, and the appetite is usually increased. The skin is dry and harsh. The temperature is generally below normal, and in the early stages the digestion may be good. The condition may be caused by damage in the brain or nervous system. There may be pains in the back and the legs or a tingling and itching in the skin.

Treatment. No attempt should be made to reduce the amount of fluid swallowed by the patient, but it is sometimes useful gradually to leave meat and salt out of the diet. Hypodermic injections of pituitary extract are very useful and sometimes have a really dramatic effect in relieving the condition. Cure sometimes takes place of its own accord. (*See also* DUCTLESS GLANDS; PITUITARY GLAND.)

DIACETIC ACID. This is an acid present in the urine in certain stages of diabetes and other diseases. If diacetic acid be permitted to continue to accumulate in the body it may lead to a very serious condition. It is important, therefore, to have a test made of the urine if there are any signs of acidosis in the body.

DIAGNOSIS. Diagnosis is the art of being able to distinguish one disease from another. When the doctor is called in to see a sick person, the first thing he does is to start finding out what is wrong with his patient; in other words, he tries to make a diagnosis. Sometimes he may require to examine the urine or the blood chemically or microscopically; sometimes the examination of the eyes or the larynx may require the help of a specialist. Sometimes X-ray or bacteriological examination may be necessary, and in obscure diseases the advice of a consulting physician or surgeon. Some diseases are very easy to diagnose, the symptoms are so definite; but there are times when it is not so easy for the doctor to arrive at a correct diagnosis without first knowing quite a lot about the patient. In nervous diseases especially, it is important that the doctor should know something of the past life of his patient and also of any inherited diseases or complications. This is known as a "history" of the case, and it is here that the patient may be of great help to the doctor.

Case History. Any past illnesses the patient may have had should be told in full to the doctor, as they might throw some light on the present condition. Residence abroad, especially in the Far East, often has an effect on a person's constitution, so such points should not be overlooked as unimportant. If the patient is a heavy drinker he should not hide this information, though as a rule, a heavy drinker shows signs of intemperance on his face. Anyone who has at any time suffered from syphilis should say so without delay, as this knowledge may be of the utmost importance.

It is not unusual for a patient to keep back information from the doctor from a false sense of modesty. Needless to say, such a situation is not only unfair to the doctor but unfair to the patient himself, because unless the doctor is in a position to make an accurate diagnosis of what is wrong with his patient he is not in a position to give the correct treatment. It is, therefore, necessary for the patient to be as truthful and as helpful as he possibly can be when the doctor is trying to make a correct diagnosis. (*See also* PROGNOSIS.).

DIAPER RASH. This occurs in children with sensitive skins, or in those who have not been properly cared for. The treatment of this condition will be found under ERYTHEMA.

DIAPHORETIC. This is the name given to any drug or treatment which causes the skin to sweat freely. Turkish baths or hot-air baths are very good examples of a diaphoretic, and certain drugs may be given which act on the nerve centers and produce an increase of sweat.

In many diseases it is desirable to make the patient sweat in order to reduce the bodily temperature; there is a loss of heat caused by the evaporation of the sweat. At the beginning of a fever the patient may be given a mixture containing spirit of nitrous ether and acetate of ammonia every three hours. This tends to cool the patient down without producing any unpleasant effects. (*See also* BATHS; SWEATING, DIS-AGREEABLE.)

DIAPHRAGM. The diaphragm is the dome-shaped muscular partition which separates the space of the abdomen from that of the chest. It is more popularly called the midriff. It is the chief muscle used in breathing, and when the diaphragm contracts, air is drawn into the lungs. Singers and athletes are trained to breathe through the diaphragm rather than the chest.

DIARRHEA. The condition in which the bowels move too frequently and the motions are of too soft a consistency is known as diarrhea. It is not a disease in itself, but rather a symptom of various diseases. It may be brought on simply by taking strong medicines or eating unsuitable food or too much fruit. Damp and cold will bring on diarrhea in some people, and various nervous conditions may be responsible for an attack. Nervous excitement, such as that experienced by students just before an examination, is a well-known cause of diarrhea.

By far the most common cause, however, is eating tainted or indigestible food. These foods set up irritation in the bowel and may be accompanied by severe colicky pains and much wind. In such a case, the first thing to do is to get rid of the irritating substance in the bowel, and this is done by taking a tepid water enema. When the bowels have been thoroughly cleansed, a chalk or bismuth mixture may be taken to clear up the diarrhea. Kaolin or china clay, given as a powder mixed with water, is very useful as it removes the poisons by "adsorbing" them. The diet for the next few days should be simple and should contain such things as arrowroot, cornflour, etc.

When treating chronic diarrhea it is important to bear in mind that it is a symptom and not a disease in itself. It is necessary that the real cause of the diarrhea should be discovered so that suitable treatment may be given as quickly as possible. Whenever diarrhea continues in spite of

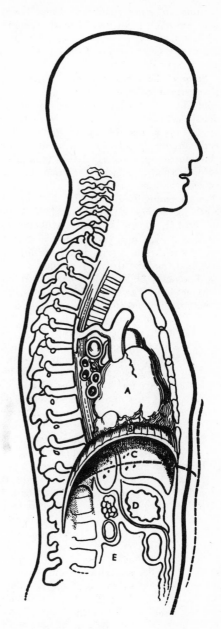

Diaphragm: A. *Heart;* B. *Diaphragm;* C. *Liver;* D. *Stomach;* E. *Intestines.*

the most simple forms of treatment, or whenever undue straining occurs, or when blood is passed, the doctor should be called in. He may prescribe sulphaguanidine or an antibiotic. Great harm is often done by treating an acute condition of the bowel with opening medicines. For diseases of which diarrhea is a symptom, *see also* CHOLERA; COLITIS; DYSENTERY; ENTERITIS; INFLUENZA; TYPHOID FEVER.

Summer Diarrhea. Summer diarrhea is also termed summer or infantile cholera, epidemic gastroenteritis, and infective diarrhea. Epidemics of this disease occur in almost every country during the summer and autumn months. Infants and young children are particularly liable to attacks of this condition, which is due to the bowels becoming infected with germs through eating bad food. In the case of bottle-fed babies, dirty milk or bottles are the greatest source of danger. Milk should be stored away in a cool place where flies are not able to get at it. It should be sterilized, and bottles and nipples should be thoroughly boiled before being used.

Symptoms. The motions are green in color, slimy, and foul, and of frequent occurrence; in severe cases there may be blood-stained mucus as well. There is usually a high fever and the temperature may be extremely high, or it may be below normal. Convulsions are common, and the child may pass into an unconscious state. An attack of this disease begins very suddenly and it is very severe while it lasts; the child quickly becomes wasted and shrunken, and in severe cases death may occur within twenty-four hours.

Treatment. As soon as the symptoms are recognized, all milk should be stopped and the child should be given cold boiled water or whey and water for twenty-four hours; this will often cut short a serious attack. If, in spite of these simple measures, the illness continues, the doctor should be called in immediately and he may prescribe a sulphonamide or an antibiotic, or other treatment. Injections of normal saline may have to be given in order to make up for the large amount of fluids which are being lost.

DIATHERMY. Diathermy is a form of electricity which is used both medically and surgically in the treatment of disease. Medical diathermy can be applied generally to the whole body, or locally to one particular part of it only. The method of its application to the patient is similar to other forms of electrical treatment; but in diathermy the electrodes which connect the patient with the electrical current must be kept in firm contact with the patient's skin, and the patient must be told never to change the position of one of the electrodes after the current has been turned on. Should he feel too much heat he must at once tell the operator, who will reduce or turn off the current. If a patient sitting on an electrode moves his position, even contact with the current may be disturbed and a burn may be the result. Or if contact is totally broken, perhaps only for a moment, a spark will jump the gap as the last point of contact is severed and cause a small, but deep and slow-healing wound. This extra care required to protect the patient makes diathermy a form of electricity which requires to be administered only by specially trained persons.

Surgical Diathermy. The surgical application of diathermy is becoming more popular every year and in many cases has decided advantages over the older method of cutting through the tissues with a knife. The diathermy knife, which is a thin blade of metal, passes through flesh with the sharpness of a knife, divides the tissues rather than cuts them and causes no bleeding, or practically none. Great advances in the use of this method of surgery may be expected. At present it is used chiefly in the removal of large growths such as cancers. One form of diathermy which works by sparking is very useful in the removal of small growths such as warts, corns, piles, birthmarks, etc.

Medical diathermy treatment is useful in chronic inflammation in the pelvis in women, and chronic prostatitis in men; also in rheumatic conditions such as gouty deposits, arthritis, and lumbago. Diseases of the nerves such as sciatica and neuritis respond very well to diathermy, and cases of pneumonia and acute laryngitis have been benefited by it. (*See also* ELECTRICITY.)

DICOUMAROL. This is an anticoagulant drug, used in the treatment of thrombosis, especially coronary thrombosis (of the heart). It is, however, a somewhat erratic drug in its action, and should be used only in hospital where the patient can be kept under careful observation, for signs of overdosage.

DIET. A diet is a specially prescribed course of food for medical purposes.

DIGESTION. The various articles of food which make up the average individual's daily diet can be divided into three main classes known as *proteins, fats,* and *carbohydrates.* Many of these substances are very complicated from a chemical point of view and are not, generally speaking, easily dissolved by the body juices, so that before they can be absorbed into the blood they must be split up into a simpler form. In the human body these splitting-up changes are brought about by chemical bodies known as *ferments* or *enzymes.* There is a special ferment for each particular class of food, and it will not split up any other type of food. The object of these ferments is to break up the food into simpler forms which can be absorbed into the system. After they have been thus absorbed, some of these simpler bodies are picked out by the various organs of the body from the bloodstream and are built up into living matter, while others are burnt up to provide heat and energy.

Proteins. From the chemical standpoint the most complicated food is the *protein.* These are the most important body-builders because they contain nitrogen and are the only substances that can be used for supplying nitrogen to build the protoplasm of the cells and tissues, which are largely composed of protein. They are built up of chains of simpler compounds called *amino acids.* About twenty of these have so far been discovered in the proteins of animals and plants. Proteins, however, are not all of equal value as foods. Some of them do not contain all the amino acids required. Many amino acids can be built from suitable materials, but there are some which the body requires and cannot itself manufacture without help.

The *essential* amino acids have to be obtained ready-made from the proteins of the food. Generally speaking, proteins from animal products such as eggs, milk, cheese, meat, and fish contain more of these than the proteins of plant products such as cereals, nuts, vegetables, and fruits, though there is no completely clear-cut distinction. The relative food value of different proteins is determined by feeding experiments, either on man or animals.

From these experiments some interesting results have been obtained. They showed, for example, that some proteins can act as supplements to one another in such a way that the biological value of the mixture is greater than would be expected from the sum of the two separate values. Cheese protein, for example, has a higher value than bread protein if the foods are eaten separately on alternate days, but if they are eaten together the value is as great as that of the cheese's protein alone. A similar result was shown to be the case with milk and potatoes.

To turn from considerations of quality to those of quantity, the accepted standard for a completely adequate supply of protein is about 3½ oz. a day, of which 1 oz. should come from animal proteins. It should be made clear, however, that these amounts refer to the *actual* protein: it would, for example, take nearly 10 oz. of boiled egg to provide 1 oz. of protein.

Carbohydrates. The next general class of food is the carbohydrate. These are the chief fuel of the body, and more than two-thirds of the required energy is supplied by their oxidation. They are taken in as sugars and starches and come mainly from plant products. Except for the sugar of milk (lactose) and a small amount of animal starch known as glycogen (found in shellfish and liver), animal products contain no carbohydrates at all.

Carbohydrate digestion is rather simpler than protein digestion in that all forms have to change into a simple sugar known as *glucose* before they can be absorbed. The various sugars in ordinary use, such as cane sugar from the sugarcane, lactose, etc., all have their special ferment which will break them down to a still simpler sugar. The last and simplest form of sugar into which the carbohydrates are changed before being absorbed into the bloodstream is *glucose.*

Fats. These are the best heat-producers, and apart from the fats actually built into the tissues, as in the nerve sheaths, for example, they are stored in greater or smaller quantities as reserves, much of them in the subcutaneous tissues. There they are available for the production of heat when the intake of food material is diminished or the expenditure of energy is increased. Fats act as carriers for several of the vitamins, and by their presence in the subcutaneous tissues protect the body from excessive loss of heat. Of the fats we take as foods, dripping and lard contain practically 100 per cent true fat, butter and margarine about 85 per cent, the rest being water. Besides these, a number of foods contain less obvious or *invisible* fats: some nuts, for instance, have 60 per cent of invisible fats, and meat contains both kinds. Fish vary very much in this fat content: fatty fish, such as herring, mackerel, sardines, and salmon, may contain up to 30 per cent of fat, while fish such as cod, haddock, or whiting may contain hardly any fat in their muscle or flesh. It is generally accepted that the daily intake of fat should be about 3 oz.

Alimentary Canal. The digestive tube as a whole is known as the *alimentary canal*. It starts at the mouth and ends at the anus; it is divided up into many different portions.

The mouth is the first portion of the alimentary canal to be considered. It is a cavity containing teeth and saliva. The teeth are primarily meant to bite into the food and to grind it into small particles so that the saliva can come into contact with as much of it as possible. The teeth in the front of the jaw are provided with sharp, chisel-like edges which are well adapted for biting or cutting. Biting a piece out of an apple illustrates the duties of the front teeth (incisors) very well. Farther back the teeth have large grinding surfaces between which the food is reduced to a finely divided state so that it can readily be mixed with the various digestive fluids.

Mastication. The jaws appear to move freely during the chewing process, but actually it is only the lower jaw which is movable. The upper jaw is part of the face and only moves with it. The lower jaw, however, is so attached that it can move·up and down and from side to side. The up-and-down movement enables the front teeth to bite into the food, while the side-to-side movement enables the food to be ground between the back or molar teeth. During this chewing process there is also a forward and backward movement of the lower jaw.

The broad and rough surfaces of the molar teeth are made to slide over each other, thus thoroughly grinding the food which may be between them. Flesh-eating animals have not got broad molars like those of human beings: they bite and tear the flesh on which they feed, generally giving the jaw an up-and-down movement only. On the other hand, the vegetarian or herbivorous animals have very large and perfect molars, and they give to the lower jaw much greater variety of motion, than we do. This is readily observed in the cow, sheep and the horse.

During the chewing or mastication, the food is continually being moved about by the tongue so that every portion of it is brought between the molar teeth. The muscles of the cheeks and lips also help.

Digestive Juices. The digestive juices of the body (enzymes and ferments) are prepared by means of various glands: a gland is a structure which has the power of separating or forming certain materials from the blood which is flowing through it. Many of the membranes which line the hollow organs of the body also have the power of forming special materials, and therefore they are called "secreting membranes."

Mucous Membrane. The whole of the interior of the digestive tube or alimentary canal, from the mouth to the rectum, is lined with a soft kind of skin known as *mucous membrane*. At the margins of the lips and of the anus this membrane merges imperceptibly into the skin which covers the external surface of the body. The mucous membrane is richly supplied with minute glands called mucous glands. These glands separate from the blood a slimy fluid called *mucus* which serves to keep the membrane moist and at the same time acts as a very efficient lubricant.

The Salivary Glands. In addition to the mucous glands, the structures surrounding the cavity of the mouth are provided with the special salivary glands. These are big glands, and there are three pairs of them: the parotid, the submaxillary, and the sublingual. The parotid glands are placed, one on each side, just below and in front of the ear. They are the largest of the salivary glands, and it is these which become so inflamed and tender in an attack of

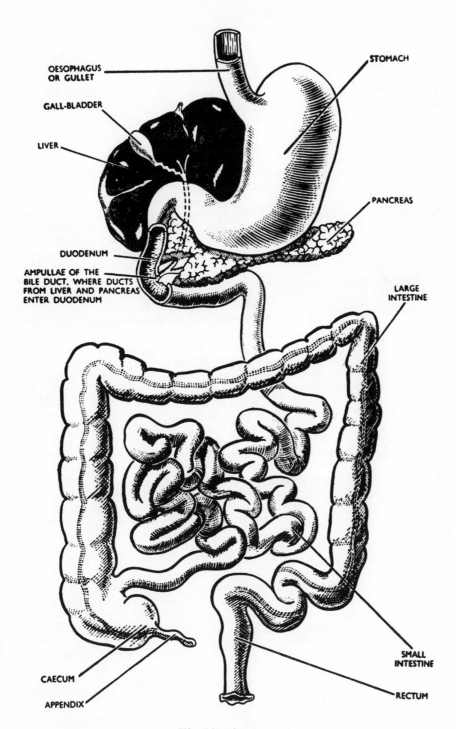

OESOPHAGUS
OR GULLET

GALL-BLADDER

LIVER

DUODENUM

AMPULLAE OF THE
BILE DUCT, WHERE DUCTS
FROM LIVER AND PANCREAS
ENTER DUODENUM

STOMACH

PANCREAS

LARGE
INTESTINE

SMALL
INTESTINE

CAECUM

APPENDIX

RECTUM

The Digestive System.

mumps. The saliva they make is passed along a tube known as Stenson's duct, which is about ⅛ in. in diameter, and this opens into the mouth through the cheek, just opposite the second molar tooth of the upper jaw.

The submaxillary glands are about the size of plums. They are placed beneath the lower jaw, one on each side. The ducts of these glands, known as Wharton's ducts, open into the mouth under the tip of the tongue at the side of the bridle of tissue which binds the tongue down to the floor of the mouth. They can easily be seen with a looking-glass.

The outlines of the sublingual glands may also be seen by means of a looking-glass. They are no larger than almonds, and are situated on each side of the bridle forming the ridge between the tongue and the gums of the lower jaw, and are covered only by mucous membrane. Each of these glands has several ducts or channels to carry their juices away. The mixed fluid produced by these different glands is called the saliva, and is a clear, thin, transparent fluid. In the mouth it is always mixed with the fluid from the mucous glands, and this makes the saliva found in the mouth thicker and stickier in character.

Salivary Digestion. As is the case in all the fluids of the body, most of the saliva consists of water—just over 99 per cent of it. The remaining very small fraction consists of mineral salts and organic matter.

The substance in saliva which takes an active part in digestion is one of the ferments known as *ptyalin*. Many of the foods we eat contain a large proportion of starch (such as bread, rice, potato, etc.), which will not dissolve in water. No food is of any use to the body until it has turned into a state in which it can be dissolved. Starch therefore, as such, is useless as a food. This ferment or enzyme, known as ptyalin, has the power of doing this: it converts the insoluble starch into a soluble variety of sugar known as maltose. In the mouth this change begins as soon as the saliva mixes with starchy foods. The unchanged starchy substances are swallowed, together with some saliva, and the change of starch into sugar is continued in other parts of the digestive tube for a short while

in the stomach, but completely in the intestines, where it is reinforced by a powerful ferment from the *pancreas*—a gland, incidentally, which is very similar to a salivary gland in structure. The saliva acts only on starchy foods.

In addition to the action of the saliva just mentioned, it is useful as a mechanical agent and general solvent. Together with the mucus it moistens the mouth and thus makes it easier to chew the food. It dissolves substances which are savory, and thus enables us to taste them. In animals which live in water there are no salivary glands, and those in flesh-eating animals have no chemical action, so that it would appear that the mechanical action of the glands is their more important duty. It also assists in forming the food into a soft mass known as a *bolus* before it is swallowed. The sticky mucus is very useful in preventing any friction.

A feeling of hunger, or the presence and sight or smell of savory foods, will cause a flow of saliva. This flow of saliva is not due to any chemical reason, but simply to the stimulus of the senses and is known as "reflex." The greater the hunger or the more attractive the food the greater the amount of stimulation of the senses affected and the greater the flow of saliva. This illustrates the importance of attractively cooked meals.

Quite a large quantity of saliva is produced during the course of a day, the amount being from a pint and a half to two pints. The outflow is more or less continuous, but is increased by the presence of any object in the mouth. This object need not be food, a glass bead or pebble will do, and often on a long march soldiers will suck a pebble to prevent the mouth from getting too dry. The thought of food when one is hungry will produce saliva, and also the smell of food will make the mouth water. On the other hand, a powerful emotion, such as that of fright, will stop the flow. One of the old tests of guilt in a suspected person was to give rice to eat. This, of course, requires a great deal of fluid to swallow it, and the guilty person, being rather afraid that he would be found out, could not produce sufficient saliva and so was unable to swallow the rice. This rough-and-ready test, which was merely based on observation, is seen to have some scientific foundation.

It is interesting to note that the salivary glands of children do not contain any ferment during the first four months or so of existence. Breast milk does not contain any starch at all. Patent foods for children, therefore, should not contain any starch when they are meant for children under four months, and a guiding principle is not to allow any starch, in the form of potato or bread, etc., until the child has cut a few teeth.

The Act of Swallowing. Food, then, is masticated in the mouth and thoroughly mixed with saliva. It is collected into a mass known as a bolus by the muscles of the tongue and of the cheeks, and then passed between the tongue and the roof of the mouth until it reaches the back of the mouth. So far all these arrangements are "voluntary," that is to say, they are under the control of the conscious will and can be stopped at any time. Once the food reaches the back of the mouth, the presence of the food will cause the swallowing machinery to come into play, and thereafter the passage of food and its further digestion is entirely beyond the control of the will.

The food has to pass into the esophagus, or gullet, without touching the back part of the nose or entering the windpipe. The back of the nose is shut off by means of the soft palate. The contraction of the muscles at the back of the throat forces the food over a flap of cartilage at the entrance to the windpipe directly into the esophagus.

As soon as the food enters the upper portion of the esophagus, the circular muscles in the walls of that tube contract just above it and force it downwards. In front of the mass of food the muscle becomes relaxed by means of a nervous reflex which is aroused by the presence of the food, so that a regular wave-like motion is set up, a narrow portion being behind the mass of food and pushing it down, and a wider part in front into which the food is forced. The force of gravity affects the passage of food into the stomach but little, and it is owing to the muscular contrac-

tion that one can swallow solids, and even liquids such as water, when standing on one's head.

When the esophagus is not engaged in swallowing, it is not a hollow tube, but is flattened, its front and back walls being in contact. In order that the act of swallowing may take place with regularity and ease, the mass of food must be sufficiently large to be within the grasp of the contracting muscles; it is on this account that some people find difficulty in swallowing a pill unless food or drink is taken at the same time.

The Stomach. The stomach is a membranous and muscular bag, about 10 in. in length from right to left, situated against the front wall of the abdomen and just beneath the partition which separates the abdominal cavity from the chest. This partition is a muscle known as the diaphragm. The shape of the stomach is very variable. The larger portion, just next to the heart except for the diaphragm, is known as the cardiac portion. When an individual is standing up, the shape of the stomach is roughly that of the letter "J." The food-pipe enters the stomach at the top of the letter "J" which is known as the *cardiac orifice,* and the narrow end of the stomach joins up with the intestines by a narrow entrance known as the *pylorus.* Food enters the stomach by means of the upper opening, the cardiac orifice, and after being thoroughly mixed with the digestive fluid of the stomach, passes through the lower opening into the small intestine.

Gastric Juices. The only important ferment in the stomach itself is *pepsin,* which acts on the complex protein foods. Pepsin is only active in the presence of acid, and in the stomach this acid is that known as *hydrochloric acid.* The pepsin does not break down the protein entirely, and more changes have to take place in the small intestine before the protein is ready to be taken into the blood-stream.

The digestion which takes place in the stomach chiefly prepares the protein part of the food for the further action of the much more powerful ferments of the pancreas and intestine. The only other important ferment in the stomach is *rennin,* which has the property of clotting milk.

Commercially this ferment is sold as "rennet." It is prepared from the stomach of a calf and is used to make junket.

The walls of the stomach are capable of being stretched a great deal. It can thus adapt itself to the quantity of food it receives and at the same time be always in contact with the food so as to act upon it.

Peristalsis. Regular wave-like or rhythmical muscular contractions pass down the walls of the stomach. These regular waves of contracting are known as "peristalsis," and by means of them the food is forced all the way down the intestinal canal. It is only in the large intestine, under normal conditions, that waves of contraction are seen to pass backwards, i.e., towards the small intestine, and these movements are referred to as "antiperistalsis."

The walls of the digestive tube consist in the main of four layers: the inner one is a mucous membrane which contains the mucus-making cells and the mouths of the various glands which are present in the next layer. Then come the *muscular coats,* circular muscle fibers on the inside and muscle fibers placed lengthwise on the outside. Even further outside still is the smooth lining of membrane known as the *peritoneum.* This makes a watery fluid which moistens and lubricates the surfaces of the organs, which can thus glide freely over each other.

The Sphincters. At each end of the stomach the circular muscles are thickened and contracted. These areas of circular muscle are known as *sphincters,* and they serve as doors to keep the cavity of the organ closed. The lower sphincter, situated at the pylorus and known as the *pyloric sphincter,* is firmly closed during digestion at first. It relaxes at certain intervals and thus allows some of the digested portions to be passed into the intestine.

The time during which substances remain in the stomach varies from one to four hours. It depends partly on the nature of the food and the method employed in the cooking. Normal people will also vary; in some the stomach will empty much more rapidly than in others.

Gastric Glands. The mucous membrane or lining of the stomach is smooth and soft when the organ is moderately distended; but it is drawn up into folds when the stomach is empty. It is covered with cells which make mucus to keep the surface moist, and its thickness is due to the fact that it is made up of glands which are like a long tube in shape. Their duty is to make gastric-juices, and they are accordingly known as *gastric glands.* When the stomach is empty the lining membrane is pale in color; but as soon as it contains some food, or even something which is not food and which cannot be digested, the supply of blood increases and the mucous membrane becomes bright pink in color, and the making of gastric juice immediately begins. It can be truly said that the stomach "blushes" during and after a meal.

Gastric juice consists of water, to which are added the pepsin, rennin, hydrochloric acid and various salts such as phosphates of calcium, magnesium and iron, and the chlorides of sodium, potassium and calcium.

Pepsin is the active part of the gastric juice. It can be obtained in a dissolved state by washing the lining membrane of the stomach with water, or it may be bought in the solid form from the chemist. "Peptonized milk" is milk which has been in contact with pepsin for some time at body temperature. The protein part of the milk is thus partially broken down or "digested," and so it becomes more suitable for invalids in whom the powers of digestion are weak owing to their illness.

Gastric fluid has no action on starchy foods, neither does it act on fats. Starchy foods, as was seen above, are dissolved in the stomach by the swallowed saliva. The rennet part of the gastric juice acts upon milk and clots it.

Fatty tissues consist of fat cells, and each cell consists of a particle of fat surrounded by a cell wall made of protein. When fatty tissues pass into the stomach, the cell walls are dissolved and the fat is set free in the form of minute globules, giving the contents of the stomach a grey appearance.

Chyme. The fluid contents of the stomach are known as "chyme," from the Greek word meaning "I pour," because it is "poured" into the intestine and bowel. It consists of saliva and starchy foods in various stages of digestion; protein food in various stages; undigested fat in the form of globules; mucus from the mucous glands, and a residue of indigestible substances.

Much information as to the processes which take place in the stomach has been obtained from chemical examination of stomach contents aspirated through a stomach tube. This method is used to analyze gastric function in disease.

The shape and outline is studied by X-rays using what is known as a "barium meal." This is a material which contains a great deal of a barium compound which will not allow X-rays to pass through it, and so the outline of a hollow organ containing it is shown up on a screen when examined with the aid of the X-rays.

There is very little material absorbed into the body directly from the stomach. Even water passes through the stomach practically without diminishing in quantity. Alcohol, on the other hand, is readily absorbed, and this is the reason for the rapid effect of alcohol when it is swallowed on an empty stomach.

How Digestion Starts. The flow of gastric juice is usually started by the mental effect of seeing, tasting, and smelling appetizing food. The next important thing in stimulating digestion is the actual presence of food in the stomach. Some foods are more active than others in this respect: meat extracts and meat juices are very active; while others, such as milk, bread, white of egg, etc., are much less active.

As the most active substances appear to be present in meat extracts and meat juices, it is obvious that in the case of people suffering from indigestion associated with excess of acid (acid dyspepsia), meat juices can only make the trouble worse.

Intestines. The intestines are made on the same general plan as the rest of the digestive tract. They have an outer layer which is made by the peritoneum; the duty of this is to anchor the intestines to the front of the backbone and to convey blood vessels and nerves to the walls of the intestine. The muscular coat has fibers of muscle arranged lengthwise on the outer surface and round and round on the inside: then a layer of loose tissue between the

muscle and the mucous coat. In this layer are found the blood vessels and nerves which supply the glands, etc., of the mucous coat, and finally the inner mucous layer which contains the various digestive glands.

The mucous membrane of the small intestine is thrown into folds like that of the stomach. Their duty is to increase the area of the secreting surface; to prevent food from passing too rapidly through the intestine, and to assist in the mixing of food with digestive fluids which are poured into the intestine.

There are various types of glands: all of them open on the inner surface of the intestine. The collected juices of all these glands is called the *succus entericus*. This is a yellow alkaline fluid, which consists of several ferments whose function it is to act on certain classes of food substances.

Digestion in the Duodenum. The inner side of the small intestine is covered also with a multitude of very small projections known as *villi* which give the surface a fine, velvety appearance. Their duty is to absorb food rather than to change food into a form which can be dissolved.

As soon as food has passed from the stomach into the first portion of the intestine—known as the duodenum—it mixes with the very important fluids known as the bile and the pancreatic juice. The bile is made by the liver and the pancreatic juice is made by a gland known as the pancreas. The pancreas (or sweetbread) is a large gland partly placed within the curve of the first part of the intestine—it lies within a curve made by the duodenum. The juices made by the pancreas have a very powerful digestive effect. The chief of them are "trypsin," a ferment which will act on protein; "amylase," which acts on starches, and "lipase," a ferment which acts on fats.

Digestion in the Small Intestine. The intestinal juice, the *succus entericus,* is made from the glands from the whole length of the small intestine. It is an alkaline fluid containing many ferments, which bring the now largely broken-up food to the final stages of digestion, ready for absorption into the blood. All kinds of food are dissolved in the small intestine and the mass as a whole is slowly urged on. The dissolved portions are rapidly absorbed by the mucous membrane, while the unabsorbed parts pass onwards to the large bowel.

The *chyme,* which is the name given to the mixture of food and digestive juices in the stomach, passes into the small intestine and is then changed in appearance by the addition of the bile and pancreatic fluids; the fats in it make it look like milk. The term *chyle* is applied to the contents of the small intestine.

Digestion and the Large Intestine. After the chyle has passed along the whole length of the small intestine it enters the large intestine through an opening which is guarded by two folds of mucous membrane. These folds prevent, to some extent, the flow of the contents of the large intestine back into the small one. They form a kind of valve which is known as the *ileo-caecal* valve.

The movements of the intestine are of two distinct types: one is *peristaltic* and consists of waves of contraction passing progressively and slowly down the intestine. The effect of these waves is to drive the contents slowly onwards. The other type of movement is known as *rhythmic segmentation*. A short length of intestine suddenly breaks up into a number of small segments or portions, and each segment undergoes a similar change. This happens many times and their combined effect is to produce a thorough mixing and absorption.

In the large intestine practically no digestion occurs, but there is a large absorption of fluid, both from the food and the watery and unused portions of the digestive juices. At the end of the small intestine the bowel contents are very watery, but the action of the large intestine makes the residue more and more solid.

Putrefaction. Putrefaction occurs only in the large intestine, which acts mostly as a storehouse. Some absorption however, does take place as is shown by the absorption of water.

The contents of the large intestine are bacteria, bile, mucus, unabsorbed food and excess of digestive juices. The bacteria form nearly half of the solids excreted.

The feces are the excretions of the large intestine. Their color is mostly due to the bile in them, and the mass should be semifluid in consistence. The presence of food in the stomach has a marked reflex action in making the rectum contract. This tendency is most marked when food is placed into a stomach which is completely empty, hence the most suitable time to empty the bowels is directly after breakfast. The bowel is a creature of habit and is far more likely to work efficiently if it is made to contract and expel its contents at the same time every day.

As regards the absorption of food into the bloodstream, it is certain that little or no absorption takes place in the stomach. Water apparently undergoes no absorption at all in the stomach. Under normal condition of digestion, neither fats nor proteins are sufficiently broken down to undergo any absorption in the stomach. The real and important site of absorption is the small intestine. Here all the products of digestion rapidly pass into the bloodstream and thence to the various organs of ·the body, which pick out the materials they require and build them up into the substances required.

DIGITALIS. This is the name of a powerful medicine obtained from the leaves of the purple foxglove plant which is to be found growing in woods and hedgerows. Nowadays it is grown specially because of the digitalis obtained from it.

It was not until about 1860 that it was used as a heart tonic. At first it was hailed as a cure for all heart conditions, but owing to the work of the great heart specialists, Sir James Mackenzie and Sir Thomas Lewis, it has been proved that the drug is only of use in certain conditions. In the condition known as auricular fibrillation digitalis is capable of giving immense relief and of prolonging life for many years. This drug, however, should only be given under medical supervision. It is usually prescribed in pills of the powdered leaf or as a tincture. When a rapid action is desirable, the pure active principle of the White Foxglove known as digoxin can be given by injection into a vein.

Poisoning by Digitalis. Digitalis is known as a cumulative drug, which means that it is not given off by the body as rapidly as it is absorbed and therefore its concentration builds up in the tissues. Its use, therefore, has to be carefully regulated by adjusting the dose from time to time so as to keep the heart beating at its most efficient rate of 70 to 80 a minute.

Vomiting is one of the most common symptoms of overdose, but the most important symptom is the slowing of the pulse below 60 beats a minute. A patient on digitalis who develops symptoms of overdosage should discontinue taking the drug and call in his doctor.

DILL WATER. This is an extract which is sometimes given to relieve flatulence and pains in the stomach. It may be given to the smallest child without any danger. A teaspoonful of dill water, slightly warmed, will be found to give considerable relief in flatulence (wind) of young infants.

DIPHTHERIA. Diphtheria is a very infectious disease which attacks the throat, and sometimes the nose and larynx. Not only does the germ of this disease cause the lining of the throat to become inflamed and swollen, but it manufactures poisons which are carried by the bloodstream to the rest of the body. These poisons may set up dangerous conditions, such as heart weakness and paralysis. The chief characteristic of the disease, however, is the formation of a "membrane" at the back of the throat, which is caused by the lining of the throat becoming so inflamed that it dies and forms an extra covering, as it were. This membrane is grayish or yellowish-white in color and is very firmly fastened to the throat. Other inflammations of the throat may look like diphtheria, but true diphtheria is diagnosed by the presence of a germ which has the special name of Klebs-Loeffler bacillus. This germ is named after two German doctors who were the first to discover, at the end of the nineteenth century, that diphtheria was actually caused by its presence.

Diphtheria was known in the East for centuries, and it is referred to in the Babylonian Talmud. "Throat Pestilences" are also mentioned as occurring in the Middle Ages. George Washington is said to have died of this disease. Diphtheria seems to be much more common on the Continent than it is in the U.S. and Great Britain, and it never seems to develop very seriously in tropical countries. The majority of cases of diphtheria seem to break out during the late summer months, especially if the weather has been dry. It will be found that by about the beginning of September the number of cases will begin to increase, and the highest peak is reached in November. After that, a fall in the number of cases takes place and between the months of May and July there may be very few cases recorded.

How Infection Is Carried. The germs of this disease are conveyed from one person to another, and the disease is so infectious that even doctors and nurses may become infected from their patients. There is a case on record where a child coughed into the doctor's face while he was examining the throat, and the doctor died within twenty-four hours from diphtheria. Infection may be spread by those cases where the disease is in the nose or ear instead of in the throat. In these cases a chronic catarrh, containing the particular germ, may be the only sign of the presence of diphtheria, and the infected person may still pass on the disease even though he does not suffer from any general poisoning himself.

"Carriers." In a large percentage of cases of diphtheria, the germs simply disappear after the patient recovers from the disease, but there are still a great number of patients who harbor the germs for long periods. These people are called convalescent carriers, and in this way it is possible for the germs of the disease to be passed on. Another type of carrier is the person who, while enjoying perfect health, is "carrying" a germ of the disease. Different people vary in the readiness with which they succumb to disease; this is known as susceptibility, and in the case of diphtheria this degree of susceptibility can be found out by means of a test called the Schick Reaction. This test is dealt with fully under its own heading.

The Importance of the Membrane. The membrane in diphtheria is formed by changes in the tissues as they are killed by the activity of the growing germs. It is firmly attached to the back of the throat; and it is from the firmness of its adherence that the true diphtheria membrane can be distinguished from the membranes that are not due to diphtheria. These can be pulled off the throat without causing any bleeding. In the worst cases of diphtheria the membrane becomes so extensive that the vocal cords are covered, and great difficulty in breathing occurs so that the patient may die unless an operation called *tracheotomy* is performed. Tracheotomy consists in making an opening in the front of the throat by means of which a tube can be passed into the windpipe to enable the patient to breathe.

The Antitoxin Treatment. It needs little imagination to realize what a horrible disease diphtheria was in the old days when the formation of the membrane had to be allowed to run its course, and all that could be done was for some heroic and devoted person to attempt to suck the obstructing matter out of the throat. Fortunately, if the disease is treated in time, and nowadays it nearly always is, there is no need for it to be such a dreadful illness. The treatment by early injection of antitoxin has worked wonders. Diphtheria antitoxin is now administered by the doctor as soon as he sees a case that looks as if it might be diptheria, while at the same time, he takes a specimen of the matter at the back of the throat and sends it to a bacteriologist to be examined, to see if the special germ of diphtheria is among it.

The reason for this haste is that the membrane grows with great rapidity, and the day, or even few hours, required for the examination of the specimen will make a great difference to the patient's chances of recovery. The importance of this early antitoxin treatment is shown by the fact that nearly half of all the cases of diphtheria used to die, whereas nowadays, only eight or nine out of every hundred cases die, and these could have been saved if treated in time.

Penicillin is now used as an adjunct to treatment by antitoxin, but it in no way replaces it. Penicillin is able to destroy the germ of diphtheria, but it is without effect on the terrible toxin which the germ has already produced and which is circulating through the tissues. Only antitoxin will "fix" this poison.

Symptoms. The period between catching the disease and the time when the symptoms first show themselves (the incubation period) varies from two to seven days:

more usually two. At first the patient has the usual feverish symptoms of chilliness, and aching pains in the back and limbs. The temperature does not usually rise above 102 deg. A young child may have convulsions at the beginning. The throat at first is only slightly sore and there is little difficulty in swallowing. The membrane usually appears first on the tonsils at the sides of the throat. Later, all the structures at the back of the throat, the tonsils, the uvula, the mucous membrane of the throat, all become swollen, and by the third day the membrane may have reached the back wall of the throat. The glands of the neck are usually swollen and tender. Gradually, in from seven to ten days, the throat becomes clear and convalescence begins.

General disturbance of health, due to the poisoning effect of the diphtheria germ, is usually slight when treatment is begun early; but when it is not the poisoning is severe and the heart affected, so that death may ensue. These serious symptoms are more common when the throat infection is extensive. The glands become greatly enlarged, the patient becomes ashen-gray in color, the pulse is rapid, and later the temperature sinks below normal.

Nasal Diphtheria. The disease can attack the nose in two ways. Either the passages of the nose become full of thick membranes but the disease remains very mild—this is called *membranous rhinitis;* or there may be true nasal diphtheria, which is very serious and the general symptoms are very grave.

Laryngeal Diphtheria. This is described separately, as the narrow entrance to the air passages—the glottis—is affected, and this leads to hoarseness and difficulty in breathing. The attack begins with a slight hoarseness and a rough cough. After a day or so the child suddenly becomes worse, usually at night, and breathing becomes difficult. At first the difficulty only comes on at times, but later it becomes continuous. The color gradually changes and the the lips and fingertips become livid. The child becomes restless and tosses vainly from side to side in his efforts to breathe. Occasionally, in a severe paroxysm, portions of membrane are coughed up. As a rule the fever is not marked, and the condition of the child is good at the beginning. In unfavorable cases the difficulty in breathing becomes more and more urgent, the blueness becomes more marked, and after a period of intense restlessness, the child sinks into a semiconscious state, and death finally occurs from poisoning of the nerve centers. In these cases of laryngeal diphtheria, the tonsils are usually covered with membrane as well.

Treatment. Measures must be taken to prevent the spread of the malady. Diphtheria is best treated at hospitals; but if the patient remains at home, the room in which the patient is kept should be clear of carpets, curtains and superfluous furniture. The room must be kept warm (67 deg. F.) and well ventilated. A steam kettle is useful. Only the nurse, the child's mother, and the doctor should visit the patient. The strictest quarantine should be employed against the other members of the household.

The local treatment is not so important now that antitoxin is used, but the mouth should be frequently rinsed out with an antiseptic mouth wash.

When the larynx is involved, a steam kettle or vaporizer is essential, and when there is obstruction the operation of tracheotomy must be performed; or intubation, in which a tube is inserted between the vocal cords, thus keeping them permanently apart. Hot applications to the neck are very comforting in the case of young children; in older children, ice poultices may be found to be preferable.

Diet and General Treatment. Food must be liquid, such as milk, beef broth, barley water, ice cream, soups, etc. If swallowing is too difficult, the fluid must be given in a tube. As much water as possible must be drunk, and the bowels must be kept open by means of a dose of calomel at night and salts in the morning. If the circulation fails, it must be stimulated by drugs such as coramine or camphor, and an injection of salt solution into the bowel, which is allowed to remain there instead of being passed out again, is very useful.

Complications. The kidneys may be damaged to some extent by the general poisoning of the system, and this is shown by the presence of albumin in the urine; this may also occur as a result of definite inflammation of the kidneys. Dropsy, however, is rare as a complication.

Paralysis. This is the most important of all the complications. The poison appears to affect the nerves directly, and paralysis of some sort is present in about fifteen out of every hundred cases. It may occur after the mildest of cases; in fact, some are so mild that the first thing which makes a patient realize that he has had diphtheria is when his coffee or tea suddenly comes back out of his nose, owing to paralysis of the muscles of the throat. This paralysis usually disappears after two or three weeks. Next to the throat the muscles of the eye are commonly affected, and this is shown by the development of a squint. Any nerve may be affected, and this will be shown by paralysis of the part supplied by the nerve.

Heart. Heart symptoms in diphtheria are not uncommon. The heart weakness is mostly due to degeneration of the heart muscle due to the poison of the disease.

Prevention of the Disease. All cases of diphtheria must be notified to the medical officer of health, and the person suffering from diphtheria must be isolated. All clothing and everything that has been in contact with the patient must be disinfected. All cases with a mild sore throat must be carefully examined for the germ of diphtheria. The chief danger is not from a well-marked case, when these precautions are carried out, but from the milder forms which are not suspected.

Active Immunization. Diphtheria formally was an important cause of death in late childhood, and a steady toll of those between the ages of one and five as well. It is now largely preventable by artificial immunization, and it is the duty of parents to ensure that their children are immunized as soon as possible after the first birthday. The procedure is to give two injections of toxoid at intervals of four weeks which confers immunity for some years. A further "boosting" dose is recommended at the age of five. Occasionally there is a small, painful swelling at the site of injection, but as a rule there is little discomfort.

Convalescence. Because of the liability to serious complications, convalescence from diphtheria requires special care, particularly if the heart is affected, in which case absolute rest in bed for a long period will be necessary. No patient should be discharged from quarantine until the throat and nose have been found free from diphtheria germs on two examinations two days apart. This is because of the likelihood of the patient becoming a "carrier" and spreading the germs of this dangerous disease further.

DIPLOPIA. This is the medical name for the condition more commonly known as double vision. (*See also* DOUBLE VISION.).

DIPSOMANIA. Dipsomania is a condition in which there is an intense craving for drink at intervals, leading to a drinking bout lasting a few days. During this time the patient is seldom sober. The advice and treatment of a psychiatrist should be sought.

DISC, SLIPPED. A common cause of pain in the back, which is often called lumbago or sciatica, is the protrusion of a portion of an invertebral disc into the canal of the vertebral column. This is the cartilaginous structure that lies between the vertebrae and allows the vertebral column to bend. The condition is usually due to injury, either acute and isolated, or mild and recurrent. The commonest site is the lumbar region or small of the back, and pain may be severe and be refined down one or both thighs. Treatment may consist of a local anesthetic; or it may require skilled manipulation, or even an operation.

DISCHARGE. The word discharge may be applied to many normal functions of the body. For instance, sweat is discharged from the sweat glands, and urine is discharged from the bladder; but, as a rule, when we speak of discharges from the body we do not refer to these but to others that occur as a result of disease.

When we are suffering from a common cold, there is usually an increase of discharge from the nose and there may be a discharge of water from the eyes. Another kind of discharge is that which comes from an ulcer or some skin diseases. Wounds or fistulae may discharge pus as well as natural fluid.

It should be remembered that most discharges are of an infective nature, so that dressings which are removed should be destroyed by burning. People suffering from a cold should be very careful with used handkerchiefs; they should soak them in an antiseptic solution. It is a very good thing to use soft paper handkerchiefs when suffering from a cold; in this way they can be burned immediately after use.

DISEASE. Disease is commonly used to mean that one, or some, of the organs or systems of the body are not working properly. This may be because the part was ill-formed or deficient in some way from birth, in which case the disease is called *congenital*. Congenital diseases are also often *hereditary*, that is, they descend from generation to generation in the same family. A *constitutional* disease is one in which the whole body or the whole of one of the systems of the body is involved, such as anemia. An *idiopathic* disease is one for which the cause is unknown, and a *veneral* disease is one which is acquired during sexual intercourse.

Symptoms of disease may also be the body's natural reactions. For instance, a sneeze is a symptom of approaching influenza, but it is also the body's way of getting rid of a piece of dust which has lodged on the lining of the nose. The same is true of conditions like diarrhea and sickness. In diarrhea the bowel is trying to get rid quickly of something that is hurting it, and vomiting is the stomach's way of returning quickly something that is irritating it, but repeated sickness and diarrhea over days or longer means that the irritating substance remains there or that disease exists.

Organic and Functional Disease. Disease may be organic or functional. An organic disease is one in which some change has taken place in an organ whose working is upset, and the change can be seen by the naked eye or by a microscope. A functional disease is one in which the working of the organ is upset but nothing can be seen to account for it. An ulcer of the lining of the stomach is an organic disease, but for some reason the stomach may be producing a different sort of gastric juice and therefore not be working well, and this is functional disease of the stomach. Long-continued functional disease of an organ is very likely to cause organic disease of that or some other organ, so it is just as important to treat the functional disease as the organic. Unfortunately it is not so easy, as the cause of the functional disease is not obvious and may be in some distant part such as the glands or the nervous system.

Causes of Disease. The causes of disease are manifold. First there are congenital diseases and hereditary diseases. Of diseases accquired later, the commonest cause is the entry into the body of germs which become too powerful for the bodily defences to deal with. Strain—either physical, where the body or some part of it is always being overworked, or mental, where the mind becomes fatigued through overwork or worry—undermines the power of the body to hold its own against infection and poisoning. Excessive cold and starvation, also extreme heat and overeating on the other hand, cause disease. Physical violence, too, either in the form of accident or otherwise, can be the starting point of disease.

Occupational Diseases. By occupational diseases we mean diseases which would not have been contracted by the individual if he had not been following that particular trade or occupation. In some occupations there is a definite danger from certain diseases, as, for instance, lead-poisoning among painters, anthracosis or silicosis among coal miners, a certain sort of cancer among cotton-spinners, etc. These are dealt with again under the heading OCCUPATIONAL DISEASES.

DISINFECTANT. Any substance which is able to kill the germs of disease is known as a disinfectant. Many people refer to antiseptics as disinfectants, but an antiseptic does not kill germs—it is used to prevent their growth. When treating a wound, an antiseptic is used to keep the wound clean and to prevent the growth of any germs. The use of disinfectants is not in the treatment of disease, but in its prevention and in the routine hygiene of the home. Thus the clothes used by the patient and all utensils used in the sickroom should be thoroughly disinfected.

There are many well-known disinfectants which can be relied upon to act properly if they are used in sufficient strength for whichever purpose they are required. Among the more common disinfectants are Lysol, chloride of lime, formaldehyde, Chlorox and potassium permanganate.

DISINFECTION. By the word "infection" we mean something catching, like influenza, or mumps, or smallpox—something that goes through the house, the school, the office, so that one after another goes down with it until it has run its course. But possibly not so many people would go down with an *infection* if everyone used common sense about *disinfection*. Apart altogether from any of the ordinary chemical disinfectants, the most powerful disinfectant we have is sunlight. It is well for us that not many germs can live in sunlight even for an hour. We should, therefore, have as much sunlight in our houses as we can. It is most unwise, for example, to pull the curtains to keep the carpet from fading. Far better have a faded carpet and good health than a bright carpet and bad health! So open up the windows, let in as much sunshine as there is and, in any case, plenty of fresh air.

There are certain precautions that must be taken after an infectious illness, when the isolation period is over. First of all, the patient himself must be disinfected: then the sickroom and anything that has been in contact with the patient must be dealt with; and, lastly, there are certain precautions which the nurse herself will have to take.

The Patient. The best means of disinfecting the patient is to give him a hot bath at a temperature of between 100 and 112 deg. F. For children, however, the temperature should be between 95 and 100 deg. F. While the patient is in the bath his clothing should be taken back to the sickroom, where the nurse should leave her overall, wash her hands, and return to bathe the patient.

If desired a disinfectant may be put into the bathwater, but soap and water are usually considered to be sufficient. Fresh towels and a new toothbrush should be provided. Towels used during the illness should be boiled, and the old toothbrush should be burned. The patient's hair should be thoroughly washed and dried with clean towels.

After the bath, the patient should be dried and dressed in clean pajamas or nightgown, taken to another room and put into an entirely clean bed. Nothing used in the sickroom must be taken out of it, and the patient should not be permitted to return to it until it has been disinfected.

The Sickroom. Disinfection of the sickroom should take place as soon as possible, and it is advisable to ask the local sanitary authorities for assistance in the matter. If, however, fumigation has to be carried out by the nurse, a formalin lamp should be obtained. This liberates formaldehyde gas and is much better than the older sulphur-candle method as it does not damage fabric or paintwork. The lamp should be placed on a metal tray raised off the floor as a precautionary measure against fire.

When preparing the room for disinfection, all sheets, pillowcases, towels, personal linen, etc., should be put into a carbolic solution made up of 1 part of carbolic to 60 parts of water. They should be left soaking for twelve hours and then washed out in the usual way. If the linen is sent to the laundry, the laundry must be notified that disinfected linen is being sent.

Blankets, eiderdowns, and anything else that cannot be treated in a similar manner, should be hung over the ends of the bed or the backs of chairs, or a line may be stretched across the room. The mattress should be stood on its side on the floor and rugs hung up so that the disinfecting fumes can get at both sides. All crockery should be boiled. Finally, all drawers and closets should be opened, and the crevices round the windows should have paper pasted over them.

When everything is ready the lamp should be lit and the room vacated. Paper strips should now be pasted down the cracks on the outside of the door, and over the keyhole, and the room should be left for twenty-four hours.

In cities, the mattress and bedding can be sent to a steam disinfector, but in country districts this is often not practicable, and they should be taken out into the garden and exposed to sunshine and fresh air.

The Nurse. After the nurse has finished nursing an infectious case, she should carefully disinfect herself by washing her hair, taking a hot bath and putting on a complete fresh set of clothes. She should do this before attending her patient again after he has been disinfected.

Excreta. Feces and urine in such cases as typhoid fever and dysentery must be disinfected by mixing them thoroughly with a strong disinfectant such as carbolic lotion, 1 part to 20 parts of water. They should be allowed to stand for four hours before being disposed of, otherwise the germs will not have been safely destroyed.

Sputum. The best means of disposing of sputum is to have the patient use paper handkerchiefs, which should be burned. It is advisable to give the patient a paper bag in which he can put these handkerchiefs so that they are not left on or in the bed. (*See also* ANTISEPTICS; ASEPSIS; DISINFECTANT; INFECTIOUS DISEASES.)

DISLOCATION. Dislocation usually refers to the displacement of a joint from its natural position. This may be caused by injury to the bones and ligaments which keep the joint in position, or it may be due to disease. Tuberculosis, for instance, is a disease in which the ligaments and bones may be gradually worn away, sometimes giving rise to dislocation. In some cases the bones may never have developed at birth, and any strain may cause dislocation. Like fractures, there are two types of dislocation, simple and compound. In the first type there is nothing but a straightforward dislocation, while in the second the skin is broken and a part of the bone may protrude through. Surgeons usually divide dislocations into two classes: (1) congenital, which means present at birth, or (2) acquired later in life as the result of an accident.

The parts of the body which are most liable to become dislocated are the shoulder, the hip, the jaw, the kneecap, the finger joints, and the elbow. The jaw may be dislocated as the result of a blow, or it may occur after a yawn. The collarbone or shoulder blade is very commonly put out as the result of a fall from a horse or during games and so on.

Once a joint has been dislocated, it is very apt to slip out again, and it is not unusual for a person to become quite expert at readjusting his own particular dislocation; but this should never be practiced on another by an amateur.

Symptoms. The symptoms of a dislocation are loss of movement of the particular joint, but much depends on the type of dis-

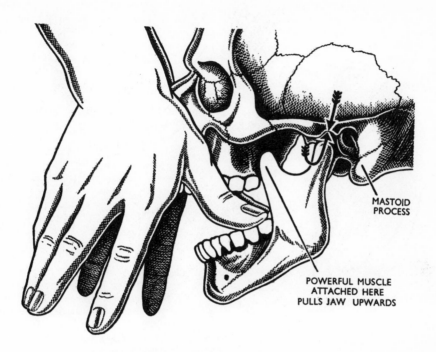

MASTOID PROCESS

POWERFUL MUSCLE ATTACHED HERE PULLS JAW UPWARDS

Dislocation of Jaw, showing method of reducing. In practice, thumbs should be protected with towel. Hard downward pressure on back teeth makes top of jaw follow curve of lower arrow, so that it slips back into its socket.

location which takes place. As a rule, it will be found that when the injured limb is compared with the normal one there is some difference in length. Sometimes shortening takes place, while in other cases the limb may have lengthened. There may be some pain and swelling around the joint, especially if the dislocated bone is pressing on some nerve.

Treatment. Immediate treatment consists of applying cold-water cloths to the part in order to relieve the pain, and absolute rest until the proper medical advice can be obtained. It is unwise for an unskilled person to attempt to put the dislocated bone back into place, as great damage may be done by tearing nerves and vessels. After the limb has been adjusted to its normal position, care must be taken in using it.

DISPLACEMENT. Displacement of various organs of the body often occurs through injury or disease, or, in some cases, the bones of the body may become displaced through the habits of standing and

walking badly. The stomach may become displaced owing to weakness of the supporting muscles, and the kidneys may be very movable and descend lower than they should do normally.

Displacement of the womb is a fairly common complaint in women especially in women who have had children. It may be displaced in several different ways; it may be bent on itself very acutely either backwards or forwards, or the whole womb may be tilted backwards (*see diagram*). In a certain number of women the womb is tilted backwards from birth, but the condition is not serious. In fact, it is less often the cause of backache, sterility, or painful periods than is commonly believed. It may, however, matter if pregnancy occurs, when it may have to be replaced to the forward position, as the congestion induced on account of the backward tilt may be a cause of miscarriage. In pregnancy the womb softens as it enlarges, due to the increased blood supply, and it is then that

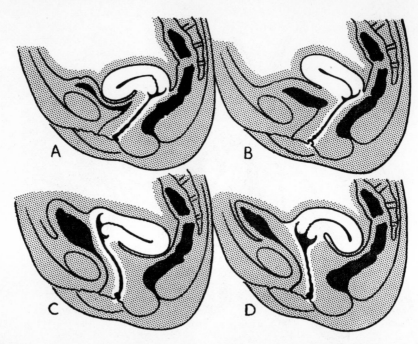

Displacement of Womb: A. *Normal position;* B. *Bent acutely forwards;* C. *Bent acutely backwards.* D. *Whole womb tilted backwards.*

the position becomes easier to correct. A displaced womb can be corrected by operation, or it may be held in its correct position by wearing a special belt or by the use of a special vulcanite support introduced into the vagina. Certain exercises, known as "restoration exercises" are also sometimes recommended.

DISSEMINATED SCLEROSIS. This is a common disease of the nervous system, and certainly the most common one in people between the ages of twenty and thirty-five. The exact cause is still unknown, but what occurs is a scattering of patches of changed nervous tissue throughout the brain and spinal cord. The changes in these patches of nervous tissue do not all take place at one and the same time; first one patch is attacked, and then another, so that the symptoms from which the patient suffers depend, practically by chance, on whichever part of the nervous system is first stricken.

In actual practice, however, it is found that certain parts tend to be involved with a remarkable regularity. The earliest effects of the disease which take the patient to the doctor are very often seen in the eyes. A very large number of patients with this disease complain first of rapid loss of vision in one eye. This may produce complete blindness in that eye for a short time, but it is good to be able to reassure such a patient that the vision will return, in nearly every case to normal, within a few weeks. The incident of the loss of vision in one eye often occurs years—even as many as twenty years—before any other signs or symptoms of disseminated sclerosis appear, and very often the patient, when seen with the fully developed picture of the disease, has completely forgotten that such an incident ever happened. Similarly, a patient may for a short time see two things instead of one, years before the apparent onset of the disease.

Other early incidents (the word "incidents" best describes these symptoms, because they are fleeting, a feature which is almost peculiar to this disease) are sudden loss of power in a limb, which returns within a week or two; sudden attacks of numbness and tingling in an arm, which last for a week or so and then disappear; prolonged attacks of giddiness or vomiting, for which no ascertainable cause is present.

Any of these may be one of the modes of onset of disseminated sclerosis. When the disease is advancing, stiffness of the legs and difficulty in walking become noticeable. This stiffness varies from time to time; it may be so severe one month that the patient is forced to keep to his bed, but within a month he may be walking again. This variation in severity is one of the chief characteristics of the disorder. The speech becomes altered, and the patient begins to speak in a jerking, "staccato" manner, but this type of speech is only heard in advanced cases. Most victims of this disease develop a trembling of the arms, which is most marked on movement towards an object, and is often noticed first in performing such fine movements as threading a needle. This trembling increases as the disease advances. The mental outlook of the patient is a happy one. The patient with disseminated sclerosis is surprisingly cheerful; even when unable to walk, he does not seem to suffer mentally. A frequent and favorite expression of these patients is: "Well, what's the use of being anything else but cheerful, doctor?" Although periods of improvement lasting sometimes for many years occur, there is at present no known cure. The periods of improvement may be so long, however, that a patient may go for ten or fifteen years between his attacks. Where there is much stiffness of the limbs, massage is of great service, and where walking is clumsy and stiff, much benefit may be obtained by special exercises and re-education under the supervision of a skilled physiotherapist.

Patients with disseminated sclerosis should avoid overexertion, but should not stay in bed as long as walking is possible. The vaccine treatment which was once hailed as a cure for this disease is discredited; it has been suggested that the disease may be due to some lack of vitamins, but this has yet to be proved.

DISTENTION. It is not unusual for the stomach to become distended or blown out with food and with gases, or for the bladder to become distended with too much urine. As a rule, these states of distension do not last very long, and they can be relieved quite quickly. Should distension of the stomach or any other organ persist for any length of time it is advisable to consult the doctor.

DISTILLED WATER. To make distilled water, ordinary tap water is heated and the vapor is collected drop by drop as it condenses. Distilled water is used if any chemically pure substance is required; for example, a chemist always uses distilled water for doing accurate scientific work. It is rather unpleasant to drink, as it has a flat, mawkish taste.

DIURETIC. A diuretic is a drug which increases the flow of urine from the kidneys.

Water is one of the best diuretics if only a mild stimulant to the kidneys is required. Many people do not drink sufficient water during the day to allow the kidneys to be well flushed out. Of course, if the kidneys are diseased, more complicated measures have to be taken, and diuretics should be given with great caution and only under medical supervision.

Caffeine, which is contained in coffee and tea, is a good diuretic and it is especially valuable in heart diseases where there is an excess of water in the body (dropsy). Theobromine is a more powerful diuretic and it is not so likely to keep the patient awake as caffeine. It may be given in capsules in doses of 1 to 5 grains.

The most powerful diuretics used in medicine are derived from mercury and are invaluable in getting rid of the dropsy found in heart failure. Very often a single injection once a week is enough to keep such a patient in health.

DIVERTICULITIS. A diverticulum is a blind pocket which sometimes forms in the walls of the soft organs of the body

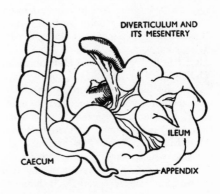

Diverticulitis.

such as the large bowel (colon) or bladder. These pockets or pouches are quite common and in a great many cases give rise to no discomfort or symptoms of any sort. Occasionally, however, they may get inflamed through the collection of waste materials in them, thus giving rise to the condition known as diverticulitis. This may be serious enough to require an operation. (*See also* INTESTINE.)

DIZZINESS. Dizziness in itself is not a disease, but it is a symptom of which patients frequently complain to the doctor. The term is used very loosely, but it should mean a slightly disturbed sense of equilibrium and perhaps loss of *full* consciousness, but not the sensation that things are spinning round—which should be called "giddiness"—nor the feeling of impending loss of consciousness, which is best called "feeling faint."

Dizziness in the above sense may have many causes, the most common of which, is, perhaps, due to a momentary partial failure of the blood supply to the brain, such as may occur on standing up suddenly after stooping or lying down, getting up after an illness, overventilating the lungs by repeated blowing, standing still after violent exercise, and such other things as make it hard for the circulation to adjust itself to sudden change.

Much the same sensation occurs at the onset of any feverish illness and from a slight overdose of alcohol or any hypnotic drug, also in the state of mild shock following a sudden fall, a painful injury or a blow on the head not severe enough to cause concussion. Dizziness can occur in the course of heart disease, but it is very rarely the symptom which calls attention to unsuspected heart trouble and, as a rule, it has nothing whatever to do with the heart.

DOGBITE. *See* BITES and HYDROPHOBIA.

DORSAL. Dorsal is the adjective applied to the back. The word is also used in connection with the back of any other part of the body. For example, the back of the hand is the dorsal part of the hand.

DOUBLE VISION. The ordinary act of seeing, which takes place whenever we look at anything, is the result of the two eyes working exactly together. It happens in certain diseases, and sometimes as a result of alcoholic excesses, that when one thing is looked, at, two images of it are seen, that is, each eye has its own vision of the object and the two are not merged into one image as they are in healthy sight. This condition is called double vision or diplopia. (*See also* DISSEMINATED SCLEROSIS; ENCEPHALITIS LETHARGICA.)

DOUCHE. A douche is an application of a stream of water to the whole or part of the body. It may be applied outwardly in the form of a jet or jets of water as in the Vichy douche and Aix douche, so called after the two famous spas, or inwardly into various cavities of the body such as the ears, nose, and vagina. The external douches are mostly used together with massage for chronic diseases of the joints and muscles, and to stimulate the flow of sweat.

Internal douching is used for purposes of cleanliness and disinfection and to relieve congestion in the neighborhood of the part which is douched. Of these douches the most generally employed is the vaginal douche for conditions in which there is a discharge or where the organs are congested and painful. These douches should be used at a fairly hot temperature, 100 deg. F. being about right. A tepid douche may give rise to a chill and so do more harm than good. The antiseptic used should be very weak, as the purpose of the douche is to wash away germs and the mucus which is always present in inflamed conditions, rather than to kill the germs. For slight irritations two tea-spoonfuls of bicarbonate of soda, added to each pint of warm water, will be found soothing.

Douching, although practiced habitually on the Continent, is seldom done as a routine in the U.S. unless the woman is wearing an internal support or is suffering from a vaginal discharge. When a pessary is worn, it is customary to douche two to three times a week to prevent the accumulation of secretions round the appliance.

For normal vaginal douching, the douche-can should be about 3 ft. above the vagina so as to deliver the fluid at the correct pressure. After pregnancy, however, the height should be reduced to about 2 ft. It is dangerous to douche during or after a miscarriage: if undertaken during a period, care must be taken to see that the water pressure is kept low.

DOUCHE CAN. The can used for ordinary douches is of glass or white enamel, and holds two or three pints of fluid. It is open at the top, and at the bottom has an outlet to which a tube can be attached. Different nozzles are used according to what part is to be douched, and if there is no tap on the nozzle for turning off the flow of fluid a clip of some sort should be provided to clip on the tubing when required to stop the flow.

All apparatus should be kept perfectly clean, and if used by different people must be boiled well between times.

DREAMS. These are more than vivid experiences we have while we are asleep. They bear a definite relationship, often obscure, but always to be found, to our waking lives. In childhood, dreams are simple and uncomplicated; what the child wishes or longs for while he is awake he obtains during his dreams. Only children often dream that they have many brothers and sisters, a realization in their dreams of the companionship they long for during the daytime. The child's mind is like a canvas on which certain impressions from the world it lives in are painted. These impressions are stored up, and if they are unpleasant ones they may be forgotten in the sense that they are not remembered when adult life is reached, but the impressions are there and may appear in dreams.

If the meaning of such dreams is not clear at first, by carrying the mind back to incidents which may have occurred in childhood the meaning may suddenly dawn on the dreamer. Here is an example: An Englishman dreamt that he was watching a funeral procession; as in most dreams, he felt no emotion, but was merely interested. Even when he realized that the funeral was that of the late Queen Mary, he felt no sorrow, but took off his hat because he saw other spectators doing likewise. When his dream was related by the dreamer, he was asked who the late Queen reminded him of. Immediately he said "My mother!" He then said, "Oh, but how awful to think of my mother dying!" (His mother was alive and well, and he was devoted to her.) But subsequently it turned

out that as a child he had been a "Mother's darling," and had secretly wished that his mother could somehow be removed so that he might have some freedom like other boys. A few days before the dream he had read a discussion in the paper on the value of learning self-reliance in youth, and his old secret resentment at having been deprived of this through excessive mother-love had caused the "death dream." Because it would have been too painful for him to have consciously wished for his mother's death, even in a dream, the mother was represented by the late Queen, a Queen being to her people what a mother is to her family. There is always a central idea in a dream which conceals an unexpressed or forgotten wish on the part of the dreamer. But because this wish is often of an unpleasant or antisocial character it is "wrapped up," so to speak; the central idea becomes a framework, on which the dream as experienced and related by the dreamer is built up. In trying to find the real meaning of a dream, it is necessary to take it to pieces, bit by bit, and gradually work back till we find the central idea, which is usually something that the dreamer does not like to face in his actual waking life.

One of the most interesting things about dreams is that nothing we do in them seems absurd. We journey round the world, we fly without wings or any other obvious means of transport, we appear to converse with famous historical characters long since dead, and in our dreams these things seem perfectly right and natural. Very often a dream forms a continuous story or drama, but it is seldom as clear-cut, as for instance, a story that we tell or read. Thus, a dream-scene may be a mix-up of many known places, and a dream-person may be built up out of the features, mannerisms, and personal peculiarities of many known persons. This mix-up takes place in order that the central idea of the dream, which we unconsciously wish to conceal, may be disguised. Only when we "take the dream to pieces" do we begin to recognize the meaning of it.

DROOPING EYELID, or PTOSIS. This is the name given to abnormal drooping of the upper eyelid, caused by some defect of the muscle which raises the upper eyelid.

Congenital Ptosis. This is due to some error in development. It may be due to absence or paralysis of the muscle. It may be on one side only, but is generally on both; and may be found in several members of the same family.

A person afflicted with drooping eyelids wrinkles up his brow, raises the eyebrows, and carries his head as far back as possible. The condition is readily diagnosed by the marked contrast between the wrinkled anxious brow and the calm drooping eyelid. Where the eyelids have drooped from birth, operative treatment is the only way to give relief.

"Jaw-winking" is the name given to a curious variation on natural ptosis. In this the patient droops the eyelid *except* when he is moving his jaw. It is due to an "error in the coupling up of the nerve supply to the various muscles," and cannot be remedied.

Drooping eyelids which only droop later in life are due to very many causes, tuberculosis paralysis of one or more of the eye muscles being the most common in childhood, and syphilitic paralysis, intracranial aneurism, tumor, or other diseases of the brain being the most common in adult life. It may occur also after some infectious fevers, shingles, certain poisons, and in neurasthenia, where there is weakness, but not actual paralysis, of the muscle.

There is a form occurring usually in delicate women of middle age; it is most marked in the morning, and gradually improves as the day goes on. It is probably due to debility, as it passes off when the system is toned up.

Treatment. The primary treatment of drooping eyelids, other than the congenital type, is that of the cause; until this has been done nothing further should be attempted. If, however, it is found to be incurable by ordinary means, an operation is performed. There are several methods, all of which have their adherents, but the principle in all is not completely to *cure* the ptosis. When this is done, i.e., if the condition is so altered that the patient's eye is wide open when he is awake, the lid will not close completely during sleep, and the sight would sooner or later be

damaged or destroyed by excessive exposure to the light. Hence what is aimed at is to *improve* the condition, but not to raise the lid so high that it cannot be lowered easily and completely.

Senile Ptosis. This occurs as a normal condition, to a slight degree, in old age; it is caused by gradual diminution of the fatty tissue at the back of the eye, and a consequent falling back of the eyeball into its socket. A more marked form is sometimes seen. These cases need not be treated.

"False Ptosis." This is the term given to drooping of the eyelids from other causes than that of paralysis of the muscle. In cases of the serious eye disease called trachoma, for instance, the patient gets into the habit of keeping the lid half-closed, to avoid the discomfort of moving the roughened granular surface over the eye. As, too, the lid is thickened and stiffened by the disease, it is all the more difficult to raise. In cases of eye disease, where light is painful to the eye, the patient again gets into the habit of keeping the eyelid down to protect the eye. This habit continues for a long time afterwards, and may be most difficult to cure; but the condition is not a true ptosis.

DROPSY. Dropsy describes an accumulation of watery fluid in the tissues, often accompanied by free fluid in the peritoneal and pleural cavities, i.e., between the abdominal wall and the intestines or between the chest wall and the lungs. The condition is fully described under the heading EDEMA.

DROWNING. In drowning, water fills the air passages so that no oxygen can enter, nor carbon dioxide leave the blood through the lungs. For a moment the breathing center at the base of the brain is stimulated by the rise of carbon dioxide, but this only makes matters worse. The lack of oxygen quickly puts the nerve cells of the brain out of action, causing unconsciousness, and very soon after this the breathing center also fails. The heart, however, is not so sensitive and will for a time continue to beat regardless of what is happening elsewhere in the body, although it becomes increasingly difficult for it to send the blood through the lungs or to obtain the fuel for its own consumption.

The arteries and capillaries lose their

tone and become overfilled with blood, so that neither the blood pressure nor the heat of the body can be maintained. Soon afterwards the heart itself will cease to beat. All this happens in a very few minutes, and if the life of a drowning person is to be saved, action must be prompt.

It is essential to empty the water out of the victim as quickly as possible. Artificial respiration should be started the moment the water has been emptied from his larger air tubes. The victim should be kept as warm as possible and above all, these efforts should be persisted in until it is certain that life is extinct. (*See also* ARTIFICIAL RESPIRATION; ASPHYXIA; FIRST AID.)

DROWSINESS. Drowsiness is a natural state when we are feeling tired, and it is not unusual for people to feel drowsy on a hot day after they have eaten a heavy meal. In normally healthy people the feeling of drowsiness should only be there for a short time before going off to sleep, but there are some people who feel drowsy during the day when the mind should be feeling fresh and active. Living in a badly ventilated room will cause a feeling of heaviness and drowsiness, because the body is gradually being poisoned through lack of fresh air. Overindulgence in alcohol may also induce drowsiness, as also does exposure to extreme cold, and, of course, the use of narcotic drugs.

Persistent and unusual drowsiness should be looked upon as a sign that the bodily health requires attention, and a doctor should be consulted. (*See also* COMA.)

DRUGS. Drugs are substances which are used to help the body to fight disease, or which help the body to carry out its normal work. Many people are afraid to use drugs because, they say, they are unnatural and dangerous; but they forget that the disease is just as "unnatural," and the knowledge of drugs which has come down to us through the ages should be looked upon as an important advance towards the happiness and well-being of mankind. Certainly it is unwise to indulge in drugs when the body is in a perfectly healthy state, and it may cause serious damage to do so; but there are many cases where the administration of the right drug at the right time may save a great deal of needless pain and worry.

The number of drugs in everyday use is very great. Many of them have been known for centuries. It is a comfort to us to know that when we are given medicine to take, the doctor is almost certain of the result it is going to have on us. Science has done much towards finding out the exact drug to use in each disease. New drugs are constantly being discovered or evolved, and by means of highly equipped laboratories and organized research modern medical science gives every hope that all diseases may be successfully treated by means of drugs, and much unnecessary pain done away with.

Drugs are obtained from several sources; some come from plants, some from molds, some from minerals, and some from animals. Many important drugs are now made artificially in the laboratory; these are termed *synthetic* drugs and they are just as effective as drugs obtained from their original vegetable or animal source. A good example is salicin, which used to be extracted from the bark of willows and poplars; it is no longer used, because sodium salicylate, from which aspirin is made, is now manufactured artificially.

Drugs from Common Plants. The majority of drugs are obtained from plants, many of our most important preparations being obtained from flowers and trees grown in our meadows. The common foxglove gives us a most valuable and widely used substance from its leaves, known as digitalis, which is used in the treatment of diseases of the heart. An extract from the male fern, which is to be found growing in almost every wood, is one of the best cures for tapeworm. The meadow saffron gives us a drug known as colchicum, which relieves the pain of gout. From the plant known as deadly night-shade many preparations of belladonna are made, and it also yields atropine, a valuable drug in the examination and treatment of the eye.

Diuretics (drugs which are given to increase the flow of urine) are obtained from broom and from juniper. Creosote, which is used as an antiseptic and as an inhalant in bronchitis, is obtained from beech trees. Oil of rosemary, distilled from the flowering tops of the rosemary plant, is commonly used to give a pleasant scent to hair lotions and other preparations.

The leaves of the henbane, collected

from the flowering plant and dried, give us a drug known as hyoscine, a powerful narcotic; it is used to soothe patients suffering from delirium tremens or insanity.

Castor oil comes to use from the castor-oil plant grown in India; jalap is grown in South America; opium, from which very many important preparations are made, is obtained from the opium poppy cultivated in the East. Rhuabarb root is grown in China and Tibet, and is commonly given to children as a purgative; cascara sagrada, another useful purgative, is prepared from the dried bark of the California buckthorn. These are but a few of the enormous number of drugs obtained from plants. Most of the more important ones will be described under their own headings throughout this book.

There are also many mineral substances, such as iron, arsenic, radium, mercury, copper, and lead, from which drugs are obtained. Coal deposits, which are the remains of ancient forests, give us some disinfectants such as carbolic acid, etc., and many important aniline dyes.

The sulphonamides are a group of synthetic chemical drugs derived from sulphanilamide—they number hundreds, but only a few are of medical value, chiefly sulphapyridine, sulphathiazole, sulphadiazine, and sulphaguanidine, used in various infections. The antibiotics like penicillin are extracted from the solution produced by the growth of living molds and are active against a wide variety of diseases.

Extracts from the glands of various animals now supply us with some of our most valuable drugs. From the pituitary gland, situated at the base of the brain, we obtain pituitrin. This drug is used a great deal in circulatory failure and it is able to act within a minute or two of injection.

An extract is also obtained from the thyroid gland in the neck which cures cretinism in children, and is also used with benefit in myxedema and other diseases.

Insulin, which is obtained from the pancreas of sheep and oxen, is of great use in the treatment of diabetes; but as insulin does not cure diabetes, the treatment must be carried on all the time.

The adrenal glands supply us with several principles used in medicine, the most recent of which, cortisone, is known to arrest the progress of rheumatoid arthritis.

Many drugs are in a *crude* state, which means that they are not pure, but are mixed with other substances. Chemists have now found means by which they can separate in a pure state the active principle of a drug from a crude preparation. In this way the treatment of a disease is made safe and efficient because the doctor is able to tell just how much active principle of a drug is suitable for his patient.

Valuable Properties of Certain Drugs. Many of our most useful drugs owe their value to the presence of a property which is known as an alkaloid. Drugs such as morphine, quinine, atropine, and strychnine all contain alkaloids and all are obtained from plants.

Volatile oils are thick oils which do not leave a greasy mark on paper; they are usually prepared by distillation. Gums are extracted from the stems of trees and plants.

Vitamins are chemicals which chemists are now able to isolate in a pure state; they are to be found in various forms of food, and are most essential to our diet.

Vaccines, sera, and antitoxins may be described as drugs which are used to protect the body against disease.

Drug Habits. The habit of taking drugs regularly is a very widespread one, but such substances as tobacco, tea, coffee, etc., are harmless if not taken to excess. The drugs which have the most harmful effect upon people are narcotics, such as cocaine and morphia, and once these drugs get a a hold on their victims the habit of taking them can only be broken with difficult.

The habit of smoking is one which the majority of people all over the world indulge in, and it can be a very pleasant and soothing habit, if kept within reasonable limits. If indulged in to excess it causes indigestion, irritability and sleeplessness. Prolonged excessive smoking may lead to blindness. (*See also* BLINDNESS, TOBACCO.)

Caffeine, which is found in tea and coffee, is very stimulating, but excessive tea-drinking may cause indigestion, probably owing to the tannin in the tea.

Opium and its derivative morphia can

be taken by eating it, by smoking and so inhaling it, or by injecting solutions of it under the skin. The type of person who eventually becomes a morphia addict is usually temperamentally unstable, but there are often circumstances which lead to the taking of drugs which one finds it very hard to condemn. It is not unusual for patients who are suffering from a prolonged and painful illness to find refuge in drugs; and such a habit pleads its own defense. But there are certain people who take morphia purely for the delight it gives them. These are often persons who have taken to it through sheer boredom and degenerates to whom excess in alcohol or any other similar drug seems to be natural and inevitable.

The results of taking cocaine are even more disastrous than those of taking morphia, and one of the most unfortunate things about the cocaine-taker is his ignorance of his state. Cocaine at first relieves fatigue, and this is followed by a delightful sense of vigor and mental well-being. But in the course of time the habitual taker of "snow," as it is called, suffers from many mental and physical disorders, and eventually insanity may develop. The only cure is to cut off the supply of the drug and to place the patient under the care of a skilled attendant.

Cannabis indica, which is also called hashish, Indian hemp, and bhang, is a drug which is used extensively in the East. Under the influence of this drug all sense of time seems to disappear and the most exciting dreams and visions occur. Taken to excess, this drug usually leads to insanity.

Other drugs which sometimes give rise to unpleasant consequences are chloral, sulphonal, veronal, and trional. The habitual use of these drugs is usually acquired in the treatment of sleeplessness. (*See also* ALCOHOLISM.)

Drug Rashes. Occasionally, after a patient has been taking a drug, he is horrified to find that shortly afterwards he "breaks out in a rash." He finds that this occurs each time he takes that particular drug, and quite rightly blames it as being the cause of his eruption. He is, however, only partly correct in assuming this: if the drug alone were to blame, *every* person taking it

would be similarly affected; as it is, only one or two in a hundred suffer. There is, therefore, the peculiarity of constitution, or idiosyncrasy, as it is called, of these patients to be taken into consideration as well as the nature of the drug itself.

The number of drugs that have been blamed at various times as being the cause of an eruption on the skin is so great that it would be impossible to give a complete list of them.

Drug eruptions are found in very many different forms; there is no class of eruption that has not its counterpart among the drug rashes. They are generally "spotty," and often resemble measles, scarlet fever, smallpox or German measles. Sometimes they are like hives but literally anything in the nature of a rash may be found, from a simple pink spot to hemorrhage or even gangrene.

Only rashes associated with the more commonly used drugs are here described in their more common forms. They are, naturally, of considerable practical importance, since not infrequently, in ignorance, a patient may continue to take as a cure for his "skin trouble" the very drug that is its cause!

Antipyrine (phenazone). This drug is calculated to produce a rash in 2 per cent of men and 7 per cent of women. There are various forms, the commonest being the "measly" variety, which lasts for three or four days, and is followed by peeling. The face and neck are seldom, if ever, affected. Weals and blisters are also seen; all these forms are accompanied by itching.

Arsenic. Eruptions can be produced either by local contact, or by taking the drug internally. The former is seen in workers in artificial flowers, cardboard boxes, and aniline dyes, of which arsenic is a frequent impurity; and "beautifying" skin lotions are a not infrequent cause nowadays. The most typical chronic eruption affects the palms of the hands and soles of the feet: these either become unnaturally pink (the so-called "pink palm"); or small areas become hardened and horny. In due coarse the skin of the legs becomes inflamed. The most remarkable eruption associated with arsenic is shingles, which is very apt to occur in those patients having injections of salvarsan and other drugs of which arsenic is a contituent.

Barbital. Commonly used in "sleeping-powders," this may produce a "scarlet fever" or blotchy rash.

Belladonna. This produces a bright-red "scarlet-fever" rash. It is usually only on the face and neck, and is very itchy, but soon fades, and there is no peeling.

Boric Acid. Sometimes produces a pink spotty rash, but the more usual form is a crop of pimples, each pimple becoming scaly at the top. It may be seen when boric acid has been used as an antiseptic wash, or when taken internally. It may, in rare cases, produce so great a skin disturbance as to be fatal.

The Bromides. These very often produce a rash. It may occur as a pink spotty rash, or as hives, or as blisters; but the most typical form is the so-called "bromide acne," which consists of little pustules, or pimples containing pus. This at first sight looks like common acne, but there are no blackheads; and unlike acne proper, "bromide acne" occurs all over the body—even on the roof of the mouth. It is well known among epileptics who have been in the habit of taking large doses of potassium bromide for years; here the eruption is very chronic. It is also common in children who have been ignorantly dosed with "teething powders"; or it may occur in infants whose mothers are taking the drug.

It is treated by withdrawal of the drug.

Ergot. Ergot, which was much used in midwifery to prevent hemorrhage after birth, has been known to produce rashes of varying severity, or even gangrene of the extremities, when taken in very large quantity.

Eucalyptus. This is so frequently taken for colds and chills that the possibility of its causing a rash may be overlooked. The usual form is a crop of weals, resembling those of nettle-rash, on the hands and feet, the weals may be accompanied by red "blotches."

The Iodides. These may cause a rash when used internally or externally. The general remarks on the bromides apply also to the iodides (which indeed are closely related chemically). A really wild mixture of eruptions has been noted: spots, blisters, hemorrhage into the skin, an "iodide acne" closely resembling the bromide acne, ulcers or "gummata" closely resembling those caused by syphilis, and even large, solid tumors that have at first been thought to arise from leprosy or cancer! The difficulty of diagnosis is sometimes very great. Naturally, very often the doctor knows that iodide is being taken, and is on the watch, but a great many cases follow the taking of certain patent medicines, many of which contain iodide in small amounts.

These rashes may occur from quite small doses, but usually follow a fairly long administration of the drug. They occur more commonly if the kidneys are affected in any way. If a rash occurs, iodide should be stopped at once.

Mercury. This is used in several forms, and may produce a rash when used internally or, especially, externally, calomel being the chief offender. The "scarlet fever" variety is the most common rash, but many forms have been seen.

Morphia. Not infrequently produces an intense itching before a rash is observed. The usual rash resembles scarlet fever very closely, and is followed by profuse peeling. If a sore throat occurs at the same time, the diagnosis is sometimes very difficult. Occasionally the rash may consist of pimples or weals.

Phenolphthalein. Frequently used for the relief of habitual constipation, sometimes producing a rash occurring as pink "plates" on the skin. As with antipyrine, if it is used for some time the spots may take on a brown coloration, which is permanent.

Quinine. When taken internally, this produces a large variety of rashes, the commonest being the scarlet fever type. When the rash form occurs, it may be very severe, producing so much swelling of the face that the eyes may be closed, and may also produce quinine "asthma," which gives rise to much distress in breathing. A quinine rash may be treated with calamine or lead lotion, with *liquor carbonis detergens* added to either. (*See also* OCCUPATIONAL DISEASE for an account of quinine worker's rash.)

Rhubarb. Sometimes causes a "scarlet fever" rash, which is followed by peeling.

Santonin. Used in cases of round-worm infection, often produces a "nettle-rash" eruption.

Salicylic Acid and the Salicylates. These are much used for rheumatism and produce a great variety of rashes; itching sometimes occurs, and peeling follows the rash.

Silver Nitrate. Produces a condition known as argyria, which is a permanent bluish-grey discoloration all over the body, including the whites of the eyes. This was formerly a common condition, both among workers in silver and people taking silver internally, but in its complete form it is now seldom seen. Silver staining of the eye is still seen in some cases where silver drops have been used.

Veronal. Like many other sleep-producing drugs, it causes a "scarlet fever" rash, which is itchy and followed by peeling. It is peculiar in that it almost always worsens any skin disease present, and should therefore not be taken in these circumstances.

The Sulphonamides. These drugs were introduced into medicine by Domagk in 1935, when he showed that streptococcal septicemia could be prevented by giving sulphanilamide. The ensuing years saw the addition of various new sulphonamides, such as sulphapyridine, sulphadiazine, sulphadimidine and sulphaguanidine, the earlier ones being more toxic than the later ones. They proved valuable in blood poisoning, pneumonia, gonorrhea and other infections.

The Antibiotic Drugs. The discovery of penicillin in 1929 by Fleming and its development during World War II by Florey and his colleagues opened a completely new chapter in the history of therapeutics, for it proved to be but the first of an important series of antibacterial compounds obtained from molds and bacteria. One of the most important properties of penicillin was that it could be given in very large doses generally without any ill effects upon the patient, but this is not the case in some of the newer antibiotics, such as streptomycin and chloromycetin. Some patients and some diseases become resistant to one particular antibiotic, hence the value of some of the newer ones, such as aureomycin and tetracycline.

Drug Rashes. It is sometimes very difficult, as might be expected, to distinguish a drug rash from one of the diseases it imitates, especially if the patient does not associate the rash with the drug. In general it may be said that, though drug rashes resemble those caused by disease in many cases, they do not imitate them quite well enough to deceive the careful eye. A drug eruption is often far more widespread and severe than a similar eruption from disease: antipyrine and copaiba, for instance, are far more "measly" than a true measles, and bromide and iodide acne occur over the whole body, instead of chiefly on the face.

The treatment in most cases is very simple. It consists in stopping the offending drug entirely; and in hastening elimination by the copious drinking of water and in the use of mild drugs which increase the output from the kidneys, and of purgatives.

DRUNKENNESS. The spectacle of a drunken person is known to us all, and perhaps a good definition of drunkenness would be to say that the term means all the effects of recent overindulgence in alcohol which are visible to other people. The amount of alcohol necessary to bring about a state of drunkenness differs with different people.

The chief effect of alcohol is to "take off the brakes." In ordinary life we practise a considerable amount of control over our actions in order to make our doings fit into the orderly scheme of communal existence; that is, so that we shall not be a nuisance to other people. This control is slackened by alcoholic drinks and relaxed altogether in the state we speak of as drunkenness. The drunken man is not responsible for his actions, but this does not absolve him in the eyes of the law for the crimes he commits while drunk. Legally, a man is supposed to be aware of the effect of alcohol on himself.

Alcohol has a slightly stimulating effect at first, but this is followed by depression, so it is wrong to look upon alcohol as a real stimulant. The gaiety and friendliness with which a drinking bout starts are succeeded by suspicions and quarrels. Next comes silliness and, finally, stupidity and sleepiness, followed by drunken stupor or sleep. The face flushes and the pupils of the eyes grow larger, the breathing becomes slow, loud, and irregular. The hands tremble and the speech becomes indistinct; or, if the person is aware of his state and has a powerful will, he will pronounce every word precisely with great care.

Tests for drunkenness are sometimes not very satisfactory, as other conditions, some of which are of serious importance, will produce almost the same symptoms. In many cases, for instance, of persons who are charged after an accident with being drunk while driving a car, the driver has to be given the benefit of the doubt because the shock of the accident may produce in him similar symptoms to those of drunkenness. The most accurate measure of the amount of alcohol consumed is a chemical estimation of alcohol in the blood. In some cases it is possible thus to state definitely that a person was drunk.

Treatment. It is of course necessary to see that no more alcohol is taken, and steps should be taken to get as much of the alcohol as possible out of the system quickly. This is done at a hospital or by a doctor by means of the stomach pump; but if this cannot be done, an emetic of salt and water, or mustard and water, should be given. When the patient has been sick he may be given strong black coffee or strong tea. (*See also* ALCOHOL; DELIRIUM TREMENS; DIPSOMANIA.)

DRYNESS OF THE MOUTH. The mouth is kept in a moist state by a constant flow of saliva, the fluid which is poured into the mouth from the salivary glands. These glands are to be found under the tongue and behind the jaw. Like other glands of the body, they are under the control of the nervous system. Thus the mere sight of food will cause the mouth of a hungry person to "water," and the smell and taste of food will have the same effect.

The first part of digestion of food is begun in the mouth by the saliva as it mixes with the food. Saliva is also necessary to keep the various movable parts of the mouth "oiled" as it were, and thus prevent them from damage by rubbing together.

It sometimes happens that for various reasons the flow of saliva is interrupted. The cause should be searched for and overcome. Dry mouth, or "xerostomia," is a rare nervous disease found usually in women. Mouth-breathing or taking of drying-up medicines such as atropine for any length of time will cause a dry mouth. It is

often present after operations or fevers, or any condition in which the body quickly loses moisture. These temporary conditions can be helped by sucking glycerine and borax pastilles. (*See also* DIABETES INSIPIDUS.)

DUCT. The ducts of the body are the channels or tubes by which fluids are carried from one part of the body to another. As a rule, the chemical substances, or secretions as they are called, of the various glands are poured into these ducts. For example, saliva is carried to the mouth by the salivary ducts. Other ducts are the bile ducts leading from the gall bladder and liver, the sweat glands all over the body, the lymphatic glands, and so on. (*See also* DUCTLESS GLANDS.)

DUCTLESS GLANDS. It is now well known that all the bodily functions are under the control of powerful chemicals or drugs. It has been shown that even the nerve impulses in certain nerves called the autonomic nerves actually cause the changes that occur at their nerve endings by setting free certain strong chemicals. Some of these chemicals are obtained from the food and are called vitamins, and others which are called hormones are manufactured in the body itself. All the tissues contain bodies which are able to set free chemicals which have a powerful effect. This can be seen especially in the way they behave when they are injured. There are, however, certain collections of cells in the body whose special work is to manufacture these chemicals and pour them into the fluids which circulate throughout the body, such as blood and lymph. Their action then becomes a general one involving the whole or part of the entire body. The substances which are manufactured by these glands are not collected together in a common tube or duct, but are taken away directly into the cells by the blood. In this way they are unlike the ordinary glands of the body, and so, in contrast to them, are called the *ductless glands* or *endocrine glands*.

The relations between the various ductless glands are so complicated that only parts of their fascinating story are yet clearly known. We must content ourselves, therefore, with a short description of the chief discoveries that have been made so far.

The Suprarenal Capsules or Adrenals. These are two small yellowish bodies which are found attached to the upper part of the kidneys. They consist of two parts, the *cortex* or bark, and the *medulla* or center. From the medulla a very useful substance is produced which is called *adrenaline*. It can also now be manufactured artificially by chemists. An injection of this substance has the same effect as would be produced by a stimulation of the part of the nervous system called the sympathetic nervous system. From the outer cortex, some thirty steroid hormones have been isolated, the most important being cortisone and hydrocortisone. A disease of the adrenals called Addison's Disease is apt to be fatal and is associated with low blood pressure, great weakness, and a peculiar bronzing of the skin. This condition is relieved by suitable treatment with cortisone. Further analysis has revealed many different hormones in the suparenal cortex, with widely varying functions. Some are essential to life, while others, like cortisone, are concerned with the protection of the tissues against damaging agents.

The Carotid Gland. This is a collection of cells lying between the fork of the carotid artery where it splits into its two main branches at either side of the neck. It is now known to have the power of affecting the blood pressure.

The Coccygeal Gland. A tiny collection of cells lying in front of the tip of the coccyx (tail) at the lower end of the backbone. Its use is still unknown.

The Gonads. These are the sex-glands— the testes in the male and ovaries in the female. They are responsible for the development of secondary sexual characteristics at puberty; e.g., facial hair in the male and breasts and menstruation in the female. They, in turn, are apparently under the control of the anterior pituitary gland. Attempts have been made to use testicular extracts to prolong the period of active sex life or delay old age. This work is, however, still in the experimental stage. The extract which was used in earlier experiments was obtained from monkeys, hence it gained the popular name of "monkey gland" treatment.

Two extracts are now obtained from the ovaries, one from the ordinary ovarian sub-stance and the other from the substance of the ovary during pregnancy.

The Pancreas. The pancreas, which in animals is called the sweetbread, contains special tissue which produces the substance called *insulin*. This substance controls the turning of sugar into energy by the tissues, and is also concerned with the storing up of sugar in the form of starch which is called *glycogen*. People whose supply of insulin is deficient are subject to the disease called diabetes mellitus, or sugar diabetes, so called from the sweetness of the urine. Such people are starved of energy because the greater part of the body's energy is obtained from the burning up of sugar, and this can only take place in the presence of insulin. The result is that the sugar is poured out from the stores of glycogen, but since it cannot be used is given off in the urine. The patient accordingly becomes very thin and weak and may die. Insulin cannot yet be made artificially.

Pineal Gland. This is a small gland situated in the brain. Tumors of this gland have been found where there is hypertrophy of the tissues of the sexual organs. Its uses are not, however, fully known.

The Pituitary Gland. This is a small gland lying in a hollow on the floor of the skull above the root of the nose, which, though small, is important enough to have been called "the leader of the endocrine orchestra." It consists of three parts: the anterior, or front, the intermediate, and the posterior or back part. The functions of the intermediate part are not clear. The anterior part is exceedingly interesting, because it is known that its products control the activity of many other ductless glands, affecting thyroid activity and growth, especially of the long bones; overproduction of its secretion leads to the person being a giant. Too much pituitary extract in adults leads to growth of the lower face bones, hands and feet, a condition called "acromegaly." In addition, it is now certain that the extract of the anterior lobe causes the development and ripening of the sexual organs. Failure of this secretion leads to the person remaining permanently in a condition of infantilism with regard to the development of the sexual organs. The pituitary extract is also associated in some way with the retaining of the fetus, or unborn baby, in the womb. During pregnancy a substance which resembles the pituitary extract is found in the urine, and at one time it was thought to be identical with it. Its presence or otherwise is used most successfully as a test of human pregnancy.

From the posterior part of the pituitary gland is obtained a secretion whose activities are well known, but whose place in the machinery of the body is not yet definitely known. Its chief activity consists of raising the blood pressure by its action both on the heart and on the blood vessels, and it is therefore very valuable in treating shock. It has also a very powerful action on the womb, causing it to contract, so it is used in obstetrics. It also has an important action in regulating the water balance of the body, especially when the water balance is wildly disturbed as it is in diabetes insipidus, or water diabetes, as it is sometimes called. It has, as well, some influence on the sugar chemistry of the body.

These extracts cannot yet be obtained in a completely pure form. They are among the most powerful of known substances.

Spleen. While the main function of the spleen is to act as a reservoir for blood, there is some evidence to show that it produces a substance which has the power of causing a rapid improvement in the condition of the blood.

The Thymus Gland. The thymus is a large gland lying in the upper part of the thorax or chest. The gland is thought to increase in size up to the time of puberty, but after about the sixteenth year is slowly shrivels up and reaches a state of atrophy by about the age of fifty. Its function is uncertain, but possibly its secretion restricts and controls the activities of the sex glands (gonads) and prevents their developing too early in life.

Thyroid Gland. The thyroid gland is a large gland situated in the neck just below the Adam's apple but extending up both sides of it. This gland in early prehistoric man actually poured its secretion directly into the alimentary canal, so it is not surprising to find that an extract from it will work almost equally well whether taken by the mouth or as an injection. This is not true of the secretions of the other glands, which only possess a feeble action, if any, when taken by mouth. An active extract has been obtained from the thyroid and can be manufactured artificially. It is called thyroxin. The manufacture of it by artificial means is one of the great triumphs of chemistry. It is peculiar in that it contains iodine. Its main effect seems to be in connection with the chemical processes of the body, including those of growth. An absence of thyroid leads to failure to develop mentally and physically, as in cretins and idiots. In older people failure of the thyroid has not quite such severe results, but it still leads to great stupidity and to various changes in the skin and hair, a condition can be relieved by taking thyroid extract or thyroxin. Too much thyroid, on the other hand, will cause a speeding up of the various processes of the body. The symptoms are loss of flesh, nervousness and flushing; the heart may be damaged. This condition is called Graves' disease or exophthalmic goitre, because there is also protrusion of the eyeballs and enlargement of the thyroid gland. (*See also* CRETINISM; GRAVES' DISEASE; MYXEDEMA.)

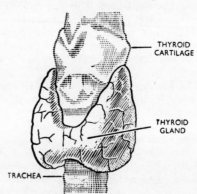

Ductless Glands: Thyroid.

The Parathyroids. These are small collections of cells situated either actually in the substance of the thyroid gland, or just outside it. They are concerned with the regulation of the level of calcium and phosphorus in the blood and tissues. Injections of the extract are able to restore to normal persons suffering from the peculiar condition known as tetany, in which there is not enough calcium in the blood. (*See also* TETANY.)

Conclusion. All these ductless glands are closely related to each other in their workings, and disturbance of one leads to disturbance of the others and to considerable confusion in the working of the body as a whole. As has been said, there is at the present time a great deal of research work being done on the subject of these glands. New discoveries have been made with results in the treatment of disease which may be described as truly wonderful; yet there is doubtless still much that is equally wonderful to be unfolded in the future. (*See also* sections on individual ductless glands, such as SPLEEN; THYROID GLAND; etc; and HORMONES)

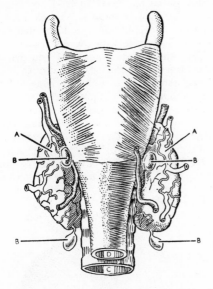

Ductless Glands: Parathyroid. A. *Thyroid Gland;* B. *Parathyroid Glands.*

DUMBNESS. Dumbness is the inability to speak or to utter any of the sounds which make up words. Most cases of dumbness are due to deafness, in which the patient is unable to speak because he has never been able to hear, and therefore imitate, speech sounds. This type is explained more fully under the heading DEAF MUTISM.

When the hearing is good, dumbness is usually due to aphasia, or loss of the function of speech. This is a disorder of the speech center in the brain, which may, however, be complex and include an inability to appreciate spoken language. In some cases it may be due to some other nervous disorder. Mentally defective people are very often dumb, and certain hysterical conditions produce dumbness. Sometimes children suffer from a slight form of dumbness due to enlarged tonsils forming an obstruction in the throat. Stammering and lisping are really slight forms of dumbness, but these can generally be cured by careful training. (*See also* DEAF MUTISM.)

DUODENAL ULCER. The duodenum or beginning part of the intestine is, like the stomach, subject to ulceration. In the case of stomach ulcers, the pain comes on after the food has been received into the stomach, that is, immediately after food; but duodenal ulcer is caused by the action of the gastric juices on the lining of the duodenum, so the pain occurs when the stomach is empty, about two hours after food, and is immediately relieved as soon as food is taken into the stomach and the gastic juices are occupied in dealing with it. Alkalis such as bicarbonate of soda counteract the gastric juices, which are acid, and render them less active, so large doses of alkalis greatly relieve the pain of duodenal ulcer.

Duodenal ulcers are much more frequent in men than in women. Duodenal ulcer may occur amongst both smokers and non-smokers, but when there is an ulcer it is advisable to give up smoking, as anything which increases the activity of the gastric juices, as tobacco does, will be bad for the ulcer.

Symptoms. Duodenal ulcer occurs at any age after childhood. It can be present for as long as twenty years without giving rise to more than a slight discomfort at intervals of months, or perhaps only for a few days in the spring and a few days in the autumn. The pain comes on a couple of hours after food, but it may only be thought of as a greater hunger than usual as the next mealtime approaches. If a definite spot of pain is present it will be just to the right of the middle line of the abdomen and above the navel. There may also be an aching pain in the right side of the back, under the shoulderblade.

It is quite usual for people with duodenal ulcers to waken in the night with a pain which is immediately quietened by taking some food or alkaline powder or mixture. The appetite is usually good with this sort of ulcer, and the patient may remain fat and well-looking, in marked contrast to the person with a stomach ulcer, who always becomes thin. The bowels are nearly always constipated, and when the ulcer is large and active there may be continuous bleeding from it, with the result that the stools will be dark in color. These dark stools, due to intestinal bleeding, are called *melaena*. The chief danger with duodenal ulcer is that the ulcer may eat its way through the wall of the bowel and "perforate," as it is called, when a very serious situation arises with dramatic suddenness.

Treatment. It has been estimated that at least 10 per cent of the male population suffer from gastric or duodenal ulcer at some time in their lives. They tend to occur in the spring and autumn and there is no doubt that they are often brought on by periods of worry. They occur in people of active and restless temperament and are one of the penalties of our highly artificial civilization.

There is no known way of preventing peptic ulcer (as ulcers of the stomach and duodenum are collectively known), and treatment cannot be said to be satisfactory. Ulcers often heal without treatment, but in those who are subject to them are liable to relapse. Management of an ulcer consists, therefore, in preventing relapses and treating symptoms as they arise, so as to avoid unnecessary loss of work.

Normally, it is possible to do this by ensuring regular meals at fairly frequent intervals and by avoiding excessive smoking and irritating, indigestible foods and drinks. Alkalis, such as magnesium trisilicate or bismuth carbonate, are necessary only when pain is present. For severe relapses a period of rest in bed on strict diet and alkalis may be unavoidable. Then it is usual for the doctor to begin by putting the patient to bed for a month on a diet called the *Sippy diet,* after its inventor. This, in its earliest stages, consists of just as little food as will maintain the patient's strength. The usual thing is a small glass of milk, which has been citrated, every two hours. Alkaline drinks are given in between times. This diet must be continued for two weeks, the patient being kept in bed.

In the third week a litle more food is added, such as a little thin bread and butter, raw egg in milk, junket, custard, and jelly. The following week potato soup, corn flour, arrowroot, sago, and tapioca may be added. In the fifth week this may be increased to a lightly boiled egg, white fish mashed up, thin toast or rusk with butter. For yet another week or two the only addition to the menu must be finely minced meat. After that there should be no more trouble from the ulcer, and in all but bad cases it should be cured sufficiently not to return, if care is taken to avoid highly spiced and very hot food, too large meals, too long an interval between meals, smoking, alcohol, and anything that is known to disagree with the individual.

The surgical treatment of duodenal ulcers is not as satisfactory as that of gastric ulcers, though it may be necessary and may result in an improvement in the patient's health and comfort. No operation, except in an emergency, should be undertaken until the medical treatment has had a thorough trial.

DUODENUM. The duodenum is the first part of the small intestine or bowel. It is connected with the stomach by a valve called the pylorus, and is from eight to ten inches long. The juices from the

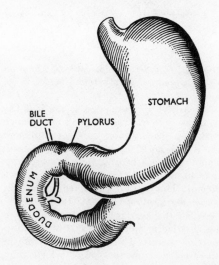

Duodenum.

pancreas and the liver empty into it, and it therefore plays an important part in the process of digestion. At its lower end the duodenum connects with the coils of the small intestine called the jejunum.

DUPUYTREN'S CONTRACTION. This is the name given to the condition commonly called "contracted fingers,' where the muscles of the little and fourth finger contract and the fingers bend over into the palm of the hand. *See also* CONTRACTED FINGERS for a fuller description.

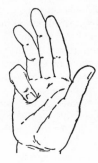

Dupuytren's Contraction.

DURAMATER. This is the name of the outer covering of the brain and spinal cord. There are three coverings altogether, of which the outer one is the strongest. (*See also* BRAIN.)

DYSENTERY. Dysentery is an infectious disease of which the chief symptom is acute diarrhea. There are several types of this disease, depending upon whether it is caused by an ameba or a bacillus, but the symptoms are all very much alike. Infection is carried by means of food and water; flies and insects also play a part in spreading this disease. Dysentery occurs in hot climates, and especially in Egypt, India, Iraq, and parts of America.

Symptoms. The disease generally begins with a feeling of illness, loss of appetite, and a certain amount of diarrhea, which gradually increases in severity and is accompanied by griping pains in the abdomen. At first the motions may be thin and watery, but very soon blood and mucus, or slime, are passed, and finally the motions consist of little else. The discharges from the bowels follow each other with great frequency, and the painful feeling of downward presure, which is always present, causes the patient to desire to go to stool all the time. Although the health may not be very greatly disturbed in a mild case of dysentery, it increases with the advance of the disease, and in severe cases the patient may die from sheer exhaustion and from loss of blood.

There is usually fever present, and the patient may suffer from thirst and scanty and painful flow of urine. At this stage the patient is usually very low and depressed and the discharges from the bowels become more offensive and are passed continually.

If, on the other hand, the course of the disease is checked before it becomes too severe, the signs of improvement are shown by the number of motions which are passed. These become less in number and more natural in appearance and the pains and straining become less severe. Convalescence is, however, a very slow business and attacks may recur.

Preventive Treatment. In countries where epidemics of dysentery occur, it is of the utmost importance that steps should be taken to prevent the disease spreading. The water supply must be properly protected, and care must be taken to see that all the excreta of persons who are suffering from dysentery or who are convalescent from the disease are properly disinfected or burnt. All food should be protected from flies by placing netting over it, and only boiled water should be used for cooking and drinking and for washing food and food utensils. Constipation should be avoided, as should also the eating of unripe fruits.

Curative Treatment. The patient should at once be put on a diet consisting of albumin-water, rice-water, or light meat broth, and then arrowroot and cornflour. He should rest in bed. Treatment depends on the type of dysentery present, and the motions of the patient are examined in order to find out the exact type of germ which is causing the disease. In amebic cases the drug which is most used is emetine, the extract of ipecacuanha. This is given night and morning for several days, the dose being lessened as the motions become more natural in appearance. The bowel is washed out with an enema containing bicarbonate of soda, and then a warm, weak solution of starch in injected into the rectum.

In bacillary dysentery, sulphaguanidine, one of the sulphonamide drugs, cures rapidly if given early.

In the general treatment of dysentery, the chief points to which attention should be given are the nourishment of the patient, and the proper care of his clothing and body, etc. During convalescence, red meat should not be given; in fact, all rich food should be avoided. A change of climate will sometimes complete the cure when all other means fail.

DYSMENORRHEA. This is the term applied to unusual pain at the menstrual periods. The complaint is a very common one and may be due to various causes. The subject is dealt with more fully under the heading MENSTRUATION.

DYSPEPSIA. By dyspepsia is meant indigestion, which includes any sort of pain or discomfort in the working of the digestive system. Dyspepsia is a symptom of the more serious stomach diseases such as ulceration, but it is also present in a great many people for some simple reason, usually a fault in their diet or mode of life, overtiredness, etc. Some people are constitutionally dyspeptic, and though the condition may do them no harm it may lead them to worry about their health more than is good for them. The subject of dyspepsia is dealt with in the article on INDIGESTION.

DYSPHAGIA. The word dysphagia comes to us from two Greek words and means difficulty in swallowing, and it is the term used whenever the act of swallowing cannot be carried out without difficulty. Dysphagia may be painful if it is caused by tonsilitis or any other throat complaint, but painless dysphagia is often experienced by people who are suffering from paralysis. Hysterical people may complain of difficulty in swallowing, but with them the condition does not usually last very long. (*See also* HYSTERIA.)

DYSPNEA. Dyspnea means shortness of breath and is an important symptom in certain diseases. (*See also* BREATHLESSNESS.)

EAR. The ear is one of the special sense organs of the body. It enables us to hear; it is also concerned with the sense of balance. It is usual to consider the anatomy of the ear under three divisions: the *external ear,* the *middle ear,* the *internal ear.* The part of the external ear which stands out from the head and acts as a collector and receiver of air waves is called the *auricle.* It is so shaped that it can bring the sound waves to the passage, or *external meatus,* which leads from the outside to the middle ear. At the far end of this passage is the eardrum, which is set in motion when sound waves strike it. It vibrates, and by its vibrations the waves are conveyed across the tiny space behind the drum, called the middle ear, to the internal ear. It used to be thought that the sound vibrations were conveyed across the middle ear by the three little bones, or ossicles, called the hammer, anvil, and stirrup. It is now considered more probable, however, that these ossicles have a damping effect upon violent sound vibrations and thus serve as a protection to the inner ear from too violent noise.

The eardrum has a much less important part in hearing than used to be imagined. A person can hear quite well with a perforation or hole in the eardrum so long as there is no suppuration; it does not damage the hearing to have an opening made in the eardrum to let out pus.

The most important part of the organ of hearing is the internal ear. The third ossicle, the *stapes* or stirrup, has its base attached to a membrane which closes the oval window of the middle ear and movements of the stapes are by this means communicated to a fluid called *perilymph,* which lies within the bony channels of the inner ear. The sound vibrations probably reach the perilymph through the membrane of another little window—the round window—into the inner ear. These movements are in turn communicated to another fluid, the *endolymph,* which is found inside the small membranous canal which lies within the long channels of the inner ear. Movements of this fluid stimulate the delicate nerve endings in the spiral, shell-like *cochlea.* The cochlea is the essential organ of hearing. It sends the vibrations on to the hearing center in the brain, where they are received and interpreted by the understanding. It will be seen from this description that the whole of the ear, or organ of hearing, is a very delicate and complicated piece of mechanism.

The Semicircular Canals. The organ of balance consists of three little canals, called the semicircular canals. They are situated deep in the temporal bone, in communication with the internal ear. These canals lie in three different planes of the body, and movements of the fluid endolymph in them, caused by alterations in the position of the head, stimulate delicate nerve endings, which help the brain to maintain the balance of the body. Diseases which affect the semicircular canals, such as Ménière's disease (q.v.), upset the balance.

Diseases of the Ear. *Wax* (cerumen) in the outer passage of the ear (external meatus) usually causes deafness as well as discomfort; it is removed by syringing with bicarbonate of soda in warm water.

A *boil* (furuncle) in the outer passage may be extremely painful, but is not serious; it is sometimes difficult, even for a doctor, to distinguish between the inflammation caused by a boil and that caused by mastoid disease; but, for one thing, the person who has a boil is not very ill, though in pain, and is usually not deaf. A boil is treated by having a gauze wick, soaked in a 10% solution of glycerine and ichthammol, pushed past it into the ear passage; penicillin is also given by injection.

Acute inflammation of the middle ear is always an extension of inflammation in the nose or throat up the little tube that communicates with the throat (the eustachian tube); it is often aggravated by that dangerous procedure, sniffing a nasal douche up the nose. The best treatment of acute inflammation of the ear is penicillin by injection or terramycin by mouth, in adequate doses. It may be necessary to have the eardrum slit with fine scalpel by a doctor; this lets out the inflammation before it bursts through the drum.

Chronic suppuration of the ear may go on for weeks, months, or years, and is a common cause of incurable deafness; it usually follows scarlet fever or measles in childhood. The most popular treatment is to drop in peroxide of hydrogen, but it

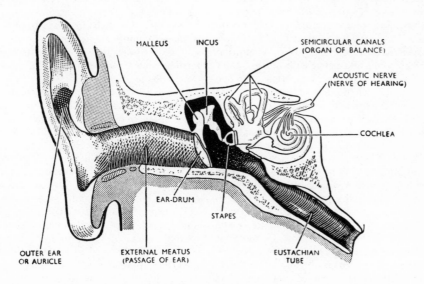

MALLEUS   INCUS   SEMICIRCULAR CANALS (ORGAN OF BALANCE)

ACOUSTIC NERVE (NERVE OF HEARING)

COCHLEA

EAR-DRUM

STAPES

OUTER EAR OR AURICLE   EXTERNAL MEATUS (PASSAGE OF EAR)   EUSTACHIAN TUBE

The Ear.

is probably better to mop out the discharge thoroughly with cotton-wool and then blow in boracic powder or 1 per cent iodine in boracic powder, though some doctors prefer an antibiotic powder. Ionization (q.v.) is another useful method of treatment.

An ear should not be allowed to discharge for more than a month without the patient's considering the advisability of having an operation to stop the discharge. Sometimes this entails merely the removal of adenoids, sometimes a modified radical mastoid operation; but either of these is better than long-continued ear discharge, which may in time even give rise to a brain abscess, and, even when it does not, is a constant worry and a cause of persistent ill health. Inflammation of the ear may lead to inflammation of the mastoid. This is a group of air cells in the bone behind the ear, which protect the delicate internal ear; these air cells communicate with the middle ear and any inflammation can easily pass on to them. Fortunately, nowadays inflammation of the ear is treated by injections of penicillin in adequate dosage, and usually settles down. The inflammation thus seldom reaches the mastoid cells, and the mastoid operation is much less often done than it used to be.

When necessary, the modern simple mastoid drainage operation, if performed early, before the inflammation of the mastoid has caused any complications, gives excellent results, and there is usually little or no pain. (*See also* DEAFNESS.)

EARACHE. Earache is a condition which should be treated with much greater care than it often is. How often does one hear that a child "has only earache"—as if earache were a thing of no importance! Far from being unimportant, earache is one of the aches of which there is almost always a cause that calls for investigation.

Many things can cause earache. In a small child it may really be the pain from teething that is worrying him, or the child may have pushed some small body such as a bead into the ear. The most serious condition is that in which the pain occurs around and behind the ear, in the part called the mastoid. This part may become infected after influenza or any of the infectious diseases, but the doctor nowadays controls it by penicillin. An infected nose

or throat, enlarged tonsils and adenoids— all may cause ear trouble of the sort that can later on lead to deafness.

Treatment. The cause of the earache must be found and treated by a doctor; but, before that can be done, the pain can be eased by lying down with a hot-water bottle, or a hot bag of salt or sand pressed to the ear, or a few drops of warm glycerine dropped in, while some simple pain-deadening tablet such as aspirin may be taken. It may be necessary for the doctor to give penicillin or one of the other antibiotics, or to incise the eardrum in order to let out pus, a small operation without ill effects.

EATING. Eating is one of the things in life that none of us can avoid. It will be evident, therefore, that like everything else which is worth doing it is worth doing well; and in order to eat wisely, care and thought must be given to the subject. Each generation in every part of the world has the experience of previous generations to guide it in its choice of food, and it is quite likely that in the end what we are accustomed to is what is best for us.

When to eat. Nature provides us with an indication of when to eat, in the form of the peculiar sensation known as hunger. The stomach, like other parts of our bodies, must not be our master, but should be trained into good habits from an early age. That the stomach can be so trained is well seen in babyhood, when the baby is trained to nurse at regular intervals, and soon ceases to want food outside its regular feeding times. An untrained baby, however, will cry for food almost every hour, and then it will take only sufficient to last another hour or so, and will again demand more. Men and women who work about the house are sometimes inclined to that themselves like these badly brought up babies and take food in the form of snacks at varying intervals throughout the day. They always pay for it in the end with digestive troubles. People who go about the business of the day at regular hours find that their stomachs adapt themselves to their hours of work, so that they just begin to feel the need for food as the next mealtime approaches.

It is found that the time of eating the heaviest meal of the day varies for people leading different sorts of lives. A rest after a heavy meal is necessary. For people engaged in heavy physical or manual labor, the heavy meal of the day comes best between midday and one o'clock, followed by the half-hour's lounge and smoke before the afternoon shift. Teachers, clerks, and other people who have to use their brains rather than their bodies during the larger part of the day find that a heavy midday meal makes them drowsy and unfit for mental effort during the afternoon, so for them the heavy meal comes best in the early evening, and a light lunch of fruit, salad, or sandwiches is all that is required during the day. Children must not eat heavily for some hours before going to bed, so midday is always, their best dinner-time. The housewife will have to choose whether she has her main meal with the children or with her husband, if he has his in the evening. Too many women, however, fall into the bad habit of having dinner with both the children and the grownups, and so grossly over-eat; or else they merely pick at their food and never eat a proper meal.

How to eat. When the appetite is ready and the well-cooked meal is on the table, it is still necessary to perform the rite of eating properly. Peace, quiet and pleasure are still as necessary for good digestion as they were in the days when Solomon said: "Better is a dinner of herbs where love is, than a stalled ox and hatred therewith." A teacher, shopkeeper or other person who has had to spend the day surrounded by people may digest his food much better if he reads a newspaper or book during his meal; while for others the cheerful domestic chatter of family or friends may be the best things. Nevertheless, the time of eating should be set aside for eating and the mind must be emptied for the time being of worries if the best result is to be obtained from the food set before us. It goes without saying that food must not be hastily bolted, but should be properly chewed. Neither should solid food be washed down with great draughts of liquid. Drink may be taken in any quantity before a meal or at the end of the meal, but if a beverage is taken with food it should be in mere sips between mouthfuls. Smoking should not be indulged in before meals or during

them. A good appetite is a very valuable possession, and it is foolish to take the edge off it and so ruin it.

EAU DE COLOGNE. Eau de Cologne, from the French, meaning "water of Cologne," is a toilet preparation or perfume containing oil of rosemary and other flower oils. It has always been popular in the sickroom because of the fresh daintiness of its smell, which has none of the heavy sickly odor of other scents. Perhaps the only rival it has in this respect is lavender water.

ECCHYMOSIS. This term is used to describe bleeding which takes place just under the skin and is often the result of a bruise. The skin usually has a purplish appearance, gradually changing to green and yellow. (*See also* BLEEDING.)

ECLAMPSIA. This is one of the serious complications of pregnancy, and is characterized by severe fits. It does not come on in the early months of pregnancy, and symptoms of it should be watched for after the fifth month; but it is not unusual for the first fit to occur actually during labor. The exact cause of eclampsia is not known, but it seems to have something to do with disordered chemistry of the body, with the result that a poison is allowed to circulate in the mother's blood instead of being got rid of in the ordinary ways by which the body rids itself of waste products.

The earliest sign of eclampsia is the appearance of albumen in the urine, so it is necessary to keep watch on the way the kidneys are working during pregnancy. This is done by examining the urine periodically.

Warning Symptoms. There are several symptoms which give warning that eclampsia may occur, and if these are recognized in time the condition may be prevented from progressing to the stage of fits. The chief of these warning signs are persistent headache and disorders of the eyesight, such as blurred vision, flashes of light before the eyes, and perhaps even blindness; or there may be a greater degree than usual of stomach upset and a lessening in the quantity of urine passed.

A typical fit. In a typical fit the muscles of the face begin to twitch. In a short time the body becomes stiff and remains rigid. The teeth are tightly clenched and the back is arched. The patient becomes blue from the inability to breathe caused by spasm of the muscles used for breathing. This spasm of stiffness may last as long as a minute, when the muscles begin to contract and relax alternately and continue to do so for some minutes, after which the patient lapses into a coma, and may remain unconscious for a few hours or even a few days. These fits recur again and again at intervals of a few hours, or they may follow in quick succession.

Treatment. Eclamptic fits are always a serious matter, and are especially dangerous if they begin in the last three months before the child is born. If the condition is discovered before the fits begin the latter may be warded off, but once a fit has occurred the only thing that can be done is to protect the patient as much as possible from harm and treat the fit. Send at once for the doctor, meanwhile endeavoring to keep the patient from hurting herself in her convulsions. Lay her on the floor, and place something, such as a spoon or piece of wood, between her teeth if they can be unclenched sufficiently. Turn her sideways so that the saliva will ooze away. When the unconscious stage arrives she may be put to bed.

The doctor in attendance will administer certain drugs and will direct his treatment towards driving the poisons out of the system, but in most cases it is necessary to hurry the birth of the child in order to save the mother. (*See also* CHILDBIRTH.)

ECTHYMA. This disease is a severe form of impetigo, in which the germ responsible for the disease makes its way into the skin and flourishes there. Echthyma is most common upon the legs, between the knee and the ankle, and always indicates that the affected person is seriously run down in health. It usually attacks neglected, ill-fed children, but is also seen in adults whose living is poor, who are unclean and below par generally. Lice and bedbugs are frequent accompaniments of the disease, and probably help in spreading it. The appearance on the legs is of small ulcers, which have a characteristic "scooped out" appearance when the scab which usually covers them is removed. Each ulcer is surrounded by an inflamed,

reddish ring of skin, and leaves a scar when healing takes place.

Treatment. This is in itself very simple. Any mild antiseptic ointment serves as a dressing for the ulcer; and under clean conditions, where the patient has plenty of vegetables, fruit and milk, and an iron tonic, he rapidly recovers. (*See also* IMPETIGO.)

ECTOPIC GESTATION. It sometimes happens that after pregnancy has taken place the fertilized ovum, instead of developing normally in the womb, begins to develop in one of the organs outside the womb. This is known as ectopic gestation. The ovum may be arrested in the Fallopian tube and begin to grow in this small cavity; such a condition is very serious indeed.

The cause of the arrest of the passage of the fertilized ovum may be some obstruction in the Fallopian tube due to adhesions or possibly due to some former inflammation. As a rule abortion takes place between the sixth and twelfth weeks of pregnancy and there may be serious internal hemorrage.

Generally there is a history of one menstrual period being missed, followed by severe attacks of abdominal pains and later a continuous flow of blood from the vagina.

It is important that the doctor should be consulted at once, as an operation may be necessary in order to save the woman's life. The condition is a very serious one and always requires surgical treatment.

ECTROPION. Ectropion is a condition in which the eyelids turn outwards. It is a fairly common condition, and is due to a number of causes.

The mildest and simplest variety is that frequently occurring in elderly people whose tissues are lax, so that the lower eyelid hangs down. It always occurs in both eyes, and the lower lids only are affected. As a result, the tears begin to drain away down the check. The skin becomes irritated, red and raw, and then contracts, so that the condition of ectropion is made worse than ever. This copious watering of the eye is generally the most troublesome symptom in this eye condition of old age, and may result in the complete turning out of the whole of the lower lid.

When the lining of the eyelid is swollen

for any reason the lid margins are mechanically pushed out; this form may occur in both lids. Again, the tears tend to flow over the cheek, and the other results usually follow as in ectropion due to lax tissues.

Treatment. Both these forms are successfully treated by slight operation; but when the conjunctiva is thickened, treatment aims at reducing its bulk, and astringent or contracting drugs such as zinc chloride or silver nitrate are employed in the form of drops.

A similar form of ectropion occurs when the facial nerve is paralyzed. When this occurs the muscle which opens and shuts the eye is quite lax, so that the lower lid hangs down. In cases where the paralysis is likely to be cured, the lid may be temporarily supported by strapping, covered with a pad and bandage; but if the paralysis is likely to be permanent an operation is the only hope of curing this form of ectropion. (*See also* ENTROPION; EYE; EYELID.)

ECZEMA. This very familiar word is derived from a Greek word meaning to boil over, burst out, or erupt. Any skin disease may be called an "eruption" or "eczema," using the word in its widest sense, but it really does not mean any one definite type of skin disease; in fact, calling any skin rash "eczema" is much the same as calling any pain of unknown origin "rheumatism."

The more recent practice is to discard the term "eczema" for the term "dermatitis," which means inflammation of the skin. (*See also* DERMATITIS.)

EDEMA or DROPSY. This is the name given to an unusually watery state of the tissue of the body. In every healthy person there is a leakage of the watery part of the blood into the flesh, but when dropsy occurs, this normal state is very much exaggerated. The fluid in the tissues is controlled by a complicated system of tiny vessels known as the lymphatics, and if obstruction takes place in any of these vessels it is obvious that swelling is bound to appear. Another cause of swelling is too great a flow of fluid out of the blood-vessels, in which case the lymphatics are not able to pass it along quickly enough, and dropsy takes place.

Edema a Symptom, not a Disease. There are very many causes of the state of edema in the body, and it is not a disease in itself, as many people seem to think, but merely a sign that something is wrong in the body somewhere. There are also various forms of this condition, which may range from a small swelling caused by a bee sting, to the great swellings which cover the whole of the body; but both states are true dropsies, the only difference being the quantity of swelling. In the case of a bee sting, the poison causes the blood vessels to open more widely than usual, and a greater amount of fluid is poured out into the skin, thus causing a swelling (or edema) to appear over the place stung.

In very hot weather it is not unusual, in health, for the feet to swell up; this is caused by an extra flow of fluid from the blood vessels which the lymphatic glands are not able to carry away at once.

Dropsies of Heart and Kidney Disease. In certain diseases of the heart, dropsy occurs all over the body. There are several explanations for this excessive watery state of the body, but there is no doubt that slowing of the blood-flow owing to the inability of the weakened heart to do its usual pumping, may cause this excessive swelling to take place. It is no unusual thing for a person to become intensely dropsical owing to heart disease, and when the heart condition is restored to normal, the swellings may soon disappear.

The dropsy caused by disease of the kidneys is not so severe as that caused by heart disease, and it seems to appear in certain parts of the body instead of all over. The legs very often become swollen, and the face, especially the eyelids, is largely affected.

Treatment. The same treatment will obviously not apply to all cases of edema. The cause of the condition will have to be taken into consideration, but the edema itself may be so distressing as to require special treatment apart from the disease which is causing it. For the slighter degrees of dropsy no special treatment need be given beyond treating the cause of the condition. Once the cause is removed, the dropsy will naturally disappear.

When the dropsy is due to heart disease,

complete rest in bed is absolutely necessary, and such drugs as digitalis or Salyrgan, which tend to increase the flow of urine, are usually given. No salt should be allowed on the table or in cooking as this accumulates in the tissue fluid. The total daily intake of fluids is usually restricted to two pints.

The treatment of the dropsy caused by disease of the kidneys is usually the same as the disease. (*See also* NEPHRITIS.) Some of the excess fluid may be taken off by the operation of tapping, and this may require to be done repeatedly. It is often inadvisable to give drugs which increase the flow of urine when the kidneys are diseased, as this may set up irritation.

The general treatment of edema depends on the cause, and a doctor should be consulted without delay in order that the cause may be discovered.

EFFERENT. This is a term used to describe motion away from a center, such as the course of a blood vessel leading away from an organ or that of a nerve proceeding from a motor center in the brain to the limb it moves.

EFFERVESCENCE. The brisk bubbling caused by the escape of carbon dioxide into a liquid is called effervescence. When effervescent drinks are drunk they have a sharp tingling effect on the back of the throat which is very refreshing. For this reason soda water, which is the simplest form of effervescent drink, appears cooler and more refreshing than ordinary still water. Various flavors, such as lemon, are added to make cool summer drinks. When an effervescent drink reaches the stomach it increases the flow of gastric juices.

An effervescent mixture can be made up of powdered bicarbonate of soda mixed with citric acid or tartaric acid. The two powders can be added separately, as in Seidlitz powders, or they can be contained in the same mixture, as with fruit salts. The well-known sherbert is composed of citric acid and carbonate of soda in a powder which effervesces when it mixes with the saliva in the mouth.

EFFLEURAGE. This is the name given to the "stroking" movement used in massage. It is described under the heading MASSAGE.

EFFORT SYNDROME. This condition,

also called Da Costa's syndrome, is characterized by breathlessness, palpitation, fatigue, giddiness, and pain in the left side of the chest. These symptoms limit the person's capacity for effort, and the condition was formerly thought to be a disease of the heart. It has, however, been proved to be due to an emotional upset, and is one of the many forms in which anxiety appears in the disguise of organic disease.

EFFUSION. The word effusion (which means a pouring out) is used in medicine in connection with the pouring out of fluid from the normal stream into some other part of the body. One of the most common types of effusion is that which occurs in "housemaid's knee" (q.v.), in which there is usually a large swelling which is filled with fluid. The same condition occurs in "miner's elbow." Treatment of effusions will naturally depend on which part of the body they appear in, and their type. (*See also* ASCITES; BURSITIS; EDEMA; PLEURISY.)

EGG. When we realize that a young chick lives on the contents of an egg until it is hatched out, it is reasonable to suppose that an egg must contain the necessary type of food for bodybuilding. But the young chicken lying in its shell does not require any energy-making food, and, as nature is never wasteful in her methods, we find that eggs lack carbohydrates. Carbohydrates are energy-makers and not bodybuilders; but since other essential ingredients of human diet are present, such as fat, protein, and some very valuable mineral salts, eggs from one of our most important and adaptable articles of food.

Because eggs are easily digested they form a particularly valuable food for children, especially those suffering from rickets.

ELBOW. The elbow is the hinge joint formed by the bones of the upper and lower arms, that is to say by the *humerus* (the single bone in the upper arm) and the *ulna* and *radium* (the bones of the forearm). The ulna is on the inner side of the arm and the radius on the outer side when the palm of the hand is uppermost. The ends of the three bones of the arm are covered with smooth cartilage or gristle, and the upper ends of the radius and ulna together form a cup-shaped socket into which the rounded end of the humerus fits snugly. The cartilage and lubricating fluid in the joint enable it to turn easily in the socket. The sharp point which is felt at the tip of the elbow when the arm is bent is the projecting end of the ulna, known as the *olecranon process.*

Injuries of the Elbow. The elbow is a part of the body which is in almost constant use, and is therefore very liable to be accidentally hurt. A fall on the hand may dislocate the elbow. A common fracture of the arm is that of the humerus just above the elbow joint. In young children the ends of the bones, called the epiphyses, have not yet become joined in the same solid piece as the rest of the bone and are therefore very easily knocked off the main bone. The olecranon process, which is the most exposed part of the elbow, is easily broken across, but probably the most crippling accidents to the arm are the numerous forms of muscular injuries to which it is subject. These range in severity from simple strains to the tearing of the muscle from the bone to which it is attached, a condition which may be difficult to cure.

Almost every form of sport in which the arm is used has its own special form of injury, such as *tennis elbow* (q.v.) These terms are loosely applied to several varieties of arm injury which are apt to occur when playing games. The little bursae, or bags of fluid which act as pads or shock-absorbers to the joints, are a very frequent seat of trouble in the arm and elbow. The most usual form of tennis elbow is due to chronic irritation of the bursa just above the elbow. (*See also* BURSITIS; EFFUSION; MINER'S ELBOW.)

Treatment of elbow injuries. A stiff elbow is a frequent result of injuries of the arm and, as well as being very inconvenient to its owner, is also a danger to him if his work takes him among machinery, so above all things treatment should be directed towards restoring or preserving the movement of the arm. Massage, remedial exercises and electricity are all of use in these injuries. Since the elbow is concerned with turning the hand, lifting, and raising and lowering the forearm, these movements may be seriously impaired by what may appear a trifling injury. If the damage is allowed to become chronic a long spell of

treatment may be required to restore the joint to health, so that it is wise to attend to a slight injury when it appears, even if it means giving up tennis or any other activity for the time being. So-called "playing-in" a sore arm or "working-off" a muscle strain may make matters worse if real injury is present.

The elbow joint is subject to all the diseases that attack other joints, of which the commonest is arthritis. The arthritis may be simply inflammation of the joint due to infection or injury, or may be due to tuberculosis. It is important that this should be treated as soon as it appears, lest serious crippling result from letting the disease get a firm hold. (*See also* ARTHRITIS.)

ELECTRIC SHOCK. When a current of electricity of shock-producing strength flows through the body it produces electric shock. The electricity must necessarily enter the body at one point and leave it at another. If there is no point of departure no current can flow. For this reason it may be safe to touch or grasp something electrically charged, or through which a current is passing, if the rest of the body is separated by some insulating, non-conducting material, from the ground or from anything by which the current can complete its circuit.

Strong electric currents damage the body in two ways—by burning and by shock. Death from lightning is believed to be due to sudden violent heating of the body tissues by the current, and electric burns on the hands are a danger familiar to those who have to handle "live" electric cables. Electric shock, however, is not a burn but a temporary paralysis of certain nerve cells, especially of the breathing center at the base of the brain, by the passage of a current not of a kind to cause death.

As water is a good conductor, care is needed when it is present, for insulators may be ineffective.

The chief feature of electric shock is, therefore, absence of breathing and, after first having cut off the current and got the patient away from the source of it, the one essential treatment is effective artificial respiration. Electric shock, perhaps even more than apparent death from drowning, demands persistence in artificial respiration until either the patient revives or it is quite certain that life is extinct. Many lives have been saved by continuing what seemed a hopeless task. Mouth to mouth breathing is specially suitable. (*See* ARTIFICIAL RESPIRATION.)

ELECTRICITY IN MEDICINE. It is frequently said today that we live in an electric age. We light our houses, clean them, cook our food, and move from place to place by means of electricity. It is not surprising, therefore, that in recent years the use of electricity in medical treatment has made great strides. The changes that different sorts of electric currents can bring about in the human tissues are now well understood, and it is recognized that a large number of human ailments can be prevented, cured, and relieved by suitable and timely electric treatment.

The effects of electricity upon the body are various, but they may be divided into physiological, chemical, physical, and mental effects. Sometimes they are a combination of all of these.

A simple example of a purely physiological change is the destruction of the cells of cancer by exposure to X-rays. Medical ionization, by which is meant the introduction of drugs into the body by means of an electric current, illustrates its chemical effect, while the heating of the tissues by diathermy is purely physical.

Varieties of Electricity. Electricity is either *static* or *dynamic*. *Static electricity,* as its name implies, does not flow in a current. It is given for nervous disorders where there is no organic disease, such as hysteria, insomnia, or nervous headache. In the form called the Morton Wave, it produces massage of the muscles, and can be used in diseases of the prostate to empty the crypts of the gland.

Dynamic electricity may be described as electricity flowing in a current along suitable conductors. The sources of such electricity are the electric mains, generators, or batteries of cells. The mains current may be direct or alternating—that is to say, the direction of the flow may be constant or it may be reversed periodically. Generally speaking, the direct current is more suitable for medical purposes.

The current amperage may be small and working at a high pressure (voltage), or it may be large and working at a low pressure.

How the Currents Are Applied. In order to treat a patient by means of electric currents passing through the body it is obvious that the patient must be brought into contact, in some safe manner, with the wires carrying the current, since electricity is dangerous when unskillfully or ignorantly applied. To provide this safe contact, appliances called "electrodes" are used, which are placed on the part of the patient's body which is to be treated. They must be made of some conducting material —that is, a material which allows electricity to pass along it. Since conductors which can be easily bent to the shape required are the most suitable, sheets of lead or wire gauze are the usual materials employed.

Pain and even burning will result from concentrating the current over too small an area of skin. Electrodes should, therefore, be as large as possible. For stimulating individual muscles and nerves special small round electrodes are used.

Electrodes are covered with several layers of lint soaked in warm saline solution, which is a good conductor of electricty. Except when a very short application is intended, care should be taken that the electrode comes *evenly* into contact with the skin; otherwise the current will concentrate at the points of good contact and burning may result. For this reason any cuts in the skin must be closed with collodion before treatment.

Another method of connecting the patient to the current is to immerse his limbs or whole body in baths of water containing electrodes. These baths distribute the current evenly and are therefore very convenient for applying current over a large area. It is important to note that, owing to the large element of danger involved when this method is practiced by inexperienced persons, particularly when the apparatus is connected with the mains, this form of treatment should *never* be employed save by a trained medical expert and with a properly designed apparatus, kept in correct working order. This warning applies, in fact, to *all* methods of applying electricity medically. They should never be employed except under trained medical supervision.

For the treatment of the hands or feet,

any vessel of a suitable size and shape, and made of a nonconducting material, may be used.

Types of Current. *Galvanism* is the name given to current that is direct, or flows constantly in one direction, when used medically.

The *faradic* current is an alternating current of small amperage but high pressure (voltage). It is derived from a faradic coil.

The *sinusoidal* current is derived from a special motor-generator or coil. It is an alternating current of very low periodicity —not more than 20 periods per second. The alternations are rhythmical and gradual, not abrupt, as in the ordinary current from the mains.

The *high frequency* current is a complicated one, in which the alternations are so rapid as to be more appropriately termed oscillations. The rapidity of alternation does not stimulate sensory or motor nerve-endings, and consequently neither pain nor muscular contractions are produced.

Diathermy is another form of high-frequency oscillating current, of which the pressure is comparatively low (about 2,000 volts) and the amperage high (2–3 amperes). The uses and methods of application of these types of current are discussed separately below.

Galvanism. This form of electric treatment is often of benefit in joint disorders, such as the following:

Arthritis.—Galvanism of the part in gouty or rheumatic arthritis may relieve pain and sometimes overcomes the inflammation.

Neuritis.—In cases where the condition is comparatively recent, mild galvanism is very beneficial, particularly in sciatica and neuritis of the arm, and sometimes in shingles. The positive electrode is placed centrally, so that the current flows outwards along the nerve. Long sittings are generally needed in these cases.

Stimulation of Muscles.—Interrupted galvanism is very valuable in maintaining the nutrition of muscles whose motor nerve has been damaged.

Faradism. Injured nerves or muscles are treated by faradism, and it is in this connexion that the electric current is so useful an aid to diagnosis. The injured muscle will respond to galvanism, but not to faradism. Therefore, if the response to a faradic current is normal it proves that the motor nerve of the muscle is unbroken and undamaged. If, however, the response is abnormal, then it is known that the nerve is injured. This is known as the "reaction of degeneration." The reaction of degeneration will show by the form it takes what the extent of the injury to the nerve is. If the nerve has been rendered entirely useless there will be no response at all to faradism and only a feeble response to galvanism. Lesser injuries will produce a feeble response to both currents.

Faradism has been found helpful in the cure of many different conditions. The chief of these is perhaps where there is a degree of paralysis. Here the faradic current is invaluable for maintaining the nutrition of muscles which have to remain inactive because the nerve which controls them is impaired. If nothing were done for them and they had to remain inactive for a considerable time they would grow feeble and flabby. Let us take the case of paralysis of the forearm and hand due to an accident in which the motor nerve of the upper arm has been injured. Daily applications of faradic electricity are given at the motor points of the muscles of the forearm and hand, with the result that these muscles are prevented from degenerating while the real damage in the upper arm is being repaired by rest and other treatment.

In cases of paralysis of the muscles of the vocal cords which is not due to any definite disease, but to some such condition as overuse or nervous fatigue, "aphonia" or loss of the power of speech may have resulted. A strong, unexpected faradic shock will usually bring about a cure.

In cases, too, of muscular atrophy, faradism can sometimes be very useful. If, for example, a limb has been fractured and for this and other reasons the muscles have become atrophied through disuse, stimulation by faradic current will be of the greatest benefit. Faradism is also frequently useful in the treatment of the tiresome condition known as incontinence (q.v.) of urine during the night, or bedwetting. Here electricity may be useful if there is no organic cause of the condition, such as stone in the bladder, inflammation of the urinary tract, worms in the intestine, bad nervous disease, or defect in the bladder itself.

An interesting use of faradic electricity is in educating muscles which have undergone the operation of transplantation to another part of the body to take the place of more important muscles which have been rendered useless.

High Frequency. The high-frequency current is a very useful form in which electricity can be administered for medical treatment, as it obtains its results almost entirely by giving rise to heat in the tissues under the skin. It requires special methods of applying it to the patient. These, like other forms of electricity, may be applied generally all over the body, or locally to one particular part.

The electrodes for high-frequency treatment are mostly made of glass tubes which vary in size and shape according to the purpose for which they are to be used. The one used by hairdressers for high-frequency treatment of the scalp is in the form of a large glass comb with a handle. When the glass tube which forms the electrode is brought into contact, or nearly into contact, with the skin it fills with a violet light.

Simple galvanic and faradic currents give rise to a slight degree of heat in the skin over the tissues through which they pass, but owing to the danger of pain and shock the amount of these currents used must be so limited that the tissues below the skin cannot be heated by them. Owing to the rapidity of its oscillations, however, a much heavier high-frequency current can be used with comfort. The heat generated by such a current during its passage is very considerable and is evenly distributed throughout the tissues through which it passes. High frequency, therefore, seems to be valuable in the treatment of disease largely, though not solely, through its power to produce heat.

Effects of High-frequency Treatment. The most noticeable effect of this treatment is a speeding up in the working of the organs of the body, as shown by an increased elimination of carbon dioxide from the lungs.

When the electrode is kept in contact with the skin only prolonged and heavy currents are felt and the sensation is one of warmth. The sweat glands and mucous glands are stimulated, and the blood vessels of the area under treatment dilate.

A very important use of high frequency is to relieve pain in conditions of inflammation, whether it be long-continued and chronic pain, or a sharp, short attack of the acute variety. The relief obtained is usually immediate, although it may not last long unless a course of treatment is taken. The usual treatment is twenty to thirty minutes three times a week, or a local application of from five to ten minutes may be given daily.

Sinusoidal Currents. Electricity in the special form known as sinusoidal currents is used in a few cases where other forms of electricity would be dangerous, such as certain heart conditions and infantile paralysis.

The important subjects of IONIZATION and DIATHERMY are discussed under their own headings.

ELECTROCARDIOGRAPHY. The electrocardiograph is an instrument for magnifying and recording on photographic strip the electrical changes which occur in the heart muscle each time it beats. The patient is connected to the electrocardiograph by means of metal electrodes which are strapped on the limbs. The very small changes of electrical potential which are produced at each heartbeat cause deflection of a fine fiber of silvered quartz which is stretched between the poles of a powerful electromagnet.

The name given to the photographic record obtained is "electrocardiogram." In health this shows three well-marked deflections with each contraction of the heart. The first deflection coincides with contraction of the auricles and the last two with contraction of the ventricles. Each person has a characteristic electrocardiogram, and it is said that people can be identified by this method as certainly as by taking their fingerprints.

This instrument has taught doctors a great deal about disorders of the heart, and in particular about irregularities of the heart's rhythm. It is sometimes a great help in arriving at a diagnosis. Alterations in the shape of the tracing occur in cases in which the blood supply to the heart is deficient—when, for instance, the coronary arteries are narrowed or when they are completely occluded by clot in coronary thrombosis. Evidence that the heart is affected in diphtheria or acute rheumatism may be obtained from the electrocardiogram when it remains undetectable by other means. The method is also invaluable as a means of investigating cases of congenital malformation of the heart, in order to determine whether they are likely to benefit from operation.

ELECTROENCEPHALOGRAPHY. It has been known for many years that tiny electrical discharges occur in the brains of animals in response to various forms of sensory stimulation, but it was only as recently as 1924 that Berger was able to demonstrate such discharges in man. By applying electrodes to the unshaved scalp, he showed that rhythmic waves with a frequency of about ten a second occurred when the eyes were closed and that they were abolished by any form of mental activity. These waves are found normally in health and their form alters in sleep and under the influence of various drugs. The apparatus devised for recording the pattern of these waves in the brain is known as the electroencephalograph, while the permanent record traced by the apparatus is called an electroencephalogram.

Several patterns of abnormal discharge are found in epilepsy, and their recognition has been of great value to doctors in the diagnosis of obscurer forms of this disorder. Each abnormal pattern has been found to respond best to treatment with a particular drug. Abnormal electroencephalograms have been found in some problem children and many delinquent adults and thus may afford important confirmatory evidence of disordered brain function; they have been so used and accepted in courts of law. By altering the position of the electrodes on the scalp it has been possible to demonstrate a focus of abnormal electrical waves over an underlying brain tumor, and thus guide the surgeon to the site of operation.

ELECTROCOAGULATION. This is another name for surgical diathermy. (*See* DIATHERMY.)

ELECTROLYSIS. Electricity applied to the skin can be made to destroy the little glands at the roots of hairs, and is consequently used by beauty specialists and others to remove superfluous hairs. It is, of course, accompanied by a certain amount of pain, and in unskilled hands may be dangerous and lead to disfigurement. Where there is a heavy crop of "down" on the face, electrolysis of the larger hairs may stimulate the growth of the down and so should be avoided, but for an isolated group of strongly growing hairs it is usually a successful though expensive way of having them removed. Each hair has to be operated on separately.

ELEPHANTIASIS. Elephantiasis is a very suitable name for this most uncomfortable and cruelly deforming disease. It may attack any portion of the body, but it seems to favor the legs, causing them to become huge and ungainly like those of an elephant. This disease is caused by a tiny worm which gets into the blood and then passes on into the lymph vessels. These become blocked and the result is a gradual swelling of whatever part of the body is affected. The disease is most frequently seen in tropical countries, and it never seems to develop in cold climates.

Symptoms. The skin at first is smooth, but afterwards it becomes rough, coarse, and thick and is thrown up in folds just like the skin on the leg of an elephant. Attacks of fever occur at intervals, and although there is no pain there is a good deal of inflammation and swelling. The legs, arms, scrotum, and breasts are the parts which seem to be affected more than other parts of the body. The scrotum (the bag containing the testicles) may become an immense size, reaching almost to the ground.

Treatment. Surgical treatment is usually carried out, and often this means amputation of one or more limbs. An elastic stocking should be worn and the leg should be raised up and rested as much as possible. This may help to delay the course of the disease, especially if injections of tartar emetic are given.

ELIXIR. Elixir is the name given to any sweetened and aromatic spiritous preparation which contains a small quantity of an active drug. Cascara sagrada, rhubarb, and senna are elixirs in common use.

EMACIATION. Emaciation means extreme wasting of the body. This may occur from excessive loss of fluid, in which case the wasting may take place very rapidly; slow emaciation is usually due to the body not getting proper nourishment, either through actual starvation from want of food, or because the body is using its nourishment in the wrong way.

In rapid wasting due to loss of fluid, which is a condition most commonly seen in cases of severe diarrhea or vomiting, the skin becomes shrivelled and dry and the eyes become sunken, with dark rings around them. The face usually has an anxious and pinched expression and the body is blue and cold. The patient may sink into a state of dullness, or even coma. Diseases which cause rapid wasting of the body are cholera, dysentery, and summer or infantile diarrhea.

The signs of slow emaciation are shown by a gradual loss of fat and wasting away of the muscles. The skin of the body, instead of hanging in folds as it does in the rapid form of emaciation, is drawn tightly over the bones of the body. The face becomes very sunken in appearance and all the bones of the body seem to stick out, especially the ribs. Emaciation from lack of food may be due to the inability to take food owing to some painful condition of the throat, such as cancer or tuberculosis, or to some condition of the stomach caused by an ulcer or new growth. Diseases of the pancreas or liver are often responsible for wasting of the body, because they prevent the digestive organs working properly, thus starving the body of its necessary nourishment.

In some feverish states caused by germs, the poisons which these germs produce prevent the cells of the body from getting their usual nourishment. Extreme wasting from such a cause is seen in tuberculosis. Cancer is another disease which produces a similar effect.

Failure of certain of the internal secretions of the body also causes emaciation. Diabetes is a complicated disease in which there is much wasting of the body brought about by failure of the internal secretion called insulin. Overactivity of the thyroid gland is another cause of emaciation.

Yet another cause is the excessive use of harmful drugs. Any person who is addicted to morphia or cocaine usually develops a haggard expression, and the body as a rule becomes thin and emaciated.

In some cases mental worries, overwork, overexcitement, or sleeplessness may bring about wasting of the body, and there are also certain nervous diseases in which part of the brain or spinal cord becomes destroyed, which are responsible for emaciation. Thus it will be seen that there are many conditions, mental, physical, and mechanical, which may give rise to emaciation.

EMBOLISM. This is the term used for obstruction of a blood vessel by an embolus —a plug of any sort which is floating in the bloodstream. Most often it is a fragment of blod clot which has broken off from a larger "thrombus" in a vein, but sometimes it may be composed of other matters which are in the bloodsteam, and which have probably broken off from some diseased part of the heart or of a blood-vessel. Air which has found its way into a vein may act in the same way as an embolus, and in countries where various sorts of worms find their way into the body, and especially into the blood, they too may form a block in the circulation. Sometimes a very tiny particle of tissue from a diseased part may be infected with germs which increase in number to such an extent that they are able to dam the bloodstream. Whatever the cause of the embolism the consequences are the same. It floats in the bloodstream until it becomes arrested in a blood vessel which is too narrow to allow it to pass. The usual site of this arrest is in the arteries of the lung, but it may, of course, happen anywhere.

The two circumstances in which embolism is most likely to occur are after childbirth and after periods of enforced confinement to bed, especially following a surgical operation. After childbirth the blood in the veins of the legs is very liable to clot and form an embolus. There is no way in which this trouble can be forseen. Fortunately, in the great majority of confinements it does not occur.

The prevention of this disaster consists in the early recognition of thrombosis in the leg veins. It is usually heralded by a little pain in the calf and swelling of the foot. It is usual nowadays in such an event to give anticoagulant drugs such as heparin and dicoumarol to prevent extension of the clot. In cases where there is evidence of spread of clotting in spite of this treatment many surgeons tie off the vein nearer the heart, so as to prevent emboli from reaching the circulation. The affected limb is always kept strictly at rest. It has been found that early encouragement to exercise the legs in bed has been followed by a fall in the incidence of clotted veins.

Surgical treatment (*embolectomy*) has been carried out successfully in a number of cases of embolism, the blocked blood vessel being exposed and the obstructing embolus removed under local anesthesia.

Fat embolism may occur through fat escaping from the marrow of a long bone after fracture and getting into the blood circulation. It is then carried to a vital part of the body, such as the brain, and causes a block there.

EMBROCATION. This is the name given to medicated substances suitable for rubbing into the skin. They usually contain oil of some sort and some alcohol as well. They are now more commonly known as liniments. (*See also* LINIMENT.)

EMBRYO. By embryo we mean the fetus in the womb up to about six weeks or two months after fertilization of the female element (ovum) by the male element (spermatozoon) has taken place.

After fertilization takes place the ovum grows rapidly in the womb, until at the end of the first month it is about ¼ in. long. At the end of the second month it is over 1 in. long and the beginnings of the human shape can be seen, although it still has a trace of a tail. The eyes, ears, and nose are forming and the limbs have begun to sprout. The head is particularly large for the size of the body and the brain is beginning to develop. Shortly after this the characteristics become recognizable and the embryo is thenceforth called the fetus (q.v.) (*See also* PREGNANCY.)

EMETIC. An emetic is given in order to cause vomiting, and this is one of the ways in which the stomach can be rapidly emptied. Emetics have been in use for many centuries, and at one time they were one of the chief forms of treatment for almost any disease. Nowadays, however, emetics are chiefly used for cases of poisoning and the best ones are those which are in everyday use in the home, as quickness of action may mean the saving of a life. A tablespoonful of mustard stirred into half a glass of hot water will produce immediate and thorough results. Two tablespoonfuls of common salt in warm water will act in the same way. If it is available, one of the best emetics is ipecacuanha wine. It is particularly safe for children, and it should

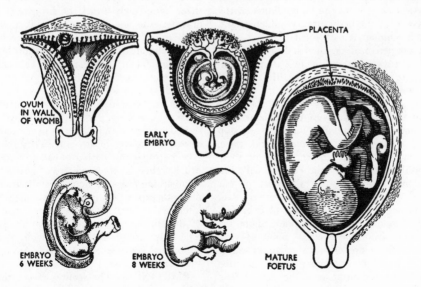

The Embryo.

be given in repeated doses of one teaspoonful until vomiting begins.

The rapid, if uncertain, method of producing vomiting by thrusting the fingers down the back of the throat must not be left out. In urgent cases this should be tried while an emetic is being prepared.

Apomorphine is an emetic which is given by injection and which produces excellent results; vomiting usually takes place within five minutes of injection, but its action generally causes nausea and prostration.

EMETINE. This is a drug which is derived from ipecacuanha and is greatly used in the treatment of amebic dysentery. It should not be taken except under medical care, as prolonged use leads to poisoning.

EMOLLIENT. Any substance which soothes, softens or protects the skin is called an emollient. Ordinary cold cream, lanolin, petroleum jelly, or olive oil are a few of the more simple forms of emollient. (*See also* COLD CREAM.)

EMOTION. By emotion we mean a feeling which moves us strongly. The chief emotions are undoubtedly fear and anger, though in cases where love and jealousy are strong enough to be classed as emotions, they too can be very strong emotive forces. In the medical sense emotions are important because they are accompanied by physical changes in the body. Think of the behavior of the body after a sudden fright. For a moment it may seem that the heart has stopped beating, then it begins to gallop, and we breathe quickly, we may tremble, the stomach may heave, the hairs of the head may rise up on end and we may have an attack of diarrhea. At the same time we do things without realizing that we are doing them. For instance, we stop dead in our tracks, we step back a pace, we may even cower down. None of these conditions is due to our express will, but is done instinctively by the part of our mind called the unconscious mind, over which we have not yet learnt to gain control. The most interesting point about the emotions from the medical point of view is that there are chemical changes taking place in the body when a strong emotion is felt—as, for instance, in the case of fear, when the tissues become flooded with the powerful chemical known as adrenalin. These chemical activities are caused by changes in the working of the ductless or endocrine glands, which are controlled by that part of the nervous system called the sympathetic nervous system. These ductless glands are explained under their own headings.

In order to be a good citizen it is necessary to exercise such control over the emotions that we do not cause any unnecessary worry or discomfort to the people with whom we come into contact. The fiery-tempered man who frequently gives vent to his fury is a bad citizen, because he robs his family and fellow workers of the peace and the ability to go about their business in an undisturbed fashion which are their right. In fact, from a health point of view, a mans' peace of mind is one of his most valuable possessions. (*See also* ADRENALIN; DUCTLESS GLANDS; NERVOUS SYSTEM; SYMPATHETIC NERVOUS SYSTEM.)

EMPHYSEMA. Emphysema is a disorder of breathing in which the chest becomes fixed in the position of "breathing in." There is very little chest expansion, so that the patient becomes breathless on slight exertion.

Common accompaniments of emphysema are asthma and bronchitis. It is a condition which is found in elderly people who have suffered from chest complaints all their lives; each attack of bronchitis aggravates the condition and makes it a little worse. Such people should live in a warm climate, or avoid attacks of bronchitis by taking great care of the chest. On no account should these people go out in cold or wet weather. Fog especially is dangerous because it irritates the airtubes.

People who suffer from emphysema should be very careful not to over-exercise or tire themselves in any way. They should take a regular rest period in the afternoons. Much relief is obtained from instruction in breathing exercises by a specially trained physiotherapist. A tight abdominal corset often assists breathing by promoting recoil of the diaphragm during expiration. It is especially useful in people with flabby abdominal muscles. (*See also* ASTHMA; BRONCHITIS; LUNG.)

EMPTINESS. The feeling of emptiness when we are hungry is a very natural one, but this feeling may occur as a symptom of indigestion, and many women experience it when pregnant.

When the feeling is due to indigestion it may be relieved by taking food in small quantities or some alkaline powder such as bicarbonate of soda; but there are some forms of indigestion in which the relief is immediately followed by a distressing feeling of fullness, even if only a small meal has been taken. Treatment of the condition lies in the proper treatment of the indigestion. (*See also* DUODENUM; INDIGESTION.)

EMPYEMA. This is a condition in which pus forms in the pleural cavity, the space between the chest wall and the lung. It is chiefly a disease of young children, although it may occur at any age. The condition may really be regarded as an abscess, and, as it is almost impossible for the pus to escape through the thick wall of the chest, it is important that the condition should be cleared up as early as possible, usually by surgical means. The condition may follow an attack of pneumonia, or it may be due to tuberculosis of the lungs. Injuries to the chest, such as a gunshot or a knife wound, or any disease in the neighboring organs may spread infection and cause empyema.

Symptoms. If, after an attack of pneumonia, the temperature of the patient does not return to normal, it is usual for the doctor to suspect that empyema is present. There may be no special symptoms at first, but a rise of temperature is a sure indication that infection has spread. Symptoms generally associated with emypema are pain in the affected side, shortness of breath, sweating, and a temperature which varies night and morning. A cough may be present, and very often the patient is irritable.

Treatment. The treatment of empyema is the same as the treatment of any abscess, namely, by opening the abscess and allowing the pus to drain away. To do this, it is necessary for the doctor to find out the exact spot in the chest where the pus is lying, and this is done by inserting a needle through the chest wall into the pleural cavity. It is often possible to cure empyema by aspirating the pus with a syringe and instilling penicillin into the pleural cavity. As soon as the pus is removed by operation

or repeated aspiration with a syringe, the lung usually resumes its normal working order. In some cases the lung may fail to expand; while in other cases, even in spite of operation, the infection may spread. Empyema is a serious condition, and much depends on early and efficient treatment.

EMULSION. Emulsions are thick liquid preparations rather like milk in color and usually consisting of oils, fats, or resins. Milk and yoke of egg are examples of natural emulsions. As a rule, substances such as cod-liver oil are emulsified by the addition of glycerine, which not only helps to conceal any unpleasant taste but makes the substance easier to digest.

ENAMEL. Enamel is the outer covering of the teeth and is the hardest tissue in the body. It is white in color, but when it is thin the yellow dentine underneath may show through. Enamel is very readily eaten away by acids, hence the necessity of cleaning the teeth after taking vinegar, certain medicines, etc. (*See also* TEETH.)

ENCEPHALITIS. This is inflammation of the brain, and it may occur in a very large number of ways. Many of the general fevers, such as scarlet fever, measles, mumps, and influenza, may be complicated by encephalitis, but fortunately this happens only rarely. Much prominence has been given to that form of encephalitis which may occur occasionally after vaccination. Much more common is encephalitis which results from extension of infection from the ear or the air cavities of the nose through the bone into the brain. In these cases, the inflammation is confined to a relatively small area of the brain, pus is produced, and an abcess forms. The danger in this form of encephalitis is that the inflammation will not remain confined to one part of the brain, but may spread to the coverings of the brain—the meninges —and so cause meningitis. While the inflammation remains localized it is possible to operate and remove the pus. But prevention of these abscesses by proper and thorough treatment of all diseases of the nose and ear should be possible if patients suffering from such troubles are seen early enough by the doctor.

Symptoms. The symptoms common to all the above forms of encephalitis are the general symptoms of any severe disturbance of the brain substance: severe headache, irritability, drowsiness, vomiting, convulsions. Later the drowsiness becomes more marked and the patient sinks into a coma from which he cannot be roused. Fever, sometimes accompanied by shivering attacks, is almost always present. Where the encephalitis is a complication of such infectious fevers as measles or scarlet fever, the signs of those diseases will be present, and the inflammation of the brain being a general one, without any pus being formed, no operation will be of any benefit to the patient.

Where the inflammation has extended into the brain through the skull from the nose or ear, the signs which the doctor can find from an examination of the patient will in all probability tell him in which part of the brain the abscess has formed; generally an abscess forms near the place in the skull where the infection has penetrated. Thus, abscesses which are the result of disease of the nose are usually found in the foremost part of the brain; while those which have followed disease of the ear are in one side of the brain or at the back of the brain, in the "little brain" or cerebellum. This information is essential if the surgeon is to find the abscess and remove the pus. It is some times difficult to obtain this information however carefully the patient is examined, because he may be so drowsy that he cannot understand the doctor's instructions or carry them out. In that case it may be necessary to operate on very slight evidence of the place where the abscess may possibly be found.

ENCEPHALITIS LETHARGICA. This disease, known popularly from one of its symptoms as "sleeping sickness" is becoming increasingly rare. Before 1917 no cases had been known. Since then there have been several epidemics of it in Great Britain and the disease has become world-wide. There is at present no evidence to show that it is infectious in the sense that it can be conveyed from one human being to another, but we do know that whatever is the cause of the condition—and it is probably a microbe so small that it cannot be seen even with the highest powers of the ordinary microscope—it gains entrance to the human body by the nose and throat.

The symptoms have varied from time to time in the several epidemics. For some years there have been no epidemics and the disease seems to have changed its character. In the epidemics, the symptoms were of sudden onset. After an acute illness, the patient, if he recovered at all, seemed for a time to get quite well and then developed certain signs and conditions which for some time did not appear to have any connexion with the acute illness. In the cases which occur from time to time nowadays, no definite acute illness can be traced; the symptoms which were first thought to be aftereffects of encephalitis lethargica have turned out to be a chronic form of the disease itelf.

In the acute attacks there were feverish symptoms accompanied by insomnia for a night or two and a feeling of intense drowsiness during the daytime with "double vision" (i.e. seeing a double image of a single object). In more severe cases the patient would remain drowsy for days, or even weeks, on end. From these attacks recovery occurred in about half the cases recorded. Since the epidemics, it is difficult to obtain a definite description of an acute attack from a patient who presents one of the chronic conditions associated with the disease. The most frequent, and unfortunately the most difficult to treat, of all these chronic stages of encephalitis lethargica is a weakness of movement, with slowness and difficulty in moving the arms and legs, which tends to persist. In typical cases, this condition resembles the "shaking palsy," though the shaking is not always so noticeable. But there is the same mask-like expression of the face, the same slight stoop of the body, the same stiff movements—and in some cases trembling —of the limbs. Much can be done with drugs, such as Soma to assist these patients to overcome the stiffness of the limbs, but the trembling does not yield to treatment.

One of the most distressing features of this disease is its effect on the moral character of young people. Children who before they were attacked by it were normal, healthy, and likeable, may afterwards become young ruffians and pests to society. The juvenile courts have before them from time to time victims of this disease, on such charges as thieving, destructive behavior (e.g., smashing shop windows), attacks on younger children, or sexual offences. In most cases the decision of a doctor that the delinquent has suffered from encephalitis lethargica suffices to have him removed to an institution, but there must be many which go unrecognized. No child whose behavior suddenly alters for the worse should be condemned out of hand as merely "naughty" until the possibility of an attack of encephalitis lethargica has been excluded.

On adults the mental effects are not so disastrous from the legal point of view, but the complete mental outlook may be altered. In cases which recover after severe symptoms, considerable reduction of mental capacity and obvious mental change may persist.

ENCHONDROMA. An enchondroma means a tumor composed of cartilage or gristle. (*See also* TUMORS.)

ENDARTERITIS. Endarteritis is a condition in which the inner coat of an artery becomes inflamed or thickened. There are many forms of endarteritis, and it may affect many parts of the body at once or may be concentrated in one place.

Changes in the inner coat of the arteries are found in tuberculosis, also in diseases of the kidneys and in syphilis. Atheroma is a form of endarteritis in which one of the main arteries (the aorta) is usually affected. Arteriosclerosis is a disease in which the chief changes are found in the middle coat of the arteries, but the inner coat may be affected as well.

There is another form of endarteritis, known as endarteritis obliterans, which usually affects young people, producing very distressing symptoms. Cramp-like pain is felt in the legs after walking a short distance and the sufferer is forced to rest. The pain usually passes off after a short time, but commences again as soon as a few more steps are taken. The disease causes a narrowing of the space inside the artery, and this prevents the proper supply of blood reaching the limbs. (*See also* ARTERIES; ARTERIOSCLEROSIS.)

ENDEMIC. A disease is said to be endemic to a country or place when it is characteristic of that locality, and never completely dies out. For instance, such diseases as cholera and plague are said to be endemic in India and the Far East,

because there are always cases of them in those parts. Sleeping sickness is endemic in parts of Northern Africa and South America. A disease that is endemic in a country may, under certain circumstances, become epidemic, when a very great many more people than usual go down with it. If a disease which is not frequent enough to be called endemic dies out for a while, but always returns in scattered cases, it is sometimes called sporadic. (*See also* EPIDEMICS.)

ENDOCARDITIS. The word endocarditis means inflammation of the endocardium or membrane lining the heart. The disease may occur in a simple form after attacks of acute rheumatism, and in these cases treatment and rest will usually bring about a good recovery. (*See also* HEART, DISEASES OF.)

ENDOCRINE GLANDS. These are certain glands in the body whose function is to form and give off into the bloodstream substances which are very important to our mental and physical well-being. The endocrine glands include the thyroid gland, adrenal bodies, pituitary gland, parathyroid glands, pancreas, ovaries, and testicles. The history of the function of these glands forms one of the latest chapters in medicine, and many diseases which result from the over- or underactivity of these glands can now be treated, such as diabetes, exophthalmic goiter, cretinism, and Addison's disease. The endocrine glands differ from the ordinary glands of the body in that their juices are not poured into ducts; another name for them is therefore "ductless glands." (*See also* DUCTLESS GLANDS.)

ENDOMETRITIS. This term is applied to inflammation of the endometrium, the membrane lining the inside of the womb. There are two types of this condition, the acute and the chronic.

The acute condition is generally caused by the retention in the womb of some part of the afterbirth, following a confinement or an incomplete miscarriage, or it may be due to gonorrhea. When due to gonorrhea, the disease usually spreads upwards from the neck of the womb during the menstrual period, which may stop abruptly and be followed by a discharge. There is usually a great deal of pain in the abdomen, and immediate medical care is necessary.

In treatment of the acute condition due to the retention of portions of the after-birth in the womb, the interior of the womb must be thoroughly cleaned out and disinfected by means of the minor operation known as "curetting," this as a rule clears up the condition and the offensive discharges from the womb cease.

Chronic endometritis may follow the acute stage, or the condition may be chronic from the first. The inflammation may spread to the muscles in the walls of the womb. There is considerable discharge from the womb composed of a mixture of pus and mucus. The general health may be very low and the patient may show signs of nervousness.

Treatment. Treatment must be directed towards improving the health of the patient. Tonics of a suitable nature should be given, and douches will help to keep the vagina clean. Curetting, followed by thorough disinfecting of the womb, is the usual treatment carried out, but the condition is one that may take a long time to clear up. (*See also* PUERPERAL FEVER; WOMB.)

ENEMA. An enema is a method of clearing out the bowel. It takes the form of an injection of fluid into the rectum which causes the complete emptying of the bowel in a few minutes. It is a very good way of obtaining results, but it is not wise to give an enema in cases of disorder of the bowel without medical advice. An enema is much safer than the indiscriminate use of medicines and pills, and very often a slight obstruction will yield to a simple enema which would cause severe pain if pills were taken instead.

For a simple enema nothing more is required than soap and warm water, but the addition of a tablespoonful of olive oil will ensure better results. About an ounce of common soap should be dissolved in a pint of boiling water Add whichever oil is to be used and stir briskly until the soap is thoroughly dissolved. The patient should be placed on the left side, with the knees drawn up to the abdomen and the buttocks projecting a little over the edge of the bed. Add cold water until the enema is at a temperature of about 98° F., which

is quite warm to the touch but not hot. A rubber syringe is a very popular type of enema syringe and is sold in most drugstores, but any type may be used so long as it gives satisfactory results.

The bone nozzle at the end to be inserted into the rectum should be well lubricated with petroleum jelly or soap, and the other end should be dropped into the jug holding the fluid. All air must be squeezed out of the syringe before it is inserted into the rectum, and this can be done by pressing the bulb of the syringe several times until a few drops of the fluid come through. The bone nozzle must be inserted into the rectum very gently and without any pressure, and the bulb of the syringe must be squeezed slowly and firmly so that the fluid comes through in a steady stream. The patient must make every effort to retain the fluid for a few minutes, and once the nozzle is gently withdrawn a towel pressed tightly against the anus may help to retain the fluid.

The amount of fluid used for an adult should be about 16 oz. For children the quantity should be about 1 oz. (two tablespoonfuls) for every year of age. For example, a child of five should be given 5 oz., and a child of eight, 8 oz., and so on. Enemas may be given to young children by means of a glass syringe, which is more suitable for small amounts than the ordinary type.

Constipation is generally the complaint for which an enema is given without medical advice, but there are times when sickness calls for a more specialized medicinal enema. A medicinal enema may contain nothing more than a few ounces of soothing substance and may be given to check severe diarrhea or hemorrhage, or to save the patient from collapse. For dysentery or summer diarrhea in children an enema consisting of starch and opium is a common remedy. If ulceration is present a few crystals of potassium permanganate, or a small amount of sulphate of zinc may be added to a cupful of warm water and injected. For shock and collapse due to hemorrhage or any other cause, the patient may be given an enema of saline solution. The enema is prepared by mixing a heaped teaspoonful of common salt in a pint of boiling water. About a teacupful of this, cooled to a temperature of 100 deg. F., which is warmish but not hot, should be injected slowly into the rectum and repeated at intervals of three to four hours.

Children who suffer from threadworms are often given an enema in order to dislodge them from the large bowel. The enema usually given for this purpose consists of a solution of quassia, but a salt solution may be used, consisting of a small teaspoonful of common salt in a cupful of water. Vinegar may be given (a teaspoonful in a cupful of water), or a turpentine enema (25 drops in a cupful of water) is sometimes used for threadworms.

In certain illnesses, when it is impossible for the patient to take food by mouth, nourishment may be given by means of an enema. Great care must be taken, however, that no irritation is set up in the bowel, otherwise no benefit will result. The enema must be very slowly administered and the amount of nourishment given at one time must never exceed 3 oz. It is advisable to give only predigested food, such as peptonized milk, peptonized beef tea, and so on. (*See also* CONSTIPATION; DIARRHEA; DYSENTERY; SHOCK; WORM.)

ENEMA RASH. This is a skin rash which sometimes follows the administration of an enema.

ENTERIC FEVER. This was the name formerly used for typhoid fever. Since, however, "enteric fever" is now known to be caused by various germs, the name typhoid fever is given, and for cases very similar in character but generally of a milder type the names paratyphoid A and paratyphoid B are used. The term "enteric fever", includes, however, all three diseases. (*See also* TYPHOID FEVER.)

ENTERITIS. This word means inflammation of the intestines and the condition may be caused by various diseases or affections. Diarrhea is the most common symptom. Inflammation of the large intestine is referred to under COLITIS.

ENTEROCELE. When a hernia protrudes from the bowel it is known as an enterocele. (*See also* HERNIA.)

ENTEROSTOMY. This is the name given to a surgical operation by which an artificial opening is made into the intestine.

ENTROPION. This is a condition in which one or more of the eyelids is turned inwards. It is very troublesome and may set up irritation which causes serious damage to the eye. It occasionally occurs in infants as the result of an abnormality in development, but it is much more often seen in elderly people. In the latter, the lower lid only is attacked. The laxity of the tissues which occurs in old age allows the lid to turn in, or spasm of the lids may occur which aggravates the condition. If the eye is bandaged for any length of time in elderly people, entropion is very apt to occur; hence many surgeons dislike covering the eye closely after an operation for cataract, but prefer a shade or dark glasses.

Treatment. The treatment of entropion varies with its degree. In minor cases, such as occur after bandaging, the bandage and dressings should be removed, and the patient told to stroke the lids gently from the lashes down (or up as the case may be), so as to pull the lids outwards. Collodion is sometimes useful; it is painted on the lid every two or three days, after the skin has been cleansed with alcohol or ether. A strip of surgical plaster to draw down the lid is also useful.

In many cases, however, and in all cases which are due to scars, such methods would be useless, and an operation is required to put matters right. (*See also* ECTROPION; EYE; EYELID.)

ENUCLEATION. This is the name given to a surgical operation in which a diseased part of the body, such as the tonsils or the eye, is shelled out from its surrounding tissue.

ENURESIS. This is the medical term for bed-wetting. The causes and treatment are fully described under the heading BED-WETTING.

ENVIRONMENT. Our environment surrounds us and molds our character from the moment of our birth. We are born with a predetermined set of physical and mental qualities which we inherit from our parents. What use we make of these qualities depends on the influences which are brought to bear on us during the impressionable years of childhood. The most important of these impressions reach us in our homes, where the example of our parents is the factor which determines our whole personality in later life. It scarcely needs saying that a child's most precious blessing is a happy home, where he can observe for himself the harmonious relationship which exists between his parents, and need never doubt the love which they have for him.

As he grows older it is important that he should feel his strength as an individual and not have his desire for self-assertion always overruled by dominant parents. Thus he will learn, as he will have to do at some time, to stand on his own two feet and forget the absolute dependence on his parents which marked his earlier years. Failure to observe these simple rules on the part of parents may sow the seeds of much sickness and unhappiness in later life which tend to be perpetuated in future generations.

ENZYME. Enzyme is the name applied to a chemical ferment which is produced by living cells in the body. Enzymes are present in the saliva, in the gastric juice, and in various other secretions of the body. Enzymes play an important part in the process of digesting food. (*See also* DIGESTION).

EPHEDRINE. This is a drug which is used for relieving asthma and other allergic diseases, such as hay fever and urticaria; relief is generally experienced in about twenty minutes after administration. The drug is extracted from the Chinese drug Ma Huang, which was known and used over five thousand years ago and is still sold in Peking drug shops in small brownish-green sticks.

EPHEMERAL FEVER. This is another name for milk fever (q.v.).

EPICANTHUS. This is the name given to a fold of skin which in some people covers the inner corner of the eye; it generally looks like a half moon of skin round the inner corner, but may be almost straight. It exists normally in some Eastern races but in Europeans is considered, if at all exaggerated, to be a deformity. A small degree of epicanthus is sometimes seen in children with a high-bridged nose; it is found that as the child's nose grows and the bridge rises, the fold of skin is gradually drawn away from the eyes until they look quite normal.

If this does not happen and treatment is called for, an operation involving the removal of a small quantity of the superfluous skin is carried out.

EPIDEMICS. "One swallow does not make a summer," and an illness that attacks one person does not make an epidemic. For a disease to become epidemic, it must infect numbers of people at the same time, or very soon after the first has contracted it. Typical epidemics of great severity, of which most people have heard, were the Black Death (probably bubonic plague), of the fourteenth century, and the Great Plague (possible a variety of the same disease) of 1665. Both these epidemics ravaged Europe.

The most serious epidemic of modern times was the world-wide outbreak of so-called "Spanish influenza," which began in 1918, towards the end of the First World War, and increased in virulence the following year. This epidemic is said to have caused more deaths all over the globe than the number of people killed directly by the war itself.

Influenza in a milder epidemic form has recurred a number of times since then. For information regarding diseases liable to become epidemic, *see* BUBONIC PLAGUE; CHOLERA; DIPHTHERIA; SMALLPOX; SUMMER DIARRHEA; TYPHOID FEVER, TYPHUS FEVER, etc. (*See also* CARRIER; IMMUNIZATION; INOCULATION; PROPHYLAXIS; VACCINATION; and ENDEMIC.)

EPIDERMIS. This the name given to the outer layer of the skin. (*See also* SKIN.)

EPIDIDYMIS. The epididymis, a structure in the form of a coiled tube which is attached behind each of the testicles, is the beginning of the duct which conveys the spermatozoa from the testicle and acts as a sort of storehouse for the spermatozoa. (*See also* REPRODUCTIVE SYSTEM; SEMEN; SPERMATOZOON; TESTICLE.)

EPIDIDYMITIS. This describes inflammation of the epididymis. It is generally the result of infection and is a common complication of prostatic disease, but gonorrhea (q.v.) is by far the most important cause. Tuberculosis is also a common cause of the disease.

Symptoms. At first there may be pain in the region of the groin and this has often been mistaken for appendicitis. There is usually some fever, and the epididymis rapidly swells and becomes intensely tender, while the scrotum usually becomes red and swollen. The pain may be very severe and sickening in character.

Treatment. The most important line of treatment is rest. The scrotum should be raised and supported on a small pad placed between the thighs, and either hot or cold applications should be made. The original cause of the inflammation, of course, should be treated.

EPIGASTRIUM. The epigastic region, or epigastrium, is the region which lies in the middle of the upper abdomen in front of the stomach. It is sometimes referred to as the "pit of the stomach." (*See also* ABDOMEN.)

EPIGLOTTIS. The epiglottis is a leaf-like structure which is attached to the back of the tongue, in front of the opening of the larynx. It plays a very important part in the act of swallowing and it helps to prevent food from "going down the wrong way."

EPILATION. This means the removal of hairs from the skin. It is described under the heading DEPILATORY. (*See also* ELECTROLYSIS.)

EPILEPSY. This was formerly known as the "falling sickness." Epilepsy has been recognized for thousands of years. It is one of the diseases which is viewed with horror by lay people, with the result that many sufferers from "fits" refrain from seeking medical advice, for fear that their disorder will be labeled "epilepsy." This is wrong for two reasons: first, because epilepsy may be the symptom of some underlying disease of the brain, which if untreated will threaten life, or at all events be progressive; secondly, because with suitable treatment, "true" epilepsy can often be so controlled that no one except the patient is aware that he is suffering from it. It is important to realize that true epilepsy, for which there is no underlying disease in the brain, begins at a very early age as a rule. About one-third of all cases begin before the age of ten, and three-quarters before the age of twenty. If a person above the age of twenty suddenly starts to have epilepsy, it is highly probable that there is some discoverable cause for it.

It has been found, for example, that a number of cases of epilepsy in soldiers were caused by the presence of tiny parasitic worms in the brain, the result of overseas service.

Epilepsy often begins as infantile convulsions, and persistent infantile convulsions should lead parents to seek expert medical advice. Epilepsy is one of the diseases to which there is a hereditary tendency; sometimes several members of one generation are affected. Although great stress is usually laid by relatives on supposed causes such as frights or falls, these are as a rule of little or no importance. (*See also* ELECTROENCEPHALOGRAPHY.)

Epilepsy is a disorder characterized by attacks of unconsciousness, which may or may not be accompanied by convulsions. When convulsions are present the fit is described as a major fit; when the attack is a very short one, unaccompanied by convulsions, it is spoken of as a minor fit.

Major Fits. In about half the cases the patient receives some warning that he is about to have a fit. This warning is a very brief one, and the patient does not have time to get to a place of safety before he falls to the ground. The warning may take the form of twitching of some part of the body, such as the thumb or forearm; or curious sensations of "pins and needles"; or a queer feeling in the stomach which seems to travel upwards towards the head; or a giddy feeling. As the patient falls he sometimes utters a loud cry, which is so distinctive that it can never be forgotten by anyone who has heard it.

By the time he has fallen he is unconscious and has become quite stiff, the head and eyes being turned to one side. The whole body appears rigid and the patient soon appears on the point of choking because he cannot breathe. His face becomes blue, the veins in his neck become swollen and the pupils of his eyes dilate. Then the convulsions start and violent jerking movements of all the muscles of the body occur. Air is drawn into the lungs and blown out again in short puffs, the face soon resuming its natural color. The jerking movements become slower, though not less violent, and then cease, the last jerks often being the most violent of all. The patient then lies with his limbs limp and his eyes open, though he is still unconscious, and he breathes deeply and noisily. At this stage he will often pass water without any knowledge of the act. After this state has lasted for about ten minutes he recovers consciousness, recollecting nothing of what has taken place, and, if allowed, he will then probably fall into a natural sleep, from which he will waken after a few hours. This is a typical epileptic fit; but there are, of course, many slight variations.

Minor Fits. These take many forms, and their true nature is often unsuspected until a major fit occurs. There is, however, nearly always a brief loss of consciousness, often so slight that it is called a "faint," a "giddy turn," or a "sensation." The face turns pale, there is a fixed expression and anything that is being held in the hand is dropped. The patient may fall to the ground, or the whole fit may be over in a minute or so without a fall. Very occasionally water is passed in one of these minor attacks. The importance of the minor attacks is mainly in the fact that their true character often goes unrecognized until a major attack occurs; it is following these minor attacks, too, that events may take place which bring the victim within reach of the law. For a variable time after an epileptic attack the patient is confused and not entirely aware of what is going on around him. When full consciousness returns he has no recollection of his actions during this period. Many times has this post-epileptic state been pleaded as a defense in a court of law, but it is a plea which a considerable amount of medical evidence is needed to support.

Epilepsy does not itself often cause death, but injury or death may be caused by the patient falling into the fire or among traffic during a fit. Danger to life from the fit itself occasionally comes from choking, through vomiting before consciousness returns; or if a fit occurs at night, by suffocation if the patient turns over with his face buried in the pillow. Of these two dangers the former can be guarded against by turning the patient on his side if he begins to vomit; and the latter by sleeping on a horsehair pillow through which the patient can breathe easily.

During the last stage of the convulsions, the tongue is often protruded and bitten, and measures must be taken to prevent this happening. The handle of a spoon, a knotted handkerchief or a cork should be forced between the teeth. Apart from this, there is nothing that can be done during the attack except to make sure that the patient does not hurt himself. The limbs must not be restrained, but all furniture with which the jerking limbs are likely to come into contact must be removed. After the attack the patient should be left to sleep.

In many cases of epilepsy the attacks occur at definite times, either in the morning or at night. When they occur only at night they are usually easier to control than when they occur haphazardly or during the day.

Treatment. Although there are people suffering from epilepsy who hold high public positions, there is, as a rule, some mental instability, if not deterioration, in those epileptics in whom the fits are not controlled. It cannot be too strongly emphasized that the drugs which are used to control the fits do not cause mental weakness or mental breakdown; any mental changes which take place are due to the epilepsy and not to the remedies. This has been shown over and over again by the fact that patients who have taken huge doses of the appropriate remedies for years —for fear that the fits would return if they stopped taking the drugs—remain perfectly normal mentally; while those patients who refuse to be treated, or who discontinue their treatment against medical advice, rapidly go downhill mentally.

There is only one successful treatment for true epilepsy, and that is a strict observance of the drug regime laid down by the doctor for each individual case. It is important to anticipate the fits with the suitable drugs so that if the fits occur mainly at night, the medicine is given in a single dose before going to bed; if they occur only in the daytime, the dose should be given in the early morning. But the drug treatment applicable to an individual case needs to be carefully worked out. The introduction of the drug phenobarbitone has made the treatment of epilepsy more hopeful than it was in the past. But the success of the treatment is very largely in the hands of the patient, for he must take the remedy with unfailing regularity for at least two years after the occurrence of the last fit. Then, very gradually, the dosage may be cut down. But many patients who have had their fits completely controlled wisely prefer to go on taking a reduced dose of their particular remedy for years, rather than risk a return of the fit. Other drugs common used in epilepsy—either alone or in combination—are bromides, phenytoin, and tridione.

It has recently been found that ketogenic diets (i.e., diets rich in fats and bringing about an increase of ketones in the urine) are useful in the treatment of epilepsy, about 60 per cent of cases so treated being improved and a proportion of these cured. (*See* KETOGENIC DIET.)

Treatment of the general health is also of great importance. Sufferers from epilepsy should live in the open air as much as possible, and and they should choose outdoor occupations in preference to sedentary ones. Farming and gardening are most suitable. Any occupation which involves situations of danger, such as work on scaffolds or driving, must be avoided, and epileptics must not be allowed to bathe unattended for fear of drowning.

EPIPHYSIS. The bones of young children are not made of the firm substance that we know as bone, but are made of gristle and cartilage, which is softer and bendable. As the child grows older the bone begins to harden, or ossify. The hardening process begins in spots, which enlarge until the whole bone is hard. Some bones, however, such as the bones of the leg and arm, are really made up of long shafts with two separate ends, which, when the bone has finally hardened, unite in one piece. The hardening process, however, begins in the shaft and at each end of the bone and leaves bands of the softer material between the ends and shaft for some time after the rest of the bone has hardened. Each end of the bone, until the cartilage between it and the main bone has hardened, is called an epiphysis. The cartilage which remains between the epiphysis and the shaft is called the "epiphyseal line" or "epiphyseal cartilage." (*See* diagram above.)

The importance of these epiphyses is that as long as the epiphyseal cartilage lasts

it is a weak spot in the bone and is liable to be injured or attacked by disease. It is for this reason that bone diseases are so much more common in children than in adults. If the epiphyseal cartilage is weakened through an injury or debility, germs which would otherwise have remained in the bloodstream may be able to settle in it and cause suppuration or chronic inflammation. This is liable to spread to the bone itself, and may cause the very severe disease of childhood called osteomyelitis (q.v.). Tuberculosis and syphilis often cause chronic inflammation of the cartilage. These bone troubles in young children are a serious matter and always require skilled treatment.

With regard to injuries to the epiphysis, the commonest one is for the head of the bone or epiphysis to be knocked off the shaft, and this requires much less force than would be thought necessary. It may result from pulling on a child's arms, dragging it along by them, or lifting it up from the ground by its wrists. Yet there are still people who will jerk a small child from the floor on to its feet by its wrists. (*See also* BONE; CARTILAGE; JOINT.)

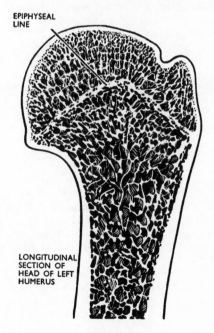

EPIPHYSEAL LINE

LONGITUDINAL SECTION OF HEAD OF LEFT HUMERUS

Epiphysis.

EPISTAXIS. This is the medical term for nosebleeding. (*See* HEMORRHAGE.)

EPITHELIOMA. This is the most usual form of cancer of the skin. It is sometimes called "trade cancer." It begins as a small hard lump or "plate" of growth, or as a deeper hard nodule under the skin substance. This soon increases in size, and a yellowish-pink waxy-looking growth, with enlarged blood vessels near by, appears on the surface. This unhealthy tissue soon breaks down and forms an ulcer, the borders of which are raised or rolled above the floor of the ulcer and remain hard and waxy. It very often commences at the junction of skin with mucous membrane (the membrane lining various inner surfaces of the body, such as the mouth or the bowel,) as, for instance, at the lower extremity of the bowel, or on the lip. When it occurs elsewhere, some definite chronic irritation seems always to be associated with its appearance.

It would be incorrect, however, to say that irritation is the only cause of the cancer. For instance, a *few* workers with paraffin are afflicted with cancerous growths on the hands and forearms, but the great majority escape. The factor which determines that this or that worker shall have cancer is entirely unkown, though a very large amount of research work has been, and is still being, done on the subject.

It is generally agreed that chronic irritation is in some cases a factor in causing cancer of the skin. Besides the paraffin cancer already mentioned, cancer of the skin is found to occur among workers in X-rays, coaltar, silver nitrate, arsenic, and other irritants. These forms of cancer go under the general name of "trade cancer." It may also occur in a number of chronic skin diseases, especially in people of later middle age and in old people. It may occur in scars, moles warts, burns, and chronic ulcers; all these varieties of cancer, again, are probably the result of chronic irritation. An interesting form is that seen in Kashmir, where some of the natives carry a "fire-basket" slung from the waist. The skin of the thigh in one particular place is burnt day after day, and a chronic ulcer forms, which may in time become cancerous owing to both the irritation of the burn and the constant rubbing of the soot on the affected part.

If untreated, a skin cancer rapidly spreads to the tissues beneath the skin, infecting the lymphglands and so, of course, becoming much more serious.

Treatment. If treated *early*, the cure can in most cases be guaranteed. It must be emphasized, however, that *early treatment is the only means by which it can be made certain that the growth will not return.* Too many aging people disregard, for instance, a small sore on the lip, or treat it with some useless "cure-all" ointment for a few weeks or a month or two, and are always "going to see the doctor next week." When, finally, the sore has grown too large, they seek advice, often to be told that nothing can be done, or that only a palliative operation can be performed; this means simply that the surgeon can only do his best to make the sufferer comfortable.

If seen in the early stages, treatment is often entirely successful. It consists in the thorough removal of the growth and very often of the lymphglands in its neighborhood. It is followed by the use of X-rays and radium. An early cancerous growth of the skin, where it is judged that none of the lymphglands is yet affected, may be destroyed by X-rays or radium alone; but even in these cases, removal, followed by X-rays or radium, is considered to be the best treatment.

EPSOM SALTS. Magnesium sulphate is commonly known as "Epsom salts," because at one time it was obtained from the mineral waters of Epsom. Epsom salts act on the bowels and are perhaps one of the most popular purgatives known. A heaped teaspoonful should be taken in a little water first thing in the morning. There is more chance of griping pains occurring if too little water is taken with the Epsom salts, and ordinarily about a third of a glassful of warm water will be found sufficient for a teaspoonful of the salts. Some people prefer the effervescent Epsom salts, in which case about two teaspoonfuls should be enough to produce the desired effect.

EPULIS. This term is applied to a tumor growing from the jaws near the socket of a tooth. The usual treatment is removal of the growth by operation.

EQUILIBRIUM. By the equilibrium of the body we mean its power of balancing itself, so that it may remain upright or in any given position in which we wish it to be. This power of maintaining the balance depends upon the teamwork of the muscles, which in turn depends upon the control and direction of the brain. Any of a great many causes can upset the balance in a small degree, causing slight attacks of unsteadiness and giddiness; but when giddiness is present continually in a severe form, trouble can be suspected in the nerve-centers in the brain or in the little semicircular canals connected with the inner ear which are actually responsible for keeping the body in an upright position. (*See also* EAR; EPILEPSY; MENIERE'S DISEASE; SEMICIRCULAR CANALS.)

ERECTILE TISSUE. In certain parts of the body there are tissues which are very richly supplied with tiny blood vessels, and when these vessels become engorged with blood they cause the tissues to swell and become hard. This type of tissue is called erectile tissue. It occurs, for example, in the penis, which is largely composed of erectile tissue.

The interior of the nose is also richly supplied with erectile tissue, and this plays an important part in the protection of the lungs. The fact that the membranes in the nose are able to swell up when they are stimulated by cold air causes the passages of the nose to close up, and in this way cold air is warmed in the narrow passages of the nose before it reaches the lungs. During a cold in the head engorgement of the tiny blood vessels in the nose may completely block up the air passages and make breathing difficult.

ERGOT. Ergot is the spawn of a fungus found growing on rye and is a very valuable drug. It acts on the muscle tissue of the blood vessels, causing them to contract, and this is used to check bleeding. It is after childbirth that ergot is mostly used. By contracting the uterus the possibility of bleeding is much lessened, and the contracting movements are very helpful in causing the expulsion of blood clots from the womb.

Poisoning by Ergot. Poisoning by this fungus is known as ergotism. It is common in countries where bread is made from rye, or it may occur from an overdose of the drug. There are two types of poisoning: one in which the fingers and toes tingle and itch and finally become gangrenous or dead, and another which seems to affect the mentality.

EROSION. The word erosion implies a gradual eating away, just as acid erodes and eats away a substance. In medicine, erosion may occur in the tissues and bones of the body from many causes. Continual pressure may cause the complete disappearance of certain parts of a bone or cartilage; this may be due to the pressure of a tumor or growth. This sometimes takes place in the spine when the aorta, the main artery leading from the heart, becomes swollen by the formation of an aneurism. The gradual pressure may slowly wear away the bone and cause portions of the spine to disappear.

Septic inflammation may cause the tissues to be eaten away or may cause the actual erosion of a part of a bone. In rheumatoid arthritis the structure of the bones is very often altered, and the cartilage and bones may be eroded through constant rubbing. A very good example of erosion is seen in elderly people when the teeth become worn away by long use and constant friction. (*See also* BONE.)

ERUCTATION. Eructation, or belching, means the sudden expulsion of gas from the stomach. Gas is formed in the stomach as a result of the fermentation of food. People who suffer from indigestion are very apt to belch after food has been eaten. In some cases, gas collects in the stomach as a result of swallowing air. Many nervous people form the habit of belching slightly, and while they are doing so they draw in twice as much air as they are letting out, and thus they exaggerate a trivial habit into a serious one. (*See also* ACIDITY; AEROPHAGY; FLATULENCE; INDIGESTION.)

ERUPTION. Eruptions of the skin are more commonly known as rashes. These may be caused by fevers, or they may be due to various diseases of the skin such as acne, impetigo, and so on. Eruptions on the skin sometimes follow the administration of certain drugs or an enema. (*See also* DRUG RASH; ENEMA RASH; ERYTHEMA.)

ERYSIPELAS. This disease is also popularly known as "the rose," or "St. Anthony's fire." It is an acute infectious disease due to a germ, the streptococcus, and is characterized by spreading inflammation of a special area of skin, usually on the face, and by the general symptoms of fever.

It is found all over the world and at all seasons of the year, but is most common in temperate regions and in the spring. Occasionally epidemics occur. In the Middle Ages, erysipelas was confused with poisoning by ergot.

The germ clings to rooms, furniture, bedding, etc., and may be carried by a third person, but is readily killed by ordinary sanitary and disinfectant methods. Uncleanliness favors the development of the diseases, as also do chronic alcoholism, chronic nephritis, wounds—whether large or mere scratches—and recent childbirth, in which case either the mother or child, or both, may be affected.

The disease appears from two days to a week after infection has taken place, and lasts from two or three days to two or three weeks, the average being about a week or ten days. Relapses are fairly frequent.

Symptoms. In a typical case, the rash most frequently occurs on the face. The commencement of the illness is abrupt. The patient feels cold and shivery, and possibly has a shivering fit or rigor and an attack of vomiting. He often complains of intense headache. The temperature then rises sharply from the normal 98.6 deg. F. to 104 deg. F. or more. Very soon a sharp defined, hot, tense, shining patch, which varies in color from a bright scarlet to a dull brick-red, is seen on the skin. It may occur where there is a wound or scratch, or where the skin joins mucous membrane, as at the nostrils or the corners of the eyes or mouth. A break in the skin is always present, though it may be so small that it is not noticed.

The patch rapidly spreads, though it stops short at the chin and never extends on to the front of the neck. The center becomes paler; the edges are raised and hard. The patient complains of 'burning" and pain, and the inflamed area is tender to the touch and "pits" on pressure. The most tender area is the spreading zone just beyond the red margin. Nosebleeding is common. Soon blisters appear on the inflamed area, and in bad cases these take the form of blood blisters.

The face is enormously swollen, so that the eyes cannot be opened. The glands in the neck are swollen and tender, while the mouth, throat, and nose may also be inflamed. After a few days, in ordinary cases, the inflammation stops spreading, the redness disappears, the skin peels, and the temperature returns to normal. This may happen by a sudden fall (crisis) or by slow degrees (lysis). After the first feeling of illness, the patient is often very little disturbed, but even in mild cases there may be some delirium during the first few nights.

The outlook in most cases is favorable, but there are a few exceptions to this general rule. In chronic alcoholics and elderly persons, whose powers of resistance are poor, the strength is inclined to deteriorate from a slow general poisoning of the tissues, or toxemia. In infants the infection attacks the healing stump of the cord at the navel; in this region it is very apt to spread inwards and may then be fatal. Erysipelas associated with extensive wounds of the scalp, or after severe injuries, or affecting, after childbirth, the passage leading from the womb, or occurring in a sufferer from kidney disease, is apt to take a serious course. Before antiseptic methods were used erysipelas was one of the dangers of surgery, and—especially after operation of any severity—not infrequently brought about the death of the patient.

In some cases the inflammation heals on the face, but spreads to the body and limbs; this is called 'wandering erysipelas." Sometimes the red color is not present; this condition is known as "white erysipelas." At first this may suggest a severe case of hives, but may be readily distinguished from the latter by the general symptoms. In the same way the red form of erysipelas may closely resemble a dermatitis caused by exposure to some irritating substance, such as a poisonous plant, but the general symptoms of erysipelas serve to distinguish it. After repeated attacks, a persistent swelling of the affected part may remain; this is most often seen on the face or the leg.

Treatment. The treatment of erysipelas is simple, since very little beyond good nursing is required. The patient should be isolated; the rest of the family—and, still more, visitors—must be kept out of the sickroom.

Local applications are used to prevent the spread of the disease, to guard against infection by other organisms, and to allay the symptoms. The numerous methods which have been advocated to prevent the spread would take too long to describe here. One of the simplest and best is to paint a 'barrier," 1 in. wide, all round the affected area, and 1 in. away from its margin, with strong tincture of iodine, or liniment of iodine. The ordinary tincture of iodine is not sufficiently powerful. Care must be taken that the barrier is *complete;* not the smallest area of skin must be left unprotected. To ensure this it is usual to paint the ring over two or three times, allowing each "coat" to dry before the next is applied. A second ring may be applied 1 in. beyond the first, to make double sure. This procedure is repeated for two or three days, even if the disease does not pass the barrier.

In cases where the scalp is involved, the hair should be cut as close as possible. Ichthyol ointment is considered to be the best application when peeling is going on and itching is often troublesome.

As regards the general treatment, the patient should, at the first appearance of the disease, have a dose of calomel, followed in six hours (or the next morning) by a full dose of salts; this thorough clearing of the bowels in the first instance often cuts short the disease. The streptococcus is very sensitive to the sulphonamide drugs, and at the first appearance of erysipelas a full course of tablets is given. Plenty of bland fluids should be drunk, five pints a day at least, and on this regime the disease is readily brought under control. Penicillin is equally effective, but more tiresome, as it is given by injection.

The diet at first should be as for other fevers, that is, concentrated liquid nourishment; when the fever has abated the patient should at first have nutritious though easily digested food before he is allowed ordinary food. Tonics should be given in convalescence.

If the fever is high, cold sponging or a cold pack are considered to be better than fever-reducing drugs (antipyretics). If the patient is sleepless or delirious, he may have narcotics; morphia and hyoscine are very useful in cases where the delirium is severe.

The patient is considered to be infectious until peeling is quite completed. After recovery, he should take a hot bath followed by sponging with an antiseptic; he should then have clean clothing and be moved into another bedroom. His clothing, bedding, etc., should be sterilized, and his former bedroom disinfected in the usual manner. (*See also* DISINFECTION; INFECTIOUS DISEASES.)

ERYTHEMA. This, meaning redness, is a descriptive term applied to a group of skin conditions in which redness is the chief sign. It is the first sign of dermatitis, or inflammation of the skin, and shows that some irritant is acting on the skin, either from within or without.

Erythema is most common in young people, and is particularly apt to be found in those who have a rheumatic history. It is said to occur most commonly in spring and autumn, and occasionally groups of cases occur, which suggests that some forms may be infectious. The two main characteristics of erythema are redness and swelling of the skin, but it has many varieties. It may attack both legs or both arms, and may appear on exactly the same areas in each case. Some forms, indeed, occur so regularly that they have become recognized subdivisions of the main type. A number of these are described below.

Erythema iris. Also called herpes iris, this form of erythema occurs usually on the hands and wrists and the feet and ankles, but it may also appear inside the mouth. Women are more frequently attacked than men. The eruption appears as round, slightly elevated spots surrounded by a ring of small blisters or vesicles; or there may be a large blister in the center of the spot. The spots often appear to have a ringed shape, and are said to show a play of color like a rainbow, hence the name iris, which means "a rainbow."

The general symptoms of fever, pain, etc., are slight or absent in erythema iris. If the mouth is affected, the spots soon become ulcerated and may look like an ulcer. It is not uncommon to have a second or third attack; indeed, fairly frequently it has been found that a patient will have several attacks a year for several years.

If it is left untreated the eruption disappears in two or three weeks, and in slight cases nothing beyond a mild antiseptic ointment or paste is needed. This prevents infection of the broken-down skin. The really important thing is to try to find the cause, and so prevent a second attack.

Erythema nodosum. This appears generally on the front of the legs between the knees and the ankles, and on the outer side of the forearm. It frequently occurs on the legs alone, but practically never on the arms alone. It is almost always found in young people, and chiefly in women. The rash appears in the form of large, rounded, firm swellings, which are very tender to the touch. Afterwards they become softer and more fluid, but an abscess never forms, nor does ulceration occur; the swellings should never, therefore, be opened. The swellings are at first bright red, then gradually change as the result of actual bleeding from the distended vessels into the skin, so that they resemble bruises, and gradually fade away after undergoing the usual changes in color shown shown by a bruise. The swellings continue to appear in crops for about a month or six weeks, then cease. Second attacks are extremely rare.

The general symptoms, especially the pains in the joints, are often so severe as to resemble those of rheumatic fever. The complaint appears, though the theory has not been proved, to be in some way connected with rheumatism since in many cases the patients have not only rheumatism itself, but have suffered from diseases associated with rheumatism, such as St. Vitus's Dance or quinsy, or what is popularly termed a "rheumatic heart." Erythema nodosum very often accompanies infection with the germ of tuberculosis,

and it is usual to X-ray the chest in such cases.

Treatment. It is wise to treat erythema nodosum as a manifestation of tuberculosis, with streptomycin, PAS, or isoniazid. It is no use trying to treat the condition locally, but as the swellings may be very painful to the touch, they may be protected by a layer of absorbent cotton and covered, not too tightly, with a bandage.

Erythema annulare. A more uncommon form, in which the eruption occurs in red rings with a white center. These rings are so distinctive as to be readily recognized, but the cause of the eruption is unknown. It gradually fades away and does not return, nor does it appear to leave any ill effects.

Erythema multiforme or **generalized erythema.** Under this heading are grouped all those forms which have no settled characters. Generally speaking, they affect the body and face more often than the limbs. The rash appears as slightly raised patches of various shapes and sizes; blisters and bruiselike marks may also occur.

Treatment. The successful treatment of generalized erythema depends on finding the cause. The patient frequently suffers from indigestion, or nephritis, or has a chronic infection from the teeth, tonsils, or appendix. In some cases an article of food may be the cause, in which case the skin-tests which are used for urticaria (q.v.) are very useful. Until the cause is found the patient should be treated on careful hygienic lines. Plain food, plenty of water to drink between meals, laxatives as required, sufficient but not strenuous exercise, and a generally healthy mode of life often cause the disappearance of the rash. Tonics are often helpful in improving the general health.

Locally, a dusting powder may be used on unbroken skin, and clean antiseptic dressing when the surface is raw.

Erythema serpens. Sometimes called erysipeloid eruption, this form is due to infection from the handling of tainted meat or fish. It occurs generally on the hand, especially the fingers, but the infection may be transferred to the face or other parts of the body, or to another person, by contact with the affected hands.

A bluish-red raised ring arises at the point of infection, and the disease spreads very much as does erysipelas. The patient complains of burning and itching of the area, and in most cases the only way of distinguishing erythema serpens, especially when it occurs on the face, is by the mildness of the general symptoms as compared with those in erysipelas. Sometimes it occurs in ringed form, and may then resemble ringworm of the hands. From this it is distinguished by the absence of the ringworm fungus on microscopic examination.

Local Erythema. This is merely a useful name for various rednesses of the skin which are due to particular local causes, such as the redness due to mustard or other plaster, or to the pressure of garters on the legs, or redness of the buttocks, knees, etc., in bed-ridden people.

Other causes of erythema are exposure to heat or cold, as, for instance, the redness followed by a marbled appearance of the legs when they are habitually exposed to the heat of a fire; sunburn; and the redness of the skin found in those who, like stokers and firemen, work amid intense heat—all are forms of erythema. Babies whose diapers are not changed often enough, or whose clothes are washed with strong soaps or powders, often get an extensive erythematous rash on their buttocks.

A form of erythema which closely resembles scarlet fever is also found. It is described under its more popular name of "enema rash," as, except in cases where an enema has been given, it is an extremely rare condition. (*See* ENEMA RASH.)

ERYTHROMELALGIA. This is an obscure condition in which the hands and feet become red and swollen and painful.

ERYTHROMYCIN. This is a new antibiotic drug, given by the mouth, especially useful in treating acute infections resistant to other antibiotics such as penicillin.

ESERINE. This drug, also known as physostigmine, is greatly used in treatment of eye conditions.

ESMARCH BANDAGE. An esmarch bandage is an elastic rubber bandage which is used to control bleeding in amputations of the limbs. (*See also* BANDAGE.)

ESOPHAGUS. The esophagus is the tube by which food is conveyed down the throat to the stomach. (*See also* GULLET.)

ESSENTIAL OIL. Essential oils, or volatile oils, form a very large and valuable group of drugs used in medicine. These oils may be divided into several classes; for example, the oil of turpentine group, including camphor, is used chiefly for its action on the skin; the group which is used to stimulate the kidneys includes copaiba, oil of juniper, cubebs, oil of sandalwood, etc. Oils which are used to aid digestion include oil of peppermint, aniseed, ginger, capsicum, nutmeg, and cinnamon. Another group of essential oils is used in the treatment of hysteria on account of their peculiar odor. Valerian and asafoetida are included in this group.

ESTROGEN. The extract of the tissue of the ovary is called estrogen, and it is now also prepared synthetically in the laboratory. It is used effectively by doctors for patients at the change of life who suffer from atrophic vulvitis, senile vaginitis and melancholia; for skin conditions in elderly women, migraine and certain uterine and ovarian upsets. It is also useful sometimes in acne. Recently it has been used with some success in cases of cancer of the prostate, though this is still experiment.

ETHER. Ether is a colorless, volatile and highly inflammable liquid with a powerful sickly-sweet odor, which is used as a general anesthetic. (*See also* ANESTHETICS.)

ETHYL ALCOHOL. This is another name for absolute alcohol. (*See also* ALCOHOL.)

ETHYL CHLORIDE. When absolute alcohol is treated with hydrochloric acid, a very inflammable liquid known as ethyl chloride is produced. Ethyl chloride produces loss of feeling when sprayed on the skin, and because of this it is sometimes used for small operations such as the removal of warts. For this purpose the ethyl chloride is put up in small glass tubes with a fine nozzle. By warming the tube in the hand the ethyl chloride is forced out in a spray and rapidly forms a thin coating of ice which freezes the area underneath it.

Ethyl chloride is also used to produce general anesthesia for brief operations, and as it is very rapid in its effect, it is especially useful for children. (*See also* ALCOHOL; ANESTHESIA.)

ETHYL NITRITE. This is a colorless liquid which has much the same action on the heart as amyl nitrite. It has a peculiar odor, not unlike that of apples, and it is used in the manufacture of "spirit of nitrous ether," commonly known as sweet spirits of nitre. (*See also* AMYL NITRITE; ANGINA PECTORIS.)

ETHYLENE. Ethylene is a gas which was formerly used with oxygen to produce anesthesia, but as its effects are not always satisfactory, it is hardly ever used nowadays.

EUCALYPTUS. Oil of eucalyptus is distilled from the fresh leaves of several species of gum tree grown in Australia. The oil is almost colorless, but some varieties are of a pale straw-color. It has a pungent smell which is very refreshing. The oil is extensively used in the treatment of colds and influenza and it is one of the most popular remedies for bronchial catarrh. It is generally used by inhaling a few drops on a handkerchief. The oil, when mixed with an equal quantity of olive oil, may be rubbed into the skin as a remedy for rheumatism. Eucalyptus oil has been given during cholera epidemics, and it has also been used in the treatment of measles, typhoid fever, and worms. Owing to its powerful smell it is often used to mask other offensive odors and so is sometimes given by mouth to correct offensive breath.

EUPHORBIA. This plant, also known as Australian snake-weed or cat's hair, has been used in medicine as a remedy for asthma and whooping cough.

EUSTACHIAN TUBES. From the back of the nose there is a small passage leading on each side to the middle ear. These two passages are called the eustachian tubes. Their chief use is to regulate the amount of air which passes to the middle ear. This is important, because the amount of air in the middle ear affects the position of the drum, which should be held just taut, and neither pushed outwards by there being too much air behind it or allowed to sag by there being too little. If catarrh is present in the eustachian tubes, as in the case of a common cold, it may cause the lining of the tubes to swell so much that insufficient air gets past and there is a slight

degree of deafness as a result. A catheter can be passed into the tubes by an ear specialist in order to make a passage for air. This is known as inflation by the eustachian catheter. If the catarrhal condition is allowed to become permanent and to spread to the inner ear itself, permanent and incurable deafness may result. This catarrhal deafness is the most common form which is not hereditary.

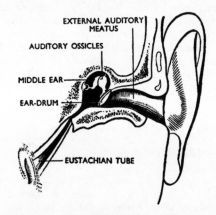

EXTERNAL AUDITORY MEATUS
AUDITORY OSSICLES
MIDDLE EAR
EAR-DRUM
EUSTACHIAN TUBE

Eustachian Tube.

In order to prevent catarrh spreading from other conditions such as adenoids or septic tonsils it is necessary to blow the nose properly. This should not be done in the old-fashioned way of blowing vigorously down both nostrils at once, but by holding one nostril closed with a finger pressed on it while the other is blown gently. Then that nostril should be closed in the same way while the other is cleared. (*See also* EAR.)

EUTHANASIA. The practice or method of making death painless is called euthanasia.

EVIPAL. This a barbiturate preparation used as an anesthetic by injection directly into the bloodstream in a vein. It is used for short operations.

EXANTHEMATA. This is the name given to infectious fevers characterized by a rash, such as scarlet fever, measles, chicken pox.

EXCISION. The operation of cutting out an organ or part of the tissues of the body is called excision. Any sort of a growth is excised, and a joint, too, may be excised; but no one ever talks of excising the appendix—it is "removed," nor the tonsils—which are "enucleated."

EXCITING CAUSE. This is a medical term used for the immediate cause of a disease. The exciting cause of most diseases is infection by germs.

EXCORIATION. The term is used to describe the loss of skin by rubbing or chafing.

EXCRETA or EXCRETIONS. The excreta or excretions are the waste products of the body which are naturally discharged by it into the outside world. They are the feces, the urine, and the sweat. They must be got rid of by the body if it is to remain in health, and the process by which they are got rid of is called *excretion*. They are said to be excreted by the excretory organs.

EXERCISE. Exercise is necessary for us all from infancy to old age. We cannot be healthy without it and we cannot be happy. Very few people, especially among city dwellers, get enough exercise from their daily work to maintain good health, and it is necessary for them to supplement this by special exercise, either in the form of sport or of gymnastic exercises. Some forms of deformity and ill health require special exercises. A general review is made of the various forms which exercise may take, both in health and disease, in the special supplement on ATHLETICS AND REMEDIAL EXERCISES.

EXOPHTHALMIC GOITER. This is another name for the disorder commonly known as GRAVES' DISEASE (q.v.).

EXOPHTHALMOS. This means protusion of the eyeballs. (*See also* GRAVES' DISEASE.)

EXOSTOSIS. Exostosis is literally a "growing-out of bone." It is an innocent bone tumor, often like a little hardcapped mushroom, growing from the surface of a bone and forming a knob which, if at all superficial, can be felt through the skin. Such tumors occur characteristically on the skull and the shoulder blade. They are in no way dangerous and never become malignant. If there are good grounds for it, they can be removed by operation; otherwise they should be left alone.

EXPECTORANT. Any drug which aids the removal of catarrhal matter and phlegm from the bronchial tubes is called an expectorant. These drugs are not all alike in their way of acting upon the body; in fact, some have a very complicated mode of action. The only direct expectorants are those which can be inhaled as a vapor, thus causing the drug to come into close contact with the inflamed bronchial tubes. In this group are included the balsams, such as compound tincture of benzoin and balsam of tolu, eucalyptus, menthol, turpentine, and benzoic acid.

An indirect expectorant is taken internally and its action is carried out by the blood circulation. Some drugs, such as senega and squills, are termed stimulating expectorants because they increase the flow of blood, and this in turn increases the amount of expectoration in the bronchial tubes and so aids its removal. Ipecacuanha is a valuable expectorant, especially in a dry cough, as it causes an outpouring of soothing sputum in the throat and gives great relief. (*See also* BRONCHITIS; COUGH).

EXPECTORATION. This is the medical term used for the act of spitting. Expectoration may vary a great deal in character and extent in accordance with the state of the lungs. (*See also* BRONCHITIS; SPUTUM; TUBERCULOSIS.)

EXTRACT. A large number of drugs in medicine are used in the form of an extract. This is a concentrated preparation of the active part of the crude drug. Extracts are made by several methods. Some drugs are treated with boiling water and allowed to evaporate until the proper strength is reached; others are treated with alcohol or ether. (*See also* DRUGS.)

EXTRAVASATION. This term means the escape and flowing over into the surrounding tissues of any of the fluids of the body that are contained in an artery, or a vessel such as the bladder. Extravasation is usually the result of a tearing of the tissues, which may be brought about by injury or disease; or the break in the walls of a vessel or organ may be due to internal pressure.

Blood is the most abundant fluid in the body and it is by far the commonest to be extravasated. A good example of this is an ordinary bruise, which shows the discoloration of the surrounding tissues owing to the blood escaping from the ruptured blood vessels. Extravasation of urine takes place when the bladder or the urethra is ruptured, and bile may be extravasated from the intestinal tract owing to perforation. (*See also* BLADDER; BRUISE; HEMORRHAGE.)

EXTREMITY. The word extremity is generally used to describe the arms and legs. The arms are termed the upper extremities and the legs the lower extremities, but the word may be applied also to the hands or feet.

EXUDATE. Exudate describes pus or matter which exudes or is poured out from an inflamed area or from a septic wound. Exudates are found in large quantities in cases of pluerisy, which is an inflammation of the pleural cavity; they are found also in the pericardium in pericarditis. (*See also* EMPHYSEMA; PERICARDITIS; PLEURISY; SEPSIS.)

EYE. The apparatus with which we see consists of the *eye* itself, the *optic nerve,* which is the special nerve supplying the eye, and the *occipital lobes* of the brain, which lie in the lower part of the back of the skull. The eye forms pictures of objects looked at, the nerve passes them on to the brain, and the occipital lobes receive the picture-messages and interpret them.

The *eyeball* (*see* illustration on page 261) lies in a bony cavity or *orbit* in the front of the skull. The eyeball is, roughly speaking, a round ball with a slight bulge in the front, known as the *cornea*. This is the membrane through which we see, the window of the eye. It covers the *pupil* and *iris*. The pupil is the round black part of the eye, and is simply a hole in the center of the iris, which is the colored part of the eye. The *sclerotic,* or white of the eye, surrounds the pupil and iris; it is formed of thick white fibrous tissue.

The cornea, in health, is a perfectly transparent membrane through which the light passes. The sclerotic and the cornea together form the first coat of the eye.

The eyeball is divided into two parts. First, a large division at the back, called the posterior chamber, which is filled with a perfectly clear jelly (*vitreous humour*), and secondly, a smaller division at the front, called the anterior chamber, which is filled with a clear watery fluid (*aqueous humour*). The division between the two

chambers consists of the *lens* and the structures which hold it in place.

The iris, or colored part of the eye, lies behind the cornea. It consists of a circular curtain of delicate muscle fibers, with the *pupil* in the middle. The muscle fibers are arranged in two layers: a circular layer, arranged in rings, which when it contracts makes the pupil smaller, and a radially arranged layer (i.e., the fibers stretch from the pupil to the outer edge of the iris) which on contracting makes the pupil larger. The function of these muscles is to permit the required amount of light to reach the eye—more in a dim light, less in a bright light—so that the delicate retina shall not be damaged. The color of the eye depends on the amount of coloring matter in the iris.

Lens. Immediately behind the iris lies the lens, which is formed of transparent crystalline material. It is convex at the front and somewhat more so at the back. It is held in place by a transparent membrane called the *capsule,* which encloses the lens and passes off as the *suspensory ligament* to be attached to the *ciliary* processes (described later). To use a rough illustration, the lens may represent a person, the capsule a hammock, the suspensory ligament the ropes holding it up, and the ciliary processes the apple trees to which the hammock is slung. To make the illustration more correct, one should imagine a circular body in a circular hammock which is slung by ropes from all sides to trees growing in a circle. The suspensory ligament and the lens form the partition between the anterior and posterior chambers of the eye. The suspensory ligament passes to the back of the ciliary body; on contraction of the ciliary muscle the ligament is relaxed and the lens becomes more convex, or, in other words, bulges more.

Choroid. The middle coat of the eye is formed of the *choroid,* which is black owing to its containing much coloring matter; it also contains a large number of blood vessels. As it passes forwards to the front of the eye, just within the edge of the white, the choroid is thickened and raised into numerous ridges called the *ciliary processes* or *ciliary body*. This forms the thickened circular front edge of the choroid coat and consists of blood vessels and circular muscles, which by their contraction tend to lessen the ring of the ciliary body, and so cause relaxation of the suspensory ligament of the lens. The iris is a continuation of the front part of the ciliary body.

Retina. The inner coat of the eye is that formed by the *retina.* This consists of a very delicate layer of cells forming the ends of the optic nervefibres. These enter the eye at the back in a fairly large bundle, and then spread out in all directions so as to cover the choroid with a pale delicate membrane. The structure of the retina can only be made out with the microscope, and is very complicated. It is in the retina that impressions of sight are started. All points on the retina are not equally sensitive to light, and one point is totally insensitive, namely, the place where the optic nerve enters. The midpoint, or very near, is the most sensitive. On examination, it may be seen as a yellowish area and is called the macula lutea, or simply the *macula.*

Eyelids. The eye is protected in front by the eyelids, which consist of a fold of skin strengthened by a very thin piece of cartilage and lined by a thin transparent membrane called the *conjunctiva.* Where this reaches the inner margins of the lids it is folded on itself to cover the white of the eye as far as the cornea. It contains many glands which produce mucus; this acts as an oiling fluid, and thus enables the eyeball to move easily and without rubbing in its socket.

Tear gland. The eyeball is also oiled by the *lachrymal gland,* or *teargland,* which lies in the outer and upper part of the orbit. The tears bathe the front of the eye, and then flow away through two little tubes called *canaliculi.* The entrances to these are situated just opposite to each other on the corner of the eyelids near the nose. They enter the side of a little bag, called the *lachrymal sac* or *tear sac,* which drains into the nose. If the tears are produced too rapidly, they flood the tubes and overflow on to the cheeks.

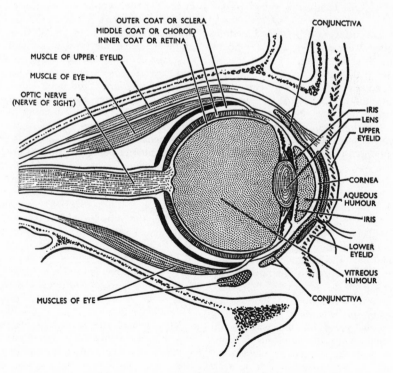

The Eye.

How the Eye Works. The work of the eye is to take pictures of external objects and convey them to the brain. It acts in the manner of a camera. The white of the eye is the box; the choroid is the black lining which prevents the reflection of light, which would spoil the clearness of the picture; and the retina is the sensitive plate which records the picture. The iris acts as the stop, which is regulated automatically; in a poor light it is opened widely to allow as much light as possible to enter; in a bright light it is made smaller. The lens collects the light rays so that they come together to a point on the surface of the retina, or "plate," and so form a clear image.

Bringing together of the light rays is done in this way: if a ray of light passes from one medium to another—for instance, from air into water or glass—the light rays are bent at an angle. (This is easily understood if a stick is held straight down in a foot or two of water. It appears to bend at the point where it enters the water.) Also, on leaving a medium the rays are again bent. This bending is called *refraction*.

If the two surfaces of the second medium are parallel to one another, as in a window-pane, the direction of the rays on leaving is also parallel. But if the glass is curved and the curves are of a different degree or are in opposite directions, the rays converge (come together), or diverge (part), as they leave the glass. Thus, in an ordinary magnifying glass the two surfaces are curved in opposite directions, forming what is called a convex lens, and it is found that if parallel rays of light enter such a lens at one surface, they tend to bend towards each other as they leave the lens from the opposite side, and meet in a point. This is known as the *focal point,* and rays of light are said to be *focused* at that point. The focal point varies in distance from the lens according to the degree of curvature of the two surfaces of the lens.

In the eye, refraction of light occurs not only in the lens itself but in all the structures it passes on the way to the retina—the cornea, the aqueous humour, the lens, and the vitreous humour. It is clear that, as the various objects seen are at various distances from the eye, a fixed

degree of refraction for these structures will not be correct for focussing all objects. In a camera, a correct focus is obtained by moving the plate or film towards or away from the lens; in the eye this cannot be done, and the only refracting medium that can be altered is the lens. The curve of this is changed by the contraction or relaxation of the ciliary muscle, to which the lens is attached. The lens is not a hard body, but pliable and elastic, so that if the capsule is tightened the lens is flattened, and if it is "slacked off" the lens consequently becomes thicker and more curved.

This alteration in the curvature, and so therefore in the length of focus, of the eye is called *accommodation;* it is accompanied by alteration in the size of the pupil, which enlarges when near objects are looked at and contracts for distant objects. If the accommodation is faulty, either myopia (short sight) or hypermetropia (long sight) occurs. Presbyopia (old sight) has the same effect as long sight; it is a perfectly normal change which comes on in middle life, and is due to gradual hardening of the lens.

The eye is moved by six muscles. Four of these, called the recti or straight muscles, arise from the back of the eye-socket and are attached respectively into the upper, lower, inner, and outer sides of the eyeball. The other two muscles are the oblique muscles, so-called because they are attached to the sides of the upper and lower parts of the eyeball. Squint is caused by one muscle being too short, by its acting powerfully, or being paralyzed.

In order that man, although provided with two eyes, shall see only one image of any object, a very exact co-ordination between the muscles of the two eyes is necessary. To ensure this, the nerve supply and action of the muscles are so arranged as to cause both eyes to move in the same direction at the same time. If for any reason this power is interfered with, the eyes move at slightly different times, and a double or blurred image is produced.

Very few of the lower animals possess this power of binocular vision, as it is called, as their eyes do not face in the same direction. The eyes of man, being slightly distant from each other, produce a slightly different image, and this gives an appearance of solidity to the object. The principle of this is shown by the stereoscope; a single photograph normally gives a "flat" effect when looked at, but when two copies of the same photograph are placed side by side and viewed independently by each eye at the same time a "solid" effect is obtained.

Binocular vision also enables man to judge distances; a man who has lost the sight of one eye suffers the handicap of being unable to do this with any accuracy.

Diseases of the Eye are described separately under the headings BLACK EYE; BLINDNESS; CATARACT; CONJUNCTIVITIS; ECTROPION; ENTROPION; EYE, INJURIES OF; EYELIDS; GLAUCOMA; IRITIS, etc.

Injuries of the Eye. *Every injury of the eye, however slight, should have immediate attention.* Strict adherence to this rule may not only prevent blindness in the injured eye, but may prevent the other eye becoming involved as well. No first-aid treatment beyond that suggested should be attempted, and hands, dressing, etc., should be scrupulously clean.

Foreign Body. The most frequent accident that happens to the eye is the entrance of a foreign body. This causes considerable pain; the eye waters freely, and sometimes, if the nose is sharply blown, the foreign body will be dislodged and washed away. The eye should not be rubbed. If it is within the lower lid, it is easily removed with the corner of a clean handkerchief.

Frequently, however, the foreign body "wedges itself" under the upper lid. One method of removal, which is especially useful in the case of children or nervous patients, is to introduce a drop of castor oil or olive oil into the eye. This may entangle the foreign body and float it out. Another method is to pull the upper eyelid gently outwards, then push up the lower lid under it and let go. As the lid descends, the eyelashes brush the inner surface of the upper lid and may dislodge the foreign body. The surgical method is that of eversion, or turning out of the upper eyelid. This needs considerable care and skill, though in expert hands, it is not an uncomfortable procedure.

A foreign body may wound the covering of the eyeball and remain there without

penetrating the eye. This is a frequent accident among coal miners and engineers. No attempt should be made to remove the foreign body; the patient should be taken to a doctor immediately.

Bruising of the Eye. In this condition the eye is red and waters copiously, while exposure to light is painful. The treatment is simple; it consists of rest and the wearing of an eyeshade for a few days.

If the bruise is severe, damage varying in severity may be done to the inner parts of the eye; therefore medical advice should be sought.

Wounds of the Eye. These are naturally of various kinds, according to what damaging agent has produced the wound, and what parts of the eye are involved.

There are two dangers which are to be feared: first, infection of the wounded eye; secondly, inflammation of the sound eye, which is most serious, as it may result in blindness. In severe cases of wounds of the eye, especially where there is injury of the surrounding parts in addition, the patient may show signs of shock.

The *first-aid* treatment is to cover the eye with a pad of boric gauze, soaked in warm boiled water, and apply a bandage. Shock, if present, should be treated, and the doctor called in immediately. The *surgical* treatment depends entirely on what part of the eye is involved; each case is treated on its merits. When the foreign body remains within the eye, it must at all costs be removed. In 75 per cent of cases the foreign body is a fragment of iron or steel, which can be removed by an electromagnet. An eye which is hopelessly damaged should be removed, or the sound eye may become inflamed and sight be lost completely.

Unequal Pupils (Anisocoria). In this condition the pupils of the eye differ in size. The causes are various: the uses of a drug which temporarily causes the pupil of the eye to expand, a marked difference in the strength of the eyes, one-sided blindness, and local injury. General causes may be aneurism or diseases of the nervous system, of which tabes dorsalis, general paralysis, and disseminated sclerosis are the commonest. It does not, of course, follow that every sufferer from one or other of these diseases has anisocoria. It may also occur in healthy people, and then has no special significance.

EYE, ARTIFICIAL. After the operation for removal of an eye has been performed it is usual for a patient to wear an artificial eye. This may first be used about a month or six weeks after the operation. If the eye has been removed because of injury or a tumor, and there has been little previous inflammation, the socket soon becomes "hardened;" but if there has been much previous inflammation, a longer time must elapse before an artificial eye can be worn with comfort. The hardening process can be hastened if the patient will—as soon as the surgeon advises it—expose the socket to the air as soon as possible.

An artificial eye is a thin shell of glass made to resemble as closely as possible the visible part of the sound eye. Not only are the size of the eye and color of the iris considered, but the exact shade of the white is matched, and the pupils are matched in size. It is advisable to choose an eye which is slightly smaller than the normal one; an eye which is exactly the same size and which for this reason looks less artificial to the patient, often produces just the very effect he desires to avoid. It tends to press the lower lid too far downwards, and to stick in the socket, instead of moving freely with the other eye.

To insert the eye, it should be held between the finger and thumb and the large portion of white passed under the upper lid; then the lower lid should be drawn down and the eye gently rolled downwards, when it will slip into place. To remove the eye, the lower lid is drawn down, a small blunt "lifter" (the bent part of a hairpin is very convenient) gently pushed underneath it, and the eye held between this and the thumb. Then by a slight rolling movement the eye is removed, the upper part last. It is a advisable to lean forwards over the bed when taking out the eye, so that it is not broken if dropped.

An artificial eye should be removed every night and thoroughly washed and dried. It should not be left to soak in water or disinfectant fluid, as is sometimes done. The socket also should be well washed out every night and a weak astringent (drying) lotion or drops inserted.

The washing of the tears over an artificial eye gradually dulls it, so that after about a year it will need repolishing. If one can afford it, it is a good idea to have more than one artificial eye in use, in case of breakage or repolishing.

Another and newer form of artificial eye is made in the shape of a hollow eyeball, flattened behind. It is said to be more comfortable than the older type on account of the rounded edge, and to look more natural since it does not present the "sunken" appearance characteristic of the flat artificial eye. The old type, however, is considered more suitable where there is still a shrunken natural eye in place in the socket, or when only a partial removal has been carried out.

EYE BATH. The best way to apply a soothing lotion to the eye is by means of an eye bath. The best type is made of glass and should be shaped to fit the socket of the eye. The glass should be filled with warm boracic lotion and applied to the eye while leaning over a basin. The eye must be kept open as wide as possible and the head tilted well back. The rim of the eye bath should fit tightly against the face so that while the head is tilted backwards no lotion is able to escape. This flushing out of the eye should be repeated several times on each occasion, the eye bath being rinsed out and refilled with lotion each time.

EYEBROW. The eyebrows consist of ridges of slightly thickened skin covered with strong hairs; the latter are so arranged that they prevent the sweat from the forehead from trickling into the eyes and obscuring or irritating them. Another useful function of the eyebrows is shown by the way they are drawn down as a protection when the eyes are exposed to strong light.

The eyebrows give much expression to the face and their movements are often an eloquent indication of our emotions or mental processes. They can, for example, express concentrated thought, incredulity, annoyance, contempt, and so on, almost as plainly as words can do. The blank countenance caused by the fashionable plucked eyebrows is a study in contrast.

The eyebrows are one of man's prerogatives. Some birds have specially arranged feathers above their eyes, and the seal has a few stiff hairs; but no animal, not even the higher apes, can lay claim to true eyebrows.

EYELID. The eyelids act as a protective covering for the eyes. They are made up of four sorts of tissue: the skin; the tarsus or cartilage, which gives strength to the eyelids; muscles, which control their movements; and the conjunctiva, the thin, moist membrane lining the eyelids.

The skin of the eyelids is finer than the ordinary skin of the body; it has no hairs (except the eyelashes) and no sweatglands. It is not firmly attached to the tissues underneath, as is the body skin, but moves easily over the tarsus. It is owing to this fact that the blood vessels below can be easily damaged, and also that the blood flows out rapidly—hence the speed with which a "black eye" appears after a blow.

At the edges of the lids are the eyelashes, which have the important function of keeping the eyes free from foreign bodies, both solid and liquid, and also from the germs of disease. To place a drop of water on the outside of a person's upper eyelid and watch it lying on the eyelashes without entering the eye is a demonstration of the perfection of the screen formed by the lashes. Behind the lashes are glands which produce an oily or waxy fluid; this does not mix with the tears, but helps to prevent them from running over the margins of the lids and down the cheeks.

The tarsus, or cartilage, of the eyelid allows the lids to be closed without puckering or turning in upon the eye. It is curved to the shape of the eye. Its importance is perhaps more readily understood in cases of disease when, owing to various causes, it presses upon the eye, or when it cannot prevent the eyelids turning outwards or inwards upon the eye. (*See also* ECTROPION; ENTROPION.)

The eyelids are moved by two muscles, one of which passes round both lids, on the outside of the tarsus, and opens and closes the lids as required. The nerve to this muscle is the facial nerve, and when this is paralysed the lower lid hangs down

and tears run over the cheek. This condition is called ectropion (q.v.). The other muscle is the muscle which carries out the involuntary blinking of the eye. This allows the moist inner surface of the upper eyelid to sweep the eye and keep it from becoming dried by exposure to the air or injured by other organisms. Since it is activated by a special nerve of its own, it will be seen that the actions of blinking and closing the eye are carried out by two different mechanisms.

When the eyelids are closed in sleep the upper and lower lids meet exactly, so that the eye is protected and kept moist. At the same time the eyeball turns upwards, still further to protect the eye from possible injury. (*See also* CONJUNCTIVA; CONJUNCTIVITIS; LACHRYMAL APPARATUS; TEARS.)

Injuries of the Eyelids. These are treated on ordinary surgical lines, great care being taken, in the repair of the lids, that as little deformity as possible is left. In every case, especially in burns, care is taken that the eyeball is not left exposed; otherwise there may be grave danger to the sight. (*See also* BLACK EYE; BLINDNESS—BLINDING FROM LIGHTNING, ETC.)

Diseases of the Eyelids. *See* ECTROPION; ENTROPION.)

Sore Eyelids (Blepharitis). A scaly, crusted, or ulcerated inflammation of the margin of the eyelids may occur in people of any age, but especially in delicate children, and seems almost invariably to be associated with a debilitated condition, either local or general. To cure this condition may require several months, and it often returns.

Treatment. The first and most important thing is to remove the cause, since local treatment alone is useless. Every effort should be made to improve the general health, which is, as has been said, invariably below par. Good food, plenty of sleep, fresh air day and night, a daily warm (not hot) bath and a brisk rubbing with a rough towel afterwards, exercise (arranged to suit the individual), regulation of the bowels, and so on should have most careful attention. Tonics are very useful, those containing iron, arsenic, and strychnine being the most valuable. Cod-liver oil is also excellent. The eyes should be examined, and glasses should be worn if necessary.

As regards local treatment, this should always be under medical direction, though the patient may help greatly by following instructions as to bathing the eyes and by perseverance in treatment. The patient should, with as great attention to cleanliness as possible, bathe the lid margins several times daily, in order to remove all crusts and scales. Warm water which has been boiled may be used, or a weak solution of bicarbonate of soda. After all crusts have been removed, apply an ointment. A stimulating ointment such as that of the yellow oxide of mercury does a great deal of good. In very obstinate cases the lid may be treated (by the doctor only) with a silver preparation, such as argyrol or protargol. Care must be taken that the lachrymal (tear) apparatus is in good order.

Chronic inflammation of the eyelids may, if untreated, lead to injury of the roots of the eyelashes, or to deformities of the lids.

When the whole eyelid is inflamed as well as the margins of the lids, the condition is called tarsitis. The whole lid is thickened, heavy and swollen. In rare cases, the inflammation grows quickly worse, and there is a danger that the cartilage of the eyelid will suppurate and slough or come away, so that the lid will remain as a lax flap. The eyelashes are generally lost in these cases. The treatment is the same as that of an abscess—opening and the application of hot boracic fomentations.

Twitching Eyelids (Blepharospasm). There is often a twitching or fluttering of the eyelid, caused by spasm of some or all of the fibers of the muscle which controls the movements of the eyelid. It is caused by irritation, such as that caused by a speck of grit in the eye, or by eyestrain, especially in uncorrected long-sight. It may also be due to irritation from decayed teeth, by ear, nose, and throat diseases, neuralgia or nerve tumors, "habit spasm," chorea (St. Vitus's dance), and, very often, by mental strain and debility.

Treatment. The treatment should aim at correcting the cause. A careful general examination should reveal any cause of irrita-

tion, and this should be treated. Faulty hygiene should be corrected, and, especially in nervous and debilitated patients, plenty of rest should be ordered. Tea and coffee are forbidden by many physicians, as they are apt to excite the nervous system.

Swelling of the Eyelids. Swelling of the eyelids occurs from many causes. Damage, acute inflammation, and other diseases in the neighborhood of the eye all cause swelling; these, however, are discussed elsewhere, and are accompanied by the other signs of inflammation, or at least of irritation—redness, heat, tenderness, and pain. Sometimes, however, the eyelids may swell without any other symptoms.

Such swelling is frequently seen in a mild form in elderly people, and is due simply to weakness and loosening of the tissues, not to any disease.

Swelling of the eyelids which occurs in the morning and gradually passes off during the day always suggests nephritis, which may occur in various forms at any time of life. A person with this form of swelling should always be carefully examined by a doctor.

"Cold edema" is a curious condition which is at present not understood. It attacks both upper and lower lids on both sides; sometimes the swelling is so great as to suggest erysipelas, but there is neither redness nor fever. It is rather like the white swelling seen in nephritis but is much greater and does not lessen as the day goes on. Sooner or later the eyes become almost closed up. No external treatment has any effect. Operations to remove some of the eyelid tissue have been performed, but are only temporarily successful. Lately, injections of alcohol into the tissues have been tried and are said to have produced a cure in some cases.

Puffy Eyelids. The tear ducts, which drain the tears away from the eye, open into the nose. If there is injury to some of the bones of the nose, so that air can pass from the nose through the tearduct and between the tissues of the eyelids, these may become puffed up with air, and on touching them a peculiar crackling sensation is felt. This generally comes on when the patient first blows his nose after the injury.

Treatment. A firm pad and bandage are

put over the eye, so that the air will be gradually pressed back into the nose; and the patient must refrain from blowing his nose for two or three days.

Herpes (Shingles). This disorder is fairly common on the face. It begins in the usual way, neuralgia, in this case on one side of the forehead and in the eye. After a day or two a crop of little blisters, or vesicles, appears on the forehead and scalp, on the eyelids, down the nose on the same side, and possibly on the cornea (the transparent membrane in front of the eye). If this is attacked, the eye may be badly damaged. (*See also* CORNEA.)

Treatment. The skin vesicles should be protected from infection by a dusting powder or ointment which contains menthol and cocaine, in addition to the usual treatment for shingles. (*See also* HERPES; SHINGLES; STY.)

Skin Diseases of the Eyelids. The skin of the eylid may be attacked by any skin disease which is present on the face; these are treated by the usual methods and only a few points need special mention.

In *eczema,* lotions should not be used on the eyelids, as they may possibly be dropped into the eyes and so cause irritation. Ointments are used instead.

Erysipelas on the face frequently causes so great a swelling of the eyelid that the eye is closed. In itself, the swelling need cause no alarm, but suppuration sometimes occurs, which may lead to sloughing or casting off of the eyelid; or it may extend to the eye and so for various reasons cause blindness. (*See also* ERYSIPELAS.)

An *abscess* may occur on the lid. This is treated in the usual way. The swelling of the lid may in this case be very great in comparison with the seriousness of the condition; but it should always be treated with care in view of the possible danger to the sight. (*See also* ABSCESS.)

Chalazion (Tarsal Cyst). This is a disease of the eyelids which is frequently mistaken for a sty. It is caused by the blockage of a gland, the contents of which are prevented from escaping, so that a cyst appears on the eyelid. It is about the size of a small pea.

It differs from a sty in that the hairbulbs on the eyelid are not affected; the cyst "points" on the under surface behind the eyelashes, and appears as a bluish inflamed spot. It is readily infected by germs, forming a tiny abscess, which bursts and then heals, but often leaves a thickened wall.

Treatment. If the cyst is small and there is no gathering it may be gently rubbed with an antiseptic ointment, such as a mild mercury or a weak iodine ointment. This is not a certain cure, but may with patience and time bring about a good result. A quicker method is to have the cyst removed by a small operation (*See also* STY.)

Eyelids Which Do Not Meet (Lagophthalmos). This is the condition in which the edges of the eyelids do not come together when the eye is closed.

It is very frequently seen in young sleeping infants, and then requires no treatment, as it passes off after the first few weeks. Care should, however, be taken that nothing can touch the eyes, or damage may be done.

Sometimes the lids are too short and cannot meet, either from an abnormality in development (which is rare), or from disease, a burn, or other injury.

Treatment. This varies with the cause of the condition. If the lids are too short, either naturally or from injury, the only treatment is to keep the eye clean and moist by regular bathing with a mild boracic lotion. If there are other conditions present, such as blepharitis (inflammation of the lid margins) or any skin disease, these should be treated, or an operation may be performed.

Distichiasis and Trichiasis. True distichiasis is a natural deformity of the eyelashes in which a second row of fine, delicate hairs is found behind the normal lashes. As a rule, they cause no trouble, and they should be left alone, unless they start growing, when the treatment should be as below.

Distichiasis is also seen in some diseases, in cases of persistent irritation of the conjunctiva (possibly after marginal inflammation), burns or injuries, but most often in cases of trachoma (granular conjunctivitis, where the fine hairs are stimulated to unnatural growth. With this is also seen *trichiasis,* which denotes a faulty position of the eyelashes: because of the scarring and shrinking of the conjunctiva, one or more of the eyelashes, perhaps the entire row, is drawn backwards till they come into contact with the eye.

Treatment. It will readily be seen that a patient so afflicted will be always, in a state of miserable discomfort. If only one or two lashes are at fault, these may be removed with forceps. If more are involved, the lashes may be destroyed by electrolysis. If the whole row, together with the lid edge, is turned in, an operation should be performed to put matters right. (*See also* ECTROPION; ENTROPION.)

EYESHADE or eyepatch. The most popular types of eyeshade are made from celluloid or from light cardboard. They can be had in various shapes and in dark-green or flesh-color. Some are made in cap shapes which fit the head, while others can be tied on with tapes. If the eye is discharging, it is not advisable to wear an eyepatch without a dressing of some absorbent material. A small shade to cover one eye can be fitted to a spectacle frame, but it must cover the eye completely.

EYESTRAIN. By eyestrain is meant simply that the eyes are suffering from extreme tiredness. This may be because they have had to do an exceptional amount of work without rest, or that there is something the matter with the eyes themselves. They may be shortsighted or long-sighted or suffering from some disease which makes their muscles less strong than they should be.

If there is anything wrong with the eyes, organic or otherwise, eyestrain is certain to result if the eyes are used a very great deal. This is of particular significance in certain trades requiring precision work, such as watchmaking, and in the printing and publishing trades.

Symptoms. The commonest symptom of eyestrain is a tired, burning, or pricking feeling in the eyes after they have been used for near work such as reading. A habit of frowning, puckering up the eyes,

blinking or rubbing the eyes should lead one to suspect that the eyes are being strained. Red eyelids are often a symptom of eyestrain, and headache over the eyes, on the top of the head, and sometimes at the back of the head on both sides is a very usual result of eye troubles.

Treatment. When it is obvious that the eyes are being strained and it is necessary to go on with close eye-work, the cause of the strain must be sought out and cured. It is not always necessary to rush to glasses for a cure, as very often the weakness of the eyes is only part of a general reduced state of health, and the eyes will strengthen as the general health improves. For a general account of the eye, its diseases and their treatment, *see* the articles ACCOMMODATION; EYE; EYE-BATH; EYELID; EYE-SHADE; VISION; and other articles referred to therein.

Some simple rules are ususally observed in offices and places where people have to do close eye-work. For instance, lights must be shaded so that the bare lights do not catch and attract the eye. This is the reason why lampshades should be used over bulbs, even in a house. The full light from a lamp should not fall on a polished surface on which writing materials or books, etc., are to be used, or the glare will impede vision. The light should, of course, fall on the book or sewing, and not on the person reading or sewing. To secure this, place the light behind one when reading. A lot of eye trouble is caused by lights which are too dim, as well as by those that are too dazzling.

EYE-TOOTH. The eye-tooth, or canine-tooth, is the third from the middle line of the upper teeth. It has a particularly long root which is directed towards the eye, and it often happens that an abscess at the point of this root causes the eye to appear swollen and bruised or discolored —in fact, not unlike a "black eye." (*See also* TEETH.)

FACE. The prominent bony parts of the face, such as the ridge which is covered by the eyebrows and the

nose, cheekbones and chin, are the means by which the character of the face varies. The square face and slanting eyes of Far

Eastern races characterize, for example, a distinct type, while the high cheekbones of the Scots are representative of another type. The shape of the face is decided by nature, but the expression or general appearance of the face can be, and is, altered by the character and circumstances of life of its owner, and in this connection health is important. Faces in which the brows are so often set in lines of pain that the lines become permanent, or which are covered with unhealthy skin, cannot be as attractive as those of normally healthy and happy people.

Skin of the Face. The skin of the face is thin and delicate compared with skin on other parts of the body, but as it has to stand constant exposure to the weather and to dust and dirt, it is well supplied with sweat—and fat—glands. These should always be kept in good working order, because when they become blocked up with sweat and oil that should have been washed away they develop acne and other disfiguring conditions. As a rule, wounds and cuts on the face heal up very quickly owing to the fact that the face is well supplied with blood vessels. On the other hand, any serious septic condition, such as a carbuncle, may have grave results, owing to the fact that the veins of the face communicate with those inside the skull. For this reason an insect sting on the face should always be carefully treated, especially if it is on the upper lip or cheek, near the nose.

Nerves and Muscles of the Face. The face is well supplied with nerves and muscle, and the interplay of these muscles causes the changing expressions of the face. The most important nerve which controls these muscles is the facial nerve, technically known as the seventh cranial nerve. It comes from the back part of the brain, passes through the skull to the ear, and continues to the face round the edge of the jaw. Injuries or wounds of this part of the face may have very serious results, as damage to the facial nerve may leave one side of the face absolutely expressionless, such as happens in facial paralysis or Bell's palsy.

Malformations of the Face. The most common malformation of the face is harelip, a condition in which the two edges of

the groove of the upper lip do not join together. This condition is congenital (present as birth), and is often accompanied by cleft palate, another common deformity.

Lupus Vulgaris, or tuberculosis of the skin, is more frequent on the face than on any other part of the body. Small tumors may also cause a great deal of discomfort, and many people are afflicted with birthmarks, such as moles or port wine stains. (*See also* BIRTHMARKS; CLEFT PALATE; HARELIP; LUPUS.)

Face Cream. Face cream is extensively used to protect the skin and to give it a smooth appearance. Cold creams may be used to cleanse the skin; as a rule they are applied at bedtime, after the face has been thoroughly washed and dried. Nongreasy or vanishing face creams are used during the day as a foundation for powder. It is advisable for every woman to find out the make of face cream suitable for her own particular type of skin.

FACIAL NERVE. The facial nerve is the seventh cranial nerve: it controls the muscles of the face, scalp, and ears. Curiously enough, one small strand of the facial nerve carries the sense of taste for the front half of the tongue. The facial nerve goes through a canal in the temporal bone, close to the cavity of the middle ear, and then spreads through the parotid salivary gland into a network that is distributed to the muscles of the face. It may be damage in inflammatory conditions of the ear or in operations, especially the radical mastoid operation on the ear. A severe chill affecting the side of the face may also cause paralysis of the facial nerve (Bell's palsy); this, however, is only temporary. (*See also* FACIAL PARALYSIS.)

FACIAL PARALYSIS. Facial paralysis, or Bell's palsy, occurs most frequently in adults, although cases in children are not unknown, especially after diphtheria. In adults the commonest cause is neuritis or some inflammation of the facial nerve at the point where it enters the skull, just behind the ear. Other cases are due to disease of the middle ear or to the radical mastoid operation. It may also be due to direct injury of the nerve or to brain diseases, such as meningitis and concussion, or to factures of the skull. Facial paralysis due to inflammation or neuritis usually comes on fairly quickly and can be readily recognized fter a few days.

Symptoms. It is possible that the patient has been sitting in a draft and begins to feel pain behind the ear. Next day, or the day after, he may find that one side of his face is stiff. There may also be a rash on the face. The condition is nearly always one-sided. On eating, the food may accumulate between the tongue and the cheek, because the muscles are not able to clear it away as they normally do automatically in eating. The inside of the cheek may also be bitten, because it falls flabbily within range of the teeth. The condition is tested by making the patient laugh, wrinkle his forehead, whistle, and close his eyes. The laugh will move the muscles of one side of the face only; the patient cannot whistle; the wrinkling of the forehead will be one-sided; the eye on the affected side will not close properly, and the eyeball will roll upwards when an attempt is made to close the eye. The senses of taste and hearing may be affected.

Treatment. Temporary facial paralysis usually clears up in about a month to six months' time. If it goes on longer it may become incurable, so that an operation should be done to give relief or cure. In the early days of the condition the patient should be kept in a warm room—though not necessarily in bed—and heat should be applied over the painful region. Massage and electricity in the form of mild galvanism are useful after the inflammation has subsided.

FACIAL SPASM. Spasms and twitching of the muscles of the face are of two sorts. The first sort are true muscular spasms, due to some irritation or injury of the facial nerve; while the other kind are nervous in origin and are called *tics,* under which heading they are described. (*See also* FIDGETS; ST. VITUS'S DANCE.)

FAINTING. Fainting implies a temporary loss of consciousness. The medical term for this is "syncope." It is due to the supply of blood to the brain becoming insufficient. This often occurs in health when we rise suddenly from a chair and for a moment feel unsteady. It happens, too, when we are compelled to stand still for long periods, as in the case of soldiers

on parade or spectators at a football match. In both cases the fainting is due to blood draining away from the brain and pooling in the abdomen or legs. It naturally happens more readily in people who are unfit from illness or sedentary habits. Very rarely, fainting attacks may be a symptom of heart disease and sometimes they are in truth epileptic disturbances, yet often pass unrecognized as such. Strong emotion, such as a great fright, is a common cause; so is physical injury or pain. The complete muscular relaxation which takes place in a hot bath is sometimes the cause of fainting, and people who are in a weak state of health should avoid taking prolonged hot baths. There are also certain drugs which have an effect on the action of the heart, and it is not unusual for excess of smoking to cause a feeling of faintness.

Symptoms. As a rule there is a warning feeling of sinking and the vision becomes blurred; finally everything becomes black and complete unconsciousness takes place. A person who is about to faint usually turns very pale and staggers a little or leans against something for support before falling to the ground. A person in a faint lies very limp and still; his skin is cold and clammy and his breathing is very feeble. As a rule a fainting fit only lasts a few moments, at the end of which the patient is seen to make slight movements of the hands and lips. The pulse recovers and a little color is seen returning to the cheeks, and in a little while the patient recovers and is able to sit up.

Treatment. The patient should be carried out into the open air if possible and laid flat on the back. Any tight clothing round the neck, such as a collar or neckband, and also any other restricting articles of clothing, such as a belt round the waist or corsets, should be loosened or removed. The blood supply to the brain may be increased by raising the patient's legs. A few teaspoonsful of brandy or other spirits may be given if the patient is able to swallow. It is not advisable to force liquid down the throat of a person in a faint unless he is able to swallow naturally, as choking may take place. Should the faint last long, or should the person be subject to frequent fainting turns, it is advisable to consult a doctor to see whether the cause of them cannot be cured.

FALLING SICKNESS. This is an old popular name for epilepsy (q.v.)

FALLOPIAN TUBES. These are two tubes, one of which is situated on each side of the upper part of the womb, the purpose of which is to conduct the ovum (which is microscopic in size) from the ovary down into the womb. Inflammation of the Fallopian tubes is called salpingitis, and is a serious condition. (*See also* SAL-PINGITIS.)

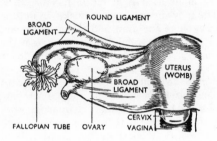

Fallopian Tube.

FALSE PAINS. A few days before child-birth takes place there may be colicky pains in the abdomen which are not true labor pains. These pains are due to contraction of the intestines and are very liable to occur if constipation is present. True labor pains are accompanied by other signs and are more regular in their occurrence. (*See also* LABOR.)

FAMILY PLANNING. Most large cities and many small communities have organizations interested in planned parenthood and if information is desired, it is suggested that they be consulted. If no such organization exists in your community, the request for information may be made directly to the Planned Parenthood Federation, 501 Madison Avenue, New York City.

FARADISM. The electricity produced by an induction coil and employed in medicine is called faradism. It is used in order to produce contraction of the muscles and stimulation of the nerves. (*See also* ELECTRICITY IN MEDICINE.)

FARINACEOUS FOODS. Dishes made from cereals are called farinaceous or starchy foods. The chief cereals are wheat, barley, oats, rye, corn, and rice, while foods such as sago, arrowroot, tapioca, and potatoes are also included. These foods contain a large percentage of carbohydrates, and need to be supplemented with other foods, such as eggs, milk, and butter, in order to provide a full and balanced diet.

FASCIA. This is the name applied to any one of the sheets or bands of tissue which surround and connect up the muscles of the body.

FAT. Fat is made up of glycerine and various fatty acids, some of which are liquid and others solid. Fats vary in consistency, some being soft and flabby, while others are firm and solid. They all melt easily when heat is applied. Alkalis split them up; and certain of the digestive juices called ferments break them down in the body into the different substances of which they are ultimately composed. The chief ferment for digesting fat comes from the gland called the pancreas; this ferment requires to be mixed with bile from the liver before it is able to do its work properly.

Fat is necessary to the body in order to produce heat and energy. Too much fat may be stored up in the tissues of the body instead of being utilized by the body as fuel; this condition is known as obesity. Obesity can be dangerous to health, as well as being a source of discomfort to the individual. Methods of treating this over-fatness will be found under the heading "Obesity."

Fat is used very extensively as a cooking agent in everyday diet. The chief animal fats used in cookery are butter, lard, suet, and dripping from meat. Cod-liver oil and cream are also animal fats. Of vegetable fats the chief are olive oil and margarine, although margarine often contains a proportion of animal fat. Nut-oils are also used, either in the form of oil or in butter form. These frying or cooking fats should be taken into consideration when the diet is being considered, because they add considerably to the amount of fat taken daily with the other food, and it is a common error to assert that no fat is being taken, while actually much of the food is being fried. (*See also* DIGESTION.)

FATIGUE. It is not possible to work

as quickly and as well when you are tired as when you are fresh, for being tired means that the human machine is running down and needs winding up. The best way to wind it up is by allowing it adequate rest. Sleep is as necessary to us as food.

Fatigue in Industry. You cannot do your best work unless you are in your best health. Your "best" is when you rise steadily to the top of your form, not when you start off with a spurt and then slacken speed. The same rule holds good for performances in sport.

The atmosphere in which you do your work is of the greatest importance. The air should be kept constantly fresh, though without drafts. It should be maintained at a moderate temperature, neither too hot nor too cold; and the humidity should be adjusted so that it is neither too damp nor too dry. The air should also be kept as clean as possible and, especially in indoor work, there should be provision for removing dust, smoke, fumes, foul odors, small particles of metals, and other harmful products.

Rest pauses are very important.

So is suitable food.

So is suitable clothing.

Monotony—in everything—is bad. Change in occupation, in temperature, in ventilation, in food, is important; so, of course, is change of posture if the work is sedentary.

Your eyes will be less tired if you look away from your work occasionally, thus giving them a change of focus.

You do better work with shorter hours, especially if there are no rest pauses. And your health is better too.

The lighting is very important. Daylight is better than artificial light. Windows should be clean so that they can let in all the light available.

A clean skin reacts better to ventilation than a dirty one.

That it is in the interests of both employer and employed to get the best output of work with the least amount of fatigue is recognized by many employers nowadays. Truly progressive commercial and manufacturing firms are careful to make proper provision for the well-being of their staff. It is usual among large firms to have rest rooms, a nurse to look after the sick

and give first aid, a cafeteria, provision for a midmorning and midafternoon coffee-break, clubs, organized games and sports grounds, etc. The object of all this is ultimately the maintenance of a high standard of health and happiness among the workers. Good employers realize that their human machines are at least as important as their plant, if not more so, and they find by experience that money spent in giving these facilities to their staff brings its own reward in better health, and therefore better and speedier work.

The study of fatigue is as important in the home as it is in the factory or office. The movements a woman makes in putting things into the oven and taking them out, in cleaning a room, and so on, may be wasteful of energy, and experiments have been made, in what is called "motion study," to find out the least number of movements needed for each operation. Since it is a truism that "a woman's work is never done," it is in each woman's own interest to think out, quite apart from labor-saving appliances, ways in which she can save herself fatigue in her daily work.

FAUCES. Fauces is the name given to the narrow opening between the mouth and the throat. On either side are the pillars of the fauces, in which the *tonsils* are embedded. Above the opening is what is known as the *soft palate,* and below lies the root of the tongue. During an attack of tonsillitis, the fauces are often blocked up by the inflammation of the surrounding tissues and the tonsils. (*See also* TONSIL; TONSILLITIS.)

FAVUS. Favus, like ringworm, is a disease of the skin and hair caused by the growth of a fungus; again like ringworm, it is most common upon the scalp, though it may be found on the nonhairy skin and affecting the nails. Its special feature is the production on the surface of rounded, sulphur-yellow, cup-shaped crusts called *scutula,* which crumble readily. When a scutulum is removed, a moist, inflamed depression in the scalp is seen.

Favus is passed on from one person to another, but it is a remarkable fact that quite often only one in a family will be attacked.

The outlook in favus depends on the treatment. Left to itself the disease goes

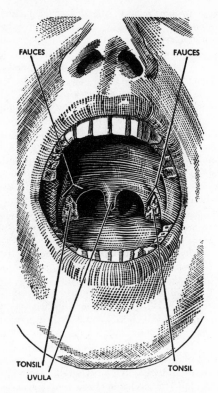

FAUCES   FAUCES

TONSIL   TONSIL
UVULA

Fauces.

on indefinitely; and even with thorough but conservative treatment a bad case may last for very many years.

Treatment. If favus attacks the nonhairy skin only, it is readily cured by the *constant* application of an antiseptic ointment, the time taken for a cure varying from one to eight weeks.

If only a small area of the scalp is affected, it can readily be cured by pulling out the hairs with forceps and thoroughly rubbing in an antiseptic ointment. In widespread cases there are only two methods which are of the slightest practical use, namely, the application of X-rays and of thallium. (*See* RINGWORM for details.)

FEBRIFUGE. A febrifuge is a drug which is given to reduce fever. Some drugs lower the temperature by increasing perspiration, while others act by preventing the body from manufacturing more heat. Quinine, salicylic acid, and aspirin are a few of the better-known drugs employed for this purpose. (*See also* ANTIPYRETIC.)

FECES. Feces is the term applied to the discharges from the bowel, consisting of the part of the food which is undigested and other substances, such as coloring matter (pigment) from the bile and large numbers of bacteria. (*See also* STOOLS.)

FEEBLE-MINDED. The feeble-minded are persons in whose case there exists from birth or from an early age mental defectiveness so pronounced that they require care, supervision, and control for their own protection or for the protection of others. This definition puts in a nutshell the whole history of those unfortunates whose brains have not fully developed, or who have, as a result of some illness or injury to the brain in early childhood, lost the power to think like normal people.

The feeble-minded are unfortunate, first, in that their brains are not normal, and secondly, because only too often the existence of an undeveloped brain is not recognized, and they are branded as lazy and unwilling. This is especially the case when, as so frequently happens, no bodily disease or deformity is present, such as occurs in persons in whom the brain is even less developed. But the trained eye can pick out the feeble-minded at a very early age. Quite often the doctor is consulted because an infant is "backward" and has not sat up, walked, or talked at the proper times. Although this backwardness in development may be due to bodily ill-health or to improper feeding, in the absence of any such obvious cause it is probable that the backwardness is due to poor development of the brain. If there is a family history of nervous or mental trouble, very marked "backwardness" in a child—especially in talking, walking and learning clean habits—must be regarded with very grave suspicion. During infancy and early childhood this "backwardness" becomes more and more pronounced in the case of the feeble-minded.

Such children do badly at school, though not every child who is an apparent dullard at school is feeble-minded; there are thousands of children who, for one reason or another—varying from enlarged tonsils to a too vivid imagination—do badly at school but in later life become excellent citizens holding responsible positions. But it is generally possible by the time a child reaches the second year of school age to find out whether he is incapable of learning his lessons because of a lack of development of his brain, or because there is something else at fault.

Those children who are not, and never will be, capable of benefiting by ordinary school teaching are sent to special schools, where the most is made of what intelligence they possess and where they are trained for such occupations as it will be possible for them to undertake after leaving school.

The type of work the feeble-minded are best fitted for is routine work which does not call for any responsibility. Unfortunately, they usually lack the common sense and self-control which most normal individuals possess, and so find it impossible to live truly independent lives; they require constant supervision all their lives.

As a rule the feeble-minded are easily managed, but a few are obstinate to a degree which taxes the patience of those who have to deal with them. In a few cases they show moral defects which may bring them within the reach of the law; petty thieving, especially of articles which have an appeal to the senses rather than a money value, is perhaps the commonest offense. They steal because "it looked pretty" or "it glittered," not because the article would be saleable. Sexual offences are not infrequent, particularly against children. It is in these cases which show moral defects that the question of diagnosis of feeblemindedness arises, for the same distressing antisocial conduct may be seen in the late stage of encephalitis lethargica ("sleeping sickness,") and in some other forms of mental disorder.

Treatment. Although feeble-mindedness is incurable in one sense, being a lack of development of an essential part of the mental equipment, yet much can be done to help these unfortunate people to make the best of what nature has given them in the way of a brain. Much is done in the schools to "sort out" the feebleminded from their normal fellows, and the institution of special schools is a step in the right direction. When adult life is reached, however, the problem is more difficult.

The feeble-minded are generally healthy physically, the bodily health being as a

rule proportional to the degree of feeblemindedness, and as most of the feebleminded are only slightly below the normal standard of mentality, their expectation of life is good, many living to fifty or sixty. The object of all treatment should be to make the best of what they can do, and for this purpose simple, nontechnical occupations are the most satisfactory. The outdoor occupations, such as farming or gardening, which can readily be supervised and in which physical exertion is required, are perhaps the most suitable. For women, domestic work in large establishments where, again, ample supervision is available, or the simpler types of handicraft are advisable. Even in adult life much may be done by skillful management of such cases and by wise training, but the earlier the training is commenced, the better will be the final result.

In childhood an intelligent mother may raise the standard of intelligence of a feeble-minded child to one little removed from the normal, and later on in adult life his difficulty in adapting himself to the normal world may be reduced to a minimum by kindly and sympathetic understanding of his difficulties. But only too often the feeble-minded are found to be "more bother than they are worth," and they wander through life bewildered and useless. (*See also* ENCEPHALITIS LETHARGICA.)

FEEDING BOTTLE. One type of feeding bottle is the boat-shaped variety which is covered at one end by a rubber nipple and at the other end by a rubber valve. This type is easily kept clean, especially if the openings are large enough to allow the passage of a bottle-brush. Care should be taken to see that the rubber nipple and valve fit on firmly at both ends, otherwise the baby may drag them off while being fed. There are now available plastic disposable infant feeding bottles.

The proper care of the feeding bottle is a very important matter, for a dirty feeding bottle may lead to infection and disease. This matter is dealt with more fully under the heading INFANT FEEDING in the supplement on CARE AND MANAGEMENT OF BABY.

FEEDING CUP. Patients who are unable to sit up in bed should be provided with a suitable feeding-cup, to enable them to drink liquid food without spilling it over themselves or the bedclothes. A feeding cup has a spout for the patient to drink from, while the opening of the cup is half covered over, so that when the cup is tilted forward the contents are prevented from spilling.

FEMORAL VESSELS. The femoral artery and the femoral vein are the main blood vessels of the thigh.

The *femoral artery*, which is a continuation of one of the two divisions of the abdominal aorta, leaves the adbomen in the middle of the groin and travels down the upper leg to the back of the knee, where it becomes the popliteal artery. After the femoral artery leaves the pelvis it can be felt as it passes into the groin and pressure can be applied at this point to stop bleeding. In the groin the artery is not situated very deeply, and so is liable to be damaged.

The vein in the leg corresponding to the femoral artery is called the femoral vein. The two blood vessels run closely together for the whole of their course down the leg to the back of the knee. The femoral vein, or one of its tributary veins, is often the site of a thrombosis or clot of blood which may follow the condition called phlebitis in which there is inflammation of the walls of the vein.

Varicose veins, which are veins in which the walls are abnormally dilated or stretched, are commonest in the leg, and many of these veins go to join the femoral vein. The condition called "white leg," which sometimes arises after childbirth, is associated with clotting of blood in the femoral vein. (*See also* PHLEBITIS; THROMBOSIS; VARICOSE VEIN; WHITE LEG.)

FEMUR. The femur, or large bone of of the thigh, is the longest and strongest bone in the body. Like other long bones of the body, the femur has a shaft and two ends. The upper end of the femur has a large rounded head which fits into the cup of the hipbone; it has also a narrower neck and two jutting-out pieces called *trochanters*.

The lower end of the femur forms part of the knee joint. It consists of two longish jutting-out pieces called *condyles*.

Fractures of the Femur. It requires a considerable amount of violence to break the femur. In old people, however, it is liable to snap near the upper end, owing to the brittleness of the bones, and in such cases a fracture here is always a serious matter. It is often fatal, owing to the complications (such as pneumonia) that may arise from the need to keep the patient lying in bed.

Treatment. Great care must be taken in setting a fractured femur, as this injury is very liable to shorten the leg and thus throw the whole body out of alignment. Setting is achieved by immobilizing the fractured limb in a special splint for periods up to 10 weeks. The patient, especially if elderly, is encouraged to sit up and carry out breathing exercises as soon as possible.

FENESTRATION OPERATION. This is a delicate operation on the internal ear, performed with the aid of a microscope, for the alleviation of deafness caused by otosclerosis, an obscure disease of the bone surrounding the internal ear. The operation does not cure the disease, but it allows sounds once more to get through to the internal ear, which is the essential organ of hearing. In otosclerosis the little ossicle called the stapes becomes fixed, preventing the sound vibrations from being communicated to the internal ear; the surgeon, by making an opening into a semicircular canal of the labyrinth or internal ear, bypasses the fixed stapes. The operation is, however, being superseded by stapedectomy, which gives relief in over 90 per cent of cases.

FERMENTATION. Fermentation is produced by the activity of minute germs and yeast plants. Probably the best-known example of fermentation is the production of alcohol. A slight degree of fermentation always takes place in the stomach, but is only significant when it occurs in an excessive degree. The formation of gas in the stomach is a sign that too much fermentation is taking place, owing to the presence of undigested foods, which should be removed by taking a suitable purge and regulating the diet. (*See also* ALCOHOL; DIGESTION; INDIGESTION.)

FERMENTS. Ferments are substances which, when in contact with other substances, are capable of bringing about chemical changes. These changes play an important part in the digestion of our food. There are various types of ferments, and each one has its own particular task of turning our food into a form suitable for easy digestion. For example, a ferment which decomposes fat is found in the pancreatic juice, while a ferment which curdles milk is found in the stomach and the intestinal juice. Ptyalin is the name given to a ferment which is found in the saliva, but similar ferments are found in the bile, blood, urine, etc. (*See also* Diges-tion.)

FERN ROOT. A preparation made from the root of the common male fern is used as a cure for tapeworms. Before taking this drug, a dose of Epsom salts should be given, and very little food should be eaten during the day, in order to starve the worm. A teaspoonful of male fern, as this drug is called, is then taken at night and followed by another dose of Epsom salts in the morning. As a rule, this cure will suffice to get rid of the worm. Castor-oil must on no account be used in con-junction with male fern, because it may give rise to poisoning. (*See also* Worm.)

FERRIC SALTS. Salts of iron are chiefly used in medicine in cases of anemia. Blaud's pills is a popular iron preparation. By far the most active salts of iron are the ferrous salts, and of these ferrous sul-phate is the most convenient.

FESTER. "Festering" is a popular ex-pression used to describe the formation of pus, or matter. (*See also* Abscess; Ulcer; Whitlow.)

FEVER. A fever is a condition in which the body temperature is raised above nor-mal. Fevers in general are discussed under the heading Infectious Diseases.

FIBROIDS. Fibroid tumors of the womb, or "fibroids" as they are called, are the commonest tumors in women. They are, on the whole, more common in young unmarried women and women who have not borne children than in mothers of families. Often they are small and cause no symptoms, so that their presence is not suspected, but they may grow to enormous sizes.

Symptoms. As has been mentioned above, fibroids often cause no symptoms, or at least no symptoms that are sufficiently uncomfortable to attract notice. When there are symptoms the commonest ones are excessive loss at the menstrual periods, and swelling and increase in size of the abdomen. Sometimes the tumor is only discovered when the patient is examined for some other reason.

Treatment. Small fibroids which are not causing discomfort or excessive bleeding require no treatment. If treatment is re-quired, the tumor can be removed by peeling it out of the womb, an operation which is simple and safe and does not disturb the functions of the reproductive organs. If the growths are very large, very numerous, or show signs of turning malig-nant, as they sometimes do at the change of life the whole womb is often removed; but this is a matter for the advice of a specialist.

FIBROSIS. By fibrosis is meant the de-velopment of a tough and leathery kind of tissue called fibrous tissue. Fibrous tis-sue develops most often when there has been some injury to the ordinary tissue of a structure to such an extent that it cannot hope to recover. If possible, it must be arrested by removing the cause. Sepsis, poisoning by germs or toxins, errors of diet, etc., may be the cause of the fibrotic process. A common form of fibrosis is that which develops in a muscle which is kept still after an injury. Massage and exercises should be used early to stop the fibrosis. (*See also* Massage; Remedial Exercises.)

FIBROSITIS. Fibrositis, or myalgia, is a condition in which inflammation occurs in the muscular tissues of the body. Tiny swellings, or nodules, appear in the mus-cular tissue. These swellings are very pain-ful to the touch, and they cause intense pain on movement. There is often a certain amount of stiffness as well. The term "muscular rheumatism" is often used for fibrositis, and it is generally considered to be due to the same causes which produce other forms of rheumatism.

When fibrositis occurs in the back, the condition is known as lumbago; this form can be very crippling. Another common type of this condition occurs in the neck (stiff neck); or the chest may be attacked (pleurodynia). There is also a very common condition of aching and stiffness of the muscles over the greater part of the body. The pain may come on suddenly and, as a rule, it recurs at intervals until the condition is cured.

Fibrositis appears to occur more often in men than in women, and it is commoner after middle life. Often bad teeth or infected tonsils are the cause. Attacks may also follow prolonged fatigue or exposure to cold or wet. Fibrositis often results, too, from minor strains and injuries.

Treatment. If the pain is very severe the patient should rest in bed, but as a rule the milder attacks are not severe enough to compel complete rest. Heat applied to the body is the most soothing way of easing the pain, and this may be given in the form of a hot bath, hot fomentations, or hot-water bottles. Radiant-heat baths or hot-air baths are very good if they can be taken.

Massage may help, as it tends to increase the circulation of the blood in the affected part. The swellings or nodules should be looked for and gently rubbed away, if possible. Liniments may be rubbed into the skin to stimulate it; a very useful one consists of methyl salicylate, menthol, oil of eucalyptus, and oil of camphor. An ointment made of methyl salicylate and lanolin is also effective.

Drugs such as sodium salicylate or aspirin may be given to help to relieve the pain. If the attack is severe, 15 to 20 grains of sodium salicylate may be given every three hours for the first twelve or twenty-four hours; then the dose should be gradually lessened.

The treatment so far has only dealt with relieving the pain, but this can in no way bring about a real cure. The cause of the fibrositis must be discovered, and this can only be done by a complete physical examination, particular attention being paid to the teeth and tonsils. (*See also* RHEUMATISM.)

FIBULA. The fibula is the smaller of the two long bones of the lower leg. It lies on the outside of the leg and meets the larger bone of the lower leg, the tibia, at both ends. The tibia and fibula curve way from each other, however, in their course between their two ends. The upper end of the fibula is not part of the

knee joint, but begins just below it and can be easily felt as a lump sticking out from the bent knee on the outside of the front of the leg. At the ankle, however, it unites with the anklebone and the tibia to form the ankle joint. (*See also* ANKLE; LEG.)

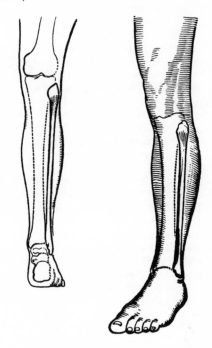

Fibula.

Fracture of the Fibula. The fibula is altogether a slighter bone than its fellow, the tibia, and is liable to be broken. But the strong tibia usually serves as a splint and saves the damaged fibula from serious displacement. By reason of the strength of the tibia the broken fibula need only be bandaged, not splinted, during the day, and it reunites very quickly. Often the weight of the body may be put on the foot as soon as three weeks after the break. Massage and passive remedial exercises may be carried out almost from the first.

FIDGETS. This denotes the jumpy and restless movements seen in children. It is always a sign that the child is in a highly nervous state, and the condition may be made much worse by allowing the child to become overtired. As a rule, these children are intelligent and a little extra care is required in dealing with them. An ordinary scolding in order to make the child sit still will only increase the state of nervousness, and a wise mother who has her child's interest at heart should give a little thought and study to the situation. Proper clothing, diet, exercise, fresh air and plenty of good, sound sleep are all necessary in the treatment of this condition.

The more regular type of jerky movement may be due to "tic" or twitching of the muscles; this ususally begins as a form of nervousness and later develops into a habit. In older people fidgets is generally a sign of overtiredness. It should not be forgotten that chorea, or St. Vitus's dance, may be mistaken for ordinary fidgetiness. (*See* St. Vitus's Dance.)

FIELD OF VISION. When a person is looking straight forward he not only sees objects before him, but also to some extent on both sides of, and above and below, the point on which his eyes are fixed. This range of sight is called his "field of vision." It may be tested by a very simple method. The surgeon faces the patient at a distance of three feet. The patient is told to look at the surgeon's opposite eye (that is, right to left, and vice versa), the other eye of both patient and surgeon being closed. The test object may be the surgeon's fingers, or a square of white paper, or, better still, a hatpin with a white head. The surgeon holds this midway between himself and the patient, and gradually moves it in from above, below, etc., towards the center, the patient giving a sign when he first becomes aware of it. (The surgeon's own field affords a standard of comparison.) A defect in the field of vision of either eye is thus easily ascertained. For exact results an instrument called a perimeter is used.

The field of vision is altered in various diseases. In disease of the nerve of the eye it lessens progressively, beginning at the outer limits and working inwards. In the disorder known as *retinitis pigmentosa* the outer portions are cut off, the central vision remaining good; sometimes a *scotoma* or "blind spot" occurs at some point. A central blind spot, which is very disabling, occurs in tobacco blindness, some forms of optic atrophy, and in neuritis of the eye. Irregular alterations may occur in *glaucoma*.

The upper part of the field is lost in *detachment* of the retina. When the nerve fibers in the brain which control the sight are abnormal, each eye may see only its right or left half of the field of vision, the other half being "blind."

In hysteria and neurasthenia the field of vision is frequently lessened to a remarkable degree. If its limits are retested at once, it will be found that the field is still further lessened in all directions. This is due to nerve fatigue, and after rest the field is found to have increased once more.

FIG. Figs, as well as various preparations made from them, act as a mild type of laxative medicine. Syrup of figs is a well known and very useful medicine for children, but the effective ingredient in it is really senna.

FILARIA. Filaria is the name given to a group of tiny worms which are responsible for producing disease in human beings. (*See also* Elephantiasis; Filariasis.)

FILARIASIS. This is a disease common in tropical and subtropical countries and caused by infection by tiny worms, especially the types known as *filaria bancrofti* and the *loa loa*. The embryos, or immature worms, are injected into human beings by the bite of the female mosquito, and they pass into the lymphatic vessels and glands (i.e., those vessels and glands which act as filters for the blood), where they grow and eventually start to breed. The female worm produces large numbers of embryos which circulate in the blood-stream. These in turn infect a biting mosquito, and, after undergoing changes in its body, are injected again into other human beings; thus the disease is spread from one person to another. A peculiarity of these tiny worms is that they stay hidden away in the lungs and kidneys all day and only enter the bloodstream at night, when the mosquito is abroad to do its deadly work. But if a person who is, for example, on night-duty sleeps during the day, the worms change their time for entering the bloodstream, and do so during the daytime.

The presence of the embryo filaria may be quite harmless while they are in the blood; it is when the adult worms cause obstruction in the lymphatic vessels and glands that serious damage takes place. The disorders produced by this blockage may include elephantiasis (q.v.). Sometimes the eyes may be affected. Lymphangitis, a condition in which there are painful red lines underneath the skin and the lymphatic glands usually become enlarged, is also caused by filaria.

Treatment. Diethylcarbamazine (Banocide) is a drug which kills off filaria, but must be started early to be effective. Injections of sodium antimony tartrate have been given, but they do not seem to have any lasting effect. In lymphangitis complete rest is indicated. (*See also* ELEPHANTIASIS.)

FILTERS. A drop of stagnant pondwater, seen through a microscope, is an amazing sight, swarming with tiny living and moving things. It is comforting, therefore, to know that the water that comes through the mains into our houses has been filtered in order to remove impurities.

For filtering large quantities of water, sand filter-beds are generally used. They are composed of a layer of fine sand at the top, then a layer of gravel, then gravel and pebbles; through these beds the water passes before being distributed to the public through the mains. The filtration beds are periodically cleaned, to get rid of the matter which is left on the sand, gravel or pebbles, and the beds are emptied and remade from time to time.

There are still some rural areas without a piped public water supply, where the inhabitants are still dependent on pumps, old and perhaps defective wells, or even ponds. Sometimes the only water available is rainwater flowing from roofs into barrels or tanks, and although rainwater is naturally pure it may collect many impurities as it passes through gutters often choked with dead leaves. For all such water, straining through several layers of fine muslin and then boiling is the best treatment. If a domestic filter is used, it should be of the type that is sterilized by boiling; this should be done every other day. Generally, however, it will be found simpler to boil the water.

Until the day when every house is provided with clean, wholesome, piped water, it is necessary that everyone should realize the importance of at least a pure drinking supply. We need only remind ourselves of some of the more serious illnesses conveyed by drinking bad water to see its urgency.

Enteric (typhoid) and cholera are among the waterborne diseases, and either may easily become epidemic.

FINGERS. One of the principal physical differences between the human being and the higher animals is the great development of the human hand, compared with the forepaw of the animal. This development is seen particularly in the fingers, which are the means by which most of us earn our daily bread. For this reason they are of immense importance, and even an apparently simple injury should be treated with great care.

The finger situated next to the thumb is known as the index finger; then comes the middle finger, followed by the ring finger and little finger. As a general rule there is a marked similarity of shape between the respective fingers of both hands. Frequently, however, the right hand is larger than the left, and the fingers are correspondingly more sturdy.

Each finger has three bones, called the phalanges (each individual bone being a phalanx). The bones in the palm of the hand are called metacarpals, and the first phalanges of the fingers join on to their corresponding metacarpals to form the knuckle-joint. The first, second, and third phalanges are, in this order, also joined to one another.

The joint at the knuckle has not only a wide range of movement towards the palm of the hand but also a more limited range of movement in a sideways direction; the other finger joints, however, can move only towards the palm and back again. The thumb has a much wider range than any of the fingers, being able to move freely in almost every direction.

There are no muscles in the fingers, but the muscles in the palm of the hand extend into the fingers in the form of strong tendons. Other tendons reach from the forearm to the fingers. Each finger is supplied with a tendon to bend it (flexor tendon) and a tendon to straighten it out (extensor tendon). The fingers are well supplied with nerves and blood vessels, and the sense of touch is very well developed, especially in the thumb and index finger, which are the two most important parts of the hand. Delicacy of touch and accuracy of movement are very necessary in some trades and occupations, and can be developed to a very high degree.

Disease of the Fingers. The fingers are so greatly used and are in such an exposed position that they are very subject to injury and infection. The bones may also become tuberculous in childhood, a condition which is known as dactylitis. Rheumatoid arthritis frequently deforms the fingers of older people. Contracted fingers, in which the little and ring fingers bend into the palm of the hand, is often a hereditary condition, but may be the result of irritation of the fingers or overuse of them. "Writer's cramp" is a condition of nerve strain in which the fingers become useless for certain movements until they have had a prolonged rest. Whitlows are painful abscesses occurring in the hand. Raynaud's disease is a disease in which the fingers go "dead" owing to defective circulation. Various skin diseases affect the fingers, such as itch, baker's itch, and cheiropompholyx. All these different conditions affecting the fingers are described under their own headings. Septic fingers are also described separately, as they are important owing to the serious results that may follow them.

Septic Fingers. A gathering of the finger pulp is known as a whitlow and usually follows infection of a prick or scratch. The most dangerous occupations, as far as hand injuries are concerned, are those of doctors, nurses and workers on the land—the first two groups because of the great danger they run of getting virulent germs into the cut, followed by rapid blood poisoning, which may mean the loss of the limb or even of life; and the land workers because of the danger of infection with the germ of lockjaw (tetanus), which lives in the soil. Septic fingers are usually due to infection entering the skin by some very small and often unnoticed opening such as that made by a thorn or splinter. A larger cut which bleeds freely is not so liable to gather, because the bleeding washes out the wound. The symptoms of a gathered finger are the same as those of any other abscess—redness, soreness, and heat concentrating in one spot and finally coming to a head with a collection of pus, or matter.

Treatment. If a splinter or piece of dirt can be seen in the sore spot or under the nail where the gathering is, it should be removed. The finger should be soaked for long periods at short intervals in water as hot as can be borne, containing some mild antiseptic. Or it may be poulticed with kaolin or hot fomentations and bandaged up until the abscess comes to a head. A tiny gathering will open and discharge of its own accord with this treatment, but any larger abscess will have to be carefully opened by a doctor. The fingers are so important that it is usual to treat infections of any severity by injections of penicillin.

If the gathering is on the front of the finger a scar may be formed by unskillful treatment which may lessen the feeling power of the finger. In some occupations this may not matter, but to some workers it may be a distinct disadvantage. For bandaging the finger *see* BANDAGES.

FINSEN LIGHT. or Ultra-Violet A form of light from which the heat rays have been excluded and only the blue and violet rays remain is known as Finsen light. It is used a great deal in the treatment of diseases of the skin, such as lupus. (*See also* LIGHT TREATMENT.)

FIRST AID. Many emergencies arise when it is not possible to secure the aid of a doctor at a moment's notice, and therefore it is often necessary to give a certain amount of treatment while waiting for medical help to arrive. This emergency treatment is called first aid, and the many aspects of this important subject will be found in the special FIRST AID SUPPLEMENT at the end of the book.

FISH-HOOK WOUND. A fish-hook wound is a very troublesome thing to deal with. The only way to extract the hook from the flesh is to push the hook *forward* until the point and barb emerge from the flesh. The whole barb should then be cut off and the rest of the fish-hook can be pulled out without further trouble. A little iodine should be painted over the wound after it has been thoroughly washed, and a dressing applied in order to prevent dirt from causing infection.

FISH-SKIN DISEASE. This is a disease in which the skin resembles the scales of a fish. It is technically known as ichthyosis. (*See also* ICHTHYOSIS.)

FISSURE. The term fissure has two meanings in medical language. In dealing with the anatomy of the body, the word

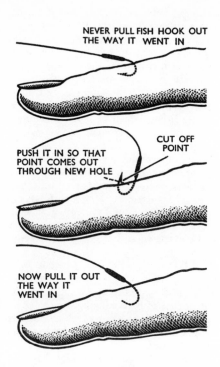

NEVER PULL FISH HOOK OUT THE WAY IT WENT IN

PUSH IT IN SO THAT POINT COMES OUT THROUGH NEW HOLE

CUT OFF POINT

NOW PULL IT OUT THE WAY IT WENT IN

Extracting Fish-hook from Finger.

fissure is used to describe various clefts which occur in the region of the brain; in surgery, the term fissure refers to cracks in the skin or mucous membranes.

Anal Fissure. The commonest part of the body for a fissure to appear in is at the margin of the *anus,* the lower opening of the bowel. The crack, which usually develops into a small ulcer, is almost always caused by the passage of hard motions.

Symptoms. Although the ulcer may be very small in size, it can create a life of misery until it is healed. Every time the bowels are opened severe pain is experienced. The pain is not only felt around the the crack or fissure itself, but may extend up the back and down the thighs and it may last for hours after movement of the bowels has taken place. As a result, anyone who suffers from an anal fissure refrains as much as possible from going to stool, thereby setting up a vicious circle.

Treatment. Constipation is usually the cause of the hard motions which cause the crack in the anus, so liquid paraffin should be given night and morning. In order to

prevent pain when movement of the bowels takes place, special suppositories may be used; these will deaden the painful area around the anus and encourage the sufferer to go to stool whenever required. After each motion the parts around the anus should be sponged with warm water. This treatment will not be found sufficient for a case that has developed into an ulcer, and it will be necessary for the patient to undergo a slight operation. It is a very simple matter for the surgeon to cure the condition, and it is advisable, at the same time, to have the condition of the lower part of the bowel investigated in case there is anything present which would cause a recurrence of the mischief.

Fissure of the Nipple. Unless due precautions are taken to harden the nipples and prepare them for suckling before the baby is born, cracks or fissures may appear and cause endless pain and trouble. The best way to prevent cracking of the nipples is to bathe them immediately after nursing, and then to dry them thoroughly. If they are at all tender, a little boric acid powder and starch should be applied at intervals. If cracks have formed, feeding from the affected breast should be stopped for twenty-four hours and the cracks dressed with comfound tincture of benzoin. (*See also* PREGNANCY.)

FISTULA. This is the name applied to any unnatural narrow channel or passage which leads from one cavity of the body to another, or which opens from a cavity

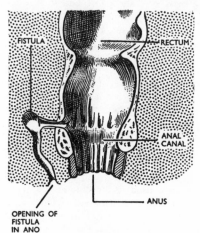

FISTULA

RECTUM

ANAL CANAL

OPENING OF FISTULA IN ANO

ANUS

Fistula.

onto the surface of the body. There are many varieties of fistula; one of the commonest is that known as anal fistula, or fistula *in ano*. The term anal fistula is usually applied to all the conditions in which chronic discharging openings are found near the anus or the lower end of the rectum. These channels or passages may spread in all directions and have many openings. Some may open on to the skin externally, or into the bowel internally, while others communicate both with the bowel and the outer surface of the body. There is more or less a constant discharge of pus or matter from these narrow openings.

An anal fistula is commonly due to the presence of an abscess which has been allowed to drain into the bowel or out on to the surface of the skin. The proper opening and draining of an abscess anywhere in the region of the anus would do much to prevent a fistula occurring.

Treatment. It is most unusual for a fistula to heal by itself without operation. Every part of the fistula must be thoroughly treated, and after the operation complete rest must be enforced.

FIT. The word fit, generally speaking, means a seizure of some kind. For example, we talk of a fit of coughing, or of weeping, or of temper, but in medicine the term fit is used to describe convulsions or any other abnormal movements of the muscles.

A fit or seizure is not a disease in itself, but only a symptom. Epilepsy is by far the most common cause and in this condition there is usually a warning (aura) which may consist of flashes of light or noises in the ears. The patient may give a loud scream before he falls to the ground. Infantile convulsions may, or may not, have some serious cause; it is quite common for a child to have a slight attack of convulsions owing to wrong diet or some infection in the bowels.

Tumors which cause pressure on the brain may cause convulsions; they may also follow large doses of certain drugs, such as strychnine, arsenic, atropine, and alcohol. The most usual is strychnine. The convulsions commence with great violence and the whole body is affected. During these attacks the hearing and sight of the sufferer are very acute and he is painfully aware of his condition. Tetanus, or lockjaw, is an infectious disease in which violent and painful convulsions occur which are very similar to those occurring in strychnine poisoning.

There is a disease of the kidneys known as uremia in which fits frequently occur, and during pregnancy some kidney trouble may arise in which similar fits take place. This condition, which is quite a common one in pregnant women, is known as eclampsia.

Many and various mental conditions are responsible for fits, and hysteria is one of the most common forms. For treatment of infantile convulsion *see* INFANTS, CONVULSIONS IN. Instructions for treating an epileptic fit are given under EPILEPSY. (*See also* CONVULSIONS; ECLAMPSIA; EPILEPSY; FAINTING.)

FLAT-FOOT. Although flat-foot in a slight degree is very common, for most people it is not serious, except from the point of view of personal appearance. There are, however, many cases in which flat feet can be a distinct handicap and lead to pain and discomfort.

The normal well-shaped foot has two natural arches: a larger arch extending the length of the foot, from the pads of the toes to the heel, and a smaller arch extending across the foot, from the ball of the big toe to the little toe. These arches may give way through weakness of the supporting muscles, thereby giving rise to flat-foot.

To tell whether flat-foot is present, wet the foot and stand on a piece of dark-colored linoleum. The outline of the foot can be plainly seen for a few minutes and can be compared with the outline of a normal foot.

Treatment. The treatment of flat-foot consists of carrying out special exercises which are easy to perform and if persevered with will give a very good result. These exercises are described and illustrated in the article on REMEDIAL EXERCISES. Any defect in the balance of the body, such as a raised shoulder, unequal length of the legs, or spinal curvature, should be corrected as much as possible. This can usually best be done by wearing specially built-up shoes. Massage of the feet may help. People with flat feet should learn to walk with the feet pointing straight ahead, instead of turning out, as so many people's feet do.

A slight degree of flat-foot may be cured by simple means, but if the condition is allowed to progress it may become a more serious matter. The weight of the body will fall on parts of the foot that are not meant to support it and bad corns will result. Also the joints of the foot will press on the ground and become inflamed until it may be agony to put the foot to the ground. The muscles of the leg become strained and pain may be felt in the calves of the legs and in the thighs. In older people it is very often necessary to support the arches of the feet by wearing a special appliance or a specially made shoe. These artificial arches give instant relief from the pain caused by flat-foot, but as they are not curative to any great extent it is better for younger people to make an effort to strengthen the arches of the feet.

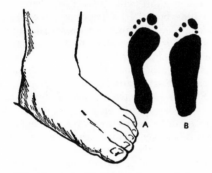

Flat Foot: A. *Imprint of normal foot;* B. *Flat foot.*

FLATULENCE. Flatulence, or flatulent dyspepsia, is a condition in which there is a tendency for wind to collect in the stomach. It may be due to intestinal, gastric or nervous causes. Intestinal and gastric flatulence usually appear together, owing to an unhealthy state of the organs of digestion, such as excessive fermentation in the bowel or stomach. This sort of flatulence is, therefore, to be treated in the same way as the indigestion which causes it. (*See also* INDIGESTION.)

Nervous Flatulence. The condition known as nervous flatulence is generally due to air-swallowing, a nervous complaint in which air is continually being swallowed into the stomach. This condition is described under its medical name of Aerophagy (q.v.).

Flatulence in Pregnancy. Flatulence is often an uncomfortable accompaniment of pregnancy, but disappears afterwards. If the discomfort is very great, retching will "bring up the wind," but pregnant women should always remember that anything in the way of straining should be avoided if possible. (*See also* PREGNANCY.)

FLEA. A flea is a tiny, brown, hard-skinned insect with a long proboscis with which it pierces the skin of its victim and sucks the blood. The bite leaves a small, red, irritable spot which fades after a few hours. There are hundreds of varieties of fleas, but for ordinary purposes we must be content to recognize two varieties only: those that live and feed on human beings and those that live on cats and dogs and other small animals. It is commonly thought that animals' fleas will not live on human beings and that fleas infesting human beings do not attack the domestic pets; but this is not so in all cases, though as a general rule it is true.

The flea that infests rats will freely attack human beings, and by this means terrible outbreaks of plague have been caused. Two of the greatest epidemics in history, the Black Death in the fourteenth century and the Plague of London in 1665, were said to have been caused by flea-borne infection. Rats coming ashore from ships may bring with them infected fleas, which by biting a human being can transmit the germs of plague to his blood. Besides plague, trench fever and typhus are known to be carried by fleas.

Exterminating Fleas. To prevent the spread of fleas the usual measures of cleanliness are sufficient in most cases. As soon as the presence of a flea on the person is suspected it is a good plan to undress in the bathroom beside a bath full of water. As each garment is removed it should be shaken over the water, and it is very likely that before the last garment is reached the flea will have been shaken into the water, where it will float on the top. A flea is, however, a very difficult little insect to kill Quite the best way is the crude and perhaps unpleasant way of cracking them between the nails of the two thumbs.

A flea-infested house presents a difficult problem, but repeated cleaning will in time usually get rid of the pest. The floors and woodwork must be thoroughly scoured, and all holes, such as mouseholes and cracks in the flooring and walls, should be blocked up. Naphthalene or D.D.T. powder may be sprinkled about and put in cracks, etc. Bedding should be washed or sent to the cleaners, and curtains, cushions, etc., should be dry-cleaned, washed, or dry sterilized. After the house has been brought to a normal state of cleanliness, the frequent use of a vacuum cleaner will keep it clean, provided the flea-containing dust is burned, and not merely thrown upon one side, thus giving the fleas a chance of breeding again.

FLIES. "All nature," said Pasteur, the great French scientist, "is a miracle." Flies are wonderfully made, and their life story is of great interest to the naturalist, but to the majority of people they are nothing but a pest and a great danger to health.

The favorite breeding-place of the common housefly is fresh horse manure that has lain for no longer than 24 hours. In this the female fly lays her eggs, perhaps as many as a hundred and fifty at once. If she cannot find fresh horse manure, she finds something else equally moist and warm, such as the contents of the outhouse or decaying refuse in an open garbage pail or on a rubbish-heap. She is a busy insect and wastes no time. It is probably that she lays at least a thousand eggs during her lifetime. In favorable cases, the egg may hatch within a few hours into a maggot. The latter is eventually transformed into a pupa or chrysalis; and from this in due time the perfect fly emerges and soon begins to lay eggs. Since the whole process of development may occupy no more than a few weeks, it is not difficult to realize how rapidly flies can breed and spread.

Invariably the fly's body is heavily contaminated with disease germs. It is not surprising, therefore, that some of the more serious illnesses are carried in this way by flies. Among these are anthrax—a disease to which butchers, shepherds, wool-sorters and others who work among animals are liable; cholera, which is common in tropical countries, where flies abound; diphtheria, one of the most deadly of children's diseases; dysentery, which, like cholera, is common in tropical countries; enteric, or typhoid, fever (also called, low, gastric, or drain fever); ophthalmia, especially the Egyptian form of it, which accounts for many cases of blindness; and foodpoisoning, which may be serious.

Just as the spider has its own ways of dealing with flies, so we, if we are to keep our houses free from this dangerous pest, must learn to be ingenious in our methods.

We can entrap the flies with one of the fly-traps now on the market, or we can make our own traps. An effective fly-trap consists of a saucer containing a solution of formalin, lime-water, and brown sugar, in the proportions of about a teaspoonful of formalin to half a pint of lime-water and a generous tablespoonful of sugar to make it palatable, for flies enjoy sweet things. Or we may prefer to "swat" the flies with a wire-gauze fly-swatter.

A point to bear in .mind is that flies dislike wind and moving air, and that a thorough draft will get rid of them for the time being. It is important, therefore, to keep windows and doors open whenever possible; it is advisable, too, to examine frequently hanging electric fittings, where flies often congregate. In a word, cleanliness is the best safeguard against the fly pest.

Flies are attracted by perspiration, and they will also settle on an open wound or sore or on a baby's sore eyes. Precautions should be taken against this when the baby is put out in the carriage.

Farmyard Flies. Where horses are kept, special care should be taken to stack the manure closely, so that the heat caused by fermentation may kill the fly maggots. The stack may be kept in a state of fermentation by moisture, or it may be broken up, scattered and dried, hard, dry lumps not being attractive for breeding.

Flies and Outside Sanitation. When fly maggots leave the egg, they burrow down into the ground and remain there for a while, perhaps a week or longer, according to climate, weather conditions, etc. When the fly is formed, it comes up through the ground, and although for another week or so it may be harmless enough, it soon becomes ready to lay its eggs. If, therefore, the house sanitation consists of an outhouse, every care should be taken to see that the floor is solid and that there are no cracks at the lower part of the walls through which these insects can creep. An old-fashioned outhouse with earthen floor and rotten woodwork may become a hotbed of disease.

It should be hardly necessary to add that garbage pails should be kept scrupulously clean, and that the lids should fit tightly, especially in summer when the flies are breeding. This applies to a temperate climate; in hot countries, flies breed all the year round.

FLOATING KIDNEY. As a general rule the kidneys are attached firmly in their normal position in the abdomen, but it sometimes happens that one or other of the kidneys, usually the right one, is more loosely attached and is able to move from its normal position. This is called a floating kidney. Floating kidneys are fairly common and usually cause no symptoms at all, but sometimes there may be pain and discomfort. (*See also* KIDNEY.)

FLOODING. This term is commonly used to denote excessive bleeding from the womb. Various causes of flooding are here outlined; further information should be sought in the separate articles on the conditions mentioned.

Flooding in Pregnancy. Flooding during pregnancy is always a danger signal and requires instant attention. It is usually the first sign of a threatened abortion, but if recognized and taken in time the abortion may be prevented. It is most liable to occur at the end of the third month of pregnancy, which is a time when special care should always be taken. Another condition which gives rise to flooding during pregnancy is conception taking place in one of the Fallopian tubes instead of in the womb (*ectopic gestation*). This is a very serious condition and calls for immediate operative treatment. There may be a misplaced afterbirth (*placenta praevia*); this also is a serious condition and requires immediate expert treatment.

Accidental Hemorrhage. In this condition there is a sudden bleeding during pregnancy, owing to the partial separation of the afterbirth, which leaves a raw, bleeding surface on the side of the womb. It is not caused by an "accident," but usually by an unhealthy condition of the afterbirth. It is a serious condition and requires immediate medical attention.

Flooding after Childbirth. Flooding immediately after, or a few days after, the baby is born is usually due to a portion of the afterbirth remaining behind and preventing the womb from contracting and sealing up the blood-vessels, as it normally does.

Treatment. The treatment is to empty the womb as speedily as possible of anything that may have been left behind. Massage of the womb through the abdominal wall may help, and drugs given by the doctor, such as pituitrin, quinine, and ergot, are helpful. In some cases hot douching of the womb may be necessary. The great danger of allowing a portion of the afterbirth to be left behind is that it may cause blood poisoning, a very grave complication of pregnancy.

Flooding after childbirth may also be caused by injury to the parts caused by the passage of the baby's head or by instruments which have been used. Such cases are usually stitched by the doctor in attendance, thus controlling the bleeding and repairing the damage. Occasionally the womb becomes partially turned inside out (inversion of the uterus) when the patient has had a very bad time during labor. This condition causes severe bleeding until it has been put right again.

Flooding Due to Change of Life. It is quite common for women to have attacks of flooding round the age of 44 years. This may merely mean that the patient is "on the change," but at the same time it is very important that every woman who experiences flooding at this age should be examined by a doctor, as it is the most common age for a cancer of the womb to develop, and bleeding may be the first sign to draw attention to it.

Puberty. Some young girls suffer from excessive bleeding at the onset of their periods. Care should be taken to ensure that too big a strain is not put on their strength until they have become more accustomed to their periods.

Tumors. Tumors of the womb are a frequent cause of bleeding. The most common are the fibroid tumors, of which there may be many or only one present, and which may grow to a very large size or may remain very small. Their removal is usually advisable. This may be done in several ways—for example, by the application of radium, by electrical treatment, or by surgical operation. Other tumors which cause flooding are polypi (which hang by a stalk from the neck of the womb), ovarian tumors and cancer.

Endometritis. This means an unhealthy condition of the womb and is usually accompanied by excessive bleeding at the periods. It is usually caused by a germ or by a misplacement of the womb.

Blood Diseases. Flooding is common in blood diseases, such as purpura and certain sorts of anemia, both primary and secondary to some other disease or to an operation. The treatment in these cases is to try to cure the original disease causing the anemia.

Gland Diseases and Debilitating Diseases. Flooding may occur in cases such as exophthalmic goiter (Graves' disease), diabetes, scurvy, heart disease, etc.

Treatment. In all the cases of bleeding the cause should be discovered and treated and, as has been said, the causes are very numerous and diagnosis is not aways easy. Blood transfusion may be required. In cases of *sudden* excessive bleeding from the womb, the patient should be put to bed, lying flat without a pillow and with the bottom of the bed raised on two kitchen chairs. While awaiting the arrival of the doctor, kettles of boiling water should be prepared ready for hot douches. Also clean bowls and towels should be placed ready, and rolls of cotton-wool and plain white gauze and any disinfectant there may be in the house, such as iodine, carbolic, or potassium permanganate. In cases where the patient is known to be pregnant a *very* tight binder round the abdomen is helpful; and so is pressure downwards, with the hand placed on the upper border of the womb.

In all cases of flooding, anything which comes away should be carefully kept for the inspection of the doctor.

FLUKE. Flukes are a kind of worm which lives in human beings or in animals. They usually occur in the tropics. (*See also* BILHARZIA; WORM.)

FLUORESCEIN. This drug is chiefly used to indicate the presence of ulcers in the cornea of the eye. A few drops of a mixture of fluorescein, bicarbonate of soda, and water, when dropped into the eye, will cause the ulcer to show up by turning it bright green.

FLUORINE. Fluorine is a mineral that is of interest in connection with dental caries. If the water contains more than one part per million of fluorine, china-white flecks appear in the teeth, and higher concentrations cause further changes. The teeth are softer than usual but are resistant to caries so that in some American cities fluorine is now deliberately added to the water supply to prevent caries.

FETUS. This is the name given to the child after the fifth week, while it is beginning to develop within the womb of the mother.

FOMENTATION. A simple means of relieving pain is by applying hot, wet flannel or lint to the part of the body which is inflamed. This is known as a hot fomentation.

In order to heat the flannel or lint, it should be cut to the required size and laid out on a small towel through which a stick has been inserted to protrude at each end to make the wringing of the towel easier. The towel and flannel (or lint) are then placed together in a basin and boiling water is poured over them until they are thoroughly soaked. The towel, with the fomentation inside it, is then wrung out very thoroughly. The fomentation is carried in the towel to the bedside in order to keep the heat in, but before applying the hot fomentation it should be opened out and shaken a little, and great care must be taken that it is not hot enough to burn the skin of the patient. The hot flannel or lint must be covered as quickly as possible with a piece of waterproof or oiled-silk which has been cut a little larger than the size of the fomentation. A large pad of cotton wool should be placed over this, and the whole kept in position by a bandage or flannel binder.

A fomentation applied in this way will keep its heat for a few hours, but if the pain is intense it may be necessary to renew the fomentation every half hour.

Wounds, ulcers, etc., are often treated by putting on boracic lint, wrung out of hot water and covered with a piece of oiled-silk or other water-proof and a bandage.

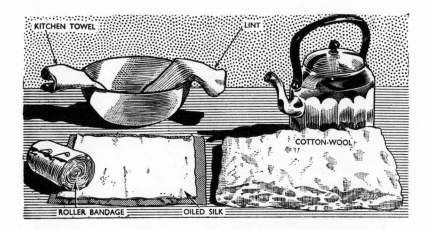

KITCHEN TOWEL   LINT

COTTON-WOOL

ROLLER BANDAGE   OILED SILK

ABOVE: *Requisites for a Hot Fomentation. Towel in basin, boiling water, bandage, lint and waterproof, cotton wool.*

RIGHT: *Boiling water poured on lint placed on towel in basin.*

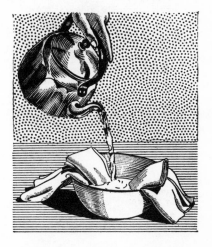

BELOW: *Towel twisted round lint, twisting out the hot water.*

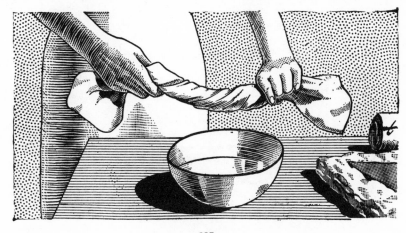

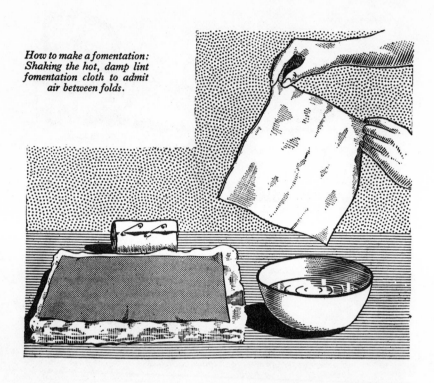

How to make a fomentation: Shaking the hot, damp lint fomentation cloth to admit air between folds.

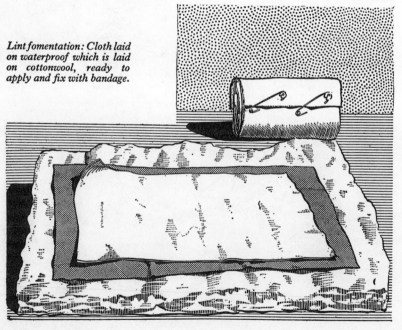

Lint fomentation: Cloth laid on waterproof which is laid on cottonwool, ready to apply and fix with bandage.

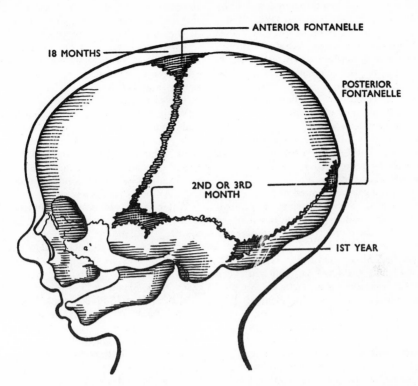

The infant skull, showing the fontanelles and their approximate dates of closure.

FOMITES. The term fomites is used to describe any article of food or furniture which is capable of harboring the living germs of disease while they are not in the human body. Infectious diseases are often spread in this way, although they are, of course, also spread by flies, fleas, etc., and human beings. (*See also* DISINFECTION; GERMS.)

FONTANELLE. The space between the bones of the head in newly born children is known as the fontanelle. Great care must be taken of the head until these bones join together, which usually happens by the age of eighteen months. Children who suffer from rickets or other wasting diseases do not develop as quickly as normally healthy children, and in such infants the closure of the fontanelle may be considerably delayed.

FOOD. Appetite assists digestion. Tasty food, carefully cooked and daintily served, stimulates the appetite. Another essential

is variety. Human beings—the so-called civilized races, at all events—soon tire of an oft-repeated dish. Changes should be skillfully made and the diet varied as widely as possible.

The function of food is twofold. It builds up and renews the tissues of the body and it supplies warmth and energy. Foodstuffs, therefore, fall into two principal classes. They are either "flesh-formers," known as *proteins* or givers of warmth and energy, called *carbohydrates* and *fats*.

Protein food is essential. Without it life is impossible, for neither carbohydrates nor fats can replace the wear and tear that takes place in the tissues of the body. On the other hand, carbohydrates and fats are not absolutely necessary, for surplus proteins, after the flesh-forming needs have been supplied, can give to the body warmth and energy. But this is a costly and unnatural method.

It is generally held that ample protein in

the diet promotes mental energy, a healthy nervous system, and high resistance to disease, and that shortage of protein causes the opposite conditions. What constitutes an adequate proportion varies rather widely according to the circumstances of life. Generally speaking, a man at rest in a temperate climate or leading a leisurely life needs one part of protein to five parts of carbohydrate and fat in his diet; but if working very hard, not only will he need more food, but he may need as much as one part of protein to three and a half parts of other nutrients.

This proportion is called the "nutritive ratio," and a diet consisting of protein, carbohydrate, and fat in quantities that are correct for the needs of the consumer is said to be a "balanced" diet.

Proteins. Most foodstuffs contain both protein and carbohydrate, but in very different and varying proportions. All proteins contain nitrogen, the element that repairs the tissue waste in the body. Proteins abound in meat, fish, milk, eggs, peas, and beans.

Carbohydrates. These are found in starch, sugar, and similar compounds. Therefore, bread, potatoes, jam and other preserves, and all cereals are rich in this food element.

Fats and Oils. Among the principal sources of animal fat are butter, bacon, pork chops, and cheese. Oils are abundant in the fruits and seeds of many plants, such as the palm nut, Brazil nut, peanut, almond, olive, etc.

Mineral Salts. The above are the principal food elements, but in addition the human body needs a small quantity of mineral salts of potassium, iron, calcium and phosphorus in order to build up the blood and brain and the bone and nerve structure. Such salts are usually present in food, and only actual starvation is likely to deprive the adult body of the necessary amount. But growing children and pregnant or nursing mothers have a special need of calcium and phosphorus. Therefore they should have plenty of milk and eggs, which contain a lot of these two elements.

Cellulose. This is the name given to the fibrous bulk of many foods. It is not digested in the human body, but is none

the less very important because of its mechanical action in helping the passage of the food along the intestines.

Vitamins. These are subtle chemical food factors, lack of which breeds so-called "deficiency" diseases, such as rickets, scurvy, and beri-beri.

The principal vitamins are:

Vitamin A, present in milk, cod-liver oil, and animal fats. Vitamin B, present in milk, the outer layers of cereals and in yeast. Vitamin C, present in fresh fruit and vegetables, especially oranges, black currants, and Vitamin D which is present in cod-liver or halibut-liver oil.

Water is an essential part of the diet. It not only keeps the digested food in solution, thus aiding its movement in the body, but it also stimulates the digestive juices and aids in flushing the intestines. Several tumblers of water per day may be taken with advantage.

Milk and its Products. Milk is a nearly perfect food. It contains protein, carbohydrate, fat, Vitamins A and B, and several kinds of mineral salt, but no iron.

Cream and Butter. Both of these contain large amounts of fat, are rich in Vitamin A, and are valuable, nourishing foods.

Margarine is made largely from vegetable fats. It is quite as valuable as butter as a fuel, though it is less palatable and lacks vitamins. In many brands of margarine vitamins are added, so as to make these products comparable to butter as a food.

Cheese is one of our most nutritious foods. It contains protein as well as fat, and may therefore take the place of meat. It is, however, deficient in carbohydrates.

Eggs are rich in protein and fat, and, like cheese, are poor in carbohydrates. They are likewise rich in iron, phosphorus, and vitamins.

The digestibility of eggs largely depends upon the individual, but to some extent upon the method of cooking as well. An egg lightly poached or boiled passes more quickly through the stomach than one that is hard-boiled or served as a heavy omelette.

Meat, like cheese and eggs, is rich in protein and often in fat, but lacks carbohydrate. If, therefore, much of it is eaten without additional vegetables or starchy foods, digestive disorders, such as constipation, are likely to ensue.

Chicken and pigeon are more readily digested than beef; but duck, turkey, and goose are not.

Beef extracts contain little protein. But they do contain most of the salts and the purines, i.e. extractives which give meat its appetizing flavor. Thus they whet the appetite and stimulate digestion.

It is recognized that meat is not a physiological necessity to man, since eggs, cheese, and milk provide proteins of animal origin, while a host of vegetables, pulses, and cereals contain this essential food element. Many races, especially in Asia, are largely vegetarian and yet are hardy and strong. Though meat is not absolutely essential to life, it is a concentrated source of proteins and vitamins in a readily absorbed form. For this reason, exclusively vegetarian diets have little to recommend them to the average American.

Fish, like meat, has a high protein, a low carbohydrate, and a variable fat content. On the whole, fish is more easily digested than meat, for which it is an excellent substitute. Whiting, sole, and cod contain little fat and are therefore more easily digested than halibut, herring, mackerel, and salmon, all of which are rich in oil.

Vegetable Sources of Protein. Protein is found in the vegetable kingdom, most richly in the pulses. Lentils, peas, beans, and in fact the grains of all leguminous plants contain an abundance of this element.

The Carbohydrates. Cereals are the most important of the group of foods in which carbohydrates predominate. Barley, wheat, oats, rye, etc., contain from 58 per cent to 71 per cent of carbohydrates and a larger quantity of mineral salts than foods rich in protein, such as eggs, meat, fish and cheese. To such foods, cereals form an excellent supplement.

In Europe and America bread is the commonest cereal food; it may be either white or wholemeal, wheat rye or corn. In Asia rice is the staple diet; in Africa, corn.

Other grain foods are barley, oat-meal, sago, tapioca, etc.

Vegetables and Fruit are both very important. They contain the precious vitamins and are rich in mineral salts and cellulose. Potatoes and beetroot are also rich in carbohydrate; but, except for the pulses, vegetables as a rule are deficient in protein.

Sugar. Cane sugar is practically pure carbohydrate, and in moderate quantities is readily digested.

Nuts have a high protein content and are widely taken by vegetarians as a substitute for protein of animal origin. It is doubtful whether these vegetable proteins have the same biological value as those contained in dairy produce.

Condiments are the spicy substances whose judicious use whets the appetite and stimulates digestion. Pepper, mustard, horseradish, and vinegar are typical condiments.

Quantity of food required. It has been calculated that a full-grown man, doing average work, needs daily about 4½ oz. of protein, 3 oz. of fat, 12 oz. of carbohydrate, 1 oz. of mineral food, and 5½ lb. of water. The total ration would weight about 7 lb., after allowing for other substances, such as cellulose and coloring matter, which are present in most foods.

As we have seen, most foodstuffs contain both protein and carbohydrate, some being rich in the former and others in the latter. For example, if the diet were confined to wheat bread, 4 lb. would have to be eaten to supply the needed 4½ oz. of protein, and then the amount of carbohydrate taken would be 2 lb., or double the quantity needed.

But if we take some other protein-rich food, such as cheese, and add ½ lb. of it to 1 lb. of bread, we get 12 oz. of carbohydrate, 4 oz. of protein, 2½ oz. of fat, and about ½ oz. of mineral salts. In this way balanced rations are planned.

As has already been said, variety is essential, and a diet of bread, cheese and water, though able to sustain life, would become deadly dull.

FOOD CONTAMINATION. By food contamination is meant the spoiling of food substances by contact with poisonous materials or by infection with germs. Since food is a necessity for us all and is partaken of several times every day by most people, it follows that food germs and poisonous substances can find their way into our bodies. We should, therefore, take precautions against food contamination. Of the food substances in everyday use, milk is probably the readiest means by which germs are carried. It may come from an infected animal, such as a tuberculous cow; or it may be handled by infected persons. Milk, moreover, provides an excellent breeding-ground for germs, so that they may actually teem in it. To prevent wide-spread disease from milk, therefore, there should be inspection of the cows, pasteurization of the milk, and sealing of the cans in which it travels.

Meat is the next best breeding-ground for germs, and many outbreaks of food poisoning have come from contaminated meat. It is wisest in warm weather, which is the weather in which germs breed most freely, to heat all meat pies, sausages, etc., to a high temperature before using them. Shell-fish are a fruitful source of infection, too, because they live at the mouths of rivers and sometimes feed on sewage.

Fruit and vegetables, especially in warm countries, are frequent carriers of germs, especially of those of cholera (*See also* FLIES.)

FOOD POISONING. "Ptomaine poisoning" was the term formerly used for foodpoisoning, as it was thought to be due to putrefaction taking place and producing poisonous substances known as ptomaines. It is now known, however, that the majority of cases are due to infection with germs actually in the food. It must be remembered that infected foods, especially meats, are not usually altered in appearance or smell. The meat may become infected from the hands of people who store and deal with it, or it may have come in contact with infected rats, mice, or flies. In cases of botulism, which is a variety of food-poisoning due to a particular germ, it is only a matter of hours before very definite symptoms begin to appear.

Cooking is not always a safeguard against poisoning, because although the germ itself may be destroyed, it may have produced toxins which remain unaffected by heat. Improper preservation of canned meats and delays in eating canned foods once they have been opened are very common causes

of poisoning. Food may also be made poisonous by coming in contact with metals such as copper, tin, or lead. Very careful attention should be given to the cleaning of all metal utensils, and food should never be left standing in them for any length of time.

There is another type of poisoning, known as *food allergy,* in which certain persons may find certain articles of food such as fish, white of egg, certain fruits, especially strawberries, and so on, definitely poisonous to them. Whenever they take such foods they develop unpleasant symptoms, such as hives irritation of the bowel, erythema, and eczema; or they may show symptoms of asthma.

Symptoms. The symptoms of food poisoning usually begin a few hours after the infected food has been eaten, but some cases may not become apparent for two or three days. The patient usually feels nauseated, and vomiting may take place. The bowels are loose, and later the motions may become very watery. The temperature is raised, and in severe cases the patient may show signs of collapse. In mild cases the feeling of illness passes off in about two days, and the majority of cases recover completely after a week or so.

Treatment. The patient should be put to bed and kept warm. Castor oil should be given, but if the diarrhea persists, a more binding medicine, such as chlorodyne, should be substituted. Precipitated chalk or kaolin mixed with water is also very helpful in soothing the stomach and bowel and stopping diarrhea. Pain in the abdomen can be relieved by application of hot-water bottles or hot flannels. In cases of collapse, hot coffee or other stimulants may be given. During the acute stages, the patient should only be given boiled water or white of egg in water. The diet should be gradually increased by adding citrated milk, glucose, arrowroot, custard, eggs, and fish. (*See also* BOTULISM.)

FOOT. The foot is made up of a framework of bones covered by tissue and muscles, with the associated tendons, blood vessels, etc. There are 26 bones in the foot proper, of which 14 form the toes, 5 are metatarsal bones joining the toes to the heel, while the remaining 7 make up the heel and take part in the formation of the

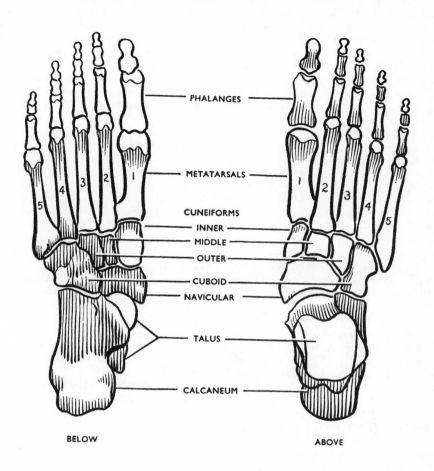

PHALANGES

METATARSALS

CUNEIFORMS

INNER

MIDDLE

OUTER

CUBOID

NAVICULAR

TALUS

CALCANEUM

BELOW

ABOVE

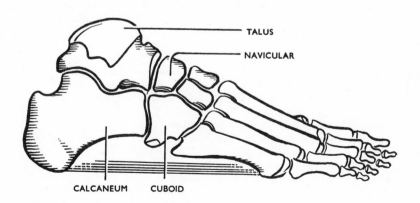

TALUS

NAVICULAR

CALCANEUM   CUBOID

The Foot.

293

ankle joint. In the part of the foot that we know as the heel, a bone called the *calcaneum* rests on the ground, with the *talus* above it. In front of the calcaneum is the *cuboid,* on the inside of the foot; the *navicular* is on the top of the foot and in front of it are the first, second and third *cuneiforms.* It will be seen that the foot has additional bony strengthening on the inside of the foot, where the central weight of the body falls.

The bones of the foot form two arches. The *lateral* arch, extending from the inside to the outside of the foot, is composed of the calcaneum, the cuboid, and the fourth and fifth metatarsal bones. The *medial* arch, from heel to toe, is made up of the calcaneum, the talus, the navicular, the three cuneiform and the remaining three tarsal bones. Either of these arches of the foot may become weakened and lose its curve, thus causing the condition called flat-foot.

The foot is supplied with blood by the *plantar arteries* (internal and external), on the underneath part of the foot, and the *dorsalis pedis* artery, on the top. There are two sets of muscles which work the foot and toes: those which have their origin in the foot, and those which extend from the muscles of the leg. Strong, tough tissue, known as the *deep fascia,* covers the muscles of the foot. On the sole of the foot this fascia is known as the *plantar fascia;* it forms a firm, supporting layer stretching all the way from the heelbone to the ball of the foot.

By our habit of wearing boots and shoes the foot is protected from many cuts and injuries it might otherwise sustain; but the pressure of footwear is largely responsible for many irritating corns, callosities, and blisters. The treatment of these will be found under the heading CORNS. Excessive perspiration from the feet is often a troublesome complaint; for the treatment of this *see* the article on SWEAT.

Swelling of the feet is due to various causes. A fluid swelling appearing after a twist or knock to the ankle may be *synovitis.* Swelling of the feet in the evening may be due to weakness of the heart. Kidney diseases also cause swelling of the feet, Varicose veins in the leg are another common cause of this condition. Many people are troubled with feet that swell when the weather becomes warm. This is merely constitutional, and the feet subside again as quickly as they swell. Chilblains in winter are another cause of swelling.

All forms of swollen feet are benefited at once by resting with the feet raised. The feet should be at a slightly higher level than the knees; therefore, if rest is being taken on a sofa or bed it is a good idea to put a pillow under the feet.

FOOT-DROP. When the foot cannot be raised from the ankle the condition is known as "foot-drop," or "dropped foot." If the muscles of the front of the leg are paralyzed, the foot may be permanently dropped as a result. Shortening of the muscles at the back of the leg will cause the foot to drop and become fixed.

Foot-drop may be due to injury of a nerve controlling the muscles of the leg or ankle, or the nerves may be diseased as a result of lead-poisoning. Disease of the spinal cord may also affect the nerves and cause the foot to drop. Some forms of foot-drop respond to exercises, some are overcome by corrective appliances, and some require surgical operation for their relief. (*See also* ANKLE.)

FOOT AND MOUTH DISEASE. This disease chiefly affects cattle, sheep and pigs, but human beings can acquire it through contact with infected animals. Infection may be spread by the discharges which come from the sores, or vesicles, which appear on the feet and mouth, or it may be carried by the milk of an infected cow.

Symptoms. The patient may have a slight fever for a few days and then sores will begin to appear in the mouth, round the lips, and sometimes on the hands and feet.

Treatment. The patient should be put to bed, and the sores must be thoroughly treated with antiseptics. A weak solution of carbolic acid with bicarbonate of soda is useful as a mouthwash or for bathing the sores.

FORAMEN. This is the medical term for an opening into a bone, through which passes a nerve, blood vessel, or similar structure. For example, the foramen magnum is a large oval opening at the base of the skull through which pass the spinal cord and many nerves and arteries.

294

FORCEPS. This is an instrument shaped somewhat like a pair of tongs or pliers and used for grasping, pulling, or compressing an object. Many types of forceps are used in surgery, a special set being required for each type of operation. Dental forceps, for example, are used for extracting teeth, artery forceps for pinching an artery in order to arrest bleeding, while delivery forceps are used sometimes when it is necessary to assist the expulsion of the infant during labor. Many other types of forceps have been designed covering a wide variety of uses.

FORCIBLE FEEDING. Forcible or forced feeding is a method of conveying nourishment to a patient who persistently refuses to feed himself in the usual way. It sometimes has to be resorted to in cases of extreme illness, but then is employed only as an extreme measure to save life.

Forcible feeding is used in cases of mental trouble, when patients refuse food, and it has been used also in prisons in cases of hunger-striking.

The method is to introduce the food by way of a soft rubber tube passed through the mouth or nose. Liquid food only is given by this means, such as milk, beaten-up egg or thin broth.

FOREHEAD. The front part of the head, just above the eyebrows, is called the forehead, the brow, or the frontal region. Wrinkling of the brow is controlled by a broad band of muscle which covers the frontal bone, the part of the skull which forms the forehead. In some people this frontal bone is prominent, but does not necessarily signify a high degree of mental capacity. A large and bulging forehead may be due to a thickening of the frontal bone, as occurs in children with rickets.

In many conditions, such as frontal sinus disease, neurasthenia, constipation, or eyestrain, it is not unusual for pain to be felt in the region of the brow. Sometimes people complain that they have a feeling as if someone was pressing a tight band across their forehead. This very often indicates eyestrain or neuralgia of the supra-orbital nerve, which passes over the forehead.

Spots on the forehead are quite common in many infectious diseases, and a seborrheic rash may spread down on to the forehead from the scalp. (*See also* FRONTAL SINUS; NEURALGIA; SEBORRHEA.)

FOREIGN BODY. The term foreign body denotes any substance or article in a part of the body where it does not naturally occur. A fish-hook in the finger or a fly in the eye furnish two common examples of foreign bodies. In the following list are given a few of the more usual places in which foreign bodies become lodged.

Foreign Body in the Ear. Insects or small seeds of grain, etc., often find their way into the ear and may be the cause of deafness.

Treatment. The head should be placed on one side and warm water very gently poured into the affected ear; or a few drops of warm olive oil poured into the ear and allowed to remain for a short time may dislodge the foreign body and cause it to float to the surface. If the foreign body cannot be removed by ordinary gentle syringing, the doctor should be called in, as it is very dangerous for an unskilled person to use instruments in the ear.

Foreign Bodies in the Eye. It is a common thing for flies or small pieces of dust and grit to be blown into the eyes.

Treatment. In some cases they can be removed by merely drawing the upper eyelid over the lower; or if the foreign body can be clearly seen it may be removed with the corner of a clean pocket handkerchief. If a sharp substance, such as a piece of glass or steel, has become embedded, castor oil should be dropped into the eye and the doctor should be sent for immediately. Very often the eye becomes so inflamed that even after the foreign body has been removed the sufferer still feels great discomfort. (*See also* EYE.)

Foreign Body in the Gullet. When a foreign body is swallowed and lodges in the gullet, the tube leading to the stomach, irritation, and inflammation may be set up immediately. A doctor must be called in at once, but usually he will have to send the patient to a specialist or to hospital for the removal of the foreign body by means of a special kind of tube.

Treatment. In the case of a small fishbone or any small, round object, it is sometimes possible to dislodge it by swallowing large quantities of bread with draughts of water. If the foreign body fails to become dislodged, it is advisable to seek the advice of a doctor as early as possible.

Foreign Bodies in the Stomach. In many cases such things as swallowed coins, pins, etc., may reach the stomach, and eventually the intestines, without any treatment whatever.

Treatment. It is not advisable to give medicines as these may do more harm than good, but eating a large quantity of new bread and fresh vegetables may assist the foreign body in its passage through the bowels. The motions should be examined to make quite certain that the foreign body has been expelled.

Foreign Bodies in the Windpipe or Lung. These are sometimes inhaled when, for instance, a screw or a pin is held in the mouth, and may either stick in the windpipe (trachea) or go down the bronchi into the lung. If a child gets an attack of coughing when playing on the floor, the possibility of such a foreign body in the windpipe must be remembered. Such foreign bodies as peas or beans are more serious than metal objects, as they set up a poisonous bronchitis, but all of them require the attention of a doctor and usually of a specialist. They are removed with the use of an instrument called the bronchoscope, but first an X-ray examination must be done.

FORESKIN. A fold of skin which covers the end of the penis is known as the foreskin. In some cases this foreskin is tight and cannot be rolled back. In such cases circumcision or removal of the foreskin is generally advised. (*See also* CIRCUMCISION.)

FORMALDEHYDE. Formaldehyde is a powerful antiseptic and disinfectant, but it is too irritating to be used on wounds and sores, except in very weak solutions. There are many preparations of formaldehyde, but the best known one is formalin, which is widely used for preserving museum specimens and many other purposes. Formaldehyde is included in many popular toothpastes and mouthwashes, since it acts as a deodorant—that is, is capable of destroying unpleasant odors. It is widely employed in sickrooms and in hospitals, and it is also very valuable for general household disinfection. It is one of the advantages of formalin that it does not destroy books or colored materials and is harmless to all metals except iron.

To disinfect a room, the walls and furniture should be first sprayed with water, and paraform tablets (a preparation of formaldehyde) are then heated over a nightlight or in a special vaporizer. If the room has been properly sealed up, by it will be found that the vapor from 25 tablets (25 grams) will be quite sufficient to disinfect a room of ordinary size in about 10 hours. (*See also* ANTISEPTIC; DISINFECTION.)

FORMIC ACID. Formic acid is found in the sting of bees and it is also present in the bodies of ants. The pure acid blisters the skin. (*See also* BITES AND STINGS; BLISTERING.)

FORMICATION. This word denotes a sensation, as if ants were crawling over the skin. This feeling, and other tingling sensations felt in the skin, are known as *paraesthesia*. Formication is a symptom of one sort of neuritis, or inflammation of the nerves, caused by alcohol and other poisons.

FOSSA. A depression or sunken place on the surface of the body is known as a fossa. There are many such depressions and each of them has its own particular name. For example, the antecubital fossa is the depression in front of the elbow, and a cranial fossa is one of the depressions in the base of the skull which holds the lobes of the brain.

FOXGLOVE. Digitalis, a drug used in the treatment of certain diseases of the heart, is obtained from the foxglove plant. (*See also* DIGITALIS)

FRACTURES. A fracture is a break in a bone, with or without damage to the surrounding tissues. Fractures are divided into various classes. If the bone is broken without any further damage it is called a *simple* fracture; if the skin is torn by the broken bone sticking through it, the fracture is a *compound* one; if the surrounding tissues and blood vessels are also injured it is known as a *complicated* fracture (there may also be a *compound complicated* type). A *comminuted* fracture is one in which the bone is smashed and splintered instead of being merely broken across. In a *multiple* fracture the bone is broken in more than one place; and in an *impacted* fracture the broken ends of the bone are driven into one another. In children the

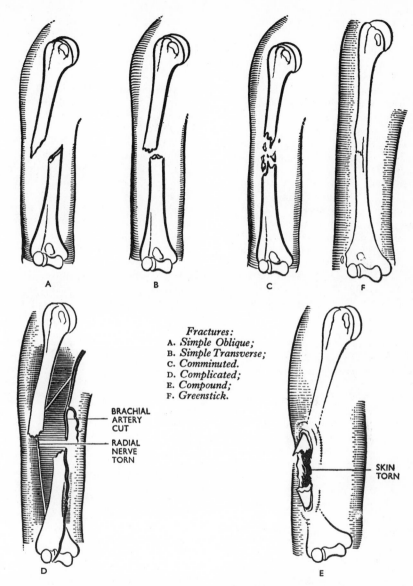

Fractures:
A. *Simple Oblique;*
B. *Simple Transverse;*
C. *Comminuted.*
D. *Complicated;*
E. *Compound;*
F. *Greenstick.*

BRACHIAL
ARTERY
CUT

RADIAL
NERVE
TORN

SKIN
TORN

bones do not snap easily, but bend, and this variety of injury is known as a *green-stick* fracture.

The diagnosis of a fracture is a matter for the expert, but in general a fractured limb is exceedingly painful and the patient is absolutely powerless to move it. Every suspected fracture should be treated as a fracture until it has been proved that it is not one. In every serious case an X-ray examination is usually carried out.

Treatment. The first consideration in the treatment of fractures is to reset the bones in their normal position. *In order to prevent any further damage, the patient must on no account be moved before the limb is secured in emergency splints of some kind.* Before applying the splint, the limb must be straightened; and if shortening has taken place, the limb should be pulled on with the greatest care and gentleness. There is great danger of a compound fracture

297

becoming infected from contact with outside materials. The bleeding must be stopped as quickly as possible, and the wound covered with a dressing of sterile gauze or lint. Failing this, a piece of clean linen is the best substitute. This dressing should be enveloped in a thick layer of cotton wool and fixed with a bandage. It is important that the splints should be long enough to extend to the joint above and joint below the fracture, and they must be carefully padded so as to fit the limb accurately.

Where there is a fracture of the spine, pelvis, or leg, the patient should never be moved except on a stretcher, as a simple fracture may be converted into a compound one unless handled very carefully. As there is always a certain amount of shock associated with a fracture, the patient should be kept as warm as possible until the doctor arrives. He should be covered with blankets and, if possible, given a hot drink of milk or broth. (*See also* HEMORRHAGE; and article on FRACTURES in SPECIAL FIRST AID SUPPLEMENT at end of book.)

FRAMBESIA. This is a tropical disease, known also as yaws and pian. (*See also* YAWS.)

FRECKLES. Freckles consist of tiny accumulations of the coloring matter of the skin. They occur most commonly on the face, neck, and arms, and are more conspicuous in the summer. Fair, and especially red-haired, people are chiefly affected. They may be looked on as a natural reaction to the sun's rays.

Freckles may be prevented by avoiding direct sunlight.

Treatment. Freckles may be removed by various applications. The mildest of these, which act by partially bleaching the skin, are buttermilk, sour milk, or lemon juice. A more elegant preparation is lactic acid, 10 per cent, in rose-water. This should be applied to the skin three times daily.

Some "freckles" are in reality small tumors. These do not fade during the winter. The widespread freckling sometimes seen in old people is of this kind.

FRENUM. This term describes any small fold of skin which restricts the movement of an organ of the body. The most common example is the short fold of mucous membrane which is found beneath the tongue. If this is unduly short in a child it may cause tongue-tie and the child may not be able to suck properly. A slight clipping of the frenum is all that is required to put matters right, but this should be done under proper medical care. Another fold of skin, or frenum, passes from the base of the thumb to the base of the first finger. (*See also* TONGUE.)

FRONTAL SINUS. The frontal air sinuses are hollows in the frontal bone of the skull; they are connected with the nose and filled with air. Their function is to give additional protection to the front part of the brain without adding to the thickness of the bone. In some people they are quite small, while in others they are so large that they extend right across the eyebrows.

Influenza and other nasal infections may cause inflammation of the frontal sinuses which may require an operation. In acute inflammation, however, operation is not usually advised, but instead hot applications to the forehead are made, with menthol inhalations (a few crystals of menthol being dissolved in boiling water) and usually injections of penicillin. Nasal douching does more harm than good in acute inflammation, but may be useful when the acute stage has been passed. (*See also* INHALATION.)

FROSTBITE. When the body has been exposed to very severe cold for any length of time, frostbite may set in. If the circulation is allowed to return too suddenly the frostbitten parts may become gangrenous, which means that they become dead. The parts of the body which seem to be attacked more than others are the fingers, the toes, the tip of the nose, and the edges of the ears. These parts lie farthest away from the heart and in consequence the blood circulation in them is inclined to be poor. People who are in a low state of health are more susceptible to frostbite than normally healthy people. This is especially true of the very young and the very old.

Symptoms. After long exposure to cold the circulation may become very sluggish and parts of the body may turn white and waxy-looking. There may be no pain while this is going on, so that a person is sometimes quite unaware of what is happening. Blisters usually form which may gradually develop into sluggish ulcers, and if the frostbite is very severe the affected parts may turn gangrenous and die.

Treatment. In the first place it must be mentioned that prevention is better than cure. Frostbite may be prevented by carefully wrapping up while in intense cold, and by keeping the circulation active by means of physical activity. However, when a part of the body does become frostbitten, it should be thawed out *slowly*. This is best achieved, not by warming the affected part, but by gradually warming the whole body.

This soon occurs at normal room temperature and can be assisted by hot drinks. The frostbitten areas should be dressed with clean lint, and then a pad of cotton wool should be placed over them. The limbs should be raised as much as possible; the leg may be placed on a pillow and the arm should be raised in a sling. This will help to relieve any congestion and pain. If the parts are already gangrenous, they should be kept absolutely dry, dusted with boric acid powder and wrapped up in cotton wool or soft flannel. At this stage in the treatment an operation may sometimes be necessary.

It must be remembered that the most important point in the treatment is to keep the patient away from heat. (*See also* CHILBLAINS; GANGRENE.)

FUMIGATION. The exposure of rooms, clothing and contaminated articles to lethal gases or chemical fumes for the purpose of destroying germs, and vermin such as insects, rats, mice, etc., is termed fumigation.

FUR DERMATITIS. A skin rash may appear in the region of the neck owing to the wearing of dyed furs. This is known as fur dermatitis. (*See also* DERMATITIS.)

FURRED TONGUE. A thin white layer on the tongue may be due to a disturbance of the digestive organs or an attack of constipation; but, on the other hand, some people seem always to have a furred tongue, even though there may be no apparent reason for it. The "fur" generally consists of bacterial growth and particles of food. Sometimes drinking too much milk will cause the tongue to appear white and furred; or it may be due to too much smoking. (*See also* TONGUE, DISEASES OF.)

FURUNCLE. This is the medical name for a boil. (*See also* BOIL.)

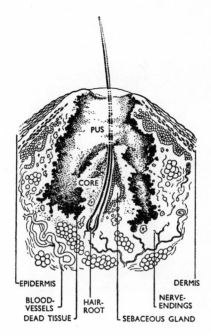

Furuncle.

GAIT. The style or manner in which a person walks gives much valuable information about the illness from which he may be suffering. The gait is especially important in cases of nervous disease, but it may be also an index of character. The man who slouches along with bent shoulders and head down, looking on the ground, is seldom one who is making a success of his life, while the man who "steps out" gaily, with head erect and shoulders well pulled back, is the man who is likely to get on in the world. The influence of gait on health is a topic on which much has been written. If the shoulders are allowed to droop and the back is bent while walking, the lungs are unable to expand properly at each breath, with the result that insufficient air is taken in to supply the oxygen needs of the body, and a body starved of oxygen cannot be a healthy one.

The correct gait is one in which the body is held erect, the head neither upturned nor with the eyes fixed on the ground, the shoulders well pulled back to allow for expansion of the lungs, the arms swinging easily at the sides and the movement of walking from the hips, not from the knees. A faulty gait may be due to a number of different causes. In children, such things as tuberculosis of the hip or knee joint, St. Vitus's dance, or acute rheumatism are to be thought of when a child begins to limp for no obvious reason. It is important that any child who develops a curious gait should be examined by a doctor, because in the early stages of such disorders the disease is curable; later on cure may be impossible. In adults, injuries to, or diseases of, the hip joint, such as osteoarthritis, may cause the gait to be altered, but the most strikingly abnormal gaits are seen in certain diseases of the nervous system.

In *disseminated sclerosis* the gait is of the "sticky" or "spastic" type; the patient has difficulty in bending the knees and drags his feet along, the toes scraping the ground at every step. The legs are moved "all of a piece" and are swung forwards, rather than raised from the ground. In people who have had a stroke and recovered, the same type of gait is seen, but in one leg only, as only one side of the brain has been damaged. The "ataxic" or "stamping" gait is best seen in people who are suffering from *tabes dorsalis* in its late stages. The patient raises his feet very suddenly, often higher than usual, and then jerks them forward, bringing them to the ground again with a stamp. He is also not quite sure where he is going to place his feet, and waves them about in the air, as it were, before putting them down, looking at his feet all this time. A "reeling" gait is often mistaken for a drunken gait, and therefore requires no other description; the unfortunate patient reels from side to side, and often falls to one side or the other. This type of gait occurs only in patients who are suffering from disease of that part of the brain which controls balance, that is, the little brain, or cerebellum. In inflammation of the nerves of the legs, such as occurs sometimes in *lead-poisoning* or in poisoning by alcohol, the gait is what is described as "high-stepping," the advancing foot hanging with the toes pointing towards the ground, the leg being lifted high so that the toes may clear the ground. In the disease known as parkinsonism, which often follows an attack of encephalitis lethargica, the gait is a peculiar shuffling one, as though the patient were chasing his own center of gravity. (*See also* DISSEMINATED SCLEROSIS; TABES DORSALIS.)

GALL BLADDER. The gall bladder is a pear-shaped vessel, about 3 in. long, which lies beneath the under-surface of the liver, in the right upper abdomen. It serves as a store for bile from the liver. The narrow neck of the gall bladder tapers to a tube called the cystic duct, and after the bile has been concentrated by having the water absorbed from it, it is passed on through the cystic duct into the main bile duct. Bile is a very important digestive substance which is manufactured in the liver and pours from it by way of the hepatic duct, gall bladder, and common bile duct into the duodenum. Some of the bile trickles from the hepatic duct directly into the common bile duct, but most of it enters the gall bladder. The signal for the gall bladder to begin pouring out its concentrated bile into the duodenum is the entry of the meal, eaten twenty minutes or so before, into the duodenum from the stomach. This food is mixed with the digestive juices from the stomach and when this acid mixture passes into the duodenum, which is normally alkaline, the effect is to bring the bile from the gall bladder and liver to mix with it.

The gall bladder is very liable to suffer from catarrh, from inflammation (cholecystitis), and from stones (cholelithiasis). (*See also* BILE; DIGESTION.)

Catarrh and Inflammation of the Gall Bladder. Catarrh of the gall bladder is fairly frequent in middle-aged persons who do not lead an active enough life and eat too much food of the starchy type. It is more common in women than in men. It is due to infection by various germs which have found their way, either directly from the bowels, or by way of the bloodstream from some distant seat of infection such as diseased teeth or tonsils. The germs which are most frequently found in the gall bladder are those which normally live in the intestine where they do no harm, such as the bacterium coli. It is a peculiarity of the gall bladder that the germs of typhoid fever will linger there for many years after a person has had an attack of it. A catarrhal state of the gall bladder, if left untreated, leads in many cases to the formation of gallstones.

Symptoms. Where catarrh or inflammation of the gall bladder is present, there is always a certain amount of discomfort after food. The stomach feels overloaded and there may be a definite disinclination to eat. A feeling of weight may be felt in the right side of the abdomen and pain just below the ribs to the right of the navel. An aching pain under the right shoulder may also be felt. Constipation is also present, and there may be a slight degree of jaundice, shown by a sallow skin and yellowing of the whites of the eyes. At intervals the condition will probably become acute, and there will then be a rise in temperature with cold shivers down the spine, and a more severe pain in the region of the gall bladder. This pain may be a steady ache or may shoot all over the abdomen and through to the back. Vomiting and nausea may be very bad.

Treatment. If gall bladder trouble is left untreated, it usually becomes gradually worse until gallstones form and an operation may be necessary. Even if the complaint is not very bad it will mean persistent ill health and a chronic feeling of being below par. Women with catarrh of the gall bladder usually aggravate the condition by putting on flesh, which again makes it even more difficult to obtain the necessary amount of exercise to keep the bile circulating. The diet should be light and as scanty as possible, with little fat and carbohydrate in it. More exercise should be arranged for, especially if most of the day is taken up in sedentary occupations.

When the disorder is of long standing, symptoms are often relieved by a morning dose of Epsom salts ,which stimulates emptying of the gall bladder. When the gall bladder is acutely inflamed the patient should be confined to bed under medical care. Then it is usual to give penicillin or one of the newer antibiotic drugs to help overcome the infection.

If the condition gets worse and the patient becomes seriously ill, it may be necessary for a surgeon to drain or (usually) remove the gall bladder.

GALLSTONES. Gallstones frequently form in the gall bladder when it has been affected by catarrh for some time. Often they are present without causing any symptoms or only the symptoms of a slight catarrh, but the moment may arise when a stone becomes dislodged from the gall bladder and begins to pass down the bile duct, on its way to the intestines. This gives rise to the condition commonly referred to as "an attack of gallstones." Intense pain is felt, which may be so bad that the patient actually rolls about the floor or bed in agony. This is called *biliary colic*. There is often vomiting and sweating. When an attack begins the patient should be put in a hot bath. This will often be sufficient to ease the pain, but in the more severe cases it may be necessary for the doctor to give morphia or a whiff of chloroform. Atropine sulphate is very useful in controlling the attacks.

Treatment. Once gallstones have developed there is no known method of dissolving them. Some people, in an attempt to do so, take large doses of olive oil, and unscrupulous persons even profess to cure the condition by giving the patient something to make him sick, and claiming that the gallstone has been vomited up. It is impossible to carry out either intention. Once the attack is over, either medical treatment is given for chronic catarrh of the gall bladder, or, more probably, the gall bladder containing the gallstones is removed by surgical means.

GANGLION. Ganglion is a misleading term, in that it has two separate, unrelated meanings. The more important meaning of ganglion is a collection of nerve cells into which other nerves run and where they join together. If the nervous system of the body is compared to a railway, the ganglia are the large railway junctions—not stations —where various lines meet together from all over the country and from which they continue on their way. The largest group of ganglia in the body is the *solar plexus,* which is situated in the middle line of the body above the navel. It is well known from the experience of boxers and others how a blow on this important junction of the nerves of the abdomen will completely knock a person out for a time. Another important ganglion is the *gasserian ganglion,* lying between the temple bone and the ear. The trigeminal, or fifth nerve, which supplies the face and is so often the seat of facial neuralgia, passes through this ganglion.

The other meaning of ganglion is a small cyst or swelling which contains fluid in the neighbourhood of a joint. These ganglia are fairly common at the back of the wrist. They are small, painless and of no importance. Sometime they disappear of their own accord, but if they do not do so the favorite treatment for them is to strike them hard with a book or give them a hard knock against a flat object. This will burst the swelling and disperse the fluid. The cyst will usually fill up again, however, and may have to be injected with a sclerosing solution, or dissected out if it is troublesome.

GANGRENE. Gangrene, or mortification, is the term used when a part of the body, usually a limb, loses all vitality and becomes dead. There are two types of this condition, "dry" and "moist." In the dry type, the dead part shrivels up, and becomes hard, dry and wrinkled, and of a dark brown color; in moist gangrene the part becomes inflamed and swollen and putrefaction sets in.

Gangrene may be due to several causes. Diabetes, and the disorder of arteries known as arteriosclerosis, are among the chief of these. Frostbite may result in dry gangrene if it has been severe. In *Buerger's disease* and *Raynaud's disease* in which the arteries are affected or after poisoning by ergot which causes constriction of the arteries, gangrene is liable to set in. Fortunately, however, all forms of gangrene are quite rare.

Symptoms of Dry Gangrene. In elderly persons with diseased arteries there may be some pain in the affected limb before gangrene actually sets in. There is no pain as a rule after gangrene has occurred and there is very rarely any fever. The gangrenous part becomes separated from the nor-

mal tissues by what is known as the line of demarcation. This line is very sharply marked by a red ring of inflammation on the healthy side. This ring gradually deepens in color, until after a month or two, the gangrenous part may drop off and leave a stump.

Symptoms of Moist Gangrene. Of the two forms, moist gangrene is the more dangerous and also more common. The part becomes swollen, and is usually greatly discolored. There are numerous blisters containing fluid on the gangrenous part and these ooze all the time and are very foul-smelling. The patient is usually in a state of high fever, and often delirious, and death may result from general blood poisoning in a few days. There is no sharply defined line of the gangrenous area, and the gangrene is apt to extend up the limb.

Treatment. Treatment of dry gangrene consists, in the first instance, of measures to prevent the part from undergoing putrefaction, or, in other words, from developing into moist gangrene. Moist dressings should never be applied and penicillin or similar powder must be used in their place. When the red line appears, amputation may be performed close above it. In the moist form of gangrene antiseptic dressings should be applied in order to keep the gangrene as dry as possible, and penicillin injected, but in rapidly spreading cases amputation may have to be carried out at an early date.

GARGLE. A gargle is a watery solution which is used to cleanse the back of the throat. Though popular, many throat specialists consider gargles of very little curative value. There are many drugs which may be used for gargling but it is always advisable to use only those which can be swallowed without any unpleasant effects. A teaspoonful of common salt with one of baking soda in a tumblerful of warm water is a very useful and handy gargle. This will help to clear the throat of any material which cannot be removed by coughing. Another common gargle is a tablet of chlorate of potash dissolved in a wine-glass of warm water.

If the throat is slightly irritated or relaxed, aspirin is a substance frequently used. Two tablets in half a glass of warm water will be found very soothing. Antiseptic gargles should be used if the throat is at all infected, or in cases of tonsillitis or bad breath. Permanganate of potassium used in a faint pink solution is one of the most common gargles. Usually one or two crystals will be found sufficient to color the water.

How to Gargle. About a tablespoonful of the solution should be taken into the mouth at one time after a deep breath has been taken. The head should be thrown well back and the solution should be made to bubble at the back of the throat. This will ensure the whole of the throat being sprayed, and will also prevent any of the solution from being swallowed. The breath should be held as long as possible in order to obtain the most benefit from the gargle.

GAS GANGRENE. This term describes the infection of a wound by gasforming bacteria, spreading rapidly and soon proving fatal unless promptly recognized and treated. It is treated by radical excision of the affected group of muscles, anti-gas-gangrene serum, and injection of penicillin.

GAS POISONING. There are many trades in which gas poisoning may occur owing to the fumes given off in the manufacture of certain materials. In the case of miners, there is always an element of danger from carbon monoxide, which is found in coal gas. Other examples of gas which may produce poisoning include the fumes from mercury, arsenic, lead, and phosphorus. During the first World War, poison gases were used which caused enormous casualties. There were many types of gases, but the most common included "mustard" gas, chlorine, phosgene, and hydrocyanic acid. Poison gas was fortunately not resorted to in the second World War. (*See also* CARBON MONOXIDE.)

GASSERIAN GANGLION. This term describes a group of nerve cells just beyond where the sensory nerve of the face (the trigeminal nerve) divides into three parts. In severe facial neuralgia the Gasserian ganglion may be injected with alcohol, giving good results in skilled hands.

GASTRIC ULCER. Gastric, or stomach ulcers are also called *peptic ulcers,* in common with ulcers situated in the duodenum. A stomach ulcer may be acute or chronic, and may occur in men or women at any age, though acute ulcerated stomachs are more common in young women than in any other class of people. Chronic ulcers of the stomach are most common in men, but are found frequently in older women. Although it is not known exactly how gastric ulcers are formed, it is believed that strongly acid gastric juices are a great part of the cause, as the ulcers always occur in situations where they are exposed to the action of these juices. Irregular meals, nervous strain, and excessive tobacco are certainly other factors.

Symptoms. In young persons the first warning that an ulcer has developed may be the vomiting up of blood from the stomach (hematemesis), an occurrence which is much more alarming than the condition warrants because these acute ulcers in young people are usually cured without much difficulty, whereas an ulcer in an older person may be a much more serious matter. There may have been preceding attacks of indigestion, pain after food, and loss of appetite caused by dread of the pain which the taking of food causes. In many cases there is vomiting of blood; but blood may be found in the stools, which become darkened in color as a result, a condition which is known as melaena. If there is any doubt about the presence of an ulcer an X-ray examination, or direct inspection of the stomach with an instrument called a gastroscope, will usually settle the question.

Treatment. The first essential in the treatment of acute peptic ulcers or chronic ulcers which have bled is rest, both for the body and for the stomach. But the psychology of the patient is also important, and to treat a busy man it may be necessary to temporize for a time, even though adequate treatment can rarely be carried out at home. To ensure the necessary rest the patient is often kept in bed for from three to six weeks, and then is only allowed to take up a strenuous life again by degrees, while treatment by dieting, etc., must be carried out for some months longer.

Diet is of the greatest importance in the treatment of gastric ulcers. Frequent feeding is the essential factor. The Sippy diet is almost universally used. This diet, or a modification of it, must be followed until there is no trace of blood in the stools and no more pain is felt. Milk is the most important item in the diet. Bicarbonate of soda, once a great stand-by, is now no longer recommended, but magnesia is a good substitute for it, and medicine containing atropine or belladonna is usually prescribed. Of course, any bad teeth or unhealthy conditions in the nose or throat must be attended to. Sufferers from long-standing gastric ulcer can often make the best of life by taking care that their meals are frequent and suitable, and by using an alkali when they are troubled by pain. If they lose much work, or their ulcers bleed more than once, they are often advised to undergo an operation. (*See also* STOMACH, DISEASES OF.)

Bleeding from the Stomach. (Hematemesis). When this occurs suddenly, lay the patient down flat, in bed if possible, and keep him quiet and motionless. When the doctor arrives, he usually makes sure that the patient will remain still by giving an injection of morphia. The mouth may be sponged out at frequent intervals with cold water, but the water should not be swallowed.

Feeding is nowadays undertaken early— as soon as the patient no longer feels sick —and is usually possible about 12 hours after a hematemesis. Cases in which there is much loss of blood need to have this replaced by transfusing, which is, of course, best carried out in hospital. Cases in which bleeding continues in spite of medical treatment will often require surgical operation. (*See also* HEMATEMESIS.)

GASTRITIS. Inflammation of the lining of the stomach is known as gastritis, and there are two stages of this condition, the acute and the chronic. The acute form usually develops as a result of taking some indigestible or some tainted food, or from drinking excessive amounts of alcohol. It may occur in influenza, bronchitis, pneumonia or at the beginning of an infectious fever. In children, acute gastritis is usually present in summer diarrhea.

Symptoms of Acute Gastritis. At the beginning of a mild attack there may be a feeling of heaviness in the region of the stomach and the tongue may be thickly coated with fur. A feeling of sickness comes on which is relieved when vomiting takes place. There may be no sign of any rise of temperature and the attack may not last

longer than from 24 to 48 hours. In the more severe forms of acute gastritis, however, these symptoms become more definite, and there may be a rise in temperature to as much as 103 deg. F. Instead of vomiting the usual stomach contents there may be a large quantity of mucus, gastric juice, and possibly some blood. The patient may suffer from collapse and faintness which may last for four or five days.

In the majority of cases, an attack of acute gastritis lasts only a short time, and apart from diarrhea there are seldom any complications; but in severe cases, the acute form may develop into the chronic condition, and in rare cases ulceration of the stomach may occur.

Treatment of an Acute Attack. The patient should be put to bed and kept warm with hot-water bottles. Two grains of calomel or a good dose of castor oil will clear out the bowel, especially if it is followed by a dose of salts in the morning. Calomel should never be given to children, as it may prove too strong for them; but castor oil will be found sufficiently powerful.

No food should be given until vomiting stops. Should vomiting persist after the stomach has been cleared, attempts to stop it may be made by giving sips of hot water. To relieve the pain in the stomach, hot flannels may be applied to the abdomen. If the condition does not clear up after the bowels have moved, or if the patient appears seriously ill, send for a doctor without further delay. For the treatment of chronic gastritis, *see also* INDIGESTION.

GASTROENTERITIS. This is an inflammation of the stomach and intestines, the main symptoms of which are vomiting, diarrhea and general weakness. Treatment is chiefly by fasting and complete rest. (*See also* DIARRHEA.)

GAUZE. This is a thin open-meshed cloth used for surgical dressings. When it has been treated with antiseptics it is referred to as antiseptic gauze. It is called gauze because it was first imported from Gaza in Syria.

GELATINE. Gelatine is a substance which is obtained by boiling down animal tissue, bone, gristle, and cartilage. It forms a colorless substance which is jelly-like when moistened, and hard and brittle when dried. It is used a great deal as a food and also in the making of pastilles and various other chemical products. Gelatine capsules are made to hold unpleasant drugs, and gelatine of zinc is sometimes poured over ulcers in order to protect them when healing. Solutions of sterile gelatine have been injected into the body in order to raise the blood-pressure after severe hemorrhage.

GENERAL PARALYSIS OF THE INSANE. This is a disease which until recently was rightly looked upon as one of the most fatal, as well as the most horrible, diseases of the nervous system. Nowadays, however, new methods of treatment, which are described later, have so changed the outlook for the unfortunate sufferers from this disorder that it is safe to say that in cases in which the disease is recognized early enough, at least one-third, and probably even more, of the cases can be so far cured that the patients can return to their ordinary work. A large number, though not curable, are enabled to live happy, useful lives instead of dying in misery a few years after the onset of the disease, which was the only outlook for them a few years ago. But everything depends on the disease being recognized in its early stages, and only too often it is found that cure is impossible because the disease has destroyed too many of the essential nerve cells in the brain for a true recovery to take place.

It is possible for a doctor to discover whether a patient has G.P.I. very early after the appearance of any symptoms whatsoever, and often before any symptoms have shown themselves. The patient is merely feeling "run down" and "nervous." This is done by an examination of the patient, and of the fluid, which is obtained by putting a needle in between the bones of the back and drawing off the fluid present in the space between the coverings of the spinal cord.

It has now been proved beyond all doubt that G.P.I. is always caused by syphilis. The germ which causes syphilis can be seen in the brains of those who have died from G.P.I., and the special test for syphilis can always be found positive in the blood and spinal fluid of patients with G.P.I. The germ in the brain manufactures poisons which destroy the delicate nerve cells, and as the most fragile nerve

cells are those which control the intellect, it is not surprising that mental changes are noticed fairly early in the disorder. In an attempt to combat the poisons which are being thrown out, the brain tissue strangles the germs by enveloping them in a new firm tissue, like delicate threads of silk; but unfortunately the firm tissue destroys the nerve cells also, thus further diminishing the number available for the patient to think with. The new treatment of G.P.I., by producing a very high temperature, kills off the germs in the brain so that they are unable any longer to produce poisons, and obviates the formation of fresh firm tissue. But once nerve cells are killed they can never re-form, so it can plainly be seen that the necessity for beginning treatment while as few nerve cells as possible have been damaged is vital for the cure of the condition.

G.P.I. occurs all over the world, and no class or race is exempt. The infection with syphilis takes place sometimes many years before the nervous disease shows itself. On an average G.P.I. occurs ten to fifteen years after the infection has taken place. It is especially likely to occur in patients in whom the syphilis has been badly or insufficiently treated. It is much more common in men than in women.

Symptoms. The first sign of the disease noticed by the relatives and friends of a patient suffering from G.P.I. is a change in his character. The affectionate husband becomes morose, depressed and neglectful, both of his own interest and of his wife. He often feels a lack of self-confidence and an apathy which is too often put down to "nerves" by his friends until more obvious changes in his personality appear. These may take one of two forms. Either the patient becomes more and more depressed, ceasing to take any interest in his hobbies and his surroundings, or he becomes more cheerful and lively, full of plans for doing impossible things, and ready with ridiculous excuses to account for his bad work and failing memory.

The latter type will make the most absurd statements, which seem to them perfectly reasonable. Thus, a man will say he possesses twenty million dollars, but in the next breath will beg the doctor to give him a cigarette as he cannot afford to buy one; or the man who claims to be a champion boxer will be unable even to assume a fighting attitude. But these false beliefs of wealth and fame are not so frequently met with nowadays as the depressed type of case, and it is certainly a common and sometimes excusable mistake for G.P.I. to be taken for simple neurasthenia in its early stages. The middle-aged man who becomes inattentive to his business or careless in his work, irritable, complaining of vague headache and sleeplessness is often judged to be suffering from overwork and sent on a vacation.

But certain physical accompaniments may make such a case suspect: any kind of attack, such as an epileptic fit, in a person who has not before suffered from epilepsy, is suggestive of some real disease of the brain which may be G.P.I. Vision may sometimes be affected, the patient either seeing two objects instead of one for a considerable time, or he may show an obvious and not previously noticed squint. Sometimes slight seizures may occur, leaving the patient more or less paralysed down one side, and the speech may alter, giving a curious slurring effect which is quite characteristic to the trained ear. This speech is difficult to describe: the patient finds it hard to say his words; he halts and stumbles over long words and may leave out, slur over, or say parts of them twice. The writing suffers somewhat in the same way; the former character of the writing is lost and it becomes tremulous, while there is a tendency to omit words or syllables. Physically, going downhill rapidly, mentally, unfit to take charge of his affairs, the plight of the patient with G.P.I. is pathetic. Before the introduction of the present methods of treatment, a year or two at home, taxing the patience and forbearance of his family, then six months or a year in a mental hospital as a wreck of his former self, saw the end of such a patient.

Treatment. At present, large doses of penicillin is the method of choice, combined with one or other method of inducing a high temperature. In the near future, possibly other antibiotics may take the place of penicillin. The induction of a high temperature is carried out by deliberately inducing malaria, either by letting the mosquito which carries the infection bite the

patient, or by the injection of the blood of another patient who has malaria.

It seems strange to give a patient one disease to cure another which is more deadly; but although malaria, as seen in tropical countries, is a very dangerous disease, there are several forms of it, and the form that is given to patients suffering from G.P.I. is a relatively mild one, which can be controlled and cured at any desired moment by a known remedy, quinine. The effect of giving malaria in G.P.I. is to produce very high temperatures in the patient's body at regular intervals, either every day, every other day or every three days, for a certain period, depending on the general health of the patient and his response to the treatment. These high temperatures kill off all, or nearly all the germs in the brain which are causing the disease and the patient is left, after his course of malaria, weak but much improved mentally. Other methods, more easily controlled, of inducing high temperatures have also been tried, a usual one being by electrical "short waves." This needs experience and a trained staff.

It must once again be emphasized that the early recognition of the disorder is all important for the success of the treatment. In advanced cases, the most that can be hoped for by any method of treatment is that the patient's life is prolonged for a few years; complete cure depends entirely on how early the case is taken in hand. (*See also* MALARIA.)

GENITALS. The genitals are the organs of reproduction. (*See also* REPRODUCTIVE SYSTEM.)

GENTIAN. This is a bitter substance much used to improve the appetite and prevent indigestion, and a favorite flavoring for tonics and other medicines. (*See also* BITTERS.)

GERM. The word germ is used in two senses, first to signify any of the bacteria or microbes. In this sense it is discussed under the heading GERMS. Secondly, the germ of a thing means the small kernel or nucleus which is the part of any living organism from which a similar new organism springs. We speak of the germ of a grain of wheat, and in this sense the nucleus of a cell is a germ; so, also, is the embryo of a human being.

GERMAN MEASLES. Also known as rubella, this is a mild infectious disease occurring chiefly in children, usually after the age of 5 years. It takes about 15 or 16 days to develop and in many communities the child is not allowed to return to school for 10 days after the appearance of the rash, or 21 days from the date of exposure to infection.

Symptoms. The child seems slightly out of sorts and develops a temperature accompanied by a slight cold, a chain of enlarged glands which feel like hard peas down the sides of the neck, and a rash which is similar in appearance to the scarlet fever and measles rashes. The rash comes out first on the face and spreads over the body, arms, and legs. It is widespread and consists of small pink spots, but scarcely raised; it has often completely vanished in 24 hours' time.

Treatment. The treatment is simple, as the disease is not as serious as ordinary measles. The child should be kept warm in bed, and the bowels kept open with syrup of figs or milk of magnesia. When the temperature has returned to normal, in a day or two, and the rash has disappeared, the child may be allowed up, but should be kept isolated in the bedroom for one week after the appearance of the rash. No visitors or animals should be allowed in the room. Although the disease is usually slight, it is necessary to send for the doctor when the rash appears, as it is extremely difficult sometimes to be certain that the rash is not that of scarlet fever, which may be a serious illness because of its complications.

German measles is not a serious or fatal disease but is known to produce deafness or eye defects in the developing child when it occurs in a mother during the early months of pregnancy. A pregnant mother should take precautions to avoid contact with the disease. An intramuscular injection of gamma globulin helps to give protection.

GERMICIDE. Any substance which is capable of destroying germs is called a germicide. Prolonged and intense heat acts as a germicide as well as many drugs. (*See also* ANTISEPTIC; DISINFECTANT; GERMS.)

GERMS. Under the heading germs are included microbes, bacteria, and yeasts—in fact, all the little living microorganisms which cause disease in our bodies. Many germs, however, have their definite use in some particular part of the body—such as the *Bacillus coli*, the germ which lives normally in the colon where it helps to break up the unwanted waste materials of food in order that they may pass on and be voided. This bacillus is useful and normal in its proper place in the lower bowel, but when it strays into other regions such as the upper bowel and gall bladder it becomes a source of ill-health.

Germs are the simplest form of life. They are minute and cannot be seen without the aid of a microscope. Each germ consists of a single cell with a nucleus. It spreads and multiplies by the division of the cell and nucleus, as is explained in the article on CELLS. Some germs have no power of movement of their own, and are simply carried about in the fluids of the body, but others can move of their own accord.

Bacteria are classified according to their shape as *cocci* or spherical germs, *bacilli* or rod-shaped germs, and twisted shapes called *spirilla*. According to the way in which *cocci* group together, they are referred to as *streptococci, staphylococci,* and *pneumococci.* Each coccus has the shape of a sphere when looked at singly, but they are more often seen in groups or strings with their sides flattened against their immediate neighbors.

The illustration commonly used to give some idea of their size is that a drop of water would contain at least one billion. The pneumococcus is the germ which causes pneumonia, the staphylococcus is the cause of boils and other skin troubles, and the streptococcus causes tonsillitis, scarlet fever, erysipelas, and various other acute infections.

Such various forms of disease as anthrax, botulism, conjunctivitis, diphtheria, dysentery, meningitis, tuberculosis, and typhoid fever are caused by separate and distinct varieties of rodshaped germs or bacilli. The germs which cause syphilis are of the twisted type called spirilla.

Many diseases are due not to a single organism but to several species attacking a weakened part such as the bronchial tubes in bronchitis. Inflammation of the gall bladder may be caused by several sorts of germs; the same is true of inflammation in the stomach, the intestines, etc. Influenza is probably one of these mixed infections, though a germ called the Pfeiffer bacillus is commonly called the influenza bacillus. The germs which cause smallpox, typhus fever, hydrophobia, mumps, etc., cannot be seen. The name of *virus* is given to a germ which is presumed to be the cause of certain diseases, but because it is so small no microscope has yet been made that will enable it to be seen. These diseases behave as if they were caused by ordinary bacteria. They can be transmitted from case to case by fluid extracts, and the virus is not held up by passage through an ordinary filter. Specially prepared filters with pores of known size will prevent the passage of many of these disease agents and are able to give us some idea of the dimensions of the tiny particles. A form of germ which is known always to cause a definite disease is called the *specific organism* of that disease, as, for instance, the tubercle bacillus which is specific for tuberculosis. Many of these specific germs, however, can be present in the body in quite large numbers without causing an attack of the disease for which they are specific, because the resistant power of the body is for various reasons too strong for them to gain the upper hand.

Aerobes and Anaerobes. Some germs cannot live without the presence of oxygen and these are called *aerobes*. Others die in the presence of oxygen and are called *anaerobes*. Typical aerobes are the germs of diphtheria, anthrax and cerebrospinal fever. Anaerobes which cannot live in the presence of oxygen are the virulent germ *B. Welchii,* which causes gas gangrene, and the bacillus of lockjaw. Many germs will thrive either with or without oxygen, such as the coccus of pneumonia and the bacillus of typhoid fever.

Fortunately, however, we are equipped with forces in our blood to render germs harmless to us except when, for some reason, our resistance is lowered, and we let them get temporarily ahead of our fighting forces.

Germs are killed off by solutions of carbolic acid, mercurial salts, and other antiseptics, but our greatest ally in germ destruction is heat. Germs die off rapidly at a temperature of 108 deg. F. or over, but as a general rule the exposure to heat must be kept up for twenty minutes at least. On the other hand, cold does not affect them much, and in laboratories and places where it may be necessary to store germs for some time, they are often kept alive in a cooling chamber and are found to be none the worse for it. Direct sunlight is a powerful agent for killing germs, but it must fall directly on them and not through window-glass, which diminishes its power. (*See also* IMMUNITY.)

GESTATION. Gestation is another name for pregnancy. (*See also* ECTOPIC GESTATION; PREGNANCY.)

GIDDINESS. Giddiness is a sensation of unsteadiness of the body which is often accompanied by a feeling of nausea. It may be due to a variety of causes, and if severe demands the attention of a doctor. (*See also* DIZZINESS.)

GIN. Gin is an alcoholic beverage made by distilling potatoes, rye, or barley and flavoring it with the juniper berry. It contains about 30 per cent of alcohol and in English gin only rectified spirit is used; in Dutch gin the spirit used is not rectified. Gin acts on the kidneys and increases the flow of urine. (*See also* ALCOHOL; CIRRHOSIS OF THE LIVER.)

GINGER. Ginger is the root of a plant which grows in India, Jamaica, and other tropical countries. It has a very agreeable smell and a hot, pungent flavor. It is given in the treatment of flatulence and dyspepsia, and is used with purgatives to prevent griping pains. Half to one dram of the syrup or of the tincture of ginger may be given.

GINGIVITIS. This is a condition in which the gums become inflamed. Mild types of gingivitis may be caused by lack of cleanliness of the mouth, or by ill-fitting dental plates. The teeth should always be brushed from the gums towards the teeth.

Treatment. Massage of the gums, painting their edges with iodine, and the use of a mouth wash of diluted hydrogen peroxide will be found effective.

Ulcerative Gingivitis. This is due to an infection. The gums become very swollen and painful and in severe cases the teeth may fall out. The infection may spread to the tonsils or the pharynx.

Treatment. In ulcerative gingivitis it is

advisable to call in the aid of the doctor so that the ulcers may be painted over with an antiseptic solution, and if necessary penicillin used locally or by injection; in addition the mouth should be washed out at frequent intervals. (*See also* PYORRHEA.)

GLANDERS. An infectious disease that occurs in horses and donkeys, but which is occasionally transmitted to man. It is characterized by swellings, which become ulcerated, in the nose or under the skin, and has been known to be mistaken for smallpox. It is treated by excision and strong antiseptics.

GLANDS. The glands of the body are organs which manufacture substances necessary to the working of the body, and which help to rid the system of harmful substances. These organs are divided into two broad classes, the ordinary glands which have a passage (duct) leading from them into which their fluids flow, and the ductless glands which, as their name implies, have no ducts. The ductless glands include many of the structures such as the thyroid gland, the adrenals, and the pituitary gland, which are now known to exercise a great influence on the health of the body by the strong action of the powerful secretions they produce. These are dealt with in a separate article called DUCTLESS GLANDS.

The ordinary glands of the body are grouped according to their use in the working of the body. There are the *lymph glands*, the *glands of elimination*, the *glands of assimilation*, and a few glands for special purposes which do not come into these classes.

Lymph glands. The lymph glands are widely scattered throughout the body. Their function is to protect the body from the action of harmful germs and substances.

The lymph glands do this by drainage and by the production of *lymphocytes*, which are one sort of white blood corpuscle. They are found in masses in such places as the armpits, the groins, the neck, under the knees and in the bend of the elbow, as well as amongst the deep tissues of the body, in the thorax and abdomen.

These lymph-glands seem to be more active in childhood than at later age. They act as the filters for the lymph—the colorless fluid which flows through the body in channels called the lymphatic channels, collecting the waste materials from the tissues.

Glands of Elimination. The glands which deal with the actual passage of waste material from the tissues of the body are called the glands of elimination. The chief of these are the sweat glands, the sebaceous glands, the kidneys, and the mucous glands which are found in the linings of all the organs of the body. The *sweat glands* are to be found all over the skin but are more plentiful in some places than in others, as, for instance, the soles of the feet and the armpits. The duty of these glands is to get rid of surplus water out of the tissues in the form of sweat, thus regulating the body temperature. The *sebaceous* glands are situated on the hairy parts of the skin and provide an oily substance which is necessary to the health of the skin.

The *kidneys* perform the greatest part of the work by clearing the body of its waste materials. They are described under their own heading. The organs of the body are lined with mucus and in this substance are numerous glands called the *mucous* glands, which provide a clear and sticky fluid which acts as a lubricating material for keeping the mucous membranes moist. They also protect the linings of the organs from attack by germs, because when germs in excessive quantity attack a part of the mucous membrane, such as the lining of the nose or bowel, a larger quantity of mucus is produced which serves to wash them away.

Glands of Assimilation. These are the glands which play a part in the digestion of food. They include all the glands of the mouth, such as the salivary glands, those of the stomach and intestinal tract, such as the glands in the duodenum, the liver, and the pancreas, all discussed under their own headings.

Glands, Diseases of. Lymph glands are liable to be overcome by the germs they deal with and become inflamed. They are also attacked, chiefly in childhood, by tuberculosis, and may become involved in secondary growths of cancer.

When a person talks of suffering from glands he generally means infected, swollen glands, especially in the neck. Such a condition used to be a very common disease, especially in children. The infection nearly always spreads to the glands of the neck from unhealthy tonsils and adenoids. These conditions are now cleared up before the glands have become infected. Tuberculosis still frequently attacks the glands in childhood, especially those in the neck and abdomen, and is usually due to infected milk. The blood condition called *leukemia,* in which the lymphglands become greatly swollen throughout the body, is discussed under its own heading. (*See also* GLANDULAR FEVER, MUMPS.)

GLANDULAR EXTRACTS. Many experiments have been carried out to make use of extracts of some of the most important glands in the body. Striking successes have followed the results of these experiments. Probably the thyroid gland preparations are the oldest and best known. The extract is prepared from the thyroid glands of sheep, and each extract is standardized to ensure absolute purity and correct dosage. These preparations have proved very beneficial in the treatment of various conditions due to thyroid deficiency, especially myxedema, which occurs chiefly in older women, and cretinism.

Extracts from the suprarenal glands are used in the treatment of Addison's disease. Adrenalin, or epinephrin, and eucortone are the names given to extracts from these glands, and they are intimately concerned with the growth and the sexual development of the body as well as the maintenance of life itself.

Extracts from the pituitary glands of animals are sold under various names such as pituitrin, pitibulin, pituglandol, etc. Injections of extract of the pituitary gland are given to stimulate the contraction of various muscles of the body, and especially to increase the contraction of the uterus so as to shorten the period of labor and to prevent bleeding after the child is born.

Injections of insulin are given as a routine treatment in cases of diabetes. Insulin is prepared from the pancreas of sheep and oxen. Extracts of ovarian and other glands are being experimented with and used at the change of life and in other conditions. It is unwise, however, for anyone to treat themselves with any any of these extracts without the advice and the supervision of a doctor. (*See also* DUCTLESS GLANDS.)

GLANDULAR FEVER. Also known as infectious mononucleosis. This is a condition in which the glands of the neck become swollen, and sometimes the glands under the arms and in the groin become affected. It usually occurs in epidemic form, especially in the autumn, and it may affect children living in one house, or children who are at school together. There is a moderate degree of fever which may last for a week or two and sometimes a rash like that of measles or German measles, or sometimes jaundice. The patient should be isolated for 7 days after the fever and swellings have gone down.

Treatment. The child should be put to bed and the neck kept warm by rolling a flannel bandage round it. Castor oil may be given to keep the bowels open. The child should not be allowed up until a few days after the temperature has returned to normal, and convalescence may be slow, as the general system may be very much depressed. Tonics and careful dieting will do much to build up the health and, if it is at all possible, a change of air is very beneficial. (*See also* GLANDS; MUMPS.)

GLAUBER'S SALT. Glauber's salt, or sodium sulphate, is occasionally used as a saline purgative. It should be taken first thing in the morning in doses of a quarter of an ounce to half an ounce in a glass of water, or repeated smaller doses may be taken if desired.

GLAUCOMA. Glaucoma is an eye disease whose special sign is a tendency to increase of pressure within the eye, resulting finally in destruction of the optic nerve fibers and blindness. There are various forms of the disease, but they differ only in the rate at which the tension increases. In some of the more acute forms the pupil is greenish, and it was to these cases that the word *glaucoma,* from the Greek word meaning sea-green, was orginally applied. The word is now used as a general term for all forms of the disease.

Glaucoma may occur in infants, owing to an error of development, and is then known as "ox-eye" from its appearance. It is, however, most common in people of fifty or more, and may follow great anxiety or emotion.

Symptoms. An acute attack usually begins at night with severe neuralgic pains in the eye and the same side of the head, which may last for two or three days. The pain may be so acute as to cause sickness, and the patient mistakenly thinks the attack to be only a sick headache. These are the cases that are so dangerous; they may destroy the sight beyond repair in a day; but an ordinarily severe case goes on for about a week, and a chronic case many months, before damage is caused.

There are all varieties between the acute and the chronic. The latter often comes on so gradually and painlessly that it is disregarded until serious damage has been done; sometimes it comes on by steps, so to speak, the patient having a series of more or less severe bouts, with clouding of vision. They pass away after some minutes or hours, each attack, however, leaving the sight worse than before. In chronic cases, artificial lights appear to be surrounded by colored haloes, and there are various other peculiarities of sight, such as lessening of the field of vision. The veins on the surface are distended, so that the eye is bloodshot. The pupil is wide and oval instead of being small and round, and may be greenish. The eye is harder than usual, and vision is hazy.

Treatment. The outlook in glaucoma is always serious as regards the sight, and the sooner treatment is commenced the better, especially in the acute cases. Formerly, the disease was regarded as incurable; but, in 1857, von Graefe introduced an operation in which a small piece of the iris was removed at one point. This is still the operation for choice in acute cases; in the less acute cases another operation is performed, where a small portion of the white of the eye is removed.

If the condition is very chronic, or if an operation is inadvisable, *eserine* drops are used. Eserine contracts the pupil and helps to open the angle of filtration.

GLEET. Gleet is the name given to a discharge from the urethra, sometimes found after an attack of gonorrhea. (*See also* GONORRHEA.)

GLOBUS HYSTERICUS. This is a common complaint in hysteria in which there is a choking sensation as if a ball were obstructing the throat. This is probably a more pronounced example of the feeling of a "lump in the throat" which is sometimes felt when the emotions are stirred. If persistent, however, a skilled

and thorough examination of the throat should always be carried out. (*See also* EMOTION; HYSTERIA.)

GLOSSITIS. Glossitis means inflammation of the tongue. (*See also* TONGUE, DISEASES OF.)

GLOTTIS. The narrow opening at the upper end of the larynx, or voice-box, is known as the glottis. It varies in width and shape with the movements of the vocal cords. During ordinary quiet breathing the glottis is open, but while the vocal cords are being used as in speech or singing, the opening is reduced to a mere slit. The narrow opening of the glottis is called in medical language the rima glottidis. (*See also* LARYNX.)

GLUCOSE. Glucose is also known as dextrose and it is the form of sugar which is found in ripe fruits, especially grapes; it is also in honey and, of course, in jam made with fruits. It is an important article in the diet as it forms a very valuable food which is easily digested. Ordinary cane sugar has to undergo a chemical change before it is digested; but glucose is what might be termed a predigested substance, so is particularly beneficial to people with weak digestions. An enema containing glucose will provide sufficient nourishment to tide a patient over a critical period, or a carefully sterilized injection may be given directly into the veins.

The body has an elaborate mechanism for controlling the level of glucose in the blood. When this mechanism is disturbed, as in diabetes, the surplus glucose spills over from the blood in the kidneys and is present in the urine. (*See also* DIABETES; URINE.)

GLUCOSIDE. There are many drugs from which glucose—and another substance which is not sugar—can be obtained. These substances are known as glucosides. The more important ones are amygdalin, arbutin, digitalin, and salicin.

GLUTEAL ARTERY. This is a large and important artery situated in the buttocks. This artery breaks up in various branches which supply blood to the lower limbs. (*See also* ARTERY.)

GLUTEUS MAXIMUS. This is the chief muscle of the buttock. It helps to join the thighbone to the pelvis.

GLYCERINE. Glycerine is a sweet, heavy fluid which is capable of absorbing water, and for this reason it is used a great deal on the hands to prevent their getting chapped. Rose-water is usually added to give it perfume. Because glycerine is so easily absorbed by the skin, it is often added to other substances such as iodine, tannic acid, salicin, etc, and applied to wounds, or to the unbroken skin through which these substances enter the body.

Glycerine has a very soothing effect on the mucous membrances, and for this reason it is used with tannic acid or iodine as a paint in cases of sore throat. Internally it has been given as a purgative in doses of 1 or 2 teaspoonfuls either by mouth or, more often, in the form of an enema. The result is prompt, usually occurring within less than half an hour, and there is very little pain or internal disturbance.

GLYCOSURIA. The presence of sugar in the urine is known as glycosuria. It is true that sugar in the urine is one of the chief symptoms of diabetes, but its presence does not always signify that diabetes is the cause. Special tests can be made to prove whether the glycosuria is due to true diabetes or whether the excess of sugar in the urine is due to some other condition.

Among the conditions which cause sugar to appear in the urine, probably the most common is faulty diet. If too much starchy food is taken, in other words, if the diet is overbalanced with carbohydrates, the excess sugar which the body is not able to deal with will be poured out in the urine. This condition is known as *alimentary glycosuria,* and it is met with in stout people and those who are overfond of the good things of the table. Any disturbance of the nervous system, or of the kidneys, may also cause sugar to appear in the urine. Occasionally during pregnancy, or after a severe mental shock, glycosuria is to be found. As a general rule if glycosuria occurs in young people it is a symptom of true diabetes, which is a serious condition, though it sometimes occurs in whooping cough and other ailments; while in people over fifty glycosuria is most commonly met with in those who eat and drink too much, and have a high blood pressure. With due care, however, the condition can be controlled to a great extent. (*See also* DIABETES; URINE.)

GOITER. An enlargement of the thyroid gland is known as a goiter or bronchocele. There are two main types of goiter, simple and exophthalmic. Exophthalmic goiter is dealt with fully under the heading GRAVES' DISEASE, and only the simple type is discussed in this article. The thyroid gland when it is working normally does not show in the neck, although there are occasions when the gland varies in size and activity quite considerably even in healthy persons.

A temporary enlargement of the thyroid gland is not unusual in women during the menstrual period, as well as during pregnancy. Such a temporary swelling is, of course, not a goiter, but at the same time it has been found that goiter is far commoner in women than in men and it is often associated with puberty, pregnancy and lactation.

Simple goiter. A swelling in the front of the neck is characteristic of this condition, and there is usually very little difficulty in recognizing that it is due to the thyroid gland. A simple goiter appearing at puberty or during pregnancy often disappears in a few months; but if it occurs in a district in which goiter is a common complaint, then it is often permanent.

Causes. There are two main theories as to the cause of goiter. It is thought that some drinking waters lack iodine, and it has been suggested that it may be due to a microorganism in the water. Certainly there is no doubt that the waters of some districts are definitely goitrigenous, and the deep valleys in mountainous districts seem to be particularly so. For example, it is very common in the Swiss Alps, the Italian Alps, and in the mountainous parts of Germany. In India it is common in the Himalayas, and in England it occurs so often in the hilly parts of Derbyshire that the condition is known by the name of Derbyshire neck. It is also very common in parts of America such as the Great Lakes, the Appalachian and Rocky Mountain states, where there is a lack of iodine in the soil. It is important to note that people may be cured of the condition by removal to another district, just as a healthy person may develop goiter by settling in a district where it prevails.

Symptoms. Swelling of the thyroid gland

may begin between the eighth and twelfth year, but as a rule its growth is at first gradual. Later on the swelling may be very marked, though there is rarely any pain. The patient is always able to swallow quite easily, and it is only when the swelling becomes very large that it interferes with breathing. During the early stages, the swelling is not hard, but in the course of time it may become firm and irregular. There are often signs of nervousness in the patient, especially if the goiter is accompanied by overactivity of the thyroid gland (hyperthyroidism). In cases of lessened activity (hypothyroidism) there may be a tendency towards fatness and sluggishness.

Treatment. In many districts in which goiter is common, it is the practice to add iodine to the drinking water at its source. If this is not possible, an iodized table salt should be used in cooking and with meals. In cases where the swelling is very unsightly, or where it is causing pressure and interfering with the breathing, a surgical operation may have to be performed. An operation is also advisable in those cases where a tumor or cyst has formed in the gland. Nowadays the surgeon never removes the whole of the gland. (*See also* DUCTLESS GLANDS; GRAVES' DISEASE; MYXEDEMA.)

GONORRHEA. Gonorrhea is a common type of infectious venereal disease and is the cause of a great deal of ill-health and chronic invalidism, especially in women. It is caused by a germ called the gonococcus, which gains entrance to the child-bearing organs and urinary tract, usually through the act of sexual intercourse, though it is said that occasionally it may be acquired from an infected towel.

Symptoms in Women. The patient complains of scalding pain on passing water, accompanied by a burning feeling and irritation in the genitals, and a thick "creamy" discharge which develops in a few days' time into a thin watery discharge which is not so irritating. Later on, there may be pain in the lower part of the abdomen and warts and sore places on the genitals. The discharge causes discomfort and soreness round the genital and on the sides of the thighs. Medical advice should always be sought though it should be noted that there are many other causes of vaginal

discharge besides gonorrhea; one not uncommon cause, for instance, is a retained and forgotten vaginal tampon.

Symptoms in Men. The disease comes on suddenly with irritation at the end of the penis, combined in a few days with scalding during the passing of water and also a thick creamy discharge which tends to persist and become worse if the condition is left untreated. There may also be pain in the groin and a painful little lump on one side or the other.

Treatment. It is of great importance to have a medical examination as soon as possible in a suspected case, so that treatment may be begun at once, for the earlier treatment is begun the less likelihood is there of complications. In spite of the revolution in treatment brought about by the introduction first of the sulphonamide drugs and then of penicillin, more general treatment is still necessary and will be described later. Sulphapyridine was the first sulphonamide drug employed, but more recently sulphadiazine and sulphadimidine, which are just as effective and less toxic to the patient, have been employed. It has been proved that sulphadiazine, or sulphadimidine, taken in adequate doses not later than the day after exposure, can actually prevent gonorrhea; but the continued employment of sulphonamide drugs causes the gonorrhea germs to become resistant to them. Since the discovery of penicillin this drug has been widely used in the treatment of the condition but it, also, has to be given in adequate large doses to prevent the development of penicillin-resistant strains of the germs. In early cases it has been shown that gonorrhea can be cured by a single injection of 600,000 units of penicillin which has been specially prepared so that it is maintained in the blood for a considerable time and not excreted as quickly as usual.

Drug-resistant Cases. Such cases have been treated successfully by artificially raising the patient's temperature to 103 deg. F. or over, for a minimum of eight hours. To do this, intravenous injections of antityphoid vaccine may be given, or an electric instrument called the hypertherm may be employed. It may be noted, however, that the treatment is not without risk and some fatalities have occurred.

General Treatment (Male). Many doctors have given up the once usual urethral irrigations on cases of gonorrhea, since the introduction of sulphonamides and penicillin; but others consider that daily irrigations of a 1 in 10,000 solution of permanganate of potash are helpful and bring about a more adequate cleansing and drainage from the crypts and ducts of the urethra, for the small foci of infection left in the urethra may cause relapses. Large quantities of bland fluids should be drunk, but absolutely no alcohol may be taken during treatment.

General Treatment (Female). So long as there is any discharge the patient should remain in bed, on a light diet, keeping the bowels open with senna or liquorice, and hot vaginal douches at a temperature of 115 deg. F. should be given. Some doctors prefer dry swabbing of the vagina, urethra, and cervix to douching; chemicals should not be used, as they are unnecessary with modern chemotherapy and may also cause irritation.

Salpingitis and Oophoritis. This is a condition in which the germ has spread from the inside of the womb along the tubes, causing inflammation in them and in the ovaries which are attached to them. This may lead to a thickening and sealing-up of the tubes (salpingitis) causing an inability to become pregnant (sterility) and also to disease and perhaps abscess of the ovaries (oophoritis).

Symptoms. The symptoms of an acute attack in a tube somewhat resemble those of an attack of appendicitis. The patient goes to bed with a pain in the lower part of the body, either on the right or left or perhaps on both sides. She is feverish and feels ill. The attack settles down in a day or two, but returns at intervals until the patient has always a certain amount of pain and tenderness in the pelvis and is never really well.

Conclusion. In all cases of gonorrhea, whether male or female, there is a risk of an attack of acute infection of the joints (acute gonococcal rheumatism). The treatment is the same as for acute gonorrhea. In addition, the joints are kept at rest in bed.

In any case of gonorrhea, great care should be taken not to spread the infection to the eyes through getting the germ on the fingers, thus causing the serious condition of gonorrheal conjunctivitis. This condition used to be the most common cause of blindness. The baby's eyes become infected from the vaginal discharge of the mother, and unless given penicillin or sulphonamides and treated at once with a silver preparation such as protargol the sight is permanently damaged.

In *all* cases of gonorrhea it is *vital* that the patient should receive medical treatment immediately.

GOOSEFLESH. This is a very common condition which is brought on by cold, fright, etc. The minute muscles in the skin contract and cause tiny raised lumps all over the skin which are called "gooseflesh" because in appearance the skin resembles that of a plucked goose. It disappears of its own accord when the fright is over or the skin is warm again.

Treatment. For gooseflesh which appears to be fairly chronic, improve the general health, apply friction to the arms and legs by vigorous rubbing with a coarse sponge soap which may be adapted to use instead of sulphur ointment by rubbing on fairly dry at night and leaving on until the morning. If the goosefleshy appearance does not clear up, a skin specialist should be consulted in good time, as the condition must be one of some definite skin trouble such as acne or dermatitis.

GOUT. Gout is a painful disease in which there is an excess of uric acid in the blood. It has a marked tendency to be hereditary. The person who comes from "gouty stock" may become typically gouty in his old age, or he may be afflicted with various degrees of ill-health in which one or other of the systems of his body is chronically below par. Such people are those who suffer from *allergic* diseases, early circulatory degeneration and so on. This tendency to inherit the liability to gouty trouble is called the gouty *diathesis*. However, in spite of family susceptibility, gout is now a rare disease.

Causes of Gout. The gouty diathesis, or hereditary predisposition to gout, is important, and men are more often attacked than women. Alcohol plays a large part in causing the condition and it is noticeable that the wines and fermented liquors are more dangerous than the distilled spirits. Rich food in excess, combined with lack of exercise and indulgence in liquor, may be said to be the root evils in causing gout.

Symptoms. In a typical attack of gout the patient may be awakened in the morning with a severe pain in a joint, usually that of the big toe or a thumb. The joint swells and becomes intensely hot and painful so that the victim cannot bear to have it touched or to move it. Any jarring of the foot will cause him to cry out with pain. A feeling of illness may also be present, such as headache, vomiting, and feverishness. If treatment is begun, the swelling and pain in the joint will subside in a few days and the joint will return to its former state; but the attack will almost certainly return perhaps in a few months' time or perhaps after a couple of years. The next attack may be identical with the first or a new joint may be affected. As time goes on the attacks become more frequent; or after a few attacks the condition may settle down and become more or less chronic.

Chalky deposits called *tophi* are found in the proximity of joints and tendons, most frequently round the joints of the large toes, and fingers, and often in the outer rim of the ear. The presence of these tophi makes the diagnosis of gout a certainty. The affected joints lose a good deal of their power. Gouty people are subject to skin diseases and frequently are asthmatical.

Treatment. Treatment must be aimed at keeping the gout at bay, and avoiding acute attacks which need never occur where a reasonable endeavor is made to counteract the gout. The rule should be to live temperately, eating moderately and restricting the diet as far as meat, liver, and coffee are concerned. Alcohol must be avoided. It is beneficial to take large quantities of water or mineral water between meals. Spa treatment is a valuable beginning to the treatment of gout, because it gives the patient an opportunity of breaking completely with the old bad habits of diet and hygiene which surround him at home. There used to be a saying "once gouty, always gouty," but this need not be so. With care, acute attacks of gout, such as were taken as a matter of course fifty years ago, can be avoided. The acute attack is treated at rest in bed with extract of colchicine. Between attacks various drugs, of which aspirin and cinchophen are examples, may be prescribed to increase the excretion of uric acid.

G.P.I. This is the abbreviation for General Paralysis of the Insane, which is dealt with under that heading.

GRAFTING. By grafting is meant the operation of removing a small piece of human skin, bone, or nerve from one part of the body in order to transplant it to another part. This operation has to be done when a vital piece of bone or muscle has been destroyed and needs to be replaced by a piece from a less vital part of the body. Skin from another part is grafted to cover unsightly injuries on the face, for instance.

Bone grafting is used to fill in gaps in the skull and thus protect the exposed brain from injury, and in tuberculous disease of the spine, to strengthen the diseased parts of the spine.

Skin grafting is the most successful form of this operation, and usually gives very good results. The attempt to graft glands of young animals (monkey glands) into human beings in order to replace the functions of glands which have become old has not been successful, as it is not known how to make a transplanted gland continue to live in the human body for any length of time.

GRAND MAL. This is a French term, meaning "great evil," used in connection with a major epileptic fit as opposed to *petit mal* or a minor epileptic fit. In *grand mal* the fit is much deeper and more lasting while in *petit mal* there may be only a transient loss of consciousness. (*See also* EPILEPSY.)

GRANULATION TISSUE. When a wound or a cut is healing, new capillary blood vessels and connective tissue cells form to connect the surfaces together. These new capillaries are called granulation tissue because the surface appears to be studded with little grains. As soon as a cut takes place, Nature begins her work of repairing the damage, and the tiny blood vessels around the cut begin to expand and develop into new connective tissue cells. Granulation tissue, when it is in a healthy state, should be of a rich, deep red color and, as healing takes place, the area should gradually become smaller, until eventually only a slight scar is left. It sometimes happens that there is an overgrowth of granulation tissue; this is called exuberant granulation. (*See also* INFLAMMATION; PROUD FLESH.)

GRANULOMA. This term means a tumor which has formed on granulation tissue. This is caused by various forms of inflammation such as occur in tuberculosis, syphilis, leprosy, yaws, and glanders.

GRAPE SUGAR. This is another name for glucose or dextrose. The name grape sugar is used because of the large quantity of glucose which is found in ripe grapes. (*See also* GLUCOSE.)

GRAVEL. Under certain conditions, stones may form in the kidneys owing to deposits of uric acid. In some cases these stones may be quite large in size and only one may form, while in others there may be a large collection of very tiny ones. Gravel is the name given to the collection of very fine stones which are so small that they are able to pass into the bladder and then through the urethra along with the urine. Gravel can be detected as a sediment

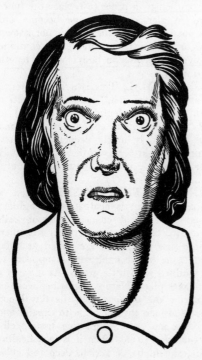

Graves' Disease.

in the urine as soon as it is passed. (*See also* BLADDER; CALCULUS; URINE.)

GRAVES' DISEASE. This is also known as exophthalmic goiter, and is a disease of the thyroid gland. It was first described by an Irish physician called Graves over a hundred years ago. It is generally found among young women between the ages of fifteen and thirty years. When men get it they are usually older, between the ages of thirty and forty-five years being the most frequent age. A sudden fright, grief, or shock, or the effects of a depressing disease or prolonged overstrain is a common starting-point for the disease, or, to be more correct, these disturbances may call it into activity. For a considerable time the patient may have had a feeling of weariness or exhaustion with no apparent cause, and have been nervous, irritable and restless.

Symptoms. As its name implies there is a goiter or enlargement of the thyroid gland which lies on the front of the neck rather below the middle. The eyes become prominent in nearly all cases, but sometimes only in a very small degree. They may, however, protrude so much that the eyelids cannot be closed over them and the patient has a staring look. The white of the eye is visible all round the iris or coloured part. Sometimes only one eye is affected.

The action of the heart is disturbed and the pulse becomes rapid with palpitation. The patient becomes nervous and irritable with tremblings of the muscles and sleeplessness. His demeanor is restless and over-active and he is the sort of person who can never sit still.

Often there is a history of other forms of nervous diseases amongst members of the family, such as hysteria, epilepsy or St. Vitus's dance. The appetite in Graves' disease is usually large, sometimes enormous, but in spite of it there is no increase of weight. When the appetite is poor, loss of weight becomes a feature, and when the illness is severe, attacks of diarrhea are fairly common. The face is inclined to flush easily, and there is much sweating and sometimes feverish attacks. In most cases the skin becomes browner than usual. It may be "tanned" all over, or there may be brown patches on the cheeks. There is always a good deal of nervousness, which may go on to serious melancholia and depression.

Treatment. The treatment of exophthalmic goiter is primarily mental and physical rest. In severe cases the patient must be confined to bed, but a warm "stuffy" atmosphere is very injurious. The room should be light, sunny, and very well ventilated. A patient who is up should rest out of doors as much as possible. The diet should be chosen from among easily digested foods and should be liberal and nutritious and attractively presented.

Any sources of poisoning such as decayed teeth, diseased tonsils, or nasal sinuses must be attended to. The drug thiouracil, in small doses and under careful medical supervision, has recently given good results. It is of especial value in rendering a severely ill patient fit for operation. The introduction of antithyroid drugs, such as thiouracil, though carbimazole is said to be even more effective, has made surgical operation less often necessary, but must be given for a long time.

The thyroid gland is treated surgically in various ways. There are two chief methods of operation; one consists in tying the arteries which supply the gland, and by thus starving it, diminishing the secretion. The other consists in removing part of the gland. Exophthalmic goiter has its ups and downs, and the operation is generally performed when the disease is fairly quiescent. Crile, the American surgeon, used to perform an operation which he called "stealing the goiter." The patient is prepared for operation for a few days, until the routine is familiar and no longer causes apprehension. Then one morning she is given a sedative, followed by an anesthetic, and recovers to find the operation over. This method is said to prevent the nervous symptoms which sometimes increase at this time.

Radioactive iodine, given by the mouth, has superseded treatment by X-rays to the thyroid. In some cases a single dose is enough. (*See also* GOITER.)

GRAVID. Gravid means pregnant. It is most commonly used in connection with the pregnant womb, which is described as a gravid uterus. It is not customary to talk of a gravid woman, but a pregnant woman.

GRAY MATTER. The gray matter of the brain is the brain tissue in which most of the nerve cells are situated, and is therefore of the greatest importance in the working of the body. (*See also* BRAIN.)

GREEN BLINDNESS. This is a form of color-blindness which also goes under the name of red-green blindness. It is the commonest form of color-blindness. In this condition there is an inability to distinguish between green and red. (*See also* COLOR-BLINDNESS.)

GREEN SICKNESS. This is a form of anemia which has the medical name of chlorosis. (*See also* ANEMIA.)

GREENSTICK FRACTURE. In a young child the bones, like the young green branches of a tree, are not so brittle as when they are fully matured, so that they are more inclined to bend than to snap in two when they receive a violent blow. This bending is known as a greenstick fracture. (*See also* FRACTURES.)

GREGORY'S MIXTURE or COMPOUND RHUBARB POWDER. This is a popular and useful purgative for small children which is made up of rhubarb, heavy magnesium carbonate, light magnesium carbonate and ginger.

GRIPING. Griping is a type of pain set up by the presence of some irritating substance in the bowel. The contents of the bowel are normally sent forward by a series of gentle motions due to the contraction of the muscles of the wall of the bowel. This movement is known as peristalsis. When some irritating substance such as poisonous food or too strong a purgative is present in the bowel, these movements become more violent in nature and the increased contractions of the muscles cause the griping pains. When strong purgatives are prescribed it is usual for the doctor to include some soothing medicine to prevent severe griping. (*See also* COLIC; FLATULENCE; INTESTINE.)

GRIPPE. This is a French term for influenza. (*See also* INFLUENZA.)

GRISTLE. Gristle is the popular name for cartilage. Cartilage in the human body is very similar in composition and appearance to the gristle of animals which is easily recognized in meat. (*See also* CARTILAGE.)

GROIN. The groin is that part of the body where the abdomen and the front of the thigh meet. It is marked by a slight groove or furrow, and in very stout people, friction may occur if absolute cleanliness is not observed. This is particularly so in fat babies, and careful attention should be given to see that the parts are washed, dried and powdered after each diaper change.

The groin is important because of the large blood vessels which lie just under the skin, and also because of the lymphglands which are grouped there. These glands frequently become enlarged in diseased conditions and are then sometimes referred to as buboes. Bubonic plague gets its name from the enlargement of these glands. Pain in the groin may occur through some other part of the body being diseased. Such a situation may arise when the spinal cord, the kidneys, or the reproductive organs are diseased.

GROWING PAINS. Many children complain of dull aching pains in the arms or legs which the mother simply puts down to growing pains. The vague term of "growing pains" has been used for years without any real basis for its use, because the progress of growth should cause no pain to a child. It is generally believed that these pains are, in fact, a form of rheumatism, and it has been found that the majority of children who suffer from such pains show other evidence of the presence of rheumatism.

A child with growing pains should be given more careful attention and not be allowed to go in for excessive exercise, because there is a distinct possibility that the heart may become affected. If the pains are bad, the child should be put to bed for a few days and the doctor should be consulted. (*See also* RHEUMATISM.)

GROWTH. The following points give a fair estimate of children's height at different ages as set down by authorities on this subject; it must not, however, be taken as an infallible guide.

Height. The newborn baby's height, or length, is about twenty inches.

Children grow more in the summer-time than in winter, probably because of the sun.

Up to the age of 5 years growth is said to be faster than at other periods of life.

From 5 to 10 years, boys grow faster than girls.

From 10 to 15 years, girls grow faster than boys.

From 15 to 20, boys grow faster than girls.

Up to 14, two and a half inches a year may be added by both boys and girls.

At 20, girls reach their full height.

At 24, boys reach their full height.

Some authorities say that soon after the age of 2 years the child is half as tall as it will be when fully grown. If this is so, we ought to be able to calculate the adult height of children at a tender age. But so much depends on food, on family characteristics, on bodily and mental conditions on health or sickness, to say nothing of those little organs of the body known as ductless glands, to which scientists are paying great attention, that no rule can be laid down at the present state of knowledge.

Weight. The newborn baby weighs from 7 to 8 lb.

Children grow in weight more in winter than in summer.

At 6 months an infant weighs about 14 lbs., and 21 lbs. at the first birthday. Thereafter, up to 10 years of age weight increases at the rate of from 4–5 lb. a year.

From 10 to 15 years it may increase from 8 to 10 lb. a year.

From 5 to 10 years of age girls weigh a little more than boys.

Up to 15 years, both boys and girls may put on from 8 to 10 lb. in one year.

From when the "growing age" stops— at 20 or even some years earlier for girls and 24 for boys—up to middle age, say 50, weight increases at something like three quarters of a pound a year.

At 50, increase in wheight should stop and even get less, if we want to keep well, lead an active life and live to a reasonably old age.

But, as pointed out above in speaking of height, so many influences must be taken into account that these figures are only rough calculations.

Keeping Records. In the days when the children's heights were carefully noted on the sitting-room door, weight was not regarded as of so much importance as it is now.

Many mothers now keep a book in which they enter the child's weight, height, and other particulars at various ages, and mount photographs showing progress in growth. This is an excellent plan.

Among influences that affect growth are housing; whether there is plenty of open space, fresh air, and sunshine; whether there has been serious illness in the family history; above all, whether the child is being brought up in happy and natural conditions, and is not forced on in mental development at the expense of health; whether it gets enough sleep in a quiet room; whether or not it is allowed to get overexcited at parties, etc. All these things are of vital importance if the child is to grow as it should.

Growing pains, as they are called, are signs that a doctor's advice is needed, for they are caused not by growth but by rheumatism, and there may be danger of heart trouble arising from them if neglected.

Giants and Dwarfs. What accounts for extremes in size we cannot say, but it is probable that the ductless glands, spoken of above, have a good deal to do with the fact that some children grow very big while others seem hardly to grow at all.

Dwarfs, of course, are people who have not grown, or grown very little, from babyhood, and when we know more about the effect on the child of food and surroundings, and of the ductless glands, it may be possible so to treat and feed unduly small babies that they will not be handicapped in this way throughout their lives. Already a great deal is being done by right feeding and treatment to overcome a bad start, and excellent work is being carried out in the children's hospitals where undersized babies born prematurely are so wonderfully cared for that they grow into normally healthy children.

Perhaps the smallest dwarf on record is a certain Jeffrey Hudson, born in the smallest county in England, Rutlandshire, who is said to have been only 18 in. high from his eighth to his thirtieth year, then to have grown to 45 in., and to have lived to the age of sixty-three. Henrietta Maria, Queen of Charles I, like other ladies of her time, was fond of having a dwarf to amuse and wait on her, and Hudson is said to have been presented to her by the Duchess of Buckingham. The Queen also had a dwarf called Gibson, whom she encouraged to marry a lady dwarf named Anne; they had nine children, five of whom were of ordinary size. Gibson is buried in St. Paul's Church, Covent Garden. Another story comes from France, where during the revolution a dwarf named Richebourg—who lived to the age of ninety years—is said to have carried dangerous dispatches while lying in the arms of his "nurse." (*See also* ACHONDROPLASIA; CRETINISM; DUCTLESS GLAND.)

Physical Development. The fact that physical dimensions have increased in recent years is reflected in the demands now made upon the various sections of trade. Larger sizes are required in footwear, hosiery, gloves, and hats, to mention only a few items of dress. Manufacturers and shops have also improved the service to their customers by catering to the small woman, who hitherto was forced to choose her clothes from the girls' sizes, with consequent difficulty in finding a style suitable for her years; by an increased range of fittings, as in corsetry, and by paying more attention to the needs of the outsize figure.

It is probable that this physical development has occurred because people have become aware of the importance of giving attention to diet, sleep, and general matters of health, as well as the popularity of "gym," physical culture and sport, and, of course, unfettered modern dress.

Growth of Animals and Insects. Compared with human beings, the growing life of the elephant and the housefly are interesting. The elephant, we are told, goes on growing up to the age of thirty, while the fly's whole life may not last, in hot weather, more than twenty-four hours.

GROWTHS. By growths we mean any abnormal formation occurring in the body and continuing to grow there. The most common growths are tumors and cysts, but corns and any sort of lumps are also growths. Growths are divided into two classes, benign and malignant. *Benign* growths are those which do not seriously interfere with the functioning of the body, whereas *malignant* growths are those such as cancer, which shorten life. (*See also* CANCER; SARCOMA.)

GRUEL. Gruel is a liquid invalid food made from oatmeal, which is of great value in sickness.

GUAIACUM. This is a resin which has been used in the treatment of chronic rheumatism and lumbago. Its contemporary use is as a test for the presence of blood in the urine or stools.

GUINEA WORM. The guinea worm derives its name from the Guinea coast of Africa where, as also in other tropical countries, it breeds in large numbers. The adult worms are found in man and cause a condition which is known as *dracontiasis*. The worms measure from 6 in. to 36 in. and are very slender. The tiny embryo worms live in water, and human beings become infected through drinking contaminated water. The worms gradually work their way into the human tissues where they grow into adults. The adult female worm bores her way through the skin, usually on the arms or legs, and then she starts discharging her embryos on to the surface of the skin for about three weeks. Whenever the skin comes in contact with water, the embryos leave the surface of the skin and pass into the water, and thus the infection is carried on.

At the spot on the skin where the adult worm is working her way to the surface, a burning sensation may be felt and a blister usually forms. When this blister bursts, the head of the worm can be seen quite plainly below.

After about three weeks, when no more embryos are produced, the worm can be extracted. This is made easier by rolling the worm round a match, giving a turn to this every day until the tail, which is recognized by its hooked form, is reached. Care must be taken not to break the body of the worm while doing this. An operation can be carried out, if desired, in which the skin is incised and the worm removed, and the incised area disinfected with a solution of carbolic acid. (*See also* FILARIA; WORM.)

GULLET. The gullet is the popular name for the ESOPHAGUS, and a full account will be found under that heading.

GUM. Gum is a heavy, sticky substance which is obtained from the trunks and branches of various trees. The two best-known gums used in medicine are gum acacia and gum tagacanth. Gums are used for throat lozenges as they are very soothing to inflamed surfaces. Gum acacia is most useful in cases of hemorrhage, and

it is given in the form of an injection in order to stop further bleeding.

GUMBOIL. Gumboil or alveolar abscess is a condition in which the gum becomes very inflamed and swollen, usually as the result of an abscess at the root of a decayed tooth.

Symptoms. Pain may be felt in the region of a decayed tooth, and matter usually collects at the root which gives rise to an abscess. After several days the abscess may burst into the mouth, or occasionally it may even burst through the cheek.

Treatment. It is better to have the abscess lanced or treated before it bursts of its own accord, and if the abscess is due to a decayed tooth or root, this matter should be attended to as soon as possible. Penicillin will usually be given by the dentist or doctor. (*See also* ALVEOLAR ABSCESS; TEETH.)

GUMMA. Gumma is the name given to a painless tumor which may appear on any part of the body as a result of syphilis. It is, however, seldom seen since the introduction of modern methods of treating that disease. (*See also* SYPHILIS.)

GUMS, DISEASES OF. Diseases of the gums usually occur through infection or as a result of irritation. Ulcers may form on the gums as a result of a badly fitting dental plate. This matter can be quickly cleared up by a visit to the dentist in order to have the plate adjusted. Small ulcers or sore spots may appear on the gums or surrounding tissues owing to some disturbance of the digestion. These usually clear up in a day or two, but the mouth should be kept clean with an antiseptic mouthwash. Gingivitis is a state of inflammation of the gums which is due to infection or irritation. Pyorrhea is one of the most important diseases of the gums, and it is a condition in which large quantities of pus are found in the sockets of the teeth. The general health should be attended to and a visit to the dentist must be made. Penicillin and other antibiotics may be used locally or by injection. Antiseptic mouthwashes, such as a dilute solution of hydrogen peroxide or chlorate of potash, should be used frequently. If the gums are soft and spongy, a daily massage with the fingers will encourage the circulation and improve their condition (*See also* DENTAL DRILL; GINGIVITIS; GUMBOIL; PYORRHEA.)

GUNSHOT WOUNDS. By gunshot wounds we usually mean all the injuries caused by explosive weapons, such as guns, revolvers, shells, bombs. The immediate treatment is nearly always a question of first aid so it is given in the SPECIAL SUPPLEMENT ON FIRST AID.

GYNECOLOGY. The study of the diseases of women, especially those affecting the generative organs, is known as gynecology, from a Greek word *gunè* meaning a woman.

HABIT. When any action has been performed several times it becomes easier to carry out, and after a time the nerves and muscles employed act with very little prompting from the person's conscious will. He may, in fact, not know that he is performing the action until it is nearly, or quite, completed. The action has then become "habitual." This habit-forming ability is of the greatest use to human beings, as it eases the burden on the hard-working executive part of the mind and leaves it free to carry out new and unaccustomed actions.

A great part of our general education is aimed at forming good habits to ease our way through life. The difference between a good craftsman and a bad one is largely the difference in the proportion of his work that has become habitual to him, leaving him with extra brain power to devote to improvement in the task. It is just as important, however, not to acquire bad habits; whereas a good habit saves mental and physical energy, a bad habit wastes it. People easily become slaves to their bad habits; there is a type of person in whom the habit-forming power is so great that if the same action is performed only two or three times it becomes a strong habit. Such people are often very difficult to live with, and their mannerisms may drive their families almost frantic; they may hum or whistle, or suck their teeth or sniff, and acquire all sorts of personal bad habits ranging from nail-biting to bad "tics." In many cases the habit has become so much a part of the person that it is an almost impossible task to cure it.

In the field of health, good habit-forming should be begun in the very earliest days of the child's life. It is most important that the working of the bowels, bladder, and the digestive system should be brought under our automatic control as early as possible. Sleep, too, is largely a matter of habit, and the ability to go to sleep the minute the head is put on the pillow is one of the most valuable faculties a hard-working man or woman can have. For this reason the sleep of the child should be safeguarded by all possible means, and it should be a rule never to disturb a child once it has been put to bed. Visitors who want to peep at it should be firmly dissuaded, because if a child has formed the habit of rapid and sound sleep, it will, with ordinary luck, be able to keep it all its life, and will be able to face each day a refreshed and renewed person.

The wise person will try to acquire useful, labor-saving habits on his journey through life, and will pull himself up sharply when he finds himself drifting into wasteful and bad habits.

Habit Spasms. Many people, especially young children, have irregular muscular movements which affect different parts of the body, such as jerking the head, twitching the shoulders, flickerings of the eyelids, grimacing, frowning, etc. These movements are perfomed unconsciously, but are under the control of the person since they can be stopped immediately if his attention is drawn to them, and they never take place during sleep. The cure for these spasms, which are really only bad habits, is for the person himself to be on the lookout for them and avoid them, or in the case of a child, careful and kindly training by the parents or teachers. Harsh measures and scolding are not of the slightest use, because the movements invariably become worse when the person is in an emotional state.

At first sight it is not easy to decide

whether the twitchings and jerkings and fidgetings of childhood are purely bad habits or whether they are due to the illness called St. Vitus's dance or chorea, in which case the child needs careful medical attention and nursing in order to save it from invalidism in the future. (*See also* FIDGETS; ST. VITUS'S DANCE; TIC.)

HAIR, THE. A hair is formed from elongated horny cells arising from the epidermis or outer layer of the skin, and grows from a tube in the skin called a hair follicle. It has a root and a shaft, which is rounded in straight hair, oval in curly hair, and varies greatly in thickness. The surface of each hair is covered with scales, arranged in overlapping fashion like tiles on a roof. The color of the hair is due to the varying amount of coloring matter in its substance. White hair occurs when numerous air spaces form in its cells. The root of the hair ends in a dented knob; into this dent fits the papilla, which is a little knot of blood vessels. This nourishes the hair, and without it the hair dies. The root is the growing point of the hair, the rate of growth being about 6 in. a year. The follicle runs at an angle into the skin, so that the hair has a natural slope; this is best seen in an animal's hairy "coat." Its use is to turn the rain.

In the true skin are small musclefibers connected with the roots of the hairs; contraction of these, as from cold or fear,

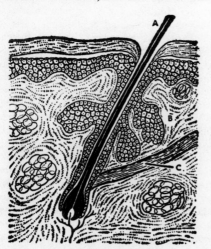

Hair: A. *Hair;* B. *Sebaceous Glands;* C. *Muscle (erector pili).*

causes the hair to stand on end, and produces "gooseflesh." This is well seen when a kitten is frightened. The hair is kept glossy by the oil from the sebaceous glands, which open into the follicle. Each gland looks like a tiny bunch of grapes.

Long hair sometimes splits at the ends, or forms greyish pointed nodules ("beaded hair"), at which the shaft kinks and finally breaks off. These conditions are due to brittleness, and are caused by removal of the natural oil by washing with coarse soaps, drying by heat, etc.

HALITOSIS. The word halitosis means a foul breath. This condition is due most commonly to septic tonsils or decaying teeth, or it may arise from constipation, dyspepsia, the eating of certain foods, or overindulgence in alcoholic beverages.

HALLUCINATION. This term is used to describe imaginary sensation, either of sight or of hearing, or rarely, of smell; that is, the person who has an hallucination sees, hears, or smells things which have no existence. Hallucinations occur in many disorders of the mind, and are of two types, pleasant and unpleasant. When they are unpleasant, as in delirium of all kinds, including *delirium tremens,* they appear to cause much terror to the patient, and those who witness his fears suffer great distress, but on recovery, usually nothing is ever remembered of the hallucinations; they are "blotted out" and should not be referred to by the patient's relatives. Pleasant hallucinations occur mainly in that form of mental trouble known as *dementia praecox,* and they are very often hallucinations of hearing which cause the patients to withdraw more and more into themselves in order to be free to indulge in listening to the voices. Imaginary voices, which tell patients that they are being persecuted, and must slay their enemies are common in *delusional insanity.* (*See also* DELIRIUM TREMENS; INSANITY; MENTAL DISEASE.)

HALLUX VALGUS. The medical name for the big toe is hallux, and hallux valgus is a condition chiefly found in growing children in which the big toe is displaced and lies either above or below the second toe. It is due to ill-fitting shoes, especially the wearing of pointed toes to the shoes at an age when the bones of the feet are still impressionable. When hallux valgus occurs it almost always forms the starting point of other foot troubles. The joint of the big toe usually acquires a bunion, and corns and callosities almost always form. The joint of the toe may become stiff, inflamed and painful.

Treatment. It is obviously better to prevent the formation of avoidable deformities of the feet than to rely upon treating them when they have arisen. Properly shaped shoes in childhood and youth are the very best preventive for such conditions. The child's foot is naturally almost a straight line from heel to the tip of the big toe in unspoilt feet, but for generations people have tried to compress their toes into a type of shoe in which the toe room corresponds roughly in amount with the heel

room, and the big toe is treated as if it were the middle instead of the outside one. When it is noticed that the child's toe is bending inwards, place a wad of cotton-wool, or a little spool-shaped plug made of rubber which is sold for the purpose, between the big toe and the second toe, inside the stocking. Continued wearing of this will do much to straighten out the toes, provided that the shoes are roomy enough. If the toe does not straighten it may be necessary to have a special shoe made with a little partition which will separate the big toe from its neighbor.

In adults, operation is the only real cure, but separating the toes and massage and exercises will help a lot to keep the condition from getting worse. Walking on tiptoes with bare feet and the toes turned in is a useful exercise that can be practised for a short time daily while dressing and undressing.

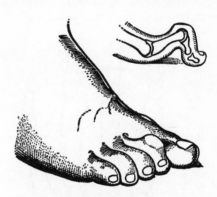

Hammer Toe.

HAMMER TOE. Hammer toe is a condition in which one or more of the toes is bent into the shape of an inverted ∧. The top of the ∨ usually presses against the toecap of the shoe and causes much distress and pain. It generally happens that a corn develops on the crown of the ∨ and others may form beneath the toe where it presses on the ground. This deformity is usually caused by wearing badly shaped shoes and is frequently associated with hallux valgus. A slight operation on the toe may be necessary to bring it down into line with the others. (*See also* BOOTS AND SHOES.)

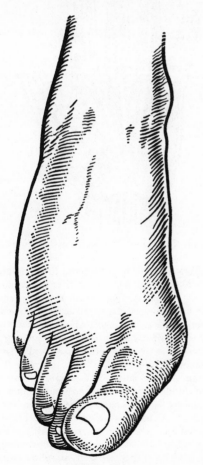

Hallux Valgus.

HAMSTRINGS. The tendons situated

at the back of the knee on the outer and inner sides are termed the hamstrings. Their action is to bend the knee and to enable the foot to turn inwards and outwards. (*See also* KNEE.)

HAND. The hand in the human being is a highly specialized tool, and therein lies one of the greatest differences between human beings and animals. Even the cleverest ape has not the delicate sense of touch and the range of fine hand movements of the human being. The difference lies in the brain, which has for generations supervised the training of our fingers and hands until they are now the means by which the majority of us earn our living. For this reason, if for no other, particular care should be taken to guard against the accidents, such as small cuts and knocks, that are almost a daily occurrence. Any sign of inflammation must be attended to at once, and it is especially necessary to take measures to keep dirt and germs away by means of a small bandage.

forearm by the wrist joint, by means of which it can move up and down, and from side to side. The normal hand turns easily from the position in which it is palm upwards to the position in which the palm faces downwards; it should also bend either up or down to the position of a right angle. With the hand held out with the palm facing the ground, it will be seen that the fingers can only be moved slightly upwards, but should bend downwards at right angles. They should be able to rotate with a complete circular movement, all except the ring finger which has not the same range. The tips of the fingers can be brought together and spread out.

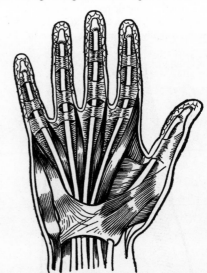

Hand: Tendons and Muscles of the Fingers.

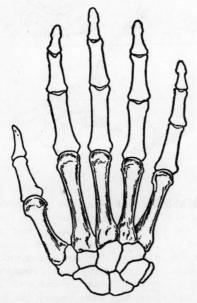

Metacarpal Bones (other bones in hand in outline only)

Insurance companies recognize the importance of the hand by usually insisting that even small accidents to the hand shall be inspected by an orthorpedic surgeon.

Structure. The hand is hinged on to the

Skeleton. The main bones of the hand are the five metacarpal bones situated in the palm and connecting the wrist bones with the finger bones. Each metacarpal bone is jointed on to a finger which consists of three small bones called the *phalanges,* except the thumb which has only two phalanges. Three principal nerves, the ulnar, median and radial, supply the hand and divide into a network of small branches radiating to the fingers. The veins on the back of the hand, which are so superficially placed that they can often be easily seen, are tributaries of the basilic and cephalic veins. The hand is well supplied with muscles and tendons which carry out the

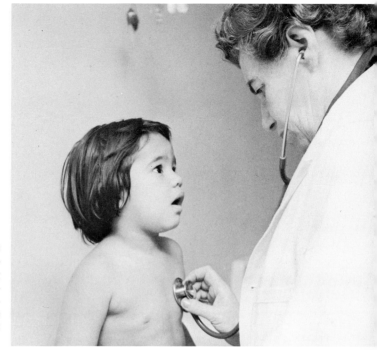

Pediatric attention acts as a strong preventive measure against crippling childhood diseases. *(Children's Bureau, U.S. Department of Public Health, Education and Welfare)*

Highly effective therapeutic measures are possible through frequent immersions in a Hubbard Tank.

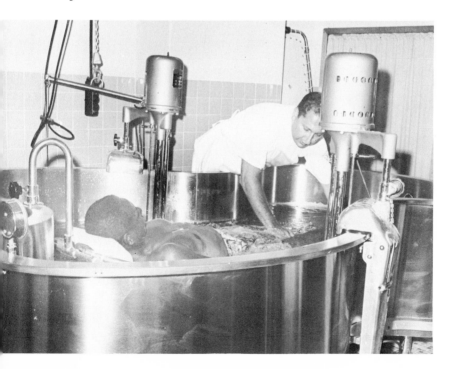

A DOCTOR'S DAY
OF HOSPITAL ROUNDS

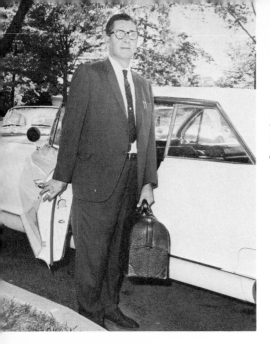

1. 8:00 A.M.: The doctor's day begins—patients to see, colleagues to consult, cases to review—a full day of hospital duties.

2. 9:00 A.M.: The doctor acts teacher as he explains a patien case to the floor nurse and h student.

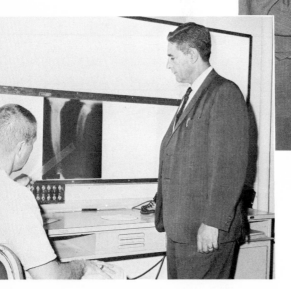

3. 10:00 A.M.: The doctor views an X-ray as the Radiologist explains a fracture.

4. 11:00 A.M.: Light moments during conferences with colleagues can brighten long mornings.

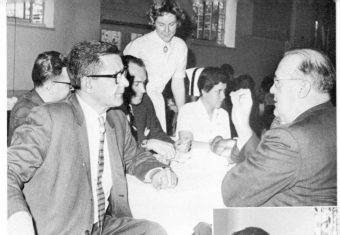

5. Noon: A chance to relax for lunch becomes an informative conversation with hospital staff.

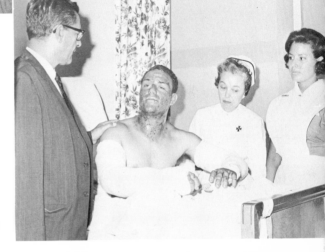

6. 1:00 P.M.: The doctor looks in on his burn case.

7. 1:30 P.M.: Hospital tour finished, the doctor returns to his office for three to four hours of seeing patients.

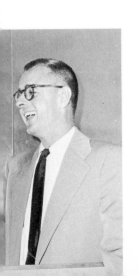

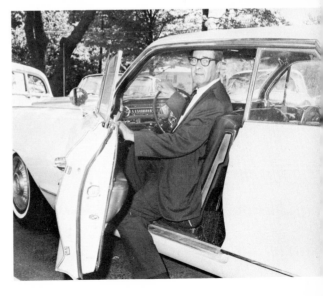

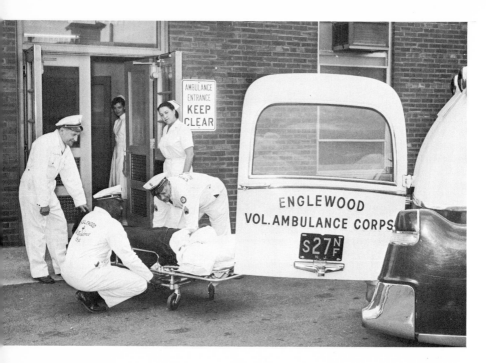

Countless near-tragedies are transformed into "happy end-ings" in the emergency room.

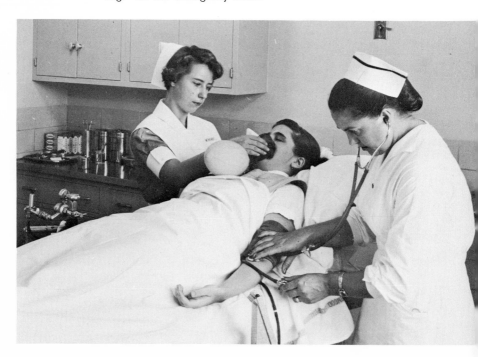

various movements required. (*See also* FINGERS.)

HANGNAIL. This unsightly and somewhat painful condition is caused by neglect. If the cuticle (the fine skin at the base of the nails) is not pushed back regularly, and in consequence overgrows, the skin will tear and in places become detached, forming hangnails.

If regular care is given the condition will not occur; but if hangnails form, they should be cut off with fine scissors, the small wound touched with a caustic stick, and covered with court plaster. A neglected hangnail has been known not only to give rise to local infection (a poisoned finger), but even to generalized blood poisoning.

HARELIP. Sometimes a baby is born with the two halves of its upper lip not joined together and this is called a harelip from its resemblance to the split lip of a hare. In the embryo the upper lip develops in three pieces; two side flaps and a middle strip, and the join in these parts— which normally takes place before birth— is represented in our faces by the two raised lines on each side of the furrow in the middle of the upper lip. Sometimes both side pieces of the lip fail to join up before the birth of the baby, but more often it is one side only. When hare-lip occurs it is usual to leave it alone for the first few weeks until the baby has learnt to suck, then an operation is performed to join the two parts of the lip. In most cases the operation is successful, and very little trace of the defect can be seen afterwards.

HARVEST MITE. These mites have many names, but the most popular ones are the harvest bug, the mower's mite, and the bête rouge. They have eight legs, while their young have only six. The adult mites are vegetarians and are to be found on gooseberry bushes, grass and other vegetation. The young burrow into the skin of human beings, particularly the ankles, arms, and neck, and set up great irritation. They are very tiny, bright red in color, whence they derive the name of bête rouge.

Symptoms. The harvest mites do not suck the blood but they cause great irritation on the skin. Scratching sets up further irritation, which may result in severe dermatitis.

Treatment. Sponging the affected parts with weak ammonia will help to relieve the irritation, especially if zinc ointment is applied freely after the skin has been carefully dried. An application of gasoline or benzine will kill the harvest mite, but care must be taken not to place these substances near fire. (*See also* DERMATITIS.)

HASHISH. Hashish is a drug which is used commonly in the East with the idea is producing pleasurable sensations. When taken to excess it is very dangerous and may lead to great depression and insanity. Other names for this drug are *ganga,* which is obtained from the dried flowering tops of the cultivated plants; *charas,* which is obtained from the resin scraped off the leaves, and *bhang,* which is the dried leaves. *Ganga* and *charas* are often smoked like tobacco. (*See also* CANNABIS INDICA.)

HAVERSIAN CANALS. These are little canals that run through the substance of bone. Each channel contains minute blood vessels and nerves which are thus distributed thoroughout the bones, and these tiny blood vessels cause a bone to bleed when it is broken. When inflammation or pressure in the bone causes these vessels to be blocked up the bone will be robbed of its food and will die, or become necrosed, as it is called. (*See also* BONE.)

HAY FEVER. Hay fever is a distressing condition which occurs regularly every summer in certain people and while it lasts, which is usually the whole of the summer, renders their lives miserable. It is one of the "allergic diseases" and attacks people who are abnormally sensitive to certain pollens. The other allergic diseases are asthma and urticaria.

Symptoms. The symptoms of hay-fever appear with great regularity in the early summer each year. They resemble a cold in the head of varying severity; sometimes there is just itching of the eyes and running of the nose, but often there are severe attacks of sneezing, great swelling of the eyes and severe nasal catarrh, asthma or breathlessness and the patient may become quite ill, even running a temperature. Hay fever is always worse in the country than in city dwellers, and it has been found that the pollen of several sorts of grass cause it in susceptible people, the most serious one being Timothy grass.

Predisposition to Hay Fever. People who develop hay fever usually come from a family where there is a history of nervous sensitivensss, and it may be found that other members of the family suffer from skin troubles such as urticaria, or are athmatic. Such people are abnormally sensitive to the introduction of any unusual substance into their systems, and great care must be taken when giving them injections of serum or drugs.

Treatment. The first step is to discover what pollen is to blame, and a simple test is carried out. A small amount of the extracts of various pollens is rubbed into little scratches on the arm. The pollen which is harmful to the patient will cause a little inflammation. It is then necessary to try to render the patient less susceptible to it by injecting an extract of the pollen in small doses into his bloodstream. This injection treatment must be begun well in advance of the hay fever season or it will not protect the patient. The usual month to begin is March or April. These courses of injections often have to be repeated, and the results are on the whole disappointing.

When an attack occurs, there are various remedies that may be used to settle it down. A spray containing adrenalin may be employed, or a soothing ointment may be used inside the nose. Some people are benefited by taking glucose or calcium, or both. Ephedrine locally or internally is a useful remedy, and some people obtain relief by light cauterization of the nasal septum. The antihistamine drugs such as benadryl, diparalene, antistin, and piriton often give good results. In some cases a small daily dose has been effective in preventing attacks during the pollen season, and in others an occasional dose has been able to control an attack as it arises.

HEAD. The head consists of the skull, or cranium, and the face. The skull contains the brain, which controls the nervous activity of the body. The face contains the organs of sight (eye), smell (nose), taste (tongue), hearing (ear). In animals the sense of touch is also largely situated in the face, but in human beings it has been almost entirely transferred to the hands.

The bony framework of the head consists of the rounded dome of bone called the cranium, with the attached cheekbones and jawbones. The nose and ears are made largely of cartilage. At the base of the back of the head are two projections called condyles, which serve as pegs to attach the head to the backbone. On these pegs the head can turn from side to side and move backwards and forwards.

Certain of the bones in the head contain air cavities which are called sinuses. These communicate with the nose and are the means by which resonance is given to the voice. They can be the seat of infection which spreads from the nose giving rise to a painful condition called sinusitis.

The shape of the head varies in individuals, but as a rule people of the same nationality have similarly shaped heads, as for example the square heads of the Teutons. People have often tried to tell fortunes and characters from the shape of the head and the protuberances on it; but phrenology, as this is called, has remained a pursuit for amusement rather than a science.

Several diseases alter the shape of the bones of the head. Of these the most important are acromegaly, osteitis deformans, and rickets, which are discussed under their own headings.

HEADACHE. Everyone is subject at some time to this complaint, but some people suffer from it to a much greater extent than others. The causes of headache are very numerous, and vary from slight indispositions in some part of the body to severe mental or physical disease. Almost any upset in any part of the body can have headache for a symptom, and people use many different words to describe their pain, such as stabbing, aching, nagging, throbbing, boring, nails being driven into the head, or tight bands being tied round the head.

Headaches in Children. When a child complains of headache it is as well to take his temperature at once, because this is usually the first symptom of any of the infectious fevers such as measles, scarlet fever, or influenza. If there is no temperature, the most likely causes are constipation or eye strain. If the headache is very severe the child should be taken at once to a doctor to be examined, in case it is the beginning of some serious trouble such as meningitis or mastoiditis.

Headaches in Adults. Some people get a headache in heavy muggy weather and can always foretell the approach of a thunderstorm by such an attack. Many women suffer from a "sick headache" each month. Other people get a bad headache when they go too long without food and it clears up immediately after a few mouthfuls of food are taken. The severe attacks of sick headache known as migraine appear to be constitutional and hereditary; they are described in a separate article. A common cause of persistent headaches is a fault in the eyesight which is not being corrected by wearing the proper glasses. Other causes of headache are defective teeth, and nose and throat troubles, stom-

ach, liver, heart, and kidney disease. It is usually a troublesome symptom in nervous diseases such as hysteria, neurasthenia, etc. Any feverish attack such as influenza, malaria, etc., usually starts with severe headache. The type of headache which might be described as a severe pain in the head rather than ache may be the result of some injury or disease of the brain itself. Neuralgia and rheumatism sometimes cause pain which is felt in the head.

Treatment. Obviously, the first thing to do towards the cure of headache is to find out its cause and clear up any underlying disease. Many of the passing headaches to which people are subject will disappear with quite simple treatment. An aperient pill at night, with a drink of health-salts in the morning, will usually clear up a "bili-

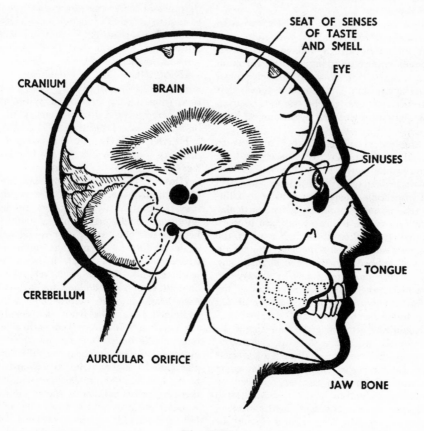

The Head.

ous" headache. There are many excellent remedies to be bought, such as phenacetin, aspirin, A.P.C., compound codeine tablets, and others. Some suit one person and some another; but when such a drug is taken it will always act better if the person lies down in a darkened room and tries to sleep while the drug is taking its effect. It is often useful to combine caffeine with one of the above drugs to counteract the depressing effect they often have on the patient. (*See also* MIGRAINE.)

HEAD LOUSE. Head lice are little grey creatures with a black line at the outer edge of the body. They are found chiefly in the heads of dirty people. The eggs of the louse are known as nits, and these are white in colour and cling firmly to the hair. One louse may lay as many as fifty or sixty eggs. These are very often mistaken for scurf, but closer inspection shows that scurf does not cling to the hair in the same way.

The lice cause considerable irritation to the scalp which is called *pediculosis,* and the scratching which follows very often sets up unpleasant skin troubles. Infection may be carried to the scalp through broken parts of the skin, and it is also known that infectious diseases can be transmitted from one person to another by means of head lice.

Absolute cleanliness is the only way to keep free of these creatures once they have been found in the head. The hair should be washed at least twice a week and careful inspection should be carried out. Children at school should be given particular attention to see if lice or nits are present. Applying paraffin oil to the head is the simplest way of killing the lice. This should be well rubbed into the head at night and left on for about ten hours. A shower-cap worn over the head will avoid soiling the pillows. This treatment should be repeated the following morning and evening, and the morning after that the hair should be thoroughly washed with soap and water. Soaking the hair in equal parts of vinegar and water is an excellent way of loosening the nits which then can be removed by means of a small-toothed comb. Medicated lethane oil is an extensively used and effective remedy. One teaspoonful should be applied to the hair and left on for 24 hours. An oily solution of D.D.T. is also effective. Any irritation on the scalp should be treated with olive oil or some soothing ointment. All combs, brushes, and caps should be disinfected before using again. This can be done by putting about a teaspoonful of lysol to each pint of water and soaking everything well before washing with soapy water.

HEALTH. When a person is enjoying good health, it is an indication that all the parts of the body are working in good order and the mental state is such that there is no feeling of strain or discomfort in carrying out the daily work. Of course, there are degrees of good health. Some days one may feel particularly energetic, the appetite is keen, and the body responds to any task without the slightest effort. This high pitch is very often reached by young people; but, unfortunately, not so often in older people. Perhaps as we get older we get lazier, and the mental effort necessary to urge our bodies to a state of better health is not made. There is no doubt that our mental attitude has a great deal to do with the state of our body.

HEARING. The internal ear is the organ of hearing, whence the sound vibrations from the air are carried by the auditory nerve to the hearing center in the brain. (*See also* DEAFNESS; EAR.)

HEARING AID. An artificial aid for deafness, usually electrical. (*See also* DEAFNESS.)

HEART. The heart is the mainspring of the human machinery. If it stops, death must follow. As it is therefore the most important single organ in the body, the heart is not only well protected by nature against injury by its position, but it is so constructed that although it never stops working while we are alive, yet a certain amount of rest is obtained for it between each beat. How this comes about will be explained later. The heart lies deeply in the chest and is covered on each side by parts of the lungs. It is roughly the shape of a pear turned upside down. The lowest part called the apex points downwards and to the left, while the thicker portion, called the base, points backwards and to the right. About two-thirds of the heart lies to the left of the middle of the breastbone, while the other third lies to the right. The size of the heart in an average adult is about 5 in. long, 3½ in. broad and 2½ in. thick. It is about 9 oz. in weight. The most important part of the heart as far as its work is concerned is the muscle of which it is chiefly made.

Once the muscle is damaged the heart is no longer a hundred per cent efficient. The walls of the heart, which are all made of muscle, enclose four separate spaces or cavities; these are two auricles, the right and the left, and two ventricles, the right and the left. The right auricle and ventricle open into each other, while the left auricle and ventricle also open into each other; but the right cavities of the heart have no communication with the left cavities in fully developed hearts. Before birth, however, the right and left auricles open into each other through a tiny hole, about the size of a goose-quill, and sometimes, though rarely, this hole does not close at once after birth, as it should, with the result that one form of heart disease is caused by some of the blood being sent directly from one auricle to the other.

The right auricle receives its blood from all the veins of the body through two large veins, the superior vena cava and the inferior vena cava. From the right auricle the blood passes into the right ventricle, whence it is pumped through a large blood-vessel, the pulmonary artery, to the lungs. In the lungs the blood takes up the oxygen which is necessary for the nourishment of the tissues of the body, and is returned to the heart into the left auricle by four large veins, the pulmonary veins.

From the left auricle the blood passes into the left ventricle, and from there it is pumped into the biggest blood vessel of all, the aorta, which distributes the blood all over the body. Both the ventricles have more work to do than the auricles, because they have to pump the blood further, but whereas the right ventricle has only to send the blood through the lungs, the left ventricle has to send it all over the body. It is not surprising, therefore, that the muscle forming the wall of the left ventricle is nearly three times as thick as the muscle forming the wall of the right ventricle, while the muscle of the auricle is very much thinner than that of either ventricle. To ensure that the blood goes

the right way in the heart, that is, always from auricle to ventricle, and not the reverse, there is a series of valves, at the entrance to each of the cavities of the heart, which shut immediately the blood has passed through them. The valve between the right auricle and ventricle has three little flaps or cusps to it, so it is named the tricuspid valve. That between the left auricle and ventricle has two such flaps to it, and looks rather like a bishop's mitre, so it is named the mitral valve. There are also valves at the junction between the right ventricle and the blood vessel which arises from it, the pulmonary artery, and between the left ventricle and the aorta. These valves each consist of three flaps or cups in the form of little pockets, the openings of which face away from the ventricles, so that when blood tries to pass back into the ventricle the pockets fill out and close the opening which they guard. From their shape, which is like a half-moon, these valves are called the semilunar valves.

How the Heart Works. The action of the heart is that of regular pumping. But the whole heart does not work at the same time. First, the muscle of the two auricles contracts, forcing blood into the two ventricles, just as water would be expelled from a rubber ball containing it by squeezing the ball. Then the muscle of the two ventricles contracts, forcing blood into the pulmonary artery and into the aorta. While this is happening, the muscle of the two auricles has become slack, or as the cavities are emptied, they are said to be at rest, or "in diastole."

When the cavities are contracting they are said to be "in systole." But as soon as the auricles have got rid of all their blood into the ventricles and had a short rest, blood commences to flow in to them again from the large veins; they become filled with blood once more; and by contracting and again forcing blood into the ventricles the whole of one heartbeat is completed. The ventricles get their rest after they have contracted, while the blood is flowing into the auricles, and the length of time they get this rest at every beat of the heart is about four-tenths of a second. When it is considered how hard the ventricles work to pump blood into the large blood vessels which carry it all over the body, it will be realized how important it is for the ventricles to get this long rest, which takes, in time, one-half of the whole time of the heart-beat. One of the signs of heart disease is a shortening of the time of rest the ventricles get at each beat, because this shows that the muscle cannot contract well enough to force all the blood out at each beat, and so must work quicker. In a healthy heart there is an excellent supply of nourishment provided for it by special blood vessels called the coronary arteries, which arise at the beginning of the aorta, so that the heart receives the blood with the most oxygen for its own nourishment. Sometimes these arteries become hardened and their openings are so narrowed that insufficient blood is pumped through for the nourishment of the heart. Then symptoms of heart disease arise, because a badly nourished heart must be a badly working heart.

The rate at which the heart beats depends on several things. One is the "pacemaker" of the heart, which is a tiny particle of tissue made partly of tissue and partly of a special kind of muscle, which lies in the wall of the right auricle and starts off the contraction of the auricles. When the auricles contract, a message is sent to another piece of special tissue, from which messages are sent out, as from a central telephone exchange, to the walls of the ventricles, to cause them to contract. Normally, this sequence of events always takes place: first the auricles contract, then the ventricles, the cycle being a regular one. When the ventricles contract, owing to the lastic tissue in the walls of the blood vessels, a wave of contraction is sent along them and this wave can be felt at the wrist in the radial artery, at each beat of the heart. This is known as the pulse. In certain diseases of the heart this normal sequence of events is disturbed and either the ventricles do not contract at every command they receive from the auricles or they may contract at every second, or third or fourth command. They may even go on strike and contract on their own, when and how they choose.

The effects of this difference in rhythm between contraction of the auricles and that of the ventricles is discussed under diseases of the heart. The rate of the heart-beat is also controlled by the nerves. Certain nerves slow the heart, others make it beat faster. If one listens over the beating heart, two sounds can be heard at each heart-beat. The first represents the contraction of the ventricles; the second, the closure of the pulmonary and aortic valves. The first sound is much longer and louder than the second, which is short and sharp. The two sounds together resemble the sound of the "lubb-dup." On an average, the heart beats seventy-two times a minute. It beats more quickly when we are standing up than when we are sitting down, and slowest of all when we are lying in bed. Hence the importance of rest in bed in the treatment of serious heart disease.

Diseases of the Heart. There are some diseases of the heart which may occur at any age; but, generally speaking, various types of disease attack the heart at certain ages and it is convenient to discuss disorders of the heart as they occur in childhood and adolescence, in adult life and in old age. Before these are dealt with, however, it must be said that many symptoms which the average persons thinks are due to heart trouble have, in fact, nothing whatever to do with that hard-worked organ. It is merely protesting as a result of some condition in another organ. For example, an overloaded stomach will, in a person who is foolish enough to go straight to bed on top of a heavy meal, give rise to a very severe attack of palpitation and pain round the heart. Similarly, a person who is suffering from anemia will often be short of breath and have palpitation, but these symptoms are only the expression of the poor quality of the blood which is sent to the heart; when the heart is supplied with richer blood, or in other words, when the anemia is cured, the symptoms of heart trouble disappear.

Fear, or a sudden fright, will also, in a nervous person, give rise to what may appear to be a quite alarming attack of palpitation of the heart, but this is a symptom only of the nervous control of the heart getting temporarily upset, and is of no consequence. The heart itself is healthy. It is possible to tell by careful examination exactly how much the heart is capable of doing, and it is found that in these "irritable hearts" the working capacity is as good as that of a normal heart.

Heart Disease in Childhood and Adolescence. It has already been mentioned that in some children the communication between the right and left sides of the heart, which is present before birth, does not close at the proper time and so there is a mixture of venous blood (which has not been sent to the lungs to pick up oxygen) with the oxygenated blood which is sent to all the other tissues of the body, and that this causes one form of heart disease in children. Fortunately this is a rare condition, like another condition from birth in which the artery which takes blood to the lungs is narrower than normal, so that less blood than usual can be oxygenated at a time. The children who suffer from these failures in development have been referred to as "blue babies.' They have bluish faces and are always short of beath, getting tired easily. They need much more care and attention than normal children as they are liable to lung troubles besides the usual childish illnesses. In addition, their shortness of breath makes general school life too difficult for them, and their education is best carried out at home, or at special schools where they are assured of help.

Up to now, it has been true to say that "blue babies" sometimes survive into adult life, but rarely live beyond middle age. It may be mentioned here, however, that although no definite cure has been found for this condition, certain important advances have been made in modern surgery which may have significant results. Operations have been performed which have, in the majority of cases, materially improved the condition of the patient, and which have increased his expectation of normal life. It has still to be discovered for how long the improvement will last, and whether it is permanent.

Although these cases are rare, it is a fact that nearly three-quarters of all cases of heart disease have their beginnings before the age of 21 years. It is in childhood and early adolescence that acute rheumatism— in one of its many forms—attacks, and unless the greatest precautions are taken, the heart is permanently affected. It cannot be too strongly emphasized to parents that a child who complains of pains in the joints (often called "growing pains"), or a sore throat, or who is "jumpy" with St. Vitus's dance, is threatened with permanent heart disease if these complaints are not taken seriously and treated. The school medical services are doing much to prevent this terrible toll of heart disease in young people, but much more could be done in early cases by the parents themselves. The germ causing the "sore throat" or other complaint poisons the lining of the heart, near the valves, and the resulting damage to the valve or valves (sometimes more than one is attacked), produces a narrowing of the passage so that the blood has to be forced through.

In other cases, the valves are stretched so that they will not close properly, and some of the blood flows back at each heartbeat into the cavity from which it has been pumped. In order to drive the blood through the narrowed valve, or to deal with the excess of blood caused by the backwash, the muscle wall of the cavities of the heart must thicken so as to become more powerful. When this happens, the damage is said to have been "compensated."

There comes a time, however, when the muscle can thicken no more, and it then begins to stretch and the cavities of the heart get larger; they dilate, but the muscle is less powerful and cannot contract so strongly. Then symptoms of distress appear, more blood gets dammed back in the cavities, from the left auricle blood gets dammed back into the lungs, and signs of congestion of the lung result. This pressure of blood is transmitted to the right side of the heart through the pulmonary artery and from there to the veins which bring blood from all the parts of the body. The swelling of the legs which is typical of dropsy is the final result of this "back pressure." But even before dropsy occurs, the heart muscle may degenerate, giving rise to irregular and valueless contractions in the auricles which the ventricles follow quite irregularly, with the result that the beat of the pulse which reflects the beat of the ventricles is completely irregular both in force and time. These happenings are the common sequels to rheumatic heart trouble in childhood, and every parent should give careful consideration to the possible damage to the heart by tonsillitis or "growing pains."

Heart Disease in Adult Life. Apart from the sequels to rheumatic infection in childhood and the same infection in early adult life, the most crippling cause of heart trouble in early middle life is syphilis. This disorder especially attacks the aorta, which supplies the smaller arteries, and which arises from the left ventricle. The valve guarding the opening of the ventricle into the aorta is also commonly attacked and, as a result, it fails to close properly at each heart-beat, allowing some of the blood to flow back into the ventricle. The muscle of this ventricle is able to thicken to an enormous size till the heart becomes as big as that of an ox; but finally it degenerates and signs of heart failure appear. It is in connection with disease of the aorta that attacks of pain occur. There may be typical attacks of angina pectoris, or milder attacks of pain over the front of the chest with a feeling of suffocation, the pain sometimes being felt, as in true angina, down the left arm.

In early middle life also, the conducting apparatus of the heart may become diseased, in some cases the cause being unknown, in others being due to syphilis. Whatever the cause, the result is the same: the ventricles no longer respond to every contraction of the auricles, since the conducting apparatus either conducts only every second, third, or fourth beat, or it fails to conduct at all, and the ventricles contract at their own rate, which as about 40 beats per minute, instead of the normal 72. This very slow beating of the ventricles sometimes produces attacks of unconsciousness with convulsions. These attacks are of serious import, as they signify that insufficient blood is being supplied to the brain.

Cardiac Catheterization. A radio-opaque catheter can be passed through a vein into one or other of the chambers of the heart, the pressure recorded, and valuable information obtained.

Heart Disease in Old Age. Heart disease in old age is either the result of arteriosclerosis or of degeneration of the muscle of the heart. Sometimes there is a combination of these two conditions, as the arteries which supply the heart itself, the coronary arteries, become narrowed through arteriosclerosis and the heartmuscle degenerates because the blood supply is not sufficient for its needs. The pumping action of the heart is thus affected and gradually it fails to be able to maintain the circulation. Occasionally, a large part of the heartmuscle is suddenly deprived of its blood supply by a coronary artery getting blocked up; it becomes so narrowed that only a small quantity of blood can pass, and then one day it gets blocked altogether. The disorders of the heart associated with disease of the coronary arteries are dealt with in the sections on ANGINA PECTORIS and CORONARY THROMBOSIS.

In simple degeneration of the heart muscle, the usual complaint is of the increasing inability to do much without getting short of breath and overtired. Pain round the heart is not common. This condition may continue for years with but few symptoms and signs, provided that reasonable care is taken of the limited capacity of the heart for work.

The Treatment of Heart Disease. In any form of heart disease, the essential treatment is to limit the patient's output of energy to that which the heart is capable of sustaining without further damage. Every case of heart trouble must be under the care of a doctor. All that can be said here is to indicate a few simple rules which will serve merely to emphasize the general line of treatment in heart disease. Rest for the heart is the most important measure by far. When rest in bed is decreed by the doctor for a patient with heart trouble, his instruction must be strictly carried out, and the patient must on no account get out of bed even to wash or to go to the lavatory.

This is especially important in the case of children with rheumatic heart disease, as a lengthy period spent in bed when the heart is first attacked may save it from serious damage. An attack of acute rheumatism in children may mean a period of up to 6 months in bed if permanent heart trouble is to be avoided. It is advisable for anyone with a damaged heart to rest in bed at least one day a week if this is at all possible, and overexertion must at all costs be avoided. Occupations should be chosen in which manual labour is reduced to a minimum. On the other hand, a certain amount of exercise should be taken unless ordered to the contrary. Easy walking, or games which do not involve too much exertion, such as bowling, for example, should be enjoyed; but any noticeable shortness of breath after exertion is a warning to "go slow." Personal hygiene is very important; the mouth should be kept scrupulously clean and the teeth must be kept free from sepsis, as septic teeth harbor germs which will attack a heart already damaged, and give rise to a very serious and often rapidly fatal disease of the lining membrane of the heart. The use of alcohol and tobacco must be regulated by the patient's medical adviser, as each individual case has to be considered separately; but generally speaking, it is possible to allow a patient who has been a heavy smoker and drinker a small amount of liquor or tobacco, though any increase in his symptoms or signs may necessitate their withdrawal.

Treatment of heart disease has been almost revolutionized by the scientifically controlled use of drugs. The salicylates are used in acute rheumatism. Digitalis in a stronger form and in large doses has saved many a life which would have been lost twenty years ago, while the onset of dropsy, formerly a dreaded sign, can now be combated with success by new mercury preparations. Another drug, quinidine, has been very successful in expert hands in restoring the normal rhythm of the heart where this has been upset. In cases of thickening or closing of one of the valves of the heart, a difficult surgical operation is now sometimes performed, to allow the blood to flow more easily through the valve. But the treatment of heart disease really lies in prevention. If the rheumatic cases can be taken in time to stop the damage at the outset; if the syphilitic cases are treated for their syphilis before the germ has time to reach the heart; and if those with a family history of high blood pressure will, in their early years, live so that arteriosclerosis does not develop, then heart disease will cease to be the commonest cause of death, as it is today, and will become one of the rarest. (*See also* ANEURISM; ANGINA PECTORIS; ARTERIOSCLEROSIS; ENDOCARDITIS; MYOCARDITIS; PERICARDITIS.)

HEARTBURN. This is the name given to a burning feeling extending up from the stomach through the chest to the mouth. It is due to the flowing back of acid fluid from the stomach—sometimes a quantity of this fluid may actually reach the mouth—accompanied by a gush of saliva. It is one of the symptoms of various disorders of the stomach. During pregnancy, heartburn frequently occurs and causes considerable discomfort.

Treatment. To remedy the condition the diet must be regulated and all rich foods should be avoided. The safest things to take are milk, eggs, fish, and other foods which are easily digested. Alcohol, spices, and highly-seasoned dishes should be avoided. As soon as an attack occurs the most effective way of gaining relief is to take half a teaspoonful of bicarbonate of soda in a little water. (*See also* DIGESTION; FLATULENCE; INDIGESTION; PREGNANCY; STOMACH.)

HEAT. Heat applied either to the body as a whole or to a particular part of it is one of the most useful treatments we have for certain conditions. Placing a hot-water bottle on a particular spot, such as an earache or a pain in the stomach, is a local application of heat. The pain is relieved by the action of the heat which causes the muscles and nerves of the affected part to relax; it also draws a greater supply of blood and of lymph to the painful area, and the antidotes to disease which they contain are brought in force to the spot where they are needed.

Heat applied to the body as a whole in the form of baths increases the activity of the skin. The whole subject of heat treatment by means of baths and electricity is discussed under those headings.

HEAT STROKE. An illness resulting from exposure to the sun. (*See* SUNSTROKE.)

HECTIC FEVER. A type of fever which may occur in advanced stages of tuberculosis, in which the temperature swings backwards and forwards, sometimes as high as 105 deg. F. in the morning and very often below normal in the evening, is known as hectic fever. The patient is usually very wasted and night sweats are frequent. (*See also* TUBERCULOSIS.)

HEEL. The heel is the hinder part of the foot and it is formed by a bone called *os* *calcis* or *calcaneum*. This bone bears most of our weight when we are standing and is raised with every step we take by the muscles of the calf, which are attached to it by the tendon of Achilles.

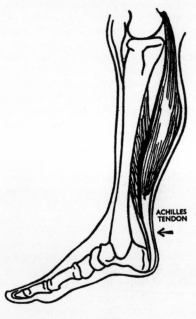

Heel.

The skin of the heel may become hard or tender from rubbing against the shoe. Pain may sometimes be a symptom of rheumatism, requiring a doctor's advice.

HEIGHT. The height of a person is to a great extent determined in advance by his parentage, though it is not an invariable rule. The length of a baby at birth is from sixteen to twenty-two inches, and in the first year growth is rapid. After that it is fairly uniform, being from two to four inches in a year until the age of puberty. A girl usually reaches to within two or three inches of her full height between the ages of twelve and fourteen, then grows slowly until about her twentieth year. A boy, on the other hand, continues his rapid growing rate until about the ages of sixteen to eighteen and will then put on another couple of inches between then and his early twenties.

Growth depends greatly upon proper feeding and proper working of certain glands, notably the pituitary gland near the brain. If this gland is not working properly the child may become either a giant or a dwarf. Apart from defects of the pituitary gland, the most important factor in promoting proper growth is a well-balanced diet with sufficient vitamins. The undersized, bent, rickety children that used to be so common are now a rarity. (*See also* BRAIN; DUCTLESS GLANDS; GROWTH.)

HEMATEMESIS. Hematemesis literally means vomiting of blood. Bleeding may occur in the stomach as a result of acute gastritis, cancer, or as a sympton of ulcer of the stomach. It may also occur in certain diseases of the blood such as hemophilia, purpura, and severe anemia. If the hematemesis is severe, the patient usually has a feeling of faintness and nausea, and then vomits up the blood. Blood brought up in this way is generally dark in color and may have the actual appearance of coffee grounds. It should be remembered that blood may be swallowed from the nose or throat, and there is also the possibility of blood being swallowed from the lungs. (*See also* GASTRIC ULCER; HEMORRHAGE.)

HEMATOCELE. The collection of blood in a cavity of the body, especially in the pelvic cavity in females or in the testicle in males, is known as hematocele.

HEMATOMA. A tumor or swelling containing blood is known as a hematoma. It is usually the result of injury, and it is very commonly found on the head of a newborn child after a long and difficult labor. At first a hematoma is rather soft to the touch, but it gradually becomes harder as the blood clots. In the course of a month or two, the whole contents of the swelling will be absorbed into the surrounding tissues and no treatment is usually required. If there is any pain accompanying the swelling, cold applications will give relief. In some cases, the swelling may become infected and an abscess may form. This should be opened as soon as any pus begins to collect.

HEMATURIA. This term signifies the passing of red blood corpuscles in the urine. *Nephritis* (Bright's disease) is one of the commonest causes of this condition, but it may result from stones, inflammation, or growths in the bladder. In tropical countries the passing of blood in the urine may be a symptom of *bilharziasis,* a disease caused by worms. If the blood is thoroughly mixed with the urine on passing, it is probably coming from the kidneys; if the blood appears only at the beginning of the flow it probably comes from the urethra, and if it noticed at the end, the site of the bleeding may be the bladder. The color of the urine depends on how much blood is passed. In some cases, if there is a large amount of blood present, the urine may be almost black or may present a smoky appearance. With small amounts it may be only faintly tinged, or may present no change at all to the naked eye. In certain cases the presence of the blood cells can only be recognized under a microscope, or by having the urine tested with chemicals. (*See also* BILHARZIASIS; BLADDER; KIDNEY; URINE.)

HEMICRANIA. This is a form of migraine in which headache occurs on one side of the head. (*See also* HEADACHE.)

HEMIPLEGIA. Paralysis of one half of the body is known as hemiplegia. It is caused by diseases affecting the central part of the brain. (*See also* BRAIN; PARALYSIS.)

HEMLOCK. This is the poison by which Socrates was put to death.

Treatment. In cases of poisoning, give an emetic. The stomach should be washed out and tannic acid given. The patient must be kept warm and artificial respiration carried out.

HEMOGLOBIN. Hemoglobin is the coloring matter in the red corpuscles which produces the red color of the blood. People with anemia are pale because of the lessening of hemoglobin in the blood. (*See also* ANEMIA; BLOOD.)

HEMOPHILIA. This is the medical term for bleeder's disease. It is a condition in which the blood does not clot in the normal time, and the patient may bleed to death unless special precautions are taken. This disease is hereditary, and it is confined almost entirely to the male members of the family, though it is transmitted through the mother. (*See also* BLEEDERS.)

HEMOPTYSIS. Hemoptysis, or the spitting of blood, is a condition which may be due to various causes; but the most common, by far, is tuberculosis of the lungs, especially when the blood is in any quantity. Another fairly frequent cause is

disease of the mitral valve of the heart, in which condition the lungs are overfilled with blood. Other less common causes of hemoptysis are bronchiectasis, growth in the lung, and blood diseases. While the nose may bleed into the throat, and the blood be coughed up, it is usually a mistake to blame blood vessels in the throat for bleeding; the blood is much more likely to have come from the lung and demands expert examination, including X-rays. (*See also* TUBERCULOSIS.)

HEMORRHAGE. By hemorrhage is meant bleeding of any description from any part of the body. The bleeding may be either external or internal. In external bleeding the blood penetrates through the skin, or gathers visibly just under the skin and is plain to see with the naked eye. In internal bleeding, however, there may be nothing showing which an unskilled person would recognize as blood. The blood will be coming from some part of the interior of the body and will eventually appear in the stool or urine, but in such an altered form that it bears no resemblance to the bright red fluid familiar to us as blood. This is called *occult blood,* meaning hidden blood. It is common in ulcerated conditions of the stomach or intestines, and if it is present in such large quantities that it darkens the color of the stools, it is known as *melena.*

External bleeding may be from veins, arteries or capillaries.

Treatment. In the case of very small cuts and scratches, the pressure of a bandage will usually be all that is required to stop the bleeding. All profuse bleeding rapidly becomes a serious matter, so the subject is dealt with in detail in the supplement on common emergencies and their First Aid treatment. In this connection it may be remarked that the time to use a first aid supplement or manual is not so much when the emergency has occurred as in the peaceful times beforehand, when the few simple devices that will save life should be memorized and practiced in preparation for the moment when the knowledge of just what to do and how to do it will possibly make the difference between life and death. The first thing to do when bleeding occurs is always to put pressure on the wound. If it is small and the finger will cover it, press hard with the finger. If it is larger, the proper pressure will have to be applied by tight bandaging or, failing this, by means of a *tourniquet*. The "pressure points" are important and are fully described in the supplement.

Internal hemorrhage will be recognized by the condition of the patient before the blood appears in the stools. A person bleeding internally becomes cold with clammy skin, pale lips and fingernails, quick and feeble pulse, quickened breathing, and sometimes breathlessness. There is usually great restlessness, a very anxious and drawn look on the face, and the patient may say that he feels his life ebbing away from him. Obviously the condition is dangerous and the bleeding must be stopped by skilled attention as soon as possible, and after the bleeding has been stopped means must be taken to restore the vitality of the patient. It is now considered that death from bleeding is due to the fact that the heart cannot work properly without a certain amount of fluid in the blood vessels, so the first thing to be done after a bad hemorrhage is to restore the proper amount of fluid to the blood vessels, so that the heart will be able to continue its rhythmical pumping. This is done by the transfusion of blood or plasma, a measure which saved countless lives during the second World War. In a very urgent case, with blood not available, the doctor may inject a quantity of the salt solution *normal saline* straight into a vein.

In surgical operations it is, of course, necessary for the surgeon to cut through at least several of the smaller blood vessels, and he will stop the bleeding from these vessels by tying their ends with ligatures or closing them with artery forceps. Bleeding from the lungs is bright red, frothy and is coughed up. Blood from the stomach is darker in color and is usually compared to coffee-grounds. It is vomited up. In both cases the patient must lie down and be kept quiet until a doctor arrives. For the emergency treatment of bleeding and a more detailed account of pressure spots, etc., *see* the FIRST AID SUPPLEMENT. (*See also* BLOOD; TOURNIQUET; TRANSFUSION OF BLOOD.)

HEMORRHOIDS. The name commonly used for hemorrhoids is *piles,* and the condition is fully described under that heading. By piles we mean a condition in which the blood vessels at the lower entrance to the bowel are dilated or varicose and cause pain and bleeding. (*See also* CONSTIPATION; PILES.)

HEMP. Extracts of Indian hemp produce a powerful drug known as cannabis indica, hashish, or bhang. (*See also* CANNABIS INDICA.)

HENNA. The hair dye known as henna is obtained from the powdered leaves of an Eastern plant, the Lawsonian Inermis. Henna has been used as a hair dye for centuries past and, as it dyes the skin as well, the women of the East make use of it to redden their fingernails, the soles of their feet, and the palms of their hands. Even the men in Mohammedan countries use it to dye their beards. Henna mixed with indigo gives varying shades of brown; the longer the dye is left on, the darker the hair will become. About one hour will give a light brown shade, but experiments should be carried out before actually trying it on the hair.

HEPARIN. Heparin is a drug derived from ox liver, used to delay the clotting of the blood. It is used, for example, in the prevention and treatment of thrombosis (clotting in a vein) and phlebitis (inflammation of a vein).

HEPATIC. Hepatic means anything pertaining to the liver. A *hepatic abscess* is an abscess of the liver. The *hepatic artery* is the artery which supplies the liver with blood, and the *hepatic ducts* are the passages by which the bile flows away from the liver. The hepatic ducts join with the cystic duct leading from the gall bladder to form the common bile duct which leads into the duodenum.

HEPATITIS. Hepatitis means inflammation of the liver. Infective hepatitis is discussed under the heading of catarrhal jaundice. (*See also* LIVER.)

HERBS. As medicines, various herbs have been used for centuries, and many people today use them for simple ailments, as their parents and grandparents did for generations back. Most herbs having a significant beneficial action on the body have been standardized so that the effects of any particular remedy can be foretold with reasonable accuracy. Thus Foxglove leaves are prepared as tincture of digitalis, which is an invaluable drug in the treatment of heart disease.

HEREDITY. This is the influence which determines inborn bodily and mental characteristics. It is a very old saying that "like tends to beget like," but why is this so? In the higher animals, reproduction takes place by the union of the male and female germ cells, the sperms with the ova, and after the union, or fertilization as it is called, the new individual develops. The whole complicated structure of the offspring is formed from these two germ cells.

The theory of heredity depends on the supposed fact that there is, in each of these parent germ cells, some substance which is not used up in the construction of the body of the offspring, but is reserved unchanged for the formation of the germ cells of the next generation. The germ cells give rise to all the body cells of the offspring and are all stored up in the germ cells of that offspring so that they may be passed on to the next generation. From this explanation it will be seen that it is very unlikely that characters in the parent which are the result of external influences or surroundings will have any effect on the offspring.

This fact disposes once and for all of the belief which has frightened so many mothers-to-be, that if a woman suffers an injury or fright while pregnant, her offspring will bear some mark of it.

The influence of inherited character as opposed to that induced by surroundings was tested a few years ago in Scotland. A number of young children from the slums of one of the biggest cities, whose parents all had bad criminal records, were transported to a peaceful fishing village on the coast where nothing was known of their history, and they were put in charge of kindly fisher-folk. But when those children grew older the influence of their criminal heredity was seen; the peaceful fishing village was peaceful no longer and the village inn resembled a thieves' kitchen. The experiment was a failure, as anyone who had studied heredity could have predicted. But it is important to note that *all* the parents had bad records, that is to say, the unfortunate children inherited badness from both sides. There is a very definite law governing the inheritance of certain bodily qualities, and there is every reason to suppose that a natural law also governs the inheritance of mental qualities.

The law which governs the inheritance of bodily characteristics is Mendel's law. This was based on plant experiments, but the principles apply to all living things. Mendel crossed dwarf peas with tall peas and found that the resulting hybrids or crossbreeds were all tall peas. When these hybrids were crossed it was found that dwarf peas appeared to the extent of one quarter. Of the remaining three-quarters, all were tall peas, one third being purebred and the rest hybrids. Mendel concluded that some characters which he called *dominant* had the power to mask others which are spoken of as *recessive,* when occurring in a crossbreed. In the example given above, tallness is a dominant and dwarfness a recessive character. This law of inheritance has been shown to operate in certain well-defined characteristics in the animal kingdom. To name but a few: the size of the comb in fowls, horned or hornless condition in cattle, the presence or absence of brown pigment in the iris of the eye in man. The new science of eugenics, which suggests selective mating for human beings so that the best characters of the race should be preserved, is only an attempt to apply the laws of heredity. Whether such a step will ever be taken cannot here be discussed. The important thing is to insure that those who suffer from known diseases which they can pass on to their offspring should be warned against marriage.

There are many disorders which are passed from one generation to the next, and families are known in which such disorders can be traced back for several generations. The one most commonly heard of is hemophilia, which is an inherited tendency in boys to bleed from the merest scratch. Unless very special measures are taken to stop the bleeding, such unfortunates bleed to death from very slight wounds; their blood has no power of clotting. This inheritance is always passed through the mother, but girls in a family never show it.

A less common but none the less terrible disease is a certain nervous trouble which afflicts children in affected families. These children—and if the family is large, several in the same generation will suffer—are born normal, and are apparently healthy up to the age of a year or so, when they "go backwards," cease to crawl or to sit up and become blind. They usually die within a few months after this has happened. This condition is especially associated with the Semetic race, though families not of that race have been known to be so afflicted.

The question of inheritance of disorders of the mind, especially the more obvious forms of insanity, is a debatable point. There can be no doubt that when there is actual insanity or definite mental weakness on both sides, some of the offspring will certainly be at least feebleminded. Some time ago, the descendants of two insane persons were traced through several generations and the proportion of idiots, feebleminded, and criminals was found to be exceedingly high. But where one partner is mentally weak or suffers from some periodic form of insanity, there is some evidence to show that the healthy partner can more than counterbalance the mental weakness of the other, and the offspring have a good chance of escaping their parent's fate, provided they are not exposed to conditions which will favor the development of mental stress. Epilepsy is one of the conditions which we know may be handed down from generation to generation; it appears to be one of those characters which are "dominant," that is, it tends to assert itself more often in the offspring than would be expected from an even chance of the mating of two individuals.

But it is not only diseases themselves that form part of our possible heredity; various tendencies to disease may be passed from one generation to the other. Certain forms of heart trouble are a case in point. High blood pressure "runs in families." One family may have a low resistance to tuberculosis and if the necessary precautions are not taken, although the disease itself is not inherited, members of one generation after another in that particular family succumb to that disease. Some diseases show a cultural preference—Jews are especially liable to diabetes; the Irish to tuberculosis. Certain infirmities depend on heredity: deaf-mutism is one of the commonest, but another form of deafness may be inherited,

nearly always through the female side. Such minor deformities as six toes or one short finger are examples of not infrequent inherited characters. The color of the hair and of the pigment of the eyes is dependent on heredity. Two blue-eyed, fair-haired parents will probably have blue-eyed, fair-haired children. Red hair tends to be a "dominant" character; it appears in more than half of the offspring if only one parent is red-haired.

HERNIA. The popular name for hernia is "rupture," and it is a common condition among men and boys and not so common among women. By hernia is meant the protruding through its covering of any organ of the body. The way hernia arises is well seen in the abdomen, where all the organs are contained in a covering called the abdominal wall. For one reason or another there may be a weak spot in this abdominal wall through which a piece of bowel or any of the organs contained in the abdomen may protrude. This protrusion will be seen as a lump under the skin which covers the abdomen.

Inguinal Hernia. The most common hernia is that called inguinal hernia. It occurs in both men and women. The wall of the abdomen is composed of a sheath of muscles in which there is an opening to permit the passage of a cord. In men it is the cord that suspends the testicle, and in women there is a cord passing from the womb to the tissues in the groin. The opening for the passage of these cords forms a weak spot in the abdominal wall, and a loop of intestine can readily protrude through it, forming an inguinal hernia.

Femoral Hernia. Another common hernia is the *femoral hernia,* which occurs at the weak spot where the great blood vessels of the abdomen pass into the thigh. The lump in this case is felt in the groin, at a spot lower down than the lump formed by the inguinal hernia, already described.

Umbilical Hernia. Hernias are also apt to occur at the umbilicus or navel. This hernia may occur at any age, but is most often found in small babies. It is also found in middle-aged women who have had several children and have grown stout.

Ventral Hernia. A ventral hernia is a hernia that occurs at the site of a former operation. The abdominal wall is often left

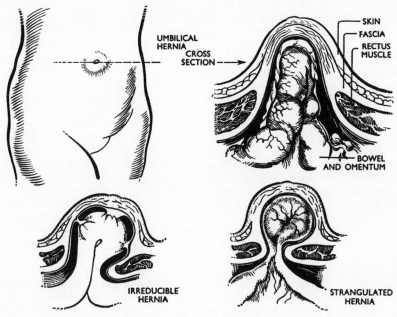

Hernia.

in a weak state after an operation, especially one in which there has been a tube for drainage purposes, and a hernia may occur here.

Treatment. Often a hernia does not cause very much inconvenience and it is sufficient to wear a properly fitting support, called a *truss,* after the hernia has been replaced in position, or reduced as it is called; but at any moment there may be further trouble especially if heavy weights have to be lifted or there is any condition which causes straining. It is usually preferable to have an operation which offers the prospect of complete cure. The great danger of hernias in the abdomen is always that the loop of intestine which has pushed into the hernia will become *strangulated,* that is, so compressed that its blood supply is cut off and it dies. A strangulated hernia is a very serious matter calling for immediate operation in order to save the patient's life. The hernias of babies and young children can nearly always be cured by wearing a small pad over the navel held on by a bandage.

HEROIN. Heroin is a drug obtained from morphine, which it resembles very much in its general action on the body. Heroin, however, acts more strongly on the part of the nervous system connected with

breathing, and because of this it is used to give relief in cases of troublesome and incessant cough. Unfortunately, as with morphine, there is a great liability to develop the drug habit, which when once formed is quite as difficult to break as the morphine habit, and leads to equally tragic results. (*See also* DRUG HABIT; OPIUM.)

HERPES. Herpes of the face occurs commonly on or near the lips. The symptoms are itching and "tightness" of the skin, followed by swollen reddish patches, which in a few hours are covered with little blisters. If uninfected they dry up in about 7–10 days. In those subject to herpes, any little "upset" to the health may bring on an attack. If cases occur persistently on the same area, infection from the teeth, nose, etc., should be suspected.

Treatment. Those who recognize the early signs may limit an attack considerably by bathing the part with very hot water, or by applying collodion. Four per cent silver nitrate in spirit of nitrous ether is also recommended. The blisters should be protected by a mild antiseptic powder.

Herpes Genitalis, which attacks the skin of the penis, resembles herpes facialis, but very readily ulcerates. It is *in itself* of small importance, but must be distinguished

339

from certain venereal diseases. In some cases also, herpes appears first, followed by a soft or hard chancre.

Treatment. In an uncomplicated case the only treatment required is an antiseptic dusting powder, such as 1 or 2 per cent salicylic acid in boric acid. All local disturbance must be avoided for at least six weeks.

Herpes Zoster, which is a ring of herpes encircling the body, is more usually called shingles, and is described under that title.

HEXAMINE. Hexamine, a drug which was formerly known as urotropine, is manufactured from formalin and ammonia. It is given as an antiseptic in the treatment of infections of the bladder, and is much more effective in the presence of acid than alkaline urine. Sodium acid phosphate should, therefore, be given an hour or two before the administration of the hexamine. Plenty of water should always be taken in order to avoid any bladder irritation.

HICCOUGH. Hiccough, or hiccup, is caused by a sudden contraction of the diaphragm due to some irritation of the nerves. The breath which is drawn in suddenly is checked midway, as it were, by the closure of the vocal cords.

Hiccough may occur as a symptom of a more serious condition than a slight attack of indigestion. In nervous disorders it may be one of the symptoms of epilepsy, encephalitis lethargica or hysteria. It often occurs in nephritis or uremia, or it may be due to tetanus, hydrophobia or strychnine poisoning.

Treatment. If the hiccoughing is due to indigestion, it is often relieved by drinking a glassful of water with a little bicarbonate of soda or bismuth carbonate. Holding the breath for as long as possible is an old and sometimes effective remedy. When the hiccoughing is due to some complicating condition it may be necessary to give soothing drugs such as chloretone or luminal.

HIP. By the hip we mean the whole region of the hip joint where the lower limb joins on to the main trunk of the body. As human beings are dependent on the hip joint for moving from place to place and for the support of the body in the upright position, it is, as might be expected, the largest and strongest joint in the body.

The hip joint is embedded in strong muscular and fatty tissues forming the buttock, the thigh and the groin in front. All this region is commonly called the hip, but for medical purposes the word hip usually is taken to mean the hip joint only.

Bones of the Hip joint. The hip joint is a ball-and-socket joint, the ball being the well-rounded head of the femur (thighbone), while the socket is a cup-shaped hollow in the haunch bone (pelvis), called the *acetabulum*. Like other bone surfaces which are exposed to rubbing, the surface of the head of the thighbone is covered with cartilage, and the interior of the acetabulum is lined with cartilage which, however, does not quite reach to the outside rim of the cup, so that it exerts a sucking action as well as preventing the rubbing away of the bone by friction. The hip has a very wide range of movement in young and supple people. It can move round from side to side, bend up and down, and swing backwards and forwards. In young infants the hipbone consists of three distinct parts, the ilium, the ischium, and the os pubis; but in adults these three parts are united to form the acetabulum, and complete union usually takes place about the age of puberty.

Hip Disease. Tuberculosis is one of the commonest causes of hip joint disease and nearly always occurs during childhood. The symptoms start quite early in life and become more noticeable as time goes on.

Symptoms. The child generally complains of tiredness, and is noticed to walk with a slight limp. He may complain of pain in the leg or the knee, and movement of the limb is usually limited in all directions. When standing or walking, the patient will make every effort to save putting weight on the affected side, and as the condition advances this limp will become more pronounced. Gradually the muscles begin to waste about the hip and the limb alters in appearance. The thigh is bent upwards, while the foot is bent outwards, and there is usually a great deal of pain and some swelling.

Treatment. The general treatment of hip joint disease is the same as for other tuberculous conditions. The child should be kept in bed and some form of splint should be used to keep the limb in a good position. He should also live in the open

340

air as much as possible, and treatment should preferably be carried out in a sanatorium. (*See also* TUBERCULOSIS.)

Hip, Dislocation of. Dislocation of the hip at birth is by no means rare, and it is due to the imperfect formation of the acetabulum. It is not usually noticed until the child begins to walk, and then it will be seen that the child walks in a curious waddling sort of way. In all cases it is desirable that an X-ray photograph should be taken to find out the exact type of the dislocation.

Treatment. The treatment of this condition is purely surgical and usually involves immobilization of the affected joints in plaster. (*See also* DISLOCATION.)

HIRSCHSPRUNG'S DISEASE. Also called megacolon, this condition of an enormously dilated large bowel is a rare disease of young children, chiefly boys, but it also sometimes affects adults. It is treated by dilating the anus and giving regular enemas. Various operations have been devised to restore the normal function of the bowel, and many give good results. (*See* SYMPATHECTOMY.)

HOARSENESS. Hoarseness or huskiness of the voice is generally the result of catarrh or inflammation of the vocal cords, but it may also result from pressure on the nerves that control the movements of the cords.

Common causes of hoarseness are small "nodes" on the vocal cords, due to overuse or bad production of the voice, or small polypi or fibromas. More serious conditions, however, are not unknown, especially in elderly men. No person should have chronic hoarseness for a month without having the larynx examined by a specialist in case any serious disease may be beginning.

HOBNAIL LIVER. This is a popular term for cirrhosis of the liver which was supposed to be due to taking too much alcohol. The term hobnail is given because the surface of the liver is studded with hard projections which suggest the appearance of hobnails. It is now suggested that catarrh or infections of the liver may be as much to blame as alcohol, and that a dietary deficiency may be the essential cause of the cirrhosis. (*See also* CIRRHOSIS.)

HODGKIN'S DISEASE. Hodgkin's disease, otherwise known as lymphadenoma

or lymphogranuloma, is a disease in which the lymph glands and the spleen become enlarged. The condition is named after Thomas Hodgkin (1798–1866), an English physician, who was the first to make records of several cases of this disease.

Symptoms. The disease usually comes on very gradually, and men are more often affected than women. The first symptom is enlargement of the glands of the neck, and there may be a great feeling of weakness accompanied by breathlessness. The glands in the groin and under the armpits may swell up, and the glands in the chest and abdomen may also become affected. These enlarged glands may cause pressure on the nerves of the various parts affected, and much pain may result. Pressure on the spinal cord may cause paralysis to take place. In about 75 per cent of cases the spleen is enlarged, but it is unusual for enlargement of the liver to occur. A slight degree of fever is generally present, and it is not unusual for the skin to turn a bronzed color. The cause of the complaint is unknown, but it is thought to be a type of growth affecting lymphoid tissues.

Treatment. There is no certain cure for Hodgkin's disease, but much can be done to arrest its progress which in any case is often slow. Injections of a chemical called nitrogen mustard may result in the disappearance of gland masses with improvement in the general condition. Deep X-rays often help too. Plenty of rest, fresh air, and nourishing food should be given. (*See also* LYMPHATICS.)

HOMEOPATHY. This is an unusual system of treating disease by drugs which produce the same symptoms as the disease. These drugs are given over a long period in very small doses.

HOOKWORM DISEASE. Hookworm disease, or ankylostomiasis as it is medically termed, is produced by the presence in the human body of a worm known as the hookworm. Another name for this condition is "miner's anemia." The worms produce thousands of eggs which are discharged from the intestine of the infected person. When these come in contact with damp soil or water, they hatch out into embryos which enter the skin of someone else and then pass by means of blood to the heart and lungs, and finally into the intestine.

They usually enter the human body through the soles of the feet, producing what is known as "ground itch." The disease is to be found particularly in warm climates such as Egypt, India, China, Ceylon, and the southern states of the U.S.

Symptoms. Small sores and swellings may occur in the feet, but these usually heal up within a week or so. Several months may pass before the patient becomes aware of any other symptoms. Later on he may complain of shortness of breath, palpitations, and general weakness. There may also be flatulence and constipation or diarrhea. The complexion may appear pale and sallow, and the temperature may be slightly raised. The disease may go on for many months if untreated, but under treatment the chance of recovery is usually good.

Treatment. In the treatment of this disease, various anthelmintic drugs are used (anthelmintic is the name given to any drug which is used in the treatment of worms). Oil of chenopodium and carbon tetrachloride are very largely used, but they should not be taken unless under medical supervision. Prevention of the disease consists in giving careful attention to the disposal of feces or excreted matter; the water supply must be pure, and shoes and stockings should be worn, especially by children.

HORDEOLUM. Hordeolums are better known to everyone as styes on the eyelids, and are described under the name STYE.

HORMONES. By hormones we mean substances which are produced by various glands of the body and poured by them directly into the bloodstream of the body. In other words, they are the *secretions* of the *ductless glands*. The study of the ductless glands and their secretions, which include substances like adrenalin, pituitrin, and insulin, is a branch of medical science in which great advances are being made, and an account of this new knowledge will be found in the article called DUCTLESS GLANDS.

HOT-WATER BOTTLE. Hot-water bottles are so well known that it hardly seems necessary to describe them, but one or two points in connection with their use should be emphasized. The first of these is to keep a hot-water bottle handy. In cases of sudden illness, especially shock, accidents, and bleeding, whether from the lungs, internally or externally, the immediate application of heat in the form of hot-water bottles may be of vital importance in counteracting the effect of shock and loss of blood on the circulation. In cases of sudden and severe pain such as gallstones, a hot-water bottle will be a great help in easing the pain until the doctor comes. Another point that is neglected sometimes with serious and even fatal results is the care that must always be taken in judging the heat of a hot-water bottle which is given to a helpless or unconscious person, whether baby or grown-up. For a small child or baby a bottle that feels hot to the hand of a working woman will be too warm. The bottle should be tested on some delicate part of the skin which is not much exposed to extremes of temperature, such as the inside of the upper arm, the breast, etc. Always examine the bottle carefully to see that the stopper is firmly in and do not fill the bottle more than two-thirds full in case it bursts. The sleep of the young is so sound that a child will sleep through a wintry night with its bed soaked in water, and of course colds and sore throats are likely to follow such an occurrence. A removable flannel cover will keep the bottle warm for a much longer period than a bottle which is uncovered and also prevent burns.

HOUSEMAID'S KNEE. Frequent kneeling may cause a swelling to appear on the knee which may become inflamed. This is known as housemaid's knee. (*See also* BURSA.)

HOUSING. The question of housing is closely related to the health, because of the great influence which the home has upon the health of mind and body. Where large numbers of people are herded together in a small area there must inevitably be a great deal more disease of an infectious nature than in surroundings where such close contact with infected persons is not necessary. It has been amply shown too, that a definite amount of breathing space per person is needed to enable people to remain healthy, and in some overcrowded districts this amount of space is not forthcoming.

Overcrowding and lack of sunshine

penetrating into the dwelling-rooms of houses and tenements promote the spread of tuberculosis and other infectious diseases, while damp and cold make it easy for rheumatism to gain a hold. Vermin-infested houses lead to the spread of infection from person to person.

The provision of proper housing accommodation for everyone is therefore a necessary part of the fight against disease.

HUMERUS. The humerus is the bone of the upper arm, extending from the shoulder blade (scapula) to the elbow. It fits into the hollow of the scapula called the *glenoid fossa* and forms a ball and socket joint, the ball-shaped head of the humerus turning easily in the socket of the shoulder blade. It has the greatest range of movement of any bone of the body at the shoulder, because of the loose way in which it is jointed. For this same reason it is very easily dislocated. At the elbow it is jointed with a hinge joint to the forearm which can only move in two directions, up and down.

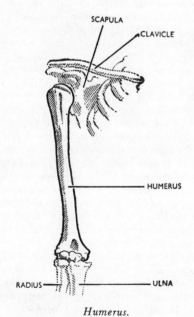

Humerus.

HUMIDITY. The amount of moisture in the air is referred to as the humidity. The question of humidity plays a very important part in connection with health. Too much moisture in the air prevents the evaporation of perspiration from the body, and in countries where the temperature is high and the humidity great, the body is inclined to feel heavy and depressed. (*See also* CLIMATE.)

HUMPBACK. Humpback, or hunchback, is caused by curvature of the spine and the typical case is usually due to tuberculosis of the spinal column (Pott's disease). The appearance of the humpback may vary from a mere roundness of the shoulders caused by standing badly, to an actual hump. Old people often become slightly humpbacked because of their inability to stand up straight, or rheumatoid arthritis may cause changes to take place in the spine. (*See also* POTT'S DISEASE; SPINE.)

HUNGER. A healthy desire for food is known as appetite, but hunger is the craving for food. Usually when a person has not eaten food for a period beyond the normal meal hours, a pleasurable feeling of hunger is experienced, but this feeling may become painful if the fasting period is prolonged.

The feeling of hunger does not always indicate that the stomach is empty, for the stomach may be full when this feeling comes on. This sensation of hunger is frequently a symptom of certain diseases. In some cases of dyspepsia, and especially in duodenal ulcer, hunger pains are felt, which are relieved when some food is eaten. In diabetes, unusual hunger is a very definite symptom, and a craving for food is also present in certain nervous diseases such as hysteria and epilepsy. In cases where it is necessary to keep the stomach empty, the feeling of hunger can be prevented by feeding the patient through the rectum. This can be carried on for several days without any discomfort to the patient. (*See also* APPETITE.)

HUNTINGTON'S CHOREA. This is a very rare hereditary disease of the nervous system in which the use of the muscles is gradually lost. The earlist symptoms are irregular muscular movements like those of the ordinary chorea (St. Vitus's Dance). The cause and cure are unknown and it is definitely of a hereditary nature.

HYDATID DISEASE. This is a disease in which cysts form in various parts of the body owing to the presence of immature tapeworms. The eggs of these tapeworms are almost always conveyed to human beings by dogs; usually through the dog licking the skin, or perhaps through licking the dishes from which food is eaten. The practice of kissing pet dogs is a highly unsanitary one.

Symptoms. A hydatid cyst produces no symptoms while it is small, but as it grows larger, which it does very rapidly, it may cause a great deal of damage by pressing on some organ of the body. In some cases a cyst may rupture with quite serious results, or again, inflammation may occur and a deep abscess appear. In a few rare instances, the cyst which is largely made up of clear fluid along with the head of the tiny worm, may dry up and gradually disappear. In many cases a secondary cyst may form inside the first; the first being termed the mother cyst while the second is termed the daughter, or there may be a granddaughter. The outside of the cyst is usually smooth and rather like elastic to the touch. Sometimes fluctuations may be felt, or on rare occasions, what is known as the "hydatid thrill," a feeling which has been compared to a quivering jelly. The commonest sites in the body for these cysts are the liver, the lungs, the brain, the kidneys, or the heart, but they may be found in any part of the body.

Hydatid cysts occur on the liver in about 60 per cent of all cases and so long as they remain small, the general health is not affected. As a cyst grows larger it may cause dragging pains in the abdomen, or pressure on the stomach may cause vomiting and dyspepsia. A cyst which spreads upwards may cause compression of the lung.

Rupture of a cyst occurs quite frequently, but the seriousness of the condition depends largely on the direction of the rupture. The most common direction for rupture is into the stomach or intestine. In this case the cyst may discharge for a few weeks and finally dry up, but fatal inflammation is not infrequent. Rupture into the peritoneum usually results in peritonitis, while rupture into the lung or a bronchus may prove fatal from suffocation. Rupture of a cyst may be accompanied by shock and by urticaria (hives).

Treatment. There is no medical treatment which can be of any use in a case of hydatid cyst, but removal of the cyst by operation may be successfully carried out.

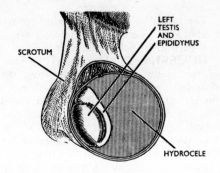

Hydrocele.

HYDROCELE. Hydrocele is a collection of fluid around the testicle or spermatic cord. This condition may occur in infants at birth, but it is most common in middle-aged men. In the majority of cases, there is no apparent reason for this accumulation of fluid, although some cases may be due to injury, or disease of the testicle.

Symptoms. A swelling is seen to form slowly on one side of the scrotum, the bag which holds the testicle. The swelling may be rounded in shape, or pear-like, and the size depends on how much fluid is present. As a rule it is quite elastic to the touch, and fluctuations or wave-like motions can be felt. In the dark, by holding a light close to the scrotum, the swelling can be seen to be translucent. This test is a most useful one in distinguishing hydrocele from other swellings of a solid nature. In cases that have been going on for a long time, however, the walls of the testicle may become very thick and the transparent appearance will be lost. There is no pain attached to this condition, but a dragging sensation may be felt if the swelling has been allowed to become very large.

Treatment. There are two courses of treatment open to a person with this condition. Either he can have the fluid drawn off by tapping, or he can have the condition cured by an operation. Tapping is done by means of a hollow needle, and as a rule, this method of treatment has to be repeated every few months. By having a surgical operation performed, the condition can be cured. Any person with hydrocele should wear a special belt which keeps the scrotum supported in a small bag, and by this means the accumulation of fluid may be lessened.

HYDROCEPHALUS. The condition of hydrocephalus, or water on the brain, occurs most frequently in children. Some cases are due to malformation before birth, but the most common cause is some obstruction of the normal flow of cerebrospinal fluid which, therefore, accumulates within the brain. Obstructions may result from adhesions following an attack of meningitis, or from the growth of tumors near the brain.

Symptoms. The head of an infant with hydrocephalus is greatly enlarged, and the forehead is seen to bulge and overhang the tiny wizened face. The skin is tightly stretched over the bulging skull, and the hair of the scalp is thin and scanty. There is usually considerable mental deficiency, which may amount to imbecility, and the child walks very badly, if at all.

When hydrocephalus commences late in childhood or in early adult life, the condition is much more difficult to diagnose, because the bones are more or less set and the skull cannot yield to anything like the same extent. The nervous signs are much more serious, consisting in severe headache, vomiting, neuritis of the eyes, and giddiness. During the earlier stages, before enlargement of the head has commenced, special tests can be carried out to demonstrate the presence of hydrocephalus.

Treatment. Treatment, either medical or surgical, is usually disappointing. In some cases the condition may become arrested and the child grow up with normal intelligence. Recently operations have been devised to by-pass the obstruction in the circulation of the cerebrospinal fluid and results have been fairly encouraging.

HYDROCHLORIC ACID. Hydrochloric acid is a strong corrosive acid produced by the gas given off when sulphuric acid is added to salt and passed through water. It is used in medicine in a very diluted form. This acid is present in the gastric juice in very small quantities. It is, therefore, of great value in the treatment of cases of indigestion due to the deficiency of gastric acid, for example, in alcoholic catarrh of the stomach. Poisonous doses of hydrochloric acid will produce severe burning in the mouth, throat and stomach, and a general state of collapse. Lime water, magnesia, or any alkali should be given, followed by milk or white of egg. Emetics should not be given in cases of poisoning by a corrosive acid. (*See also* POISONING in FIRST-AID SUPPLEMENT.)

HYDROCYANIC ACID. This acid is more commonly known as prussic acid and it is found in the oil of bitter almonds. It is an extremely powerful poison, but it is used in very small doses in the treatment of certain conditions. (*See also* PRUSSIC ACID.)

HYDROGEN PEROXIDE. This is a colorless, odorless liquid which is also referred to as peroxide of hydrogen, and consists of oxygen in solution in water. Hydrogen peroxide when it comes in contact with the tissues of the body gives off oxygen, which accounts for its antiseptic action. Because of this action it is greatly used in the treatment of sores and inflamed wounds. When sprayed on the wound, many little gas bubbles are formed which help to remove any pus there. Though ear specialists now seldom use it, equal parts parts of hydrogen peroxide and water may be dropped into discharging ears, or into an ear which has become blocked up with wax, as it helps to soften the wax and to bring away any other matter present in the ear.

Diluted with about three parts of water, it makes an excellent mouthwash, and is very soothing to painful ulcers of the mouth. It is particularly good for cleansing the mouth during fevers, as it not only disinfects the mouth but acts as a deodorizer as well, which means that it removes any unpleasant taste in the mouth and leaves the breath fresh and pleasant.

Hydrogen peroxide has also bleaching properties which are made use of for bleaching the hair. The hair should first be thoroughly washed with soap and water, and rinsed out in a weak solution of ammonia to make sure that all the grease is removed. The hydrogen peroxide is then rubbed into the roots and hair until the desired fairness is obtained. A final rinse in plain water should complete the bleaching. A few drops on the toothbrush will help to whiten the teeth, and is particularly good for removing the yellow stains which appear from too much smoking.

It is of great value in aiding the removal of dressings which have become stuck to a wound, and it is also useful in helping to stop bleeding. It can be used on the skin with perfect safety as it does not set up any irritation.

HYDRONEPHROSIS. This condition is due to a blocking in the urinary passage below the kidney which causes swelling to take place in the kidney. It may be due to a stone in the ureter, to enlarged prostate, or to pressure caused by an abdominal tumor.

The only treatment is operative, which consists in removing the obstruction or, when necessary, one of the kidneys. (*See also* OEDEMA; KIDNEY.)

HYDROPHOBIA. Hydrophobia is a very dangerous disease due to the bite of an infected or rabid dog, but other infected animals, especially wolves, may cause it. The disease is due to a virus which is present in the saliva of infected animals, and which is carried into the wound made by the teeth.

Symptoms. The symptoms do not arise for some considerable time after the bite —usually about six weeks; but the time may vary from ten days to six months. The wound, which has usually healed up, begins to look red and irritable, and the patient becomes very depressed and restless. In a few days the restlessness may give way to excitement and wildness. The patient finds pain and difficulty in swallowing, and the sight of water may cause violent spasms and contractions of the muscles of the throat; hence the name hydrophobia ("fear of water"). This stage lasts about three days. Finally, complete collapse and unconsciousness takes place and death may occur thereafter within a few hours.

Treatment. When a person is bitten by a dog, no efforts should be spared to thoroughly disinfect the wound. If the dog is suspected to be rabid the police should be at once notified so that the animal may be looked after by the proper authorities. The authorities will then arrange for the bitten person to have the Pasteur treatment, or rather, a modification of the original treatment carried out by that great scientist in 1885. This treatment consists in inoculating the person daily over a period of at least fourteen days, with gradually increasing doses of the virus which causes hydrophobia until he becomes immune. This treatment has been the means of saving thousands of lives, and there are now Pasteur Institutes in most countries of the world where treatment can be carried out under ideal conditions.

HYGIENE. Year by year, a higher standard of personal cleanliness is noticed. This is not the place to delve into the unsavory past, but it may be noted in passing that King James I had a skin as soft as silk because he never washed, and that Queen Anne, a hundred years later, showed an advance in cleanliness by washing her *hands* every morning. One hesitates to think of the habits of other classes, if these were the customs of royalty. The widespread practice of making and using perfumes was probably, in those times, not so much to add to personal attractiveness as to conceal personal odors. In these days, when the daily bath is a settled habit among a large proportion of the community, a far greater interest is taken, not only in actual cleanliness, but in what might be called the theory of cleanliness.

The skin is constantly exuding perspiration and oil, and shedding scales from the skin and the scalp. These accumulate on the skin surface, and partially penetrate into the underclothing. It follows, therefore, that the skin must be frequently cleansed, and the underclothing periodically changed, if the person is to be clean.

Moreover, a dirty skin and dirty clothes are not only offensive but also injurious to the health. If, as frequently happens, the skin is scratched or chafed, this foul matter may cause infection by absorption into the lymph vessels of the skin, and these and their neighboring glands may become inflamed. An example of this is seen in children with louse-infested heads, where the glands at the back of the neck are frequently found swollen and inflamed. Unclean people commonly "suffer from the cold" far more than those who have frequent baths, because their skins are less adaptable to changes of temperature.

Some people believe that by having a *cold* bath every morning they have therefor cleansed their skin of impurities. This is a mistake. The matter upon the skin is mainly of a fatty nature, and it is common knowledge that cold water will not dissolve grease. Hot or at least warm water, soap, and friction are all necessary to ensure true cleanliness of the skin. Soap acts chemically upon the fat and so assists in its removal. Soap is made up of an alkali and a fatty acid. The alkali combines with the grease on the skin (practically forming more soap), and so enables it to be readily washed off with water. Chemically, no fatty acid is necessary; but, practically, the alkali used alone would be too drastic, removing almost all the oil from the skin and thus causing it to be cracked and chapped by this drying action. Every one who uses fairly strong alkalis, as for instance, in washing powders, knows this effect by practical experience. Cheap toilet soaps, and most of the "household" varieties, contain more or less free alkali, which, though quite satisfactory for cleansing purposes, is injurious to the skin. This effect is seen, naturally, when the skin is "tender," either constitutionally, or in cold weather when it tends to be drier, or in very young or very old skins. A "superfatted" soap—a term frequently applied to good toilet soaps—contains no free alkali and is suitable for these types of skin. The skin is cleansed quite effectively, and a sufficient amount of lubricant remains to prevent damage. The use of superfatted soaps in this manner might be compared to the use of oil in anointing the body in tropical and arctic countries, to protect the skin from the extremes of hot sun and intense cold.

Friction is applied to the skin by the hands, rubber sponge, and so on, and finally by a towel. A rough bath towel should be used, as this removes the dead scales from the skin, increases its circulation, and thereby improves its health and appearance.

Even if the whole body cannot be washed daily, the feet should always be washed. The glands of the feet are always very active, even in the coldest weather, and this sweat, together with the dead scales, rapidly gives off an offensive odor if not removed. Other "active" parts are the armpits, the crotch, and the space between the buttocks; these likewise should have a daily wash whenever possible.

The question is frequently asked: "Should baths be taken during the menstrual period?—to which the answer is a very decided "yes." Cleanliness is, perhaps, even more important at this time than during the intermenstrual period. Cold baths may be left off if, by increasing the internal congestion, they cause more discomfort; otherwise they do no harm. A warm bath, however, is not only more cleansing, as has been seen, but is very helpful at these times in relieving pain and discomfort.

The hair should have frequent washing; its nature should be considered (*See also* HAIR, CARE OF), but generally speaking, once every week or two is quite long enough between shampoos. After a visit to the hairdresser, unless a shampoo is taken there, the hair should *always* be washed. It is very seldom indeed that the combs, clippers, and other instruments used by a hairdresser are cleansed, much less disinfected, after use. Not only is this a every unclean custom, but it is well known that many diseases are passed on in this way. Hairbrushes and combs should be as much one's private property as a toothbrush. They should be washed twice a week, or at least as often as the hair is washed. The hat-lining, too, should be regularly cleansed.

The nose is often neglected by otherwise clean people. It should be carefully cleansed at least once a day. This is generally done only in cases of disease, when syringing is ordered, but it is very necessary. The nose is a most useful organ, and does a great deal of dirty work in filtering the dust, soot, and germs from the air before it enters the lungs. Like other filters, it must be kept clean if it is to do its work well. The simplest method is to give it a good "blow," then clean it with a soft handkerchief dipped in warm water. This should be done gently, or the mucous membrane of the nose will be damaged. A clean nose is far more able to resist infection than a dirty one.

The eyes and ears require little special attention. Wax in the ears is a natural secretion, and usually comes out by the movement of the jaws. Its removal should never be attempted by the introduction of foreign bodies, such as hairpins. The ear is readily damaged in this way. If the wax cannot be removed, a doctor's advice should be asked before syringing the ears. The eyes should *never* be dried with another person's towel, especially if he is suffering from any disease. Many eye diseases are contracted in this way.

The teeth should be regularly and thoroughly brushed from the gums towards the teeth; and the bowels kept clean by suitable diet and regular habits. Teeth and bowels are fully dealt with elsewhere.

The underclothes should be changed as frequently as circumstances allow. None of the day clothing should be worn at night, and both day and night clothing should be thoroughly aired before further use.

The outer clothing should be cleaned from time to time: it is extraordinary how long some "clean" people will wear overcoats, suits, and so on, without cleaning them.

Persons whose skin and clothing are dirty are very attractive to lice and other parasites. (*See also* PEDICULOSIS.) On the other hand, both lice and fleas dislike cleanliness, especially if scented soap or other scent is used. Head and body lice are easily transferred from person to person by contact, or by the wearing of lice-infested clothes and hats; the latter mode of infection is common when children "change hats" at school. Cloakrooms become infected, so that from one dirty garment left there, even for a short time, lice may pass to many others. Hairbrushes and combs, when used in common, are very frequent sources of infection by headlice.

HYMEN. The hymen is a delicate membrane which partly closes the entrance to the vagina in women. The hymen is usually broken through at the first sexual intercourse, but this cannot be taken as an infallible sign that such intercourse has taken place, since in some women com-

paratively slight strain such as might arise in athletic pursuits or any other vigorous activities will cause it to rupture.

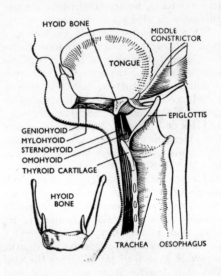

Hyoid Bone.

HYOID BONE. The hyoid bone is a U-shaped bone situated in the neck above the larynx. The important muscles of the throat and tongue are attached to it and it serves as their support.

HYOSCINE. Hyoscine, or scopolamine, is a drug which resembles atropine in its action on the nerves of the body, but it is more rapid and twice as strong. It is a powerful sleep-inducing drug and it is often used to quiet persons suffering from acute mania or delirium tremens. Hyoscine and morphia are given to achieve what is known as "twilight sleep," a state in which the memory of the pain suffered during childbirth is entirely forgotten. This condition sounds ideal, but twilight sleep requires favorable surroundings and skilled supervision and is not always free from danger. (*See also* ATROPINE; HENBANE.)

HYPERACIDITY. An excess of acidity in the gastric is medically known as hyperacidity and hyperchlorhydria. (*See also* ACIDITY; HYPERCHLORHYDRIA.)

HYPEREMIA. The excessive flow of blood to, or congestion of, a part of the body is known as hyperemia.

HYPERESTHESIA. When the skin is highly aware of the slightest touch, the condition is known as hyperesthesia. This is a common symptom in many nervous diseases, and in hysterical patients there are frequently patches of skin that are more sensitive than others. Many women suffer from oversensitiveness of the skin at the times of the menstrual periods and also at the menopause. It is often noticeable that the scalp is very sensitive, and the weight of each hair may seem to cause slight irritation. Various conditions such as influenza, anemia, and rickets may be accompanied by general or local hyperesthesia. Under the influence of small doses of drugs such as opium or alcohol, certain areas of skin may become more sensitive than others, while larger doses blunt the sensibility altogether. The condition in which the merest pin-prick feels like a violent stab is known as hyperalgesia.

HYPERCHLORHYDRIA. This term is used to describe a high acid secretion in the stomach. It is a common finding in health, but is often associated with chronic duodenal ulcer and various forms of dyspepsia. (*See also* ACIDITY; INDIGESTION.)

HYPERIDROSIS. Excessive sweating is technically known as hyperidrosis. In tuberculosis, night sweats are very common, or sweating may occur after the use of certain drugs. The parts of the body which are mostly affected are under the arms, the palms of the hands, and the feet. When excessive sweating occurs, the parts should be frequently washed and a dusting powder should be used. (*See also* SWEAT.)

HYPERMETROPIA. This is the technical term for what is more commonly known as long sight. (*See also* ACOMMODATION; ASTIGMATISM; EYE.)

HYPERPIESIA. The condition medically termed hyperpiesia is more commonly spoken of as high blood pressure, and is described under the heading BLOOD PRESSURE.

HYPERPYREXIA. When the temperature reaches 105.8 deg. F., the word hyperpyrexia is used to describe the state of excessive fever. Means should be taken to reduce the temperature by cold sponging or the application of an ice pack. Such a state is very dangerous to life and treatment should always be supervised by a doctor (*See also* FEVER.)

HYPERTENSION. This is a term often used to describe high blood-pressure.

HYPERTROPHY. This word comes to us from Greek words meaning overnourished, and the term is used to describe parts of the body which have become enlarged. It is not always an abnormal condition, but one which may occur quite normally through various means. For example, the muscles of an athlete generally become greatly enlarged as a result of strenuous exercise, and it is quite common for the right arm of a tennis player to be larger than the left, owing to hypertrophy of the muscles. In diseases of the kidneys it may be necessary to remove one of them, whereupon the other usually becomes enlarged because of the double amount of work entailed. Hypertrophy of the prostrate gland occurs in a large percentage of men over the age of sixty, and its increase in size may obstruct the outflow of urine. In the more severe cases, an operation may have to be undergone to remove the prostate gland, so as to relieve the obstruction. Hypertrophy of the muscles of the heart may cause great enlargement of that organ. This condition occurs in the hearts of athletes. (*See also* HEART.)

HYPNOTIC. Any drug which causes sleep is known as a hypnotic or soporific. It is not advisable to rush to drugs when sleeplessness occurs, as this may start a habit which is sometimes difficult to break. Very often sleeplessness is caused by indigestion, and by avoiding eating just before retiring a cure may be achieved without taking any drugs whatever. There are many ways of curing sleeplessness, which is very often caused by some trivial worry. In some cases, however, there may be actual pain which is too severe to allow the patient to sleep, and in such cases an anodyne should be given. An anodyne is a drug which relieves pain, whereas a hypnotic merely induces sleep. Of the drugs which act as true hypnotics the chief are chloral hydrate, chloralamide, bromides, the barbiturates, trional, veronal, paraldehyde, and hyoscine. The narcotic drugs morphia, opium, alcohol, etc., also act as hypnotics, but they cause a feeling of excitement first. (*See also* INSOMNIA.)

HYPNOTISM. This is a condition of sleep, artificially produced, or a trance-like state, in which the will of the person hypnotized is open to suggestions which may be made to him.

Hypnotism has been known for many hundreds of years, and a form of self-hypnotism is probably responsible for many of the extraordinary feats of endurance performed by Indians. The first physician to use hypnotism as a form of treatment was Mesmer of Vienna, who, although he undoubtedly stumbled on a valuable method of treatment, yet was scorned because he employed much ritual and apparatus which were not necessary for the real use of hypnotism. It was left to an English doctor from Manchester, Dr. Braid, about the middle of the last century, to find out the simplest way of producing the hypnotic state. He discovered that if you make a person gaze for some time at a small bright light and suggest to him that he will sleep, telling him that this will be a natural peaceful sleep, then, provided that the patient is comfortably seated, he will, within a very short time, pass into what is to all intents and purposes a restful sleep.

But this sleep differs from ordinary sleep. The patient is in a dreamy state, yet his mind is active and he will respond to any suggestions that may be made to him. For instance, if he is told, "You cannot move your hand," and then a moment later "Try to move your hands," he will be unable to do so. If his arm is stroked and he is told it has become stiff, within a moment or two the limb will actually become stiff and can be placed in any position the physician chooses. The further suggestion is then made that the limb is no longer stiff, and in a couple of minutes it ceases to be stiff. It is important that exactly what is going to happen to him should be told to the patient before the hypnotic state is produced, otherwise he may really fall asleep; he must be told that the sleep into which he will pass differs from ordinary sleep in that his mind will be very alert.

There is a popular belief that a hypotized patient is entirely under the control of the person hypnotizing him and that, for example, crimes can be committed if the physician wills the patient to commit them. Nothing could be further from the truth. No action can be suggested to a person through hypnotism which he would not carry out in his waking state. That has been absolutely proved over and over again. On the contrary, under the influence of hypnotism many people have revealed the reasons why they have felt tempted to commit certain crimes or offend the moral code in some way, and the physician has been able by suggesting that they will never think such thoughts again, to prevent what might have led to disaster. Another popular mistake about hypnotism is that a person can be hypnotized against his will. This is quite impossible, and in fact it is difficult to hypnotize anybody unless he is not only willing but anxious to be hypnotized. Once this essential fact is grasped, it will be seen that the uses of hypnotism in treatment depend to a very large extent on the cooperation of the patient. Certain disorders of the mind, especially those which result in physical symptoms, are the most satisfactory to treat by this method, but in many cases of incurable physical illness, pain can be relieved or even abolished by hypnotism. (*See also* AUTOSUGGESTION; HYSTERIA.)

HYPOCHONDRIASIS. This is a condition of misery in which the sufferer believes that there is something wrong with his health, whereas he is, as far as medical science can discover, perfectly sound in "wind and limb." Such persons make not only their own lives, but often those of their relatives and medical advisers, miserable by constant complaints about their supposed diseases. As soon as their minds are set at rest by one physician, they discover fresh symptoms, decide that their medical attendant "doesn't understand," and seek fresh advice. These unfortunate folk live in a little hell of their own making, and it is useless to assure them that they are well; in a queer way, they "enjoy bad health." The feeling of misery and depression grows so strong in these people that they may become victims of melancholia and can no longer be considered of normal mind. But the majority of those who suffer from hypochondriasis live to a good old age. (*See also* MELANCHOLIA.)

HYPODERMIC INJECTION. The method of giving drugs by injection under the skin is used because of the rapidity with which they are absorbed into the system, and also because the dosage can be judged with the greatest accuracy. Hypodermic injections are usually made into a part of the body where the skin is loose and blood-vessels are scarce. The upper part of the arm or the thigh or buttocks are the most common parts for this purpose. Great care must be taken to see that the syringe and needle are strictly sterilized, and that the surface of the skin has been cleansed with tincture of iodine, alcohol or ether before the injection is given. (*See also* INJECTION.)

HYPOGASTRIUM. For convenience of description it is usual to divide the abdomen into regions. The hypogastrium or hypogastric region is the lowest part of the abdomen, lying in the middle line below the umbilicus and above the genitals. It contains coils of small intestine and the beginning of the rectum. When distended, the bladder may protrude into the hypogastrium, as may the womb in pregnancy.

HYPOGLOSSAL NERVE. The hypoglossal nerves or twelfth cranial nerves are the nerves which work the muscles of the tongue. There are two of them and each serves one side of the tongue. They lie underneath the tongue, as their name signifies, and each is connected with one-half of the tongue, so that it is quite usual for one side of the tongue only to be paralyzed and the other to escape. When the whole tongue is paralyzed, the damage must be in the region where both nerves take their origin.

HYSTERECTOMY. This is the name of the operation for the removal of the womb, which is done for various conditions, such as prolonged bleeding from the womb, fibroid tumors, and cancer. (*See also* FIBROIDS; WOMB.)

HYSTERIA. This is a disease, mainly of young, physically healthy women, in which there is a lack of control over acts and feelings, often accompanied by certain bodily complaints. It is important to insist that although the disease exists only in the mind of the person affected by hysteria and although various extraordinary bodily illnesses may be imitated, yet to the sufferer those illnesses and symptoms are very real; she is no malingerer. This point cannot be too strongly insisted upon, because to treat a person suffering from hysteria as a malingerer, and to tell her to "pull

herself together," is not only useless but harmful. The patient has no inkling of the nature of her trouble, and it is only by very careful and wise treatment by a doctor who has had special experience in dealing with hysteria that such patients can be permanently cured. The exact nature of the changes in the mind which underlie the development of the symptoms of hysteria are not yet perfectly understood, but much has been learned about the condition from the work of Freud. According to his view of hysteria, the victims of it have at some time or another in their lives suffered from some painful mental experience, which through its unpleasant nature has become forgotten by the patient, but is still stored up, buried in the unconscious mind. The natural end of such painful mental experiences is a gradual dimming of their effects by time; but if, for any reason, the impressions are not so dimmed, the memory is apt to be only buried and not destroyed. Then, given certain circumstances, in which life is difficult or not running smoothly, these memories unconsciously influence the feelings and activities of the patient. These unconscious memories often have a sexual character and may date from early childhood. ("Sexual" is here used in the broad sense as spoken of by those who deal with disorders of the mind, not in the popular, physical sense.) As a result, the mental trouble is translated into, or converted into, the symptoms of hysteria. These may be either mental or physical. The physical ones are so striking that they nearly always call attention to themselves. Sudden loss of power in one or more limbs is a very common symptom of hysteria. The patient is apparently quite helpless to walk or feed herself. Yet the most careful examination fails to reveal any signs of disease of the structures of the nervous or muscular systems which could possibly account for such a complete paralysis. The limbs may also be held stiffly and the patient declares she is quite unable to relax them, but under an anesthetic, for example, such limbs are freely relaxed.

All symptoms of hysteria are dramatic; they ensure that attention shall be paid to the sufferer. And there is always something to be gained from the presence of a physical symptom: the unconscious memories may choose to disguise themselves as physical symptoms, but once these show themselves the patient appears perfectly happy. It might be expected that a person who had to lie in bed all day because she was unable to walk would be depressed, to say the least; not so the victim of hysteria. She has gained her object in two ways and is therefore happy; her unconscious emotional difficulties have translated themselves into something which the world can see and sympathize with, and she cannot be expected to face the battle and realities of life while she is physically incapacitated. It must be repeated that this knowledge is not possessed consciously by the hysteric. The main problem of the treatment of hysteria is to get the patients to understand how their paralysis or loss of voice (another very common symptom) has come about. It is of little use to cure the symptom by suggesting that it will get well—the underlying cause for the symptom must be threshed out with the patient. After the symptoms of paralysis have been removed by suggestion, as they can easily be by anyone with sufficient influence over the patient, fresh symptoms occur, either physical or mental, depending upon the particular type of patient. A most distressing, as well as a most difficult symptom to prove to be truly hysterical, is the fit or convulsion. These convulsions mimic those of epilepsy very closely, and no one except a doctor should attempt to distinguish between the two types of fit. The patient may cry out or roll her eyes about and then jerking of the arms and hands and legs begins. This may go on for a minute or several minutes and then the patient slides to the ground—she never falls so that she hurts herself; if she falls directly, she will find a soft place to fall on. This is characteristic of the hysteric, she never hurts herself. The most peculiar positions may be adopted; the movements of the arms and legs get more and more violent, and the patient may foam at the mouth, scream, or sob. She is never really unconscious, although she will not answer when spoken to and will deny all knowledge of what has happened during the fit. But these fits never occur when the patient is alone, or when she is in any position of danger, as do true epileptic fits. They always cease on admission to hospital if curtains are placed round the bed so that there is no audience.

One of the most puzzling of all the physical symptoms of hysteria is the loss of feeling to pain, which is often found in this condition. The loss of feeling is either on one side of the body, and on the corresponding arm and leg or it is found on both arms and hands, usually to the level of the elbows. The extraordinary thing about this loss of feeling is that a patient who suffers from it will allow a large pin to be stuck right through her arm, and even to be left sticking in, while she declares she feels nothing at all. But the most amazing feature of this loss of feeling is that it can be produced at any place on the patient's body by suggesting that she will not feel any pain if a pin is inserted in her flesh at a certain spot. And it can also be removed by suggesting that feeling has returned to that spot after a certain amount of stroking or patting, or whatever aid to his suggestion the doctor cares to use.

"Suggestibility" is one of the main features of hysteria. If it be suggested to a hysteric with sufficient confidence that she will be able to do a thing (as for example, that she will walk, although she may have been lying in bed for months), it is possible to get her to do it, but the underlying cause of the symptom remains and will find fresh expression in new symptoms whenever there is something in life she unconsciously wishes to avoid. The mental symptoms of hysteria are very numerous, but there is rather a characteristic nature associated with hysteria. The patient with hysteria is emotionally "up and down;" her moods change rapidly she takes unreasonable likes and dislikes; she is either very depressed, or "up in the clouds." But her chief characteristic is a craving for sympathy. Before so much was known about the mental side of hysteria, it was treated mainly by "wholesome neglect," that is, no sympathy was shown to the unfortunate sufferers, they were scorned and told: "Not to be foolish." Nowadays the treatment is a mental treatment which goes to the root of the trouble and frees the patients from their mental "bogies."

Hysteria may imitate in its symptoms almost any physical disease, and before the diagnosis of hysteria is even thought of, the most careful examinations are necessary to prove that no disease which can be responsible for the physical symptoms of the patient is present. There is one nervous disorder which occurs in young people with which hysteria is often confused, because this disorder can, and often does, cause loss of power in one or other limb for a short time. This disorder is disseminated sclerosis, and it is specially important to avoid such a mistake.

If by unwise treatment of a physical symptom in hysteria this symptom has been cured and no attempt has been made to deal with the underlying mental problems, it is likely that these will find an outlet in some other hysterical symptom. These are extremely varied in nature, but they all realize the same end, namely, an escape from reality. One such symptom is loss of memory. The patient may be aware that she lost herself at such and such a place and at a certain time. She may find herself at a wholly different place and be quite unaware of how she got from one place to the other. In these states the patient may wander for miles and carry on perfectly sensible conversations with others without revealing anything wrong with her. The "second personality" may be quite able to carry on the patient's affairs for a while without anything amiss being noticed.

It is interesting that this form of "escape" from reality which results in these failures of memory with the development of a "second personality" capable of carrying on a patient's affairs is much more common in men who suffer from hysteria than in women. It must not be thought that hysteria is only seen in women: it may be present in men, especially in those who have a family history of nervous or mental trouble, and it may also occur in children, in whom isolation in a hospital ward is almost essential for cure. In adults, the frank discussion of their mental troubles with a doctor almost invariably reveals the underlying cause of the hysterical symptoms and should result in

cure. (*See also* DISSEMINATED SCLEROSIS; PSYCHOLOGY.)

HYSTERICAL or SELF-PRODUCED DERMATITIS. This occurs in two classes of persons: malingerers, who are generally men, and hysterical patients, who are often girls in their teens or early twenties.

The first group are either incorrigibly "work-shy" or are trying to get compensation fraudulently. They more often try to increase or at least prevent the cure of a skin disease that already exists, than to create a new one. Such cases are often very puzzling at first sight; but a medical man is soon rendered suspicious by a dermatitis which persists in spite of suitable remedies, and shows features strange to the disease.

The patients comprising the second group, which is by far the larger, are a most interesting type. In many cases they appear to be normal in every way; not specially excitable, far less showing the signs commonly spoken of as "hysterical." They are hardworking in good general condition, and with plenty of healthy interests suited to their age. Indeed, in very many cases the patient appears to be an exemplary type; she can produce a character reference from her parents, teachers, or pastor which is unassailable.

The injuries produced on the skin are generally recognized by a trained person as being artificial. They do not resemble any known disease of the skin; they are always made on parts of the body within reach of the right hand (or left, if the patient is left-handed), and very, very rarely are seen on the face. They end abruptly in normal skin, instead of fading away into it.

Treatment. The treatment of these cases is, whenever possible, to send the patient to a hospital or nursing home. When the material cause has been discovered, an attempt should be made to bring to light the underlying mental conflict, otherwise the patient will find an outlet in some other symptom.

ICE AND ICEBAG. Ice and refrigeration are used as a means of keeping foodstuffs fresh. Apart from the importance of fresh food, ice is very useful in the treatment of various diseases. In cases of fever it is sometimes necessary to give cold applications, and these can be carried out most conveniently by placing chopped ice in what is known as an *icebag*. The bag is made of rubber and is closed by a screw cap. As a rule a piece of flannel is placed between the bag and the skin. When there is any internal bleeding from the stomach or throat, or in case of inflammation of the throat or mouth, small pieces of ice should be given to the patient to suck. This keeps the mouth fresh and moist and may help to relieve vomiting. Severe headache and delirium are often relieved by placing an icebag over the forehead. Pain is usualy relieved in the abdomen or elsewhere by a cold application, and in cases where the patient is unable to bear the weight of an icebag on the body, the bag should be suspended from a bed cradle. (*See also* HEMORRHAGE.)

ICHTHYOSIS. Ichthyosis, meaning fish disease, is so called because those suffering from it have a dry scaly skin somewhat resembling that of a fish. All varieties may be seen (the mildest fortunately being the commonest), from a mere dryness of the skin to cases where the patient is covered with "large horny masses, and the skin resembles rather that of a reptile."

Treatment. The treatment consists in supplying to the skin the fat which it so sadly lacks; the patient should take a daily bath, and afterwards grease himself thoroughly with lanolin, almond oil, etc. A diet rich in fats is also recommended.

ICTERUS. The word icterus is just another name for jaundice, the yellow coloring of the skin and "whites" of the eye caused by the presence of bile in the blood. Icterus neonatorum is a form of jaundice found in newly born babies. It usually wears away in a few days, but if it does not do so it may be due to the Rhesus factor, congenital syphilis, or infection entering the blood stream through the umbilical cord. (*See also* JAUNDICE.)

IDIOCY. This is a condition of imperfect development of the brain which exists from birth, and which is so marked that the sufferers therefrom are unable to protect themselves from the common dangers of life. As long as they live they have to be looked after and protected like young children. Fortunately, idiots rarely live to a very old age, and the more severe types die before they reach adult age. It is sometimes asked how an idiot can be distinguished from a child who is merely "backward." Apart from the fact that idiots are usually badly formed physically, it may be said that while a backward child is merely younger in mind than the normal child of the same age, the idiot would be abnormal in mind at any age. But idiots show by their vacant expressions, the way their heads roll about and their entire lack of sensible speech, that they will never be capable of normal life. Many of them show queer movements of the arms and legs, which they repeat over and over again, or they may make extraordinary noises, which may be interpreted as attempts to talk. It is difficult to train such beings to be clean in their habits, and this is one of the great trials in dealing with these unfortunates. There are many different types of idiocy, of which only two need special mention here. One is the Mongolian type, so called because they have slanting "almond-eyes" like a Chinese. The children with this form of idiocy are often the last of a large family. These children differ from the ordinary idiots in being trainable to a certain extent. They are very fond of music, and will beat time to a rhythm and can be taught to play the simpler musical instruments. They are also very quick to imitate any actions they see, and therefore do well in institutions where they can copy those whose sole duties are to train them to make the best of their limited brain power. Mongolian idiots do not often reach adult life because they are very liable to chest troubles and have little power of resistance.

The other form of idiocy is of great interest, because it is the one form which, if taken in time, is capable of complete cure. This form is cretinism, and is now known to be due to a deficient thyroid gland. The children who suffer from cretinism are dwarfs, and enormously fat. Their arms and legs are short and the skin is dry and thick. They have very little hair, and walk in a clumsy, waddling fashion. Speech consists of a few words, spoken in a squeaky harsh voice. The effect of giving these children the correct treatment, which is large doses of thyroid gland by mouth, is often little short of miraculous. They lose their fatness in a remarkable short time; they grow quickly and cease to have a dwarf-like appearance, and their mental state improves, though the amount of improvement can never be predicted in any particular case. In some cases the mental state becomes almost normal; this applies particularly to those cases in which the condition has been recognized and treated at an early age. In others, the brain power never develops above that of a feeble-minded child. (*See also* CRETINISM; MENTAL DEFICIENCY; THYROID GLAND.)

IDIOPATHIC. Idiopathic is a word used in medicine to mean a disease or symptom for which no cause is known.

IDIOSYNCRASY. By idiosyncrasies we mean individual peculiarities of constitution or temperament. Some people are more or less violently upset by contact with ordinary substances which do no harm to the majority of their fellow human beings. For instance, milk or eggs act as a poison to some people, bringing on one of the diseases which are now known as *allergic* diseases—i.e., hay fever, asthma, migraine, urticaria (nettle-rash), etc. These people are said to have an idiosyncrasy for the substance which harms them. It is very common for patients to have an idiosyncrasy in connection with some particular drug, as for instance, a violent headache may follow the taking of quinine, etc. (*See also* ALLERGY; ANAPHYLAXIS.)

ILEO-CECAL VALVE. The last part of the small intestine before it joins on to the large intestine (colon) is called the *ileum*. The cul-de-sac of intestine called the caecum joins on at this point, and the ileum acts as a valve at the entrance to the caecum in that it allows the contents of the small intestine to flow in one direction—i.e., into the caecum only. This is called the ileocaecal valve.

ILEUM. This is the name given to the lowest part of the small intestine or bowel. (*See also* INTESTINE.)

ILIAC REGION. The abdomen is spoken of as if it were divided up into compartments to simplify descriptions of symptoms, etc. The two iliac regions are the two lowest parts of the abdomen on the right and left and are so called be-

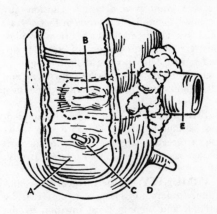

Ileo-Caecal Valve: A. *Caecum;* B. *Valve;* C. *Opening into Appendix;* D. *Appendix;* E. *Ileum.*

cause they lie in front of the *iliac bones.* These iliac bones form the two wing-like crests at the sides of the haunch bones. The caecum and the appendix lie in the right *iliac fossa,* and pain is felt there when they are inflamed. Pain in the iliac fossae in women is often due to some derangement of the female reproductive system. (*See also* ABDOMEN; GROIN.)

ILIUM. The ilium is the haunchbone. It is also called the innominate bone and is described fully under the heading INNOMINATE.

ILLEGITIMACY. It is a very noticeable thing that the death and sickness rate is far greater among illegitimate children than among the children of married parents. People have tried to attribute this to all sorts of reasons such as inherent weakness at birth and so forth, but the fact remains that the illegitimate child is exactly the same as the ordinary child, but lacks care and attention in many cases.

ILLUSION. Illusions, hallucinations, and delusions are all states in which a person misinterprets facts, and believes in his misinterpretation. The three misinterpretations differ in form. Take the case of ghosts. To see a man crossing the garden path in the twilight and mistake him for a ghost is an *illusion*. To think you see a man crossing the path when there is no one there is a *hallucination*. To see a man crossing the path and *believe* that he is a ghost is a *delusion*. Illusions are harmless mentally. They are in fact merely mistakes. Hallucinations are often harmless but are sometimes signs of mental disorder, and delusions are definitely signs of mental abnormality. HALLUCINATIONS and DELUSIONS are described under their own headings.

IMBECILITY. A form of feeblemindedness similar to idiocy, but as a rule showing a greater degree of intelligence, is known as imbecility. (*See also* IDIOCY; MIND.)

IMMUNITY. In the medical sense, immunity refers to the power possessed by animals and men to resist invasion by the germs of disease.

The normal blood contains substances which are hostile to germ life and so tend to protect against disease. Everyone knows that certain people when exposed to infection do not contract the disease. This is due to those protective qualities which constitute "natural" immunity. It is also well known that one attack of an infectious disease often protects against another attack of the same disease. In such cases, an "acquired" immunity has developed. This response on the part of the blood can be artificially produced and used to prevent possible infection. In the case of "vaccination," a mild attack of smallpox is induced and the protective powers of the blood are so stimulated that immunity to smallpox is obtained. Such an acquired immunity is not permanent, hence the need for revaccination. Vaccine treatment is the injection of dead germs with the object of increasing the resistive powers.

In the body, germs produce their harmful effects by manufacturing poisons (toxins), but the blood counteracts this by producing an antidote or antibody. It is the formation of such substances which enables a person to recover from an attack of a certain disease, and it is their persistence in the blood in some quantity which gives immunity against further attacks of the same disease. It is possible to produce antipoisons, or, as they are called, antitoxins, for diseases such as diphtheria and lockjaw and, by injecting the antitoxins into the blood of a sufferer, the disease is greatly diminished in severity. This is termed *passive* immunization as opposed to the *active* immunization of vaccine treatment. It is also possible to produce active immunity against bacterial poisons by graded injections of a suitably modified toxin.

IMMUNIZATION. With improvements in social conditions and in the general hygiene of the community many infectious diseases which were formerly common are now rare, such as typhoid fever, diphtheria, and smallpox; but when they do occur sporadically they are usually very severe and not infrequently fatal. The sulphonamides and antibiotics have changed the outlook in the treatment of many infections, though they have had little or no effect upon virus infections. Nevertheless, all mothers (and fathers as well) should be impressed with the importance of having their children immunized against poliomyelitis, whooping cough, diphtheria, tetanus, and smallpox; and expectant mothers should themselves be immunized against poliomyelitis. A combined whooping cough, diphtheria, and tetanus vaccine should be given when the child is aged 2 to 6 months, and smallpox vaccination done during the first two years of life but preferably at the age of 4 or 5 months. It is probable that poliomyelitis vaccine will in the near future be carried out by giving the Sabin (dead virus) vaccine by mouth at 4- to 6-week intervals; but at present the Salk (attenuated living virus) vaccine is being given by injection at the following intervals—first injection at age 7 to 10 months, then one month between the first and second injections, then six months between the second and third injections, and a fourth injection at school entry.

Immunization may also be carried out, when indicated, against typhoid and paratyphoid fevers, cholera, yellow fever, plague, and tuberculosis.

IMPETIGO. Impetigo is a common and infectious skin disease, in which pustules (festering spots) appear on the face and scalp and sometimes on the other parts of the body. It is extremely catching and may run rapidly through a family or school. It is most common in children and young adults, and is chiefly found in dirty, neglected children, though no class of people, however clean, are exempt from it. It very frequently accompanies lice on the head or body, and is probably carried by them from child to child. A running ear has often been noted before the appearance of impetigo, and in this case it is probably the same germ that causes the two conditions.

Symptoms. Little red patches appear first on the skin of the face or head, and turn into watery blisters. The fluid in these blisters turns yellowish and they break, leaving yellowish scabs, surrounded by a reddish ring. As these rings may run into each other and cover large tracts of the face, the condition can be most unsightly, but fortunately the scabs do not leave permanent scars. On the scalp the disease spreads even more quickly than on the face, and as the hair is all mixed up with it the picture is soon a horrible one. The blisters burst and discharge thick, sticky, and foul-smelling pus into which the hair is matted and bound down by the crusts.

Treatment. Impetigo is a very simple disease to treat, but the most important thing is to get treatment started quickly. Washing and shaving, or hair combing or brushing must be forbidden, as the infection is so rapidly spread by these means. The only thing that can be done is to facilitate the drying up of the crusts, which is best done by the use of a good drying powder, or a lead and spirit lotion. Powders that can be used are boracic, zinc, or talcum. A preparation that combines both the lotion and powder treatment and is easy to use is a thick calamine lotion. Paint on and leave to dry, renewing at intervals. See that the child does not pick the scabs, but that they are allowed to drop off when they are ready.

Impetigo on the Scalp. Impetigo on the head is much more difficult to deal with. If the condition is very bad it may be necessary to cut off the hair in the case of a girl. If, however, there are only a few spots widely separated this will not be necessary. It will be sufficient to clip the hair short in the region of the spots. Powders and calamine lotions are not suitable for the head, so a spirit lotion must be used; one with mercury being the best. When the crusts are dry on both the face or the head they can be softened by the use of a mercury ointment and this will make them ready to come off sooner. (*See also* DERMATITIS.)

IMPOTENCE. In the medical sense, this is used to denote lack of sexual power in the male. It is to be distinguished from sterility and lack of desire. Impotence means that a man, though he may desire sexual intercourse, is unable to carry out or complete the sexual act. There are many causes for this condition, some permanent, others temporary, the most common being psychological. Any exhausting illness such as chronic kidney disease or diabetes, chronic nervous diseases, and the excessive use of alcohol or drugs such as morphia will tend to produce impotence.

Deformity of the sex organs, either inherited or from disease, is liable to prevent complete sexual gratification; while excessive intellectual work may cause a temporary loss of power. Sexual overindulgence leading to exhaustion is a common cause of impotence, but the commonest cause is a psychological one, a mental conflict often due to subconscious guilt feelings related to masturbation in early life.

Treatment naturally depends upon the cause. Impotence from physical or mental exhaustion will quickly disappear under the influence of rest and tonic medicines. Alcohol must be avoided and tobacco cut down to a minimum. Psychological impotence will be benefited by a period of abstinence from all attempts at sexual intercourse, and by leading a vigorous, out-of-door life, with the mind fully occupied with useful work and recreation. If such measures fail, it will be necessary to consult the doctor. Only in a few cases will aphrodisiac (sex-stimulating) drugs be necessary, and these should be taken strictly under medical advice only. Most of the alleged remedies on the open market are useless, and some are harmful. (*See also* SEX HYGIENE.)

INCISION. This is a term which is used in surgery. It is applied to a cut or a wound.

INCISOR. The four front teeth of each jaw are called the incisors. (*See also* TEETH.)

INCONTINENCE. This describes the inability to control the passage of urine from the bladder, or feces from the rectum (back passage). It is sometimes used to denote sexual intercourse outside marriage (the opposite of continence). Very young children, up to about twelve months, cannot control the bladder and rectum at will, but gradually from that time a voluntary control is established. In children and some nervous adults, a sudden fright or shock may induce the urine to be passed involuntarily, and in certain diseased states, notably those affecting the spinal cord, these symptoms may arise. The passing of urine is a reflex controlled by the mind and is dependent upon the healthy state of the nervous system. In tabes forsulin, the spinal cord is diseased and the reflex may be lost. In consequence, the bladder gets distended and overflows, this being known as "overflow incontinence." In some spinal injuries, the bladder empties itself automatically—"reflex incontinence," while in some cases the bladder will not retain any urine, but allows it to flow away immediately—"dribbling incontinence."

Incontinence of feces may occasionally occur in nervous children under strain, but in adults it may arise as a result of injury or disease of the brain or spinal cord or as a sequence to injuries or operations on the rectum. This symptom may also arise during the unconsciousness (coma) which often accompanies severe diseases and is common in mental disorders and senility. (*See also* BEDWETTING; BLADDER, DISEASE OF; DIARRHEA; ENURESIS.)

INCUBATION. The incubation period of any disease is the time which passes between the infection and the first appearance of symptoms. In most of the infectious diseases this period remains fairly constant in each case; for example, in measles the incubation is generally around 14 days; while in diphtheria, about 2 days is the usual time. It is important to know the various periods of incubation, as a watchful eye can be kept on any suspected person during this time and further spread of the disease may be avoided. The average incubation periods of the more important infectious diseases are as follows:

Disease	Incubation Period
Chicken pox	10–16 days
Diphtheria	2–4 "
Erysipelas	1–3 "
German Measles	14–17 "
Influenza	1–5 "
Measles	10–14 "
Mumps	18–21 "
Scarlet Fever	2–3 "
Smallpox	12–14 "
Typhoid	10–21 "
Whooping Cough	10–14 "

INCUBATOR. An apparatus used for the artificial hatching of eggs is known as an incubator. Prematurely born or very delicate babies are sometimes reared in an incubator in which the temperature is regulated to maintain the desired level. Incubators are also used in laboratories for the growth of germs or bacteria.

INDIGESTION. This condition may be defined as one in which discomfort, distress, or pain is felt in the abdomen (belly) during or after a meal. It is also referred to as dyspepsia and it is distinguished as the commonest of all the ailments of civilization. Most commonly indigestion is associated with actual disorder of the stomach or bowels, but dyspeptic symptoms may arise during the course of many other diseases.

Causes. Overworking of the digestive organs is one of the most frequent sources of indigestion. Large and elaborate meals, if habitually eaten, tire the stomach. Constipation is inevitably associated with indigestion, and this further induces mechanical changes which handicap the whole digestive apparatus.

Food is often eaten too hastily, with the result that it is imperfectly chewed and mixed with saliva, so that additional work is thus thrown upon the stomach. Upsetting the natural rhythm of the stomach by taking meals at irregular times is harmful to good digestion as is also the bad habit of eating between meals. The stomach requires rest pauses just like the other vital organs. Also, eating between meals spoils the appetite and without the stimulus of appetite a meal is poorly digested and assimilated. Tea or coffee, when too strong and when taken to excess, have an astringent and irritating effect upon the lining of the stomach, diminishing the flow of juice and causing digestive trouble. Abuse of alcoholic liquids acts in the same way. Any sepsis (or poisoning) arising from the gums, teeth, tonsils, or nose is apt to cause indigestion owing to the constant swallowing of poisonous matter. Worry and anxiety, by preventing the free flow of the stomach juice, readily lead to dyspepsia.

Indigestion is more accurately to be described as a symptom and not a disease, and each requires careful investigation to determine what is causing it, and the precise nature of the disorder. One type of indigestion is associated with a functional disturbance of the stomach, i.e. there is some breakdown in the digestive mechanism without any structural defects. Too much acid or too little acid may be secreted by the stomach glands (hyperchlorhydria and hypochlorhydria.)

Another type is associated with actual disease of the stomach or duodenum, such as dilation, inflammation (gastritis), and ulceration and cancer. Severe pain immediately on taking food, along with sickness and nausea and tenderness over the stomach region, is very suggestive of stomach ulcer. Pain coming on an hour or two after a meal—often with a feeling of hunger, and therefore called "hunger pain" —is generally indicative of a duodenal ulcer.

Indigestion may also arise in connection with liver, gall bladder, heart, kidney, appendix, and lung disease. The diagnosis in this type is often difficult, as is also the case where mental causes, neurasthenia, and hysteria are the underlying factors.

Prevention. Eat such foods which will prevent constipation, i.e. those containing vitamins, mineral salts, and roughage. Do not worry or attempt any serious mental work at the table. Eat slowly, masticating the food thoroughly, and do not wash it down with mouthfuls of water. Be sparing with all condiments. Never take undiluted alcohol on an empty stomach. Be moderate with smoking, otherwise the appetite may be affected. Be careful with the hygiene of your mouth and throat. If in doubt, consult the doctor. Treat your stomach to an occasional fast. This last piece of advice is probably the most valuable of all. (*See also* APPETITE; HUNGER.)

INDUSTRIAL HYGIENE. A tired or sick worker will not do as good work, or as much work, in a given time as a fresh and fit one. This applies to the mind as well as the body. The best work is done by contented and happy people. A good deal of attention is now being given, therefore, to the problem of fitting the worker to his work, keeping him happy while there, and looking after his bodily fitness. Certain conditions must be fulfilled by the employers of labor in factories; factories are made as safe as possible for those who work with machinery, and a sufficient supply of fresh air is provided by ventilation.

First-aid boxes are installed, and often nurses are in attendance. Lighting is adapted to the work that is to be done. It is not always possible to ensure that the temperature of the room is comfortable, as many industries require heat and a few are carried on at low temperatures. The whole business of making conditions of work such that the best physical and mental results will be got from the workers is fast becoming a special science under the name of Industrial Hygiene. (*See also* HYGIENE.)

INFANT MORTALITY. The infant death rate is calculated as the number of infants per 1,000 registered births who die in the first year of life.

It can be seen from contemporary documents that in earlier times the infant death rate was frightfully high. One noble family, the Colets, in the 16th century records the birth of 23 children, 22 of whom died in infancy or early childhood. It is certain that if the wealthy suffered to such an extent, other classes would not escape. Even in the 19th century it was not uncommon in the poorer classes for the birth and death of an infant to be registered at the same time. Since then, however, the infant death rate has steadily declined.

Even in the best circumstances, some loss of infant lives is unavoidable, and so far we cannot calculate this loss. Avoidable general causes, however, are now well known to any thinking person. The chief are ignorance; carelessness; poverty; dirt; bad feeding; sanitation and air; infectious diseases; and lack of skilled care before and at confinement. The industrial employment of women before confinement does not increase the infant death rate (as was seen during the war).

The chief special causes of infant mortality are debility, wasting, congenital defects, prematurity, diarrhea, convulsions, accidents (including overlaying), bronchitis, and pneumonia. Seventy per cent of infant deaths are due to the above; 29 per cent are due to prematurity and congenital defects, and occur during the first four weeks of life.

INFANTILE CONVULSIONS. Convulsions in infants, that is, in children under the age of 2 years, must be looked upon in quite a different light from convulsions or fits in adults. They may not mean very much, or they may be of serious importance, and in any case they require the advice of a doctor. Many fevers in children, such as whooping cough or measles, may begin with a convulsion, or they may be due to such minor ailments as teething, overfeeding, indigestion, constipation, or intestinal worms. On the other hand, convulsions may be a symptom of rickets or of some serious nervous disorder. These convulsions are generally caused by some weakness of the nerve cells which in the case of epilepsy is often inherited. In cases where the system becomes poisoned, for example, in diseases of the kidney, convulsions may follow as a result of the poisoning.

Excessive or unsuitable diet, such as a highly indigestible meal of coconut or unripe fruit, may induce convulsions in a healthy child, but it should be remembered that convulsions, apart from those caused by serious brain or other disease, are rarely due to irritation alone, and even when they appear to be so, there is often an additional factor in the shape of nervous excitability, either hereditary or acquired as a result of lowered health. Other common causes of irritation are an adherent foreskin or obstruction to the airway by tonsils and adenoids.

Asphyxia or severe hemorrhage may cause such a loss of oxygen in the body that the nerve cells become weakened, and the result is seen in convulsions.

Symptoms. Typical convulsions begin with a dazed look, followed immediately by momentary pallor and dilation of the pupils of the eyes. The head falls forward, or the child sinks to the ground and becomes unconscious. Breathing is irregular; there is frothing at the mouth, and the contents of the bladder and bowel may be passed. The attack may be over in a few seconds, or last for hours with intermissions. They are nearly always followed by a period of more or less profound sleep.

"Premonitory" symptoms are rather rare; the so-called "inward convulsion" in which the infant moans, draws up its legs, distorts its face and clenches its fists is merely a sign of colic.

In early infancy frequent attacks of petit mal (minor epilepsy) consisting of momentary pallor, dilatation of the pupils, drooping of the head and loss of consciousness, suggest "fainting" or heart disease rather than epilepsy. There is no difference between the symptoms of infantile convulsions and epilepsy.

The outlook, as far as life is concerned, is usually good. Convulsions themselves are rarely fatal. With regard to recurrences, if there is an obvious cause, such as gross overfeeding or intestinal inflammation, the probability is that the fits will cease if these causes are attended to. Where there is no real cause, e.g., all that can be found is a tooth which has or has not cut through the gum when expected, the fits may recur on very slight provocation.

Permanent mental impairment, resulting from convulsions alone, is rare. If mental deficiency exists, it is probably the cause of the convulsions.

It is usually estimated that 10 per cent of infants who suffer from convulsions become epileptics in later life. There is some ground for the popular belief that children may "grow out of fits," for it is a fact that epilepsy may become latent. In 34 out of 237 cases, there were intervals of from 2 to 30 years between seizures.

Treatment. As the most common cause is improper feeding, a grain of calomel or a teaspoonful of castor oil should be given. Hot baths, so frequently advised, are of little use, but may be soothing and relieve colic when present. Ice should be applied to the head if the temperature is raised above the normal. Rectal injections of chloral are sometimes advised by the doctor; but such drugs are, of course, only given under medical advice.

Children who suffer from fits only in consequence of emotional excitement or physical fatigue should be treated by careful attention to their mode of upbringing, education, and environment. Bromides used to be given, for two or three months, but it is not much employed in medicine nowadays. Phenobarbitone (also called Luminal, a proprietary name) is much more useful in controlling a convulsion which is not due to obvious overfeeding, etc. It can be given by itself as a powder, or in solution as the sodium salt. It does not produce any skin rash or spots, and does not tend to dull the mentality to the same extent that the bromides did. This drug must never be discontinued suddenly after prolonged administration, as there is the possibility of a series of fits. (*See also* SUPPLEMENT ON FIRST AID.)

INFANTILE DIARRHEA. This is a serious type of diarrhea which affects young infants and which may leave them very pinched and ill. It is a curious fact that this condition almost always breaks out in epidemic form when the earth temperature reaches 56 deg. F. Flies play a very important part in carrying the germs of the disease, and particular care should be taken to see that the milk of bottle-fed babies is stored in a cool and safe place. The condition is discussed fully under the heading DIARRHEA.

INFANTILE PARALYSIS (Acute Anterior Poliomyelitis). This is an acute infection of the spinal cord by a virus which may cause destruction, or partial destruction, of those parts which control the power of movement. The name of "infantile paralysis" is an unfortunate one, as the majority of polio cases make a complete recovery. The disease most commonly attacks children between 1 and 3 years of age and occurs usually in August and September. It is spread by "carriers," that is to say, people who have the germ probably in their noses and throats (though this is not quite certain), although perfectly healthy themselves, are able to infect other people. It may occur in epidemics or in isolated cases, and it is interesting to note that when it occurs in epidemics the disease takes a much milder form, and may be thought to be merely a feverish cold.

The child should be isolated for 14 days after exposure to infection.

Symptoms. The illness always comes on suddenly, after an incubation period of 4–7 days, with a slight feverish attack and vomiting and perhaps stiffness of the neck. A few hours, or perhaps a few days later it is discovered that the child is unable to move one of its limbs. As a rule the onset is so slight that the mother does not think it necessary to send for the doctor until a few days later when she suddenly realizes that the child cannot move an arm or a leg. There may or may not be pain on trying to move the limb.

Infantile paralysis is sometimes confused with acute rheumatism, but an examination of the fluid from the spinal column during the acute stages will practically always reveal the true nature of the disease.

Whether the patient will recover or not depends upon what part of the spinal cord has been damaged and to what extent. The number of paralyzed cases varies greatly in each epidemic, but about one in every ten cases dies; of the remaining nine children, three or four may be left crippled to some extent. In those cases where the onset is more sudden, the recovery is usually more complete.

It is very difficult at the beginning of the illness to give any idea as to whether the affected limb will recover or will go on growing or remain permanently shortened.

Treatment. During the acute stage the child is kept in bed, lying still, as any movement of the child or the limb may make the condition much worse. The well-known Sabin and Salk vaccines are preventive, not curative.

The affected limb should be supported comfortably, in order to prevent deformity such as wrist-drop or foot-drop occurring, and as soon as the pain has eased off it should be put in splints and a cradle should be rigged up over the limb to take the weight of the bed-clothes.

In cases where the muscles used in breathing are affected, special apparatus (known popularly as an "iron lung") has been devised. This carries on artificial respiration in the hope that the paralysis will lessen or disappear and the chest muscles recover. Tracheotomy may be necessary.

The methods of treatment advocated by Sister Kenny, of Australia, in 1937, consisting of frequent hot packs for the relief of pain and spasm, and re-education movements at an earlier stage than had been usual, are still a subject of controversy among doctors.

The nursing in these cases is of the utmost importance. The bowels should be kept freely open with mild aperients such as milk of magnesia or syrup of figs and the child should be kept on milk diet with a large amount of fluid such as water, lemonade, and barley water. Sedatives may be necessary. When the acute stage has subsided and there is no more pain, usually three or four weeks from the beginning of the illness, the limb should be gently massaged to keep up the tone of the muscles, thus increasing the chance of recovery of the power of movement.

Later on light, noninflammable celluloid splints can be applied to the limb to keep it in good position, but these must be frequently removed so that the massage and electrical treatment can be continued. Operative treatment may be necessary in the later stages from time to time to divide the contracted tissues and correct deformity in the limb. At all times during the illness the limb should be kept extra warmly covered. (*See also* IMMUNIZATION.)

INFANTILISM. This is an abnormality of development which results in a failure to grow up. The individual bears into adult life many of the physical and mental characteristics of a child. In the category of infantilism, mental defectives are generally excluded, and the term is limited to certain fairly clear-cut types with definite causes. One of the commonest varieties is that which results from defects in the working of the thyroid gland situated in the neck. In extreme cases of thyroid deficiency, the child is stunted in mind and body and is called a "cretin." Lesser degrees of deficiency occur, the child showing various infantile characteristics of mind and body, and such persons have been aptly described as "pocket editions of humanity." If an extract of thyroid is given to such children as soon as the defect is discovered, a remarkable improvement takes place.

Intestinal or pancreatic infantilism arises from a deficiency of the pancreatic gland, with the result that nutrition is seriously interfered with and growth is impeded. It is often accompanied by diarrhea. If appropriate dietetic measures are adopted, this type is curable. Disorder of the pituitary gland, situated at the base of the brain, may produce infantilism and this type is often associated with marked obesity. Chronic kidney disease in early childhood leads to infantilism, but as a rule the children are so delicate that they succumb early in life. (*See also* BRAIN; CRETIN.)

INFARCTION. If a part of an organ in the body is deprived of its blood supply, *infarction* is said to have occured. Each organ is supplied with blood by an artery, which in the tissue subdivides or branches into numerous small vessels, each controlling the nutrition of a cone-shaped piece of the organ. Should one of these branches be blocked by a small clot of blood, or a fragment of growth from a heart valve (embolus), the conical part is deprived of blood and dies. This portion of dead tissue is known as an infarct. This is often seen in the spleen and kidney where an infarct is white in color. It may happen, as in the case of the lung, that blood from neighboring veins passes into the empty vessels and engorges them. In such instances, the term *red infarct* is applied, and if the blood is squeezed into the surrounding tissues, it is called hemorrhagic. Should this occur in the lung, the expectoration (spit) will be bloodstained. In some cases the clot which blocks the artery may be septic, i.e. infected with germs, and then the resulting infarct will form an abscess in the organ. Infarcts are ultimately replaced by fibrous or scar tissue.

INFECTIVE HEPATITIS. This condition is described under its popular name of catarrhal jaundice.

INFECTIOUS DISEASES. Diseases which are capable of being transferred from one person to another are termed *infectious*. If actual contact with a diseased person is required to convey it to another, the disease may be called *contagious*. The infectious diseases are numerous and include those which are popularly termed "the fevers."

How Disease Germs are Spread. Microorganisms or germs (bacteria) are the cause of the infectious diseases and their spread takes place in a variety of ways. The germs may be *airborne,* which means that infection takes place through contact with the expirations, coughs, and sneezes of an infected person. This is one of the commonest methods of infection and it is in this way that measles, scarlet fever, diphtheria, and the "common cold" are spread. Germs may also be *waterborne,* through contamination of a water supply. Typhoid and dysentry are often spread in this way.

Food may also distribute germs, particularly milk, which may give rise to epidemics of scarlet fever, diphtheria and infantile diarrhea, and is a common source of tubercular infection. Clothes, or articles used by a sufferer from an infectious disease (called fomites), may act as distributors of infection, smallpox being an example of a disease liable to be spread in this way. Another method of spread is by "carriers," i.e. persons who harbor the germs but do not themselves suffer from the disease. Typhoid, diphtheria, and cerebrospinal fever are often spread by carriers. Finally, infection may be conveyed from one person to another by the agency of insects and other parasites. Typhus, relapsing, and trench fever are conveyed by the bite of an infected louse; malaria, and yellow fever by the bite of an infected mosquito; and sleeping sickness is caused by the bite of an infected tsetse fly.

Stages of an Infectious Fever. After the invasion of the germs, a varying period of time elapses before any symptom becomes manifest. During this time germs are developing and multiplying. This is called the "incubation" period and it varies for different fevers. Then comes the "invasion" or onset of the first symptoms, which is followed by the stage of eruption shown by the appearance of the rash while the feverish symptoms are marked. Running a definite course, the fever diminishes during the stage of "resolution," and eventually reaches the stage of convalescence. At any time, however, "complications" may arise and delay the favorable course of the disease.

Nursing of a Fever Case. The nursing of a case of infectious fever is of great importance. The patient should be cared for in an open airy room, preferably at the top of the house and stripped of curtains, pictures and carpets.

Complete Isolation (except in the case of the nurse) is required until all danger of spreading the infection is passed. The bed should be freely accessible and a hair mattress is best. Feeding and other utensils should be kept quite separate. Books should not be allowed to leave the sick room. Antiseptic precautions must be adopted if any of the body discharges are infectious—as in typhoid for example. Motions and urine may be sterilized with lysol or chloride of lime; bedlinen can be similarly treated. The nurse should keep a careful note of the quantity of food given and should record on a chart, temperature, pulse and respiration rate. When the period of infectivity is over, the room and all its contents must be thoroughly disinfected. This is generally undertaken by the local public health authorities. It is to be noted that all who have been in contact with an infectious case should be isolated until the quarantine period (dependent upon the incubation period) has elapsed.

Certain infectious diseases must be "notified" to the Medical Officer of Health for the district. This is usually undertaken by the doctor attending the case. The chief notifiable diseases include: scarlet fever, diphtheria, small-pox, erysipelas, typhoid, dysentery, typhus, infantile paralysis, tuberculosis, cerebro-spinal fever and encephalitis lethargica. From time to time diseases such as mumps, measles and chicken-pox may be made notifiable in a particular locality.

The duration of the incubation and quarantine periods for the different infectious diseases are given under the heading INCUBATION. (*See also* SERUM.)

INFILTRATION. The term is used to describe the development of fat in the cells of the heart or liver. It is also used to describe the method of spread of cancer among the normal cells of a tissue.

INFLAMMATION. The reaction of animal tissues to any irritant is described as inflammation. There are four characteristic signs, viz. redness, heat, swelling and pain. Inflammation is a defensive reaction to injury from any cause, germ infection, chemical irritants, and heat, as in a burn. There is first of all a dilatation of the vessels in the area affected and flushing of the part with blood, thus explaining the heat and redness. There is also a discharge of watery fluid or lymph into the tissue spaces, distending them and causing the swelling and pain. This distension allows the drive of the heartbeat to be felt, so causing a throbbing pain.

There is a slowing down of the circulation in an inflamed area, and the white cells of the blood accumulate in large numbers and many make their way between the tissue cells. The migration of these cells and of the watery fluid is an essential part of the defensive mechanism. The lymph contains substances which are harmful to germ life, while the white cells wage warfare on the germs, eating them up when possible. Sometimes, however, the fight between the germs and the white cells results in the latter being killed. In this way *pus* cells are formed, and if this takes place on a large scale, an *abscess* results. A boil, for example, is a tiny skin abscess, the core of which consists of white cells killed by the invading germs.

Inflammation, therefore, is a defensive activity of the body and it is usually strong enough to cure the condition. On the other hand, this line of defense may fail, and the germs, gaining a temporary victory, make their way along lymphatic vessels, inflaming them and ultimately reaching the lymph glands. It is well known, for example, how a poisoned and inflamed finger gives rise to pain in elbow and armpit.

Treatment. In the treatment of inflammation three points must be observed: (1) removal of the cause; (2) rest for the inflamed part; (3) removal of the products of inflammation. Rest will lessen pain and reduce the work of the part, so permitting it to concentrate against the enemy. Occasionally it may be possible to get rid of the offending agent at once, as when a foreign particle gets into the eye, or by washing and cleaning a dirty wound. It is possible to assist nature by applying heat which increases the blood supply to the part. Also, hot applications tend to relieve the pain. If pus should form, it should be permitted to escape. This may necessitate incision with a knife. Chronic inflammation may follow in an acute form, or the intensity of the initial inflammation may be very slight and the resistance of the tissues low so that the inflammation process is long drawn out.

In these circumstances, there are some repair processes taking place alongside the destructive ones. There is a growth of new fibrous tissue cells producing hardness, but little redness, heat, or pain. This type of inflammation is often seen in the case of a chronic leg ulcer resulting from a varicose vein. Chronic inflammation is difficult to treat, but every effort must be made to stimulate the resistance of the body generally by good food, tonics, and fresh air, sunlight, and exercise. (*See also* ABSCESS; BOIL.)

INFLUENZA. This is an infectious disease, occurring in epidemic form, and from time to time ravaging the whole world. The last great epidemic was in 1918, and prior to that date, in 1889–90. It may occur at almost any time of the year, but is generally most prevalent in the colder months. It is caused by a germ or microbe, but the specific nature of this germ is still undecided. Recent research points to a filterable virus, i.e. a germ so minute that it cannot be seen by a microscope, but is able to pass through a fine porcelain filter. Infection takes place when a sufferer coughs, sneezes, or speaks loudly, emitting droplets of expectoration which are laden with germs. It is possible that handkerchiefs and clothes harbor the germs and act as distributing agents.

The symptoms of this disease are many and varied, and may show themselves in all the systems of the body. After invasion with the germs, there is a short incubation period of from one to four days and the onset is sudden and marked by shivering, rise of temperature, headache, sickness, vague muscular pains, and a feeling of exhaustion. The throat may be sore and there is often a dry irritating cough. Three main types of influenza occur: respiratory, gastro-intestinal, and nervous. In the first, bronchitis, pleurisy, and pneumonia may arise; in the second, there is catarrh or inflammation of the stomach and intestines, with sickness and diarrhea, pain in the belly, and sometimes jaundice; in the third and nervous type, headache is very severe; there may be an excessively high temperature, and occasionally meningitis may arise. Influenza thus shows considerable variation in type and in different epidemics, one or other of the types tends to predominate.

As a rule, the course of the disease is short, lasting from three to five days, but complications are very apt to arise and delay convalescence. Bronchitis may persist for some weeks and not infrequently develops into bronchopneumonia (a patchy inflammation of the lungs). In all forms of the disease, heart symptoms are common and constitute one of the major dangers of influenza. The heart muscle may be weakened, revealed by irregularity and rapidity of the pulse. Inflammation of the middle ear is not uncommon as a sequel to influenza, and occasionally the infection may spread to the brain and spinal cord. One of the most troublesome symptoms of the aftermath of influenza is mental depression which may even amount to an attack of melancholia. Even in mild cases of influenza a degree of prostration occurs which seems to be out of proportion to the severity of the symptoms and may leave behind an enfeeblement of the general health which may take some months or even years to overcome.

Treatment and Prevention. The patient should be isolated and precautions taken to avoid spread of infection. Even the mildest cases should be treated in bed, as this lessens the chances of complications arising. The room should be very airy—as fresh air is the best preventive against spreading influenza throughout a household. The diet should be light: milk, beaten-up eggs, beef tea, and fruit juices. If the throat is sore, an inhalation of compound tincture of benzoin will be of benefit, and if there is tightness of the chest a linseed poultice will relieve the discomfort. Aspirin is the drug generally used in the treatment of influenza. It is given in ten-grain doses, every four hours, during the acute stage of the illness. During convalescence, a tonic such as sylop Hypophosphetes is helpful in restoring appetite and energy, and if possible a change of air to the hills or seaside is very desirable. To avoid influenza during an epidemic, endeavor to live as much as possible in the open air. Keep away from warm crowded rooms, theaters, etc. The diet should be generous, containing plenty of raw fruit, green vegetables, and dairy produce. Every effort must be made to prevent any tendency to constipation. It may lessen the risk if the throat is sprayed or gargled every morning with a weak solution of peroxide of hydrogen. The antibiotic and sulphonamide drugs have unfortunately no effect on the influenza virus, but are effective if bronchitis or pneumonia develop as secondary infections.

INGROWING TOENAIL. This is a condition in which the outer edge of the big toenail presses into the flesh and causes a very tender spot to appear. Badly fitting shoes are very often the cause of this painful condition, but probably the chief cause is cutting the nail in the wrong fashion. The nail of the big toe should be flat and should never be cut too short. The outer edges should never be trimmed down at the sides as this induces the nail to curve instead of remaining perfectly flat; in fact, it is better to cut the nail lower at the center. Trimming the nail in this way will help to avoid the condition.

INHALATION. Inhalation is a method of treatment in which drugs can be taken into the body by the breath. In this way general anesthesia is usually carried out by means of a special inhaling apparatus. Steam inhalation is perhaps the most popular form of this type of treatment. It is used especially in cases of bronchitis and in inflammatory conditions of the nose and throat. A very simple way of carrying out this treatment is to fill a jug with boiling water into which has been placed a teaspoonful of tincture of benzoin or any other soothing volatile oil. The head is covered with a towel and held over the jug so that the fumes from the jug are not allowed to escape. The patient should breathe through the mouth as well as the nose in order to allow the soothing fumes to reach the mucous membranes of these parts. Instead of steam, liquid substances may be sprayed into the throat or nose by an atomizer, and by taking a deep breath this fine spray can be carried on into the back of the throat and the lungs. This method is particularly useful when there is a quantity of thick mucus or phlegm which the patient has difficulty in coughing up. A steam-kettle may be used in cases of chronic bronchitis or croup.

People who suffer from asthma often obtain relief from an attack by inhaling an atomized solution of adrenalin, of which there are so many patent preparations on the market. Special machines have been developed which produce a "mist" in which the individual droplets are so small that they will pass with the air currents into the tiny terminal air-sacs of the lung. These mists have been used as a vehicle to carry penicillion and other antibiotics to remote infected areas of the lung, and have achieved success in the treatment of bronchitis and also sometimes in bronchiectasis.

Inhalation may be carried out by means of sprinkling certain drugs on a handkerchief and breathing into this. A few drops of eucalyptus is often used during a cold in the head, and amyl nitrite is also taken in this way to relieve an attack of angina pectoris.

INJECTION. Medicinal remedies in solution are sometimes administered by forcing them into the tissues of the body from a syringe fitted with a hollow needle. In most cases the purpose of the injection is for speed in obtaining its effects and for accuracy of dosage. Again, this method has obvious advantages in the case of patients who are unconscious and collapsed and cannot swallow. Also, some drugs are acted upon by the digestive juices and rendered ineffective so that injection is the only method of administration.

An injection may be intradermal, i.e. into the skin, this method being used for producing local anesthesia or insensitiveness to pain. The most usual way for administration of drugs is hypodermically, i.e. under the skin. Some drugs are liable to irritate the skin (mercury and quinine), and these are given intramuscularly, i.e. deeply into a muscle, usually of the thigh. Intravenous injection, directly into the bloodstream, can be accomplished through a vein, usually one of the surface veins of the arm at the elbow. This is the most rapid way of obtaining the action of a drug.

Injections may be made into the spinal canal in order to secure insensitiveness to pain for operation purposes. An injection into the bowel is called an enema, while injections into the nose or vagina are termed douches. (*See also* DOUCHE; ENEMA.)

INOCULATION. This is the operation by which disease germs, dead or greatly reduced in virulence, are introduced into the body by injection through the skin. The purpose of this is to increase the resistance of the body to the germs inoculated and so prevent disease. The system of inoculation was founded on Jenner's experiments with cowpox, which is simply smallpox in the cow. He used material from an infected cow to induce a mild form of this disease in order to prevent the more severe ordinary smallpox. A considerable number of diseases are prevented and treated by this method of inoculation. The most important of these are typhoid, paratyphoid, rabies, dysentery, tuberculosis, and common septic infections such as boils, acne, and catarrh of the nose. (*See also* ANTIBODY; ANTITOXIN; SERUM.)

INQUEST. If there is any reason to suspect that a person has died a violent or unnatural death, the circumstances must be investigated and the matter made the subject of a formal inquiry. The inquest, as it is called, is conducted by the coroner, with or without a jury, this being left to his discretion. The same procedure is adopted if a person dies in prison. The coroner issues summonses to the witnesses to attend and failure to do so occasions a fine. The jury and coroner must "view" the body. Persons interested may attend and be represented by their attorneys. The coroner is not bound by the laws of evidence which prevail under the jurisdiction of an ordinary court of law.

It is the duty of the coroner to sum up the case and for the jury to deliver the verdict. The jury are entitled to add a "rider," if any matter has become apparent which deserves public comment. A coroner may commit a person for trial at the criminal court for murder or manslaughter.

INSANITY. This is a legal and not a medical term denoting the civil state in which a person is unable to look after himself or his affairs, and is a danger to himself or to society. It signifies that liberty must be restricted and a certain degree of legalized control must be exercised. In such a state of mind a person requires to be "certified," and this implies detention for the purposes of care and treatment in a mental hospital. Insanity is dependent upon disease of the mind, and it must always be distinguished from mental defect or feeblemindedness, which means that the mind has not developed but has remained fixed at a childish level.

There are a great many types of insanity and a great many causes. In about 40 to 50 per cent of cases, an unstable mind is inherited, but in a very considerable proportion of cases external factors, such as alcohol, syphilis, childbirth, physical exhaustion, hardened arteries, severe fevers, brain tumors and injury, diabetes, and prolonged mental stress are the direct causes of the mental symptoms. Some forms of insanity are associated with great depression and impulses to suicide, others with excitement and violence. In one type, there is tendency to a gradual breaking up of the mind (schizophrenia or dementia praecox), while in another, delusions of persecution is the chief symptom. Confusional mental disorders, or insanity, are generally due to some variety of brain poisoning.

The procedure of certification depends upon the means of the insane person. If the patient or relative can afford to pay nursing-home fees, he may be admitted to a "licensed house" or registered hospital as a "private patient." There are certain statutory documents to be filled in. These consist of (1) a petition of a near relative to the judicial authority: justice of peace, or judge); (2) a statement of particulars signed by petitioner; (3) two medical certificates and (4) the order of the judicial authority ordering the reception of the patient into an institution. These documents together constitute the *Reception Order on Petition*, and the reception of the patient must take place within seven days of the signing of the order.

If it is necessary to place a patient under control immediately, an *Urgency Order* may be used. This consists of a reception order signed by the nearest relative, a statement of particulars, and a medical certificate giving the grounds for the urgency. This permits of detention for seven days. A patient can be certified and kept under care in his private home, or in the house of a doctor or lay person, provided that the patient can be suitably nursed and that the court is duly notified.

Patients may be admitted to a mental hospital as *voluntary patients*, i.e. without certification, by the request of the patients themselves; or as *temporary patients* for six months, where recovery is likely to take place within that time.

A great deal can nowadays be done for the insane by scientific methods of treatment. The modern mental hospital is very different from the asylums of the last century. It is no longer merely a place of detention: its organization promotes the alleviation and, in many cases, the cure of the mentally sick.

A patient, though certified of unsound mind, is not debarred from making a valid will provided he possesses a "sound disposing mind," which simply means that the insane person has an understanding of the nature of the will, the extent and details of his estate, and the individuals who have reasonable claim to benefit from it. It is generally advisable to have the testimony of a medical witness to the patient's testamentary capacity, otherwise it is not likely to be upheld by law, if contested. (*See also* MENTAL DEFICIENCY; MENTAL DISEASE.)

INSECT BITES. This subject is dealt with fully under the heading BITES AND STINGS.

INSECT REPELLENTS. For many years, oil of citronella has been the principal insect repellent in everyday use. Early in the last war it was replaced for general use among the Allied troops by the chemical repellents, D.M.P. (dimethylphthallate) and D.B.P. (dibutylphthallate). When applied to the skin these substances give protection against biting insects for two to three hours. A high degree of protection was achieved in tropical warfare by wearing impregnated veils, gloves, and socks. The materials required reimpregnation about once a week. By this method troops were protected from the bites of mites and ticks carrying typhus fever and other diseases.

INSECTICIDE. A drug which is capable of killing insects is known as an insecticide. Mercury may be used as an ointment or as a lotion in order to get rid of the small insects which are parasitic on human beings. D.D.T. as a 5 per cent mixture in some inert powder or in solution in kerosene is the most effective household insecticide in use today. (*See also* BITES AND STINGS.)

INSECTS. Insects play a large part in carrying disease, perhaps more so in tropical countries than in temperate climates. Of recent years much public health work has been done towards the prevention of the spread of disease by these pests. (*See also* BED BUG; FLIES; MOSQUITO.)

INSOMNIA. Sleeplessness or insomnia is a symptom of disturbed working of the mind or body. It is, in itself, very dangerous to health, particularly in the case of growing children who suffer stunting in mind and body as a result. Among the common causes which may initiate sleeplessness are lack of fresh air from bad ventilation of the bedroom, insufficient exercise, heavy meals before retiring, late hours, and mental work carried beyond the stage of weariness. With sensitive people, a strange bedroom, unaccustomed sounds or lights, a pillow of unusual height, an uncomfortable mattress, or too-heavy bedclothes are liable to make falling asleep difficult. Bodily ill health, particularly when associated with pain, and notably in heart or chest complaints, frequently hinders sleep, while mental ill health ranks as a prominent cause of insomnia. Worry or apprehension are formidable enemies of sleep, for they tend to reach their highest pitch at bedtime.

Sufferers from persistent insomnia are apt quickly to reach the stage when they despair of ever again enjoying a good night's sleep. This hopeless attitude is very natural, but it must be fought against. The first step is to convince the mind that the disability is remediable. That accomplished, the sufferer should examine his habits of life and try to discover the cause

or causes of the insomnia. Provided there is no physical disease requiring medical attention, there are certain measures which, if persevered in, will eventually restore the sleep rhythm.

Sufferers from insomnia should spend the hours before retirement in some restful pastime and go to bed at approximately the same time every night, as habit plays a large part in the function of sleep. Late meals are taboo, as are strong coffee or tea, but a glass of warm milk is soothing and promotes drowsiness. The bedroom must be well ventilated without being cold, and the bed comfortable with light but warm bedclothing. The body should be warm before retiring. Cold feet are a common cause of sleeplessness; therefore, a hotwater bottle may be necessary. A warm bath is often valuable as it promotes relaxation of the muscles.

When in bed, it is best not to anticipate a bad night or think deliberately about getting off to sleep. The sufferer should concern himself only in making himself thoroughly comfortable and should try to *stop* thinking. A word of warning. It is most inadvisable for anyone to have recourse to sleep-producing medicines except under the personal direction of the doctor. Such drugs are dangerous when wrongly used and are seldom necessary if natural means to sleep are fully tried. (*See also* SLEEP.)

INSUFFLATION. The introduction of powdered drugs into the nose, throat or ear is called insufflation, and the apparatus, which simply consists of a rubber ball attached to a vulcanite tube, is termed an insufflator. The powder is injected in a fine cloud and insufflation is a useful means of introducing antiseptics to the' inaccessible parts of the nose and throat. Boracic powder can be blown into the ear or nose when it discharges, while iodoform can be similarly used in other septic conditions.

INSULIN. In the pancreas, one of the digestive glands in the abdomen, are groups of cells called the islets of Langerhans which produce an internal secretion (i.e., passed directly into the bloodstream), called insulin. This substance is necessary for the utilization of sugar by the body and its absence or deficiency leads to diabetes mellitus. Insulin was discovered in 1921 by Banting of Toronto, and it is prepared commercially and used extensively in the treatment of diabetes. Since its introduction the mortality caused by diabetes has been greatly lessened. It is generally given by injection under the skin, and the doses must be carefully controlled according to the amount of sugar in the blood. Insulin is particularly valuable in the treatment of diabetic coma. (*See also* DIABETES; DUCTLESS GLANDS; PANCREAS.)

INTELLIGENCE, TESTS FOR. Up to the beginning of the present century, there was no rational attempt at grading persons in terms of their intelligence. Children not quite up to the average were classed all together as "backward;" and persons, whether children or adults, still further below the average as "mentally deficient." There was no attempt at special education, and, as a result, a terrible waste of many lives which nowadays, if not reaching a high standard of intelligence, are yet happy and useful.

Alfred Binet (1857–1911) was the first to recognize this practically, and he devised, in 1905, scales and tests to measure the intelligence, which are now very widely used. They have been modified from time to time by other workers, notably Simon and Stamford, and are now known as the Binet-Simon tests. Many other tests such as the Stamford-Binet have been devised, all on the same lines.

They are used in order to find out the stage of mental development which a person has reached; they refer not to special learning, but to general intelligence or aptitude. The tests have been standardized by "trying them out" on a large number of normal children, and are arranged in a series of increasing difficulty, each year having its own tests. Then, according to the capacity a person shows he is classified as being of *mental age* 6, 10, 15, etc., regardless of his *actual age*. It is interesting to note that the tests work out very accurately for all normal children, except illiterates, irrespective of race, position, or education. As examples, the tests for children 5, 8 and 15 years are appended:

(5) 1. Tells which is the heavier of two boxes similar in size and appearance.

2. Copies a square with pen and ink.
3. Repeats a sentence of 10 syllables.
4. Counts 4 cents.
5. Puts together an oblong card which has been cut from corner to corner.

(8) 1. Compares two things from memory such as fly and butterfly, wood and glass, paper and cardboard.
2. Counts backwards from 20 to 1.
3. Points out what is missing in 4 sketches, e.g. a face without a nose.
4. Knows the day and date.
5. Repeats 5 numbers after the examiner.

(15) 1. Repeats 7 numbers.
2. Finds 3 words rhyming with "day" in one minute.
3. Repeats a sentence of 26 syllables after hearing it once.
4. Understands pictures capable of sympathetic interpretation. A description alone is not enough.
5. Completes an incomplete account such as: "My neighbor has had strange visitors today; a doctor, a lawyer, and a minister. What is happening at my neighbor's?"

The examiner should see that the child is at his ease, preferably looking upon the tests as a new game. Each child is tested separately. No help is given; it is considered that a child has failed in a particular question if he does not understand it. Various criticisms are made regarding the tests, especially that they are too easy for American children. They are not perfect; but in spite of that they are of great practical value. They are very useful in grading children, especially young children on first going to school, and those mentally deficient. Their principal value, however, is to remove from many "backward" children the stigma of mental deficiency. Such a child may even have been reported by his teacher as being deficient, but is found to be of normal intelligence by the tests. The fault sometimes lies with the teacher or the school, and when he is placed in another school, his "backwardness" disappears.

For mentally deficient adults, the tests are used in a similar way. (*See also* MENTAL DEFICIENCY.) There have been a great variety of tests devised for normal adults, but so far there are none of any practical importance. Some are very trivial; some far too difficult and complicated, requiring special apparatus, etc.; some are too liable to errors of interpretation by the examiner. After numerous experiments, however, it has finally been decided that "a man succeeds in any act requiring intelligence because he possesses both general ability and specific ability." This the ordinary person already knows, only he would say that "Brown gets ahead because he has common sense and a talent for his job."

INTERCOSTAL. This name is applied to the nerves, muscles, and vessels which lie between the ribs. The space between each rib is also known as the intercostal space.

INTERMITTENT CLAUDICATION. This condition, sometimes called intermittent limp, consists of painful cramp in the muscles of the leg. It comes on after walking and leads to a limping gait or it may cause complete inability to walk. As a rule the pain subsides rapidly, but tends to return after further walking. This affection is often associated with hardening and thickening of the arteries (arteriosclerosis) and is caused by a spasm of the narrowed arteries depriving the muscles of their blood supply. During an attack, rest followed by massage is the best means of obtaining relief. Prevention of further attacks depends upon the successful treatment of the existing hardening of the arteries, or of the block in the circulation which caused the limp. (*See also* ARTERIOSCLEROSIS; DEGENERATION.)

INTERTRIGO. This condition arises through two parts of the body coming in contact with each other and causing redness and chafiing on the opposed skin surfaces. The most common parts to be affected are the groins, the thighs, and the armpits. In infants the chafing may be caused by the diaper, and stout women may find that chafing occurs underneath the breasts. In the earlier stages of intertrigo the condition will soon clear up with the application of a good dusting powder.

Care must be taken to keep the parts clean, and on no account must the skin be scratched. Irritation of the affected parts may turn a case of simple intertrigo into a septic dermatitis which will require special treatment. (*See also* CHAFING; DERMATITIS; ERYTHEMA.)

INTESTINE. The intestine or bowel is that part of the digestive system which extends from the outlet of the stomach to the anus and it is approximately twenty-five feet in length. It is suspended in the cavity of the abdomen, or belly, by folds of tissue called the mesentery. The intestine is divided into two parts, the small and the large. The small intestine extends from the stomach to the caecum, a pouched portion of the large intestine to which the appendix is attached.

The small intestine consists of three parts, viz., the *duodenum,* consisting of the first ten or twelve inches into which open the ducts of the pancreas and the liver; the *jejunum,* extending for eight or nine feet, and continuing as the *ileum,* which opens into the large intestine. The small intestine is about one and a half inches in width. It has four coats, an outer serous or smooth glistening coat, a muscular one, a submucous one containing blood vessels and nerves, and the mucous coat, which is arranged in folds and which is covered with little projections, called villi, for the absorption of nutriment from the food. There are also some small glands in the mucous coat which produce the intestinal juice, a secretion which helps in the work of digestion. Scattered throughout the small intestine are small collections of special cells—called "Peyer's patches," and these are of interest because they become inflamed and ulcerated in typhoid fever.

The large intestine is about six feet in length and is of unequal caliber being largest at the caecum and gradually diminishing until it reaches the expanded part just before the anus, called the rectum. The large intestine has four coats similar to the small intestine, except that villi and digestive glands are absent. It is divided into caecum, ascending colon, transverse colon, descending colon, pelvic colon and rectum. The appendix is a worm-like structure about three inches long and a quarter of an inch thick, having a small canal extending through it but closed at the end.

Food is passed along the intestine from the stomach by rhythmic muscular waves called peristalsis. Segmental contraction also takes place so that the contents are broken up at regular intervals. In this way the food masses are thoroughly churned up and subjected to the action of the digestive juices. By the time the food reaches the caecum all digestion and the greater part of absorption of nutriment has taken place. Only water is absorbed in the large intestine and the food remains are hastened on to the rectum, from which they are evacuated. About five hours after taking a meal the contents of the small intestine begin to pass into the large intestine and the food remains reach the rectum in about eighteen hours. (*See also* DIGESTION.)

INTOXICATION. This term is applied to any form of body poisoning. The poisons may be taken by the mouth—e.g. alcohol, morphia, cocaine, or hashish—or the poisons may be derived from the body, as in the case of thyroid intoxication from excessive activity of the thyroid gland. The symptoms naturally vary with the intoxicating agent. The effects may be transient or permanent according to the severity of the condition.

Alcoholic intoxication produces well-known symptoms and if very intense may lead to coma (unconsciousness). The respiratory and heart centers are depressed, and this may be fatal.

Treatment. Treatment should aim at emptying the stomach either by an emetic (mustard and water) or by the use of the stomach tube. Then, a hot stimulating drink of coffee should be given and the patient kept warm with hot blankets and bottles.

INTUBATION. This term means the introduction of a tube into the larynx (throat), between the vocal cords, in order to maintain the air passage. It is most commonly done in order to give an anesthetic for a surgical operation. Formerly it was done to prevent suffocation from diphtheria, and in order to avoid the operation of tracheotomy, when an opening was made into the windpipe and a short curved tube inserted. But with immunization having become general, diphtheria is now seldom seen. (*See also* DIPHTHERIA.)

INTUSSUSCEPTION. This condition consists of the passage of a part of the bowel into the adjoining part: it is as if one part was telescoped into the adjacent part. Most often this takes place at the junction of the small intestine (bowel) with the caecum. The end of the small intestine normally projects into the beginning of the caecum, and, in the state of intussusception this portion travels along the interior of the large bowel—sometimes for a considerable distance, occasionally as far as the anus.

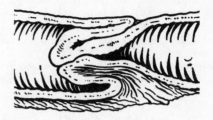

Intussusception.

Intussusception occurs most commonly in children under the age of twelve months. It arises most probably from the presence of some irritant in the food. This calls forth violent expulsive movements of the bowel and so carries the end of the small intestine into the caecum. The outstanding symptoms are vomiting, prostration and the passage from the bowel of a little blood-stained jelly-like substance.

Treatment. An immediate operation is necessary to save the life of the child, but if medical aid is not immediately forthcoming, an enema of warm water will be beneficial.

A chronic form of intussusception occurs in adults, often associated with a bowel tumor. The symptoms are not so urgent but there is some danger of obstruction of the bowels. Treatment is by surgical operation. (*See also* INTESTINE.)

INUNCTION. The administration of drugs to the body through the skin is termed inunction. The drug is mixed up with a fatty substance and the ointment so formed is rubbed into the skin, which has considerable absorptive powers. The outstanding use of inunction used to be in the treatment of syphilis with mercury ointment, but that is now obsolete. Inunction is also a valuable means of administering cod-liver oil to children.

IODINE. This is a substance, taking the form of dark lustrous scales, which is still used extensively in medical practice. Generally, the iodine is dissolved in alcohol to form a tincture, which is most often used as an antiseptic in cases of wounds of the skin, when it is painted on. It is sometimes used to prepare the skin prior to a surgical operation. If the skin is at all sensitive iodine may produce blistering, so that it must be used with caution. It should be remembered that the use of iodine for the treatment of cuts and abrasions does not exclude the need for thorough cleansing of the wound first of all with clean water.

Iodine is also given internally sometimes by doctors, in small doses, especially in the treatment of goiter and thyroid diseases. Iodine is sometimes used in ointment form for the treatment of skin affections—and for rubbing over rheumatic joints and muscles.

Iodine is normally present in the body, being an essential constituent of the secretion of the thyroid gland.

Poisoning. If the tincture is accidentally swallowed, give an emetic (salt or mustard and water), and then thin starch, arrowroot, or bread freely.

Iodized Salt. A table salt containing a small amount of potassium iodide, a salt of iodine, is now available, and it is of benefit in a certain type of simple goiter. It is believed that this form of goiter is related to a deficiency of iodine in the drinking water.

Iodism. If iodine or iodides are given in excess they may produce symptoms known as iodism. The eyes and nose run freely the saliva is increased; there is dull headache and sometimes depression. Treatment is obvious: stop the administration of the iodine preparation.

IODOFORM. This substance, made from alcohol, iodine, and carbonate of potassium, is generally available as a lemon-yellow crystalline powder. It is used as a local antiseptic, for it liberates iodine on contact with the tissues. It is used for dusting septic wounds and sores, ulcers and abscess cavities. Care has to be taken not to apply iodoform to large raw surfaces or poisonous symptoms may arise. It is often employed as a surgical dressing when applied to gauze. A paste made up of bismuth, iodoform, and liquid paraffin is still sometimes used for packing abscess cavities: this is commonly referred to as Beck's paste.

Poisoning by Iodoform. The symptoms are variable, but a quick pulse, dilated pupils, headache, vomiting, depression and collapse are generally observed. The use of the drug must be immediately discontinued and any surface to which it has been applied should be washed with a solution of sodium bicarbonate in water.

IONIZATION. Ionization or ionic medication is an electric treatment from which great things were hoped when it was first introduced. It aims at depositing curative drugs in the tissues by means of an electric current.

IPECACUANHA. This is the dried root of a Brazilian plant. It contains two alkalids, emetine and cephaeline. The drug stimulates expectoration, but in large doses is emetic—i.e., causes vomiting. Ipecacuanha has also some action in producing sweating. The drug, in various preparations, is often used in the treatment of bronchitis and other diseases of the respiratory system. It may be used as ipecacuanha wine, or as compound ipecacuanha powder.

Emetine, the alkaloid of ipecacuanha, is used in the treatment of amoebic dysentry. It is usually given hypodermically, i.e. by injection under the skin, but sometimes it is combined with bismuth iodide when it is given by the mouth. Considerable care has to be exercised in treatment with emetine, as it has a harmful effect upon the liver and kidneys. Emetine is also used as an emetic in the treatment of poisoning when it becomes necessary to empty the stomach rapidly.

IRIS. The colored part of the eye is known as the iris and it surrounds the black center part of the eye known as the pupil. Its purpose is to regulate the amount of light which enters the eye. (*See also* EYE.)

IRITIS. Inflammation of the iris of the eye is known as iritis. This is a serious infection which requires expert attention, and is now usually treated with penicillin or one of the newer antibiotics.

IRON. This metallic element is normally found in the body, chiefly in the red pigment or hemoglobin of the blood. It is the iron pigment which enables the blood to absorb and carry oxygen to the cells of the body.

Iron is primarily obtained by the body from the vegetable kingdom, and as there is a small but constant destruction and excretion of this element, it is essential that the stock should be replenished regularly by eating food containing iron.

Iron deficiency may lead to a form of anemia, most often observed in young girls living under unhygienic conditions, which is called chlorosis. In such cases, prolonged administration of iron in medicinal form (as well as by eating foods rich in iron) is necessary.

Iron can be given in a great variety of ways medicinally. One of the most popular and useful is in the form of Blaud's Pills, which are not proprietary articles, but the name given to an old formula. These are given in 5–15 grain doses twice or three times daily, after each meal.

The most active iron preparation is ferrous sulphate, which will cure iron-deficiency anemia in a daily dose of 9 grains. As iron is astringent, it may be necessary to give some aperient at the same time. Iron preparations may not agree with certain people, causing upset of digestion, and occasionally it may be necessary to give the iron by hypodermic injection. Apart from anemia, states' of exhaustion, convalescence after feverish diseases, or nervous breakdowns will benefit from iron combined with some stimulating drug such as strychnine. If iron is taken in liquid form, it is well to remember that it may stain the teeth. To prevent this, the dose may be sucked up through a straw or glass tube and the mouth well rinsed with water afterwards.

IRRIGATION. Irrigation of the bowel is carried out in the treatment of mild types of dysentery and colitis (inflammation of the colon). A rubber tube is inserted into the rectum and several pints of fluid are slowly allowed to run in. Various types of antiseptics may be given, but as a rule, what is known as a normal saline solution is used for this purpose. Irrigation is also a valuable means of cleansing cavities such as the vagina, etc. This is done by means of a douche; but irrigation of the womb,

which is a much more difficult procedure, can only be carried out by a doctor. Irrigation is also a valuable way of removing pus and then impurities from a septic wound. (*See also* DOUCHE; ENEMA.)

IRRITABILITY. To the physiologist, the property of all living cells to respond to a stimulus is termed irritability. It is this property which, for example, enables muscles to contract and glands to secrete. The responses are increased or depressed according to the health and nutrition of the cells concerned. Nervous irritability occurs in neurasthenia and anxiety neuroses. In these conditions there is often an underlying exhaustion of the nervous system. Overfatigue and poisoning from any cause may also lead to nervous irritability.

ISCHEMIA. A localized area of bloodlessness or anemia is referred to as an ischemia. When there is a general state of bloodlessness, anemia is the term used. Ischemia is most often due to a stoppage of the blood flow in an artery by some external pressure—e.g., splints too tightly applied to a limb in a case of fracture. In the arm, this accident leads to malnutrition of the muscles, which in turn causes them to contract, a condition known in the forearm as *Volkmann's ischemic contracture*. The fingers become fixed (bent) and almost impossible to straighten, while the hand is often pulled backwards.

Treatment. Massage may improve the condition, but not infrequently a surgical operation may be necessary. When splints are applied, the state of the circulation should always be tested. Overtightness is evidenced by "pins and needles," coldness, and blueness of the fingers or toes. A severe ischemia may lead to death of the tissue concerned. (*See also* ANEMIA, LOCAL.)

"ITCH, THE" (Scabies). The itch, or scabies, is an infectious disease of the skin produced by the Acarus scabiei, an insect just visible to the naked eye. It lives upon the skin, and the female burrows into it to deposit her eggs. At the point of entrance is a tiny blister, and from this a greyish line or burrow is seen. The parts generally affected are the skin between the fingers, the front of the forearms and elbows, the armpits, the nipples, the lower part of the abdomen, the genitals, and the buttocks. The face seldom suffers. In infants, the whole body, including the scalp, may be affected.

"Norwegian scabies," as it is called, is a severe inflammatory type found among the very poor and dirty, those suffering from wasting diseases, and lepers.

Treatment. Sulphur used to be the great stand-by in treatment, especially thorough rubbing in of sulphur ointment, and this is still effective, though it may cause dermatitis through overuse. In recent years a number of new drugs and methods have been introduced. A very effective preparation is an emulsion of benzyl benzoate made in water with a 2 per cent lanette wax, the proportion of benzyl benzoate being 25 per cent. The patient should first have a hot bath, in which he soaks for thirty minutes, meanwhile scrubbing himself vigorously with a nailbrush and soap in order to remove the roofs of all the burrows made by the scabies parasite. The emulsion is then thoroughly rubbed in all over the body from the neck downwards. The emulsion should be used on three successive days, though it has been stated that two applications at one sitting can effect a cure.

ITCHING. For itching due to general causes, *see* PRURIGO; PRURITUS.

JACKET. The term straitjacket is used in connection with insane people who have become so violent that they have to be restrained. The jacket is made of very strong material, usually leather. The sleeves are made to come well below the hands so that the extra length of material can be crossed in front of the body and tied behind the back; in this way the violent motions of the arms are under complete control. The term jacket is also used in connection with spinal supports, or a pneumonia jacket may be meant. This is worn to protect the chest.

JACKSONIAN EPILEPSY. Described by John Hughlings Jackson, an English physician who was born in 1834 and died in 1911, this is a form of epilepsy in which the spasm is limited to a single group of muscles in the face, arm, or leg. (*See also* EPILEPSY.)

JAUNDICE. Jaundice is due to the presence of bile in the blood which causes the skin to turn a yellowish color. There are many different causes of this condition, and naturally the symptoms vary with the cause. The commonest form is that known as *catarrhal jaundice,* or infective hepatitis. It is an infectious disease due to a tiny germ known as a virus. Cases often occur among several members of a family or among troops living at close quarters. Jaundice may also occur in almost any general fever, or it may result from obstruction caused by gallstones passing down the bile duct.

Symptoms. Catarrhal jaundice starts with a feeling of nausea and depression for a few days and the skin may feel irritable and itchy. The whites of the eyes turn yellow, and the skin also becomes a bright yellow. The tongue is furred and the temperature may rise to 99 or 100 deg. F. The part of the body over the liver and gall bladder may feel very tender to the touch. The urine is dark in color, and motions are rather offensive, large, and pale or putty-colored. The jaundice generally takes about two or three weeks to disappear, and as a rule the skin gradually regains its normal color.

Treatment. The patient should be kept in bed until the coloring matter has disappeared from the urine. The bowels should be kept open with salts and, if necessary, an enema should be given. The diet should have very little fat in it; in fact, it would be better to exclude fat altogether. Liquid or semisolid food should be given, such as barley water, meat extracts, toast, and about a half-pint of milk daily. If the skin is very irritable it should be bathed with a weak solution of carbolic acid or bicarbonate of soda.

Obstructive Jaundice. Obstructions which may bring on symptoms of jaundice include gallstones, a tumor or cancer arising in the gall bladder, the presence of round worms, or a hydatid cyst. Obstruction may also be caused by pressure on the bile duct owing to enlarged glands or a growth in any of the surrounding organs.

Infantile jaundice. Jaundice is very often seen in newborn infants, appearing during the first two days of life. Mild cases are usually the result of destruction of the infant's blood by circulating rhesus antibodies derived from the mother. It clears up after a week or two without any treatment whatever. More severe types may be due to absence of the bile duct or some other form of obstruction, and the outlook may be very serious indeed. (*See also* GALL BLADDER, DISEASES OF.)

JAW. The jaws or jawbones are two sturdy bones of the face into which the teeth are fitted. Of the two jaws the lower is by far the stronger—and it is a much harder task to extract the teeth from it. The lower jawbone is angular in shape and fits into the temporal bone at a point in front of the ear, forming a hinge joint. The upper jaw is altogether a slighter one, and is composed of two bones which are firmly atached to the other bones of the upper part of the face. The teeth fit firmly into sockets in the two jaws which are called *alveoli.*

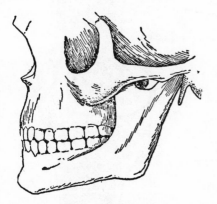

Upper and Lower Jaws.

Dislocations of the jaw are of fairly frequent occurrence but can be easily replaced. Between the ends of the two jaws are little pads of cartilage, each of which is called a meniscus. These serve as shock absorbers and relieve the wear

and tear of friction between the two jaws. These menisici sometimes get jerked out of place, causing great pain until they are replaced.

JEJUNUM. This is the name given to the middle portion of the small intestine. The word comes to us from the Latin. meaning empty of food, and it is applied to this part of the intestine because it is generally found to be empty on examination after death.

JOINTS. Joints or articulations in the body are formed when two bones or cartilages meet. The joints of the body are divided into two groups: the fixed joints, which have limited movement, and the movable joints.

Fixed joints. This is the name given to joints like those between the bones of the skull and the vertebrae of the spine. There is a layer of cartilage between the two bones, binding them together, but not permitting movement to any noticeable extent. In the spine, the result of a long series of little bones with flexible cartilage joints between them is to make the whole spine slightly flexible, but this is not true movement as understood medically.

Movable Joints. To make up a movable joint four different structures are necessary: the two bones, the layer of cartilage which covers the end of each bone, a capsule of fibrous tissue which holds the bones together and, lastly, the lubricating fluid—called *synovial fluid*—which oils the movements of the joint.

Varieties of Joints. Movable joints are divided into groups according to their range of movement. The most freely movable joint is the *ball and socket*—like the hip or shoulder, in which one bone has a rounded head like a ball which fits snugly into a cup-shaped socket in the other bone and allows movement in every direction. Joints in which the movement is mainly in one direction, as in the wrist and ankle, are called *gliding joints. Hinge joints,* which include the knee and the the elbow, move chiefly round one axis like a hinge.

Joints, Diseases of. Joints are very subject to injury and strains, and dislocations are frequent. These injuries always require careful treatment, as when once

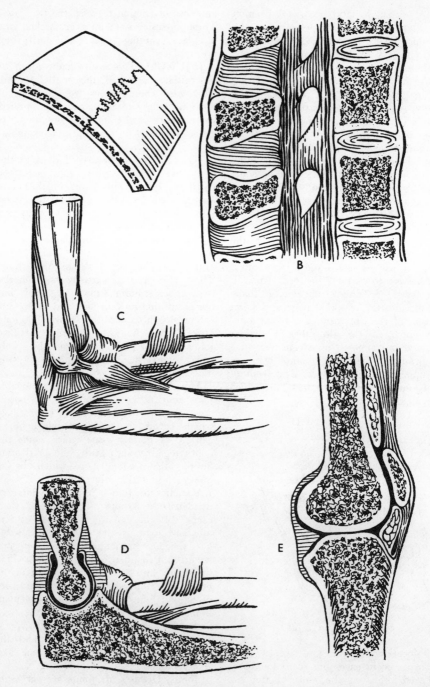

Types of Joints.—A. *Immovable Joint (between bones of skull).* B. *Intervertebral Joints (between the vertebrae of the spine).* C. *Elbow joint (hinge joint) showing ligaments holding bones in place.* D. *Section of elbow joint, showing joint cavity and synovial membrane lining.* E. *Section of knee joint, showing patella, or kneecap, on the right.*

infection gets into the cavity of a joint it is very difficult to treat.

Inflammation of the lining of the cavity of a joint is called synovitis. Inflammation of a joint as a whole is known as arthritis. (*See also* DISLOCATION; ELBOW; KNEE; SYNOVITIS.)

Tuberculous disease of a joint. Tuberculosis may attack a joint and is characterized by a stiff swelling of the joint, which is sometimes called "white swelling." It is much commoner in children than in adults. Hip-joint disease is often tuberculous in origin; gout, rheumatism, rheumatoid and osteoarthritis are all important causes of joint disease and stiffness. Hysterical states affecting such joints as the knee and hip are not uncommon. These diseases will be found described under their own headings. (*See also* TUBERCULOSIS.)

JUGULAR VEIN. There are three large veins on each side of the neck, known as the anterior, external, and internal jugular veins. It is the duty of these veins to carry blood from the head and neck regions to the heart. The most important of the three is the internal jugular vein, which collects the blood from the brain and part of the face and neck. The anterior and external jugulars lie very near the surface of the skin, and wounds of the neck may involve these veins and cause severe bleeding. (*See also* BLEEDING FIRST AID SUPPLEMENT; HEMORRHAGE; NECK.)

JUICE. The fluids produced by organs of the body are popularly called juices. For example, gastric juice is made by the stomach and it contains ferments which are necessary to the proper digestion of protein food and the clotting of milk. Intestinal juice contains ferments which deal with the digestion of carbohydrate foods; while pancreatic juice, by means of its ferments, assists in the digestion of starches and fats. The three types of foodstuffs, carbohydrates, proteins, and fats, are all dealt with and digested in the course of their journey from the mouth. (*See also* DIGESTION; FERMENTS.)

JUNIPER. The juniper is an evergreen shrub from which is obtained an oil not unlike turpentine in smell. The flavor of gin is due to the small quantity of juniper it contains and is responsible for the increased flow of urine familiar to those who take this drink. Juniper was at one time extensively used medicinally for this diuretic effect.

KALA-AZAR. Kala-azar is a tropical disease characterized by enlargement of the spleen, wasting, and intermittent fever. The infection is due to a very tiny parasite which is transmitted to human beings by the bite of a sandfly. The condition seems to flourish in warm, moist climates, especially in parts of India, China, and West Africa. Infantile kala-azar is found along the shores of the Mediterranean.

Symptoms. In some cases the onset of the fever is very suggestive of malaria, while other cases may resemble typhoid fever. The disease usually starts insidiously with a gradually increasing feeling of weakness, and the body becomes wasted in appearance. Diarrhea and sweating may be present, also bleeding from nose and gums. The spleen is enlarged and the temperature very irregular.

Treatment. The morbidity has been greatly lowered by injections of pentavalent antimony or pentamidine in freshly prepared sterile water. An untreated case may go on for as long as two years, when death usually takes place from wasting and weakness, or some septic complication arising directly from this illness.

KAOLIN. Kaolin is also known as china-clay or white clay. It consists mainly of a natural silicate of aluminium which is powdered and freed from gritty particles. It is sometimes used as a protective application in cases of eczema or other skin diseases and it is also used as an ingredient of the modern type of poultice like antiphlogistine. Internally it is an excellent remedy, mixed with water, for diarrhea, food poisoning, and dysentery, one or two tablespoonfuls taken every hour until the symptoms abate.

KELOID. An overgrowth of tissue at the site of a scar is known as a keloid. The scar does not shrink in the ordinary way but tends to remain raised up, and the surrounding tissue becomes wrinkled. The raised surface may be white, but more often it remains pinkish in color. The best way to remove the disfigurement is by exposure to sunlight, X-rays, or radium. Surgical excision may be carried out, but it is quite likely that the fresh scar will also become keloid.

KERATITIS. Inflammation of the part of the eye known as the cornea is termed keratitis. In the form known as interstitial keratitis, there is a gradual mistiness of vision until the entire cornea presents an opaque appearance. Later, blood vessels dilate and the cornea may become cherry-red in color. Another form of this condition is known as keratitis punctata, in which opaque dots make their appearance on the back of the cornea. These dots generally appear in an easily recognized triangular formation. (*See also* CORNEA.)

KERATOSIS. The term keratosis is used to denote any overgrowth of the horny layer of the skin. Ordinary corns or callosities may be looked upon as an exaggerated example of this condition. Keratosis senilis is the term applied to the roughening of the skin which occurs in elderly people. (*See also* CALLUS; CORN; SKIN.)

KETOGENIC DIET. The ketogenic diet was designed for the treatment of epilepsy. It arose from the observation that fits in epilepsy were often lessened by starving the patient and so causing "starvation acidosis;" similar acidosis was brought about, with chemical changes ("ketones" in the urine and breath) by putting the patient on a diet very rich in fats and low in carbohydrates and proteins. It was also found that the increased acidity and the ketones in the urine brought about by this diet stopped the growth of colon bacilli in the urine and so cured infections of the kidney and urinary tract caused by these germs. The diet is still sometimes used for this purpose, though the required acid reaction of the urine can be more simply achieved by drugs such as mandelic acid.

KIDNEYS. The kidneys are a pair of glands placed in the back of the abdomen just below the waistline on either side. Their function is to collect certain waste materials from the blood and the spare water from the tissues in the form of urine. The urine is then passed by way of the two tubes called the ureters to the bladder and thence by the urethra to the exterior. It is obvious, therefore, that the kidneys must be kept in good working order if the body is not to be poisoned with waste materials.

The kidneys are usually described as bean-shaped, being slightly narrower in the middle with bulging ends, much the same shape as a bean. Each kidney is about four inches long, a couple of inches across, and an inch thick. On the inner border there is a crack called the *bilum* where the renal vein and artery and the lymphatic glands and nerves that supply the kidney enter and leave it. The tough coat of fibrous material which covers the kidney is called the *capsule*. The kidney itself is made up of two distinct layers of tissue, the outer being called the *cortex* (bark) and the inner the *medulla*. At the upper portion of each kidney a small gland called the *suprarenal* gland or *adrenal* is attached. These are ductless glands and are of great importance in the correct working of the body. (*See also* DUCTLESS GLANDS.)

Position of the Kidneys. The kidneys lie on each side of the backbone on the back wall of the abodomen under the waistline. As a general rule, the large mass of the liver pushes the right kidney father down into the abdominal cavity than the left kidney. This does not interfere with the working of the organ in normal cases.

Displaced and Floating Kidney. One or both kidneys may become displaced from their normal position, usually as a result of general laxness of the front wall of the abdomen in women who have had several pregnancies. As a general rule the condition causes no inconvenience. Sometimes there is a kidney which is insecurely attached to the neighboring organs, and sudden acute pain with perhaps sickness and faintness may occur from time to time owing to its displacement.

Treatment. Often it is sufficient to change position and the pain passes off.

A great deal of unnecessary fuss is made by nervous people about these so-called floating kidneys. The best cure for them is to fatten up, so that the pads of fat may keep the kidneys more securely anchored. This treatment, unfortunately, is often scorned by the thin, nervous type of person who is the most inclined to worry.

Kidney Diseases. The pain from kidney troubles is felt very typically in the back of the loins, and pressure there will sometimes relieve the pain temporarily. Perhaps the most common disease of the kidneys is the inflammation known as Bright's disease or nephritis. This is described under its own heading. The kidneys are very subject to stones or calculi. The presence of a stone may pass unnoticed until it begins to move and pass towards the bladder, when there may be attacks of excruciating pain as it passes down the narrow ureter. The remedy is to have the stone removed by operation, as it does not pass naturally. Where there is any tendency to kidney stones, the kidneys should be kept well flushed by drinking copious amounts of water between meals. It should be ascertained, as well, whether the water of the district is suitable for kidney cases. In some neighborhoods kidney trouble is much more common than in others, and it is customary to blame the water for the increased number of people who suffer from "stone."

Tuberculosis may affect the kidneys, and if only one is affected it may be removed with benefit to the patient. (*See also* CALCULUS; NEPHRITIS.)

KLEPTOMANIA. This is the name given to a mental state in which the patient is unable to resist the temptation to steal. Very often the articles which are stolen are of little value. The treatment of kleptomania lies in a mental analysis of the individual, and the modern treatment by psychoanalysis may do much to bring to light the underlying motives which cause the impulse to steal. (*See also* PSYCHOANALYSIS.)

KNEE. The knee joint is the joint between the upper and lower bones of the leg, that is, the thighbone or femur, and the shinbone or tibia. The other and smaller bone of the leg, the fibula, does not come into the joint but becomes associated with the shinbone below the knee.

Unlike other joints, the bones that are connected by the knee joint are not fitted into each other. The thighbone has two knobs which rest on flat places on the end of the shinbone. Cartilage covers the ends of the bones, and there is a large pad of fat in front of the joint and a small plate of bone called the kneecap or *patella*. Between the knee and the smaller leg bone, the tibia, there are two pads of cartilage called, from their shape, the *semilunar cartilages*. The strength of the joint depends very largely upon the firm binding of muscular tissues and strong ligaments. Behind the knee the muscles of the leg, coming down the thigh and up the leg, leave a small diamond-shaped space between them called the *popliteal* space.

Movements of the Knee joint. The movements of a normal knee are those of an ordinary hinge joint, with a little additional movement made possible by the fact that the tibia is detached from the joint. When the knee is straightened, the whole leg forms a straight and rigid column, and the tibia, by a separate movement of its own, locks the limb in position. When the knee is bent backwards and forwards it is an ordinary hinge joint, the locking movement of the tibia coming into play only at the moment of the complete straightening of the limb. This complicated mechanism is to provide a strong support for the body's weight. Like other joints, the knee in health is well provided with the lubricating fluid called synovial fluid, which enables easy movement without undue wear and tear.

Diseases and injuries of the knee. The knee is the most complicated joint in the body and it is very difficult to get at it for treatment purposes. As the knee is essential in our movements of walking and sitting, it is obvious that a small injury to it may cause a large amount of disability. The joint may become infected with germs whose rapid spread may cause very serious illness. The diseases that affect other joints of the body also affect the knee joint. These are found under their own headings, such as ARTHRITIS; SYNOVITIS; TUBERCULOSIS.

Injury to the semilunar cartilage causes

a great deal of pain and temporary disablement. It is a very common thing for the semilunar cartilages to be dislocated in games such as football. The kneecap, too, is readily dislocated, but total dislocation of the knee is very rare and is only the result of great violence.

Housemaid's Knee. The condition commonly called housemaid's knee is a swelling of the bursa or sac of fluid in front of the knee. The swelling is due to continual pressure on the bursa caused by kneeling. In order to prevent housemaid's knee it is wise to use a mat when kneeling for any length of time. (*See also* BURSITIS.)

KNEE JERK. If the knees are crossed and a light tap is given with the tips of the fingers on the front of the knee just below the kneecap, the leg is seen to make a sudden jump forward. This is known as the knee jerk. In certain diseases of the nervous system this reaction does not occur, and it is very often of great importance to the doctor when he is making his diagnosis.

KNOCK-KNEE. This is a deformity of the lower limbs medically known as *genu valgum*. When the feet are placed together it will be found that the space separating the ankles is abnormally wide, and as a result the knees knock together when walking. Sometimes the inner part of one knee may be more prominent than the other, but as a rule both knees are equally affected.

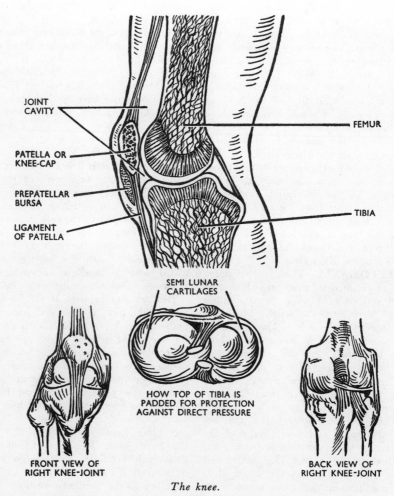

JOINT CAVITY

FEMUR

PATELLA OR KNEE-CAP

PREPATELLAR BURSA

TIBIA

LIGAMENT OF PATELLA

SEMI LUNAR CARTILAGES

HOW TOP OF TIBIA IS PADDED FOR PROTECTION AGAINST DIRECT PRESSURE

FRONT VIEW OF RIGHT KNEE-JOINT

BACK VIEW OF RIGHT KNEE-JOINT

The knee.

In young children, knock-knee is often due to rickets, owing to weight being put upon the soft bones. Prolonged standing in a rapidly growing child will often bring about a condition of flatfoot, resulting in knock-knee. The condition may also be seen in young boys who, in the first place, do not possess a strong constitution, but whose work compels them to carry heavy weights.

Treatment. In young children the treatment is, first, the general treatment for rickets. Exercises and manipulation of the limbs are helpful in young children whose bones have not yet hardened. In more advanced cases splints may need to be worn. In very severe advanced cases, operative treatment is the only cure. (*See also* KNEE.)

KOCH'S BACILLUS. Robert Koch, a German bacteriologist (1843–1910), was the first to discover the germ which causes tuberculosis. After years of patient research work he found that tiny rod-like organisms were present in every case of consumption, and as a result of his discovery many diseases which were then unnamed were able to be classed definitely as tuberculosis. The term is now applied to the tuberculosis germ. (*See also* TUBERCULOSIS.)

KYPHOSIS. Kyphosis means hump-back or curvature of the spine, with the prominent part of the hump directed upwards. A slight form of this condition is more commonly known as round shoulders. This condition is usually due to faulty habits of standing and can easily be corrected by the mother or teacher. It may also be found in rickety children or in children afflicted with adenoids; or sometimes bad eyesight will cause a child to stoop and peer.

In adults, round shoulders may occur in those who have to stoop constantly over their work. Rheumatism, especially rheumatoid arthritis, is a common cause of this condition. When children are born, the spine is shaped in a very definite curve which disappears as growth proceeds, but in old age it is seen that the spine again reverts to its curved position.

Treatment. In young children the defect can be prevented by insisting on correct posture, and by seeing that stooping is avoided when the child is sitting down. Any underlying condition such as rickets, adenoids, or bad eyesight should be given attention, and the general tone of the system should be stimulated by plenty of fresh air, good food, sleep, and sufficient exercise of the right sort. Once curvature of the spine has become established it must be treated regularly and continuously by special remedial exercises.

L ABOR. Labor is the name given to the act of childbirth, and is usually looked upon as divided into three stages. The *first stage* begins with the onset of regular, rhythmic contractions of the muscular walls gradually dilating the mouth of the womb; at first the contractions come on about every quarter of an hour or twenty minutes, but the interval gets shorter and shorter and the contractions become stronger and stronger; this stage may last for 24 hours or more in a woman who is having her first child, but usually lasts a much shorter time in a woman who has previously borne children.

The *second stage* is one in which the mouth of the womb has become fully dilated and the child is being expelled from the womb to the exterior; this stage usually lasts about three or four hours in a first childbirth, but lasts a much shorter time—sometimes only a minute or two—in a woman who has previously had a child; during this stage the contractions become more and more forceful, and it is at this stage that chloroform or another anesthetic is usually administered in those cases which seem to warrant it.

After the child is born the doctor or nurse cuts and ties off the umbilical cord, which connects the navel of the child to the afterbirth or placenta, the structure which is attached to the mother's womb and supplies the infant with nourishing blood while it is still in the womb. The *third stage* of labor consists in the delivery of the afterbirth or placenta, which usually comes away, accompanied by a few slight contractions and some bleeding, within half an hour of the birth of the child.

Complications of Labor. Complications of labor are not very uncommon, the most usual being a "breech presentation" of the child; i.e., the child is born buttocks first, instead of head first. This happens rather less than about once in every twenty labors, and while there is no increased danger to the mother there is an increased danger to the life of the child. Other complications consists in other abnormalities of position of the child, such as a "face presentation" or a "cross-birth," but these are very rare. *Hemorrhage* or bleeding during the third stage of labor, may be unduly severe, and if so, in the absence of expert assistance an attempt should be made to stop it by kneading the womb through the abdominal wall and raising the foot of the bed on a chair; no stimulants should be given. *Convulsions* during or immediately after labor ususally denote "eclampsia," which is a serious complication, requiring immediate attention by a doctor. *Fever* after labor may be due to blood poisoning, and in that case is very serious; a doctor must be called immediately. (*See also* CHILDBIRTH; PREGNANCY.)

LABYRINTH. The labyrinth comprises not only an essential part of the organ of hearing, the internal ear or cochlea, but also the sense organ of balancing, in the three delicate semicircular canals. The labyrinth consists of two parts: the *osseous labyrinth* and the *membranous labyrinth*. The osseous labyrinth is a series of cavities hollowed out of the temporal bone, comprising the vestibule, the semicircular canals and the cochlea. The membranous labyrinth consists of a series of communicating sacs and ducts enclosed within the bony labyrinth, containing within them the delicate sense organs. (*See also* EAR.)

LACERATION. A laceration is a tear in the flesh such as may be produced by injuries from machinery, etc. The more clean-cut type of wound is called an incision and it is not such a complicated type as a laceration. (*See also* WOUND.)

LACHRYMAL APPARATUS. The tears and watery secretions of the eye come from the lachrymal gland which is situated behind the outer part of the upper eyelid. By means of the lachrymal

ducts or canals excess moisture is drained away into the passages of the nose.

LACTATION. Lactation is the period during which the child is suckled at the mother's breast.

LACTEAL VESSELS. The lymphatic vessels of the intestine are referred to as the lacteal vessels because of the milky appearance of their contents. (*See also* DIGESTION; INTESTINE.)

LACTIC ACID. This is a colorless, thickish, sour liquid which is produced by the action of certain germs upon milk. It is in this way that milk becomes sour.

Lactic acid, or soured milk, is very often of use in the treatment of disorders of the intestine, such as diarrhea and colitis.

The lactic acid germs can be procured in suitable tablets for use when required. These are added to freshly-boiled milk which has been allowed to cool, and in a little time a junket will form. This can be eaten with cream and sugar, or with sugar and a little powdered cinnamon or ginger as flavoring. (*See also* MILK.)

LACTOSE. Lactose is the technical name for the sugar of milk.

LAMELLA. A thin small disc or wafer made of gelatin and glycerine which contains an active drug for application to the eye, is known as a lamella. The lamella is placed over the white of the eye, the eye is then closed and the disc allowed to dissolve. The four usual lamellae are those containing atropine, cocaine, homatropine and physostigmine.

LANGUOR. Languor is a state in which the body feels listless, and there is a decided disinclination to take any bodily exercise, or to exert oneself. It may be a symptom of illness and it is often present in anemia and early tuberculosis. After any serious illness, the patient is usually in a languorous state for a week or two during convalescence. A feeling of listlessness may be brought on by lack of fresh air or insufficient sleep, or it may be temporarily produced by overeating or hot weather. If, however, the feeling of languor is a persistent one, a change of surroundings with plenty of fresh air and good food may do much to stimulate the system. (*See also* CONVALESCENCE.)

LANOLIN. A fat obtained from the

wool of the sheep is known as lanolin, and it is a useful and soothing ointment. When rubbed on the skin it is believed to be more quickly absorbed than most fats, and because of this, it forms a basis for other substances such as mercury, etc. It may be kept over a long period of time as it does not turn rancid.

LAPAROTOMY. The operation of cutting through the abdomen for the purpose of dealing with any of the internal organs is technically known as laparotomy.

LARD. Lard is the purified fat of the pig, and it is contained in many ointments; but in India, prepared suet is used in its place. Like lanolin, it penetrates the skin easily and is non-irritating, but it has the disadvantage that it is liable to turn rancid on keeping. Lard is very useful as a cooking fat and is very cheap to buy. (*See also* LANOLIN.)

LARVA. When the egg of an insect hatches out it is called a larva. For example, the egg of the common housefly hatches out into a maggot, and a caterpillar is the larva of the butterfly. This larva is more popularly known as a grub.

LARYNGISMUS STRIDULUS. This is a spasmodic condition of the larynx in which the breath is suddenly caught, followed by a loud crowing noise as the breath comes back. It is most common in children with rickets, but may also occur as a symptom of laryngeal catarrh. (*See also* CROUP.)

LARYNX. The larynx is the organ of speech in man though in primitive beings it was used as a valve to prevent anything other than air from entering. The position of the larynx is at the Adam's apple in front of the neck; it consists of a large *thyroid cartilage* (the part which projects as the Adam's apple), a ring cartilage, or *cricoid* below it, a pair of tiny *anytenoid* cartilages placed on the edge of the cricoid at the back, and the *epiglottis,* which sticks out above the larynx and protects it. Various ligaments bind the cartilages together, and there are several small muscles situated within it which have the important function of moving the vocal cords, under the control of the *recurrent laryngeal nerves,* which are branches of the important *vagus* nerve. The *vocal cords* are tense ligaments at-

tached to the arytenoid cartilages, and as they move to and fro and vibrate, sound is produced by air passing through the space between them.

Larynx, Diseases of. Disease of the larynx usually shows itself first by hoarseness, which may be so marked that the voice completely lost. The usual cause of *acute laryngitis* is the extension downwards of a cold or influenza, and it may be accompanied by severe pain deep in the throat; it is best treated by keeping the patient in bed (if the temperature is raised) and giving him ten grains (two tablets) of aspirin every four hours, also inhalations of compound tincture of benzon (one teaspoonful in a pint of boiling water, the steam being inhaled). *Chronic laryngitis* is usually caused by over-use or bad production of the voice, and happens most often in professional singers, actors or actresses, clergymen, or school teachers. The essential in treating *chronic laryngitis* is to rest the voice—if necessary by keeping silent altogether for a time. Smoking should be avoided. A throat specialist can spray the larynx with weak cocaine or with adrenaline, and paint the vocal cords with weak perchloride of iron solution, weak silver nitrate solution or an oily prepara-

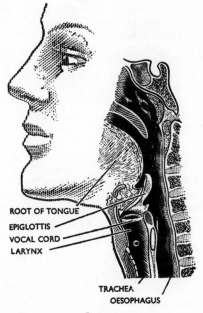

ROOT OF TONGUE
EPIGLOTTIS
VOCAL CORD
LARYNX

TRACHEA
OESOPHAGUS

Larynx.

tion like gomenol; but such methods require special skill and experience.

If a person loses the voice for more than a month the larynx should *always* be examined by a throat specialist; it may only be a simple chronic larygitis, but it may be something more serious, for the larynx is sometimes affected by tuberculosis or by cancer, which can only be treated successfully at an early stage. (*See also* BRONCHITIS; INFLUENZA.)

LASSAR'S PASTE. This is a paste used in the treatment of eczema, etc., composed of salicylic acid, zinc oxide, powdered starch and petroleum jelly. It was named after Oscar Lassar, a German skin specialist. It is a very soothing and antiseptic paste, and other ingredients such as sulphur can be easily added if necessary to meet specific conditions.

LASSITUDE. This indicates a state of weakness or exhaustion, arising from causes other than fatigue. Any source of infection, such as bad teeth or tonsils, or an infection of the ear or nose, may give rise to a state of poisoning which brings with it a decided feeling of weakness. Many diseases which cause changes in the blood, thus bringing on a condition of anemia, will also cause a very great lowering in the vitality and the patient may feel in a permanently exhausted state. This feeling is very promient during the onset of typhoid fever, and again, it is very marked after an attack of influenza. It is also a symptom of certain nervous diseases. (*See also* ANEMIA; DEBILITY; FATIGUE; LANGUOR.)

LAUDANUM. This is a popular name for tincture of opium, though the origin of the name seems to be obscure. It is a drug which should never be given to children as they are very easily poisoned by it. (*See also* OPIUM.)

LAUGHING GAS. Nitrous oxide, which is used as an anethetic for slight operations, was commonly referred to as laughing gas, because of the laughter it may produce in those who inhale it. (*See also* ANESTHETICS.)

LAVAGE. Lavage, from the French word *laver,* to wash, is a term applied to the washing out of the stomach or other organs. This process is carried out in cases where the stomach is dilated owing to fermentation of the food contents, and also in cases when certain poisons have been swallowed, and in various other circumstances. Special rubber tubing is used for this purpose, and the stomach contents are run off by siphonage. Bicarbonate of soda, boric acid or other substances are very often dissolved in the water if required.

Lavage of the bowel is very often carried out in the treatment of colitis by means of irrigation. Lavage of the bladder is carried out in the treatment of chronic cystitis by means of a rubber tube attached to a catheter, which is inserted into the bladder. (*See also* DOUCHE; ENEMA; IRRIGATION.)

LAXATIVES. Laxatives are medicines which produce an action of the bowels, and they are given in the treatment of slight constipation. Aperient is another name for this type of drug, and it is the mildest form of purgative. (*See also* APERIENT; CATHARTIC; CONSTIPATION; PURGATIVE.)

LEAD. The salts of lead are used a great deal in medicine because they have a powerful astringent (drawing together) action on the skin. The most important salts are the acetate, the iodide, and the oxide; the acetate is the only one given internally. Lead acetate is sometimes used in cases of severe diarrhea. The subacetate of lead may be used as a throat gargle, or painted on with glycerine, in cases of relaxed throat.

Solutions of lead salts, when applied to broken skin, to sores, and to ulcers, are particularly beneficial because they form a protective coating over the wound, and they contract the tissues, which helps to stop any further bleeding. Too strong a solution should be avoided as it may do harm by causing irritation; any salt is irritating if used in too concentrated a form. Sugar of lead, which is the name for the dilute solution of subacetate of lead, is used in the treatment of bruises, sprains and any local inflamed part of the skin. Lead can also be used in ointment form for application in diseases of the skin. Diachylon ointment, also know as lead plaster, which contains lead as well as other substances, is very good for chronic eczema, and for relieving itching of the skin.

Lead poisoning. At one time, lead poisoning was very common in industry among people who came in contact with the metal, but government regulations have been introduced which afford a great deal of protection. Nevertheless, chronic poisoning is very liable to affect those who deal with lead, such as lead-smelters, painters, glaziers, plumbers, and so on. On the other hand, lead may be introduced into the system by means of our food or our drinkingwater.

Symptoms. In cases of acute lead poisoning where a large dose of lead has been taken either accidentally or with suicidal intent, the patient suffers from burning in the mouth, vomiting, cramps in the legs, severe pains in the belly, and convulsions. Cases of acute poisoning are rare, but cases of chronic lead poisoning are very common.

In chronic cases, the earliest symptoms are constipation and intestinal colic. The worker complains of lassitude and tiredness, and of vague pains in the arms and shoulders. Cramps may occur in the legs, and he may lose his power of concentration. The lead circulates through the blood and produces a state of anemia which leaves the patient very pale, and the skin takes on a grayish tinge. A blue line may be seen on the gums at the base of the teeth, which is due to lead sulphide being formed by putrefaction in the mouth. Lead very often produces chronic inflammation of the nerves which control the muscles, and any part of the body may be paralyzed. It is very common for the muscles of the hand to be affected in this way, producing a condition known as wrist-drop. Inflammation of the nerves of the eye, or optic neuritis, may be present, and gout is common.

Treatment. In the treatment of lead poisoning the stomach should be emptied by an emetic such as mustard and water. Salts should be taken every four hours until the bowels are thoroughly cleared out. Chronic local poisoning is treated with ammonium chloride. The diet should be controlled by a physician, as it is necessary to regulate the calcium in the system. The anemia which results from the poisoning should be treated with an iron tonic. The intestinal colic is treated by hot fomentations, and if necessary the doctor may give an injection of morphia or some other soothing drug.

After the patient has been cured, he should, if possible, seek employment in some other type of work, especially if there is any sign of a recurrence of the symptoms. In cases of poisoning from contaminated drinking water, every effort must be made to remove the source of the poisoning. (*See also* INDUSTRIAL HYGIENE; OCCUPATIONAL DISEASES.)

LEG. Most people when they refer to the leg include the whole of the lower extremity; but, medically speaking, the leg extends from the knee to the ankle, the upper part of the limb being the thigh. (*See also* ACHILLES' TENDON; BONES; BOWLEG.)

LEG, ARTIFICIAL. *See* article on ARTIFICIAL LIMBS.

LEISHMANIASIS. A group of diseases due to infection with certain parasites known as protozoa of the Leishman-Donovan type is called leishmaniasis. The group includes kala-azar and oriental sore (Aleppo button). In South America the oriental sore is known as espundia, and it is a condition in which ulcers may form inside the mouth and nose as well as on the skin. (*See also* KALA-AZAR.)

LEMON. The juice of the lemon contains a large percentage of citric acid and other acids which are very valuable in preserving the alkalinity of the blood. It will be found that many people who suffer from indigestion obtain great relief after taking the unsweetened juice of a fresh lemon. This occurs when indigestion is due to overacidity of the stomach, which is immediately rendered alkaline by the lemon juice. The lemon also contains Vitamin C which is used in the prevention and cure of scurvy.

LENS. The lens of the eye, which is situated behind the pupil, acts, by the bulging or flattening brought about by the ciliary muscle, by focusing objects at varying distances upon the retina. Over the age of about 40 it begins to lose its power of focusing and spectacles may be needed to help it. The disease called cataract is due to the lens becoming hardened and opaque. (*See also* Eye; Spectacles.)

LEPROSY. Leprosy is a chronic wasting disease caused by a germ which affects the skin, mucous membranes, and nerves, and results in mutilations and deformities. It is infectious, and though nowadays rare in the U.S., is still found in many other countries.

Symptoms. Its onset is insidious, four-fifths of the cases taking any time up to five years to develop. The patient may have intermittent attacks of fever, with aching of the bones, headache, and sometimes nose-bleeding. Finally, the spots on the skin, by which the disease can be recognized, appear. There are two types, the nodular and the maculoanesthetic (macula, a spot), which are often found together.

The nodular form appears as little yellowish brown lumps or nodes, generally on the face, the backs of the hands and wrists, and the feet and legs. The nodes grow in number and size, and spread, until the face assumes a hideous, lion-like appearance. The mucous membranes of the mouth, nose, and throat are also affected, and the eyes. The voice becomes hoarse, and breathing may be difficult. The fingers and toes are first deformed and later drop off. This form generally lasts about 8 or 9 years, and ends fatally.

The maculoanesthetic type is much milder. It appears as reddish-brown spots usually on the back and the limbs. At first there is increased sensitiveness and neuralgic pains, but as the disease progresses, anesthesia of the affected skin develops. The hair and nails come off, the fingers and toes amputate, and the muscles shrink. This form may last 10, 20, or 30 years, and may pass into the nodular form and end fatally, or, quite commonly, recover, though the patient may be only a miserable remnant of a human being.

Treatment. The treatment is still on the whole unsatisfactory, and too large and too frequent treatments with special drugs may do more harm than good. Many remedies have been tried, the most useful being chaulmoogra oil, hydnocarpus, promine

and other sulphones, and sustained injections of Vitamin B_1.

Remedies may be given to help such symptoms as ulceration, but surgical methods are often required. The most important thing, however, is to *prevent* the spread of the disease by raising the standard of personal and household hygiene, and to recognize early cases as soon as possible.

LESION. A lesion is a wound, injury, or sore which causes changes to take place in the tissues of the skin. In many diseases the first symptoms are recognized by lesions on the skin.

LETHARGY. This is a condition of drowsiness or stupor which may be due to disease or physical fatigue. The most prominent disease which induces this feeling of drowsiness is encephalitis lethargica. (*See also* Coma; Fatigue; Lassitude.)

LEUCOCYTE. The colorless or white cells of the blood are known as leucocytes. By means of microscopic examination (after staining with certain dyes), it is possible to pick out the different varieties of white cells, or corpuscles, as they are called. All leucocytes are able to move about, and they are formed in the lymphatic tissues (lymphocytes) and in bone marrow. The normal number of leucocytes in a healthy person is from 7,000 to 8,000 per cubic millimeter of blood (i.e., in a space the size of a pin's head) and very important information can be gained by noticing changes in the proportions either one way or the other. An increase in the number of white cells in the blood is called leucocytosis, and a lessening of the number is technically referred to as leucopenia.

LEUCOCYTOSIS. This term means an increase in the number of white cells in the blood. In health this occurs after every meal and after taking a cold bath or exercise. In children it is normal to find more leucocytes in the blood, especially in the first few days of life, and the same pertains in pregnancy. Leucocytosis is not a disease, but it is an indication that the blood is in a state of defense, ready to do battle and attack any invading germs of disease. The leucocytes, or white cells, do not live in the tissues but are found in the blood vessels; yet when any septic or inflammatory condition arises, the leucocytes find their way to the spot and begin their job of destroying the invading germs. As soon as these leucocytes leave the blood vessels, the bone-marrow immediately begins to manufacture a fresh supply. During many acute infective diseases the number is largely increased.

This protective habit which the body has developed of rushing white cells to the area of septic infection gives a great deal of aid to the doctor in diagnosis. For instance, an abscess may form in the abdomen where it cannot readily be examined, but the examination of a drop of blood may point out the necessity of an operation. There are a few conditions in which the blood does not respond and manufacture fresh white cells, such as typhoid fever, measles, mumps, malaria and influenza, but if any increase in the number is found to be present, it is an almost sure indication that there is an infection or abscess forming in some part of the body.

LEUCODERMA. A condition of the skin in which whitish patches appear is known as leucoderma. There may be no obvious cause for the condition; on the other hand, it may result from other skin diseases, or syphilis. The white patches are due to absence of coloring matter (pigment) in the skin. If a patch of leucoderma develops on the scalp, the hair growing on that area loses its color, and the same applies to the hair on any part of the body where these whitish patches appear. The condition is incurable and treatment is not very satisfactory, but much can be done to hide the white patches with the aid of cosmetics. (*See also* ALBINISM.)

LEUCOPENIA. A decrease in the number of white cells in the blood is known as leucopenia. This occurs normally in old age, and it also occurs after long exposure to cold or heat, and particularly after prolonged starvation. It is also met with in tuberculosis, influenza, typhoid fever, and malaria. A degree of leucopenia is found in splenic anemia and pernicious anemia. Exposure to X-rays or radium leads to a destruction of the blood-forming tissues, so it is important that technicians as well as patients undergoing a course of treatment should be examined at frequent intervals. Many drugs used in medicine are known to depress the formation of white blood cells. The sulphonamides, amidopyrine, and thiouracil are well known to have this effect, and their use needs expert supervision.

LEUCORRHEA. Any discharge which comes from the female genital passage which is not blood is termed leucorrhea. It is usually of a whitish color and is more commonly referred to as "the whites." The condition may occur in females of all ages.

In children, there may be inflammation and redness around the opening of the front passages as well as a discharge. The condition is usually caused by lack of cleanliness, or irritation from threadworms. Fortunately, the condition is easily cleared up. The parts must be thoroughly washed several times a day for a few days with some antiseptic lotion. Boric acid will be found very soothing, or a solution containing enough potassium permanganate to color the water a faint red, may be used with good results.

In adults, unless the discharge is excessive, no special treatment is necessary, but the general health should receive attention. The condition may be associated with rheumatism or anemia, and once these conditions are attended to, the discharge may completely clear up. The bowels must be regulated, as constipation tends to aggravate the condition.

It is always advisable for anyone suffering from a distressing discharge to consult a doctor as soon as possible and have a local examination carried out so that the right sort of treatment, local and internal, can be instituted

Treatment. When the discharge is due to weakness and debility much can be done by toning up the system with iron, proper diet and fresh air. It is important that the bowels should be regulated, and a soothing douche carried out every day to cleanse the parts will be found very beneficial. At least a quart of water should be used to each douche, and antiseptic substances such as potassium permanganate (sufficient to tint the water a pink color), boric acid, hydrogen peroxide, or tannic acid may be added to the water. If the condition is very severe or due to some definite disease, these measures will not effect a cure, and some special form of treatment may have to be carried out under the doctor's orders.

LEUCOTOMY, PREFRONTAL. A surgical operation for division of certain nerve fibers in the front of the brain, is called prefrontal leucotomy. It is also called frontal lobotomy. This sometimes transforms an unstable (or even maniacal) patient into a dull but useful and reliable individual.

LEUKEMIA. This is a serious disease in which there is a persistent increase in the white cells of the blood. There are many other symptoms which accompany this condition, such as enlargement of the spleen and changes in the marrow of the bones, or enlargement of the lymph glands all over the body. There are two main types: lymphatic leukemia and myeloid leukemia, according to the type of white cell present in the blood. The cause of the disease is not known and the diagnosis depends on a microscopic examination of the blood.

Myeloid leukemia usually occurs after the age of twenty. The onset is very insidious and the condition may be quite advanced before it is noticed. Sometimes the enlarged spleen attracts attention by causing enlargement of the abdomen, but there are few cases that come under observation in the early stages. The changes in the blood are so characteristic that a diagnosis can often be made after a single examination. The leucocytes in the blood increase enormously in number. Hemorrhages may occur from the gums and nose or sometimes from the stomach and other sites.

Lymphoid leukemia is a much rarer disease, which appears to affect middle-aged or elderly people. The symptoms are very similar to myeloid leukemia, but enlargement of the lymphatic glands is often the first symptom which attracts attention. Examination of the blood shows a very increased number of the leucocytes, consisting almost entirely of lymphocytes (*see* article on LEUCOCYTE). No cure for leukemia is at present known. The synthetic steroids prednisone and prednisolone sometimes bring about temporary improvement, and blood transfusions may help for a time. (*See also* ANEMIA; LEUCOCYTE.)

LEUKOPLAKIA. A condition in which there are whitish patches on the surface of the tongue and inside the cheek is known as leukoplakia. It usually affects middle-aged or rather elderly men, and although the cause of the disease is unknown, it is thought to be due to excessive smoking or spirit drinking. As the condition advances, these raised-up patches may cause a considerable amount of pain, and the mouth and throat become dry. The disease is important because it very often leads to cancer. Antiseptic mouth washes should be used, and some cases have been satisfactorily treated with radium.

LEVATOR. Any muscle whose action is to raise or elevate a part of the body is termed a levator. For instance, with the help of the levator anguli oris we are able to raise the mouth when we smile, and there are many such muscles all over the face which alter our expression. (*See also* FACE.)

LICHEN PLANUS. Lichen planus is an inflammation of the skin and mucous membranes characterized by papules or pimples. On the skin these favor the flexures or "bends," especially the wrists, the thighs, above the knee, and the back of the neck. They are grouped into irregular, ringed, or linear patches. The pimples are flat, small, shiny, and mauve in color. Older patches are brownish and scaly, except at the margins, where the characteristic pimples are seen. Several varieties of the disease are described. It is found equally among men and women, and most often in middle life.

The patient often feels very ill, though feverish symptoms are rare. His chief complaint is itching, which may be so severe as (literally) to drive him nearly mad. At times this seems to be out of all proportion to the small area of skin affected.

The cause of the disease is unknown. Some experts say that nervous strain is a factor in its production. The outlook varies, some cases recovering rapidly, others, more commonly, are prolonged. A widespread case may take six months; the patchy variety, especially on the legs, may persist for years.

Treatment. The internal treatment is principally by arsenic and mercury, in the former cases with great care as to dosage. These cure successfully in many cases. An ointment containing carbolic acid and mercury perchloride is often very helpful; it tends to prevent the severe itching. X-rays in careful hands give good results. The diet should be simple, and alcohol and tobacco avoided.

LIGAMENT. A ligament is a structure which serves to bind together the bones at the joints. Some ligaments are made of white fibrous tissue which, although they are unstretchable, are so arranged as to allow free movement. Other ligaments, formed of yellow elastic tissue, are able to stretch, and are found in those parts of the body where a considerable amount of movement is required. For example, these elastic ligaments serve to bind the back parts of the vertebrae and are stretched when we bend forward, and their tension helps the muscles to straighten the back from the stooping position. If undue strain is put upon the muscles, the ligaments then come in for their share of the strain, which often causes them to be torn or ruptured. The term ligament is also used in connection with certain folds of the peritoneum which bind various internal organs together; for example, there is the ligament of the liver, also the ligament of the womb. *(See also* JOINT.*)*

LIGATURE. When a blood vessel is cut, the thread-like material which the surgeon uses to tie it together is called a ligature. The material used for ligatures is usually catgut, but for very fine vessels, linen thread or silk may be employed. *(See also* CATGUT.*)*

LIGHT TREATMENT; ARTIFICIAL SUNLIGHT. The sun is not only the source of all light, but also maintains all animal and vegetable life.

In 1893 the genius of a Danish doctor, Niels Finsen, gave to the world the first artificial source of ultraviolet rays. In November, 1895, he began to treat his first patient by means of his electric carbon arc lamp. The case was one of long-standing lupus (tuberculosis) of the face, and in four months was completely cured.

Since Finsen's epoch-making discovery much progress has been made. Modern *mercury-vapor, tungsten,* and other lamps are richer in ultraviolet rays than actual sunlight—as it reaches this earth—and are also poorer in certain other rays, which are not beneficial. Furthermore, the different types of lamp give off invisible rays in different proportions, one type being more suitable than another for a particular case.

Indications for Light Treatment. Light treatment has become the recognized treatment for certain diseases and a help in treatment for certain diseases and a help in treatment of many others.

Artificial ultraviolet rays must never be given except on medical advice and under medical supervision.

The following is a list of the principal conditions in which ultraviolet rays are used.

Tuberculosis. For all forms of tuberculosis, *except* of the lungs (phthisis), ultraviolet rays, natural or artificial, are often useful.

Chilblains (pernio). Along with electrical treatment, twice-weekly general body and local light treatment is given.

Bronchitis. The general raising of the body's resistance to infection explains the improvement brought about by light treatment in cases of chronic bronchitis. The amount of phlegm in the throat is lessened, the cough becomes less troublesome, and thereby the sleep less disturbed.

Whooping Cough. This disease may benefit very much indeed by light treatment. The fits of coughing become rarer and milder. Children are less irritable, eat and sleep better, and gain weight.

Diseases of Nutrition. *Rickets.* Ultraviolet radiation is now an acknowledged treatment for this disease. There is improvement in sleep, color, appetite, activity, and general fitness, probably due to an increase of calcium and phosphorus in the blood. The children gain height and weight, and marked improvement of the bony structures is shown by the X-rays.

Some authorities advise light baths for the expectant and nursing mothers, in view of the heavy calcium demand during this period.

Diseases of the Skin. The powerful germ-killing action of the ultraviolet rays is used with excellent results in such diseases as *alopecia, eczema, erysipelas, impetigo,* and *ringworm.* Light treatment is also successful in treating septic wounds, ulcers, boils, and carbuncles. Its outstanding success in *lupus* has already been mentioned.

Diseases in which the treatment should

not be used. Light treatment should *not be given* in the following cases.

Albinos. Owing to the absence of melanin there is no protection against an overdose.

Pulmonary Tuberculosis. Radiation is likely to induce hemoptysis (spitting of blood) and increases the activity of the disease.

Radiant Heat. So far we have been chiefly concerned with the properties of the ultraviolet rays, but the infrared rays, occurring at the other end of the spectrum, are also used in medicine.

Ordinary glass, which does not allow the ultraviolet rays to pass, allows the infrared, or heat rays, to pass. Special lamps for this treatment are not, therefore, needed.

The treatment consists of local or general light baths with a number of incandescent electric lights. These are of suitable size and shape for different parts of the body.

Local treatment is beneficial in synovitis, muscular rheumatism, and sciatica.

X-rays. X-rays are used for the treatment of such parasitic diseases as ringworm and favus, and for destroying tumors. They are also used with ultraviolet rays in cases of stubborn ulcers and similar lesions, and in such skin diseases as acne and eczema, and to help to get rid of the disfiguring scars left by boils and carbuncles. (*See also* X-RAYS.)

LIGHTNING. The effect of lightning is similar to that of a severe electric shock. A person may be killed immediately, or he may escape with his life but be severely burned or paralyzed. There is a case on record where a man was struck by lightning while crossing a field and every bit of his clothing was torn, even his boots, but he himself was quite unhurt and had no mark of any kind on his body. (*See* SPECIAL SUPPLEMENT ON FIRST AID, at the end of this book.)

LIME. Lime is often referred to as calcium, and it is present in the body, especially in the bones and teeth. There is a small amount in the tissues and blood, and it is essential for the maintenance of life. Prepared chalk or calcium carbonate is used extensively as a dusting powder, and also for making up tooth powders.

Slaked lime, or calcium hydroxide, has been used in the form of Vienna paste to destroy warts. Lime water mixed with olive oil or linseed oil is known as carron oil, used in the treatment of burns. Lime water is also given to infants along with their bottle as it makes the milk more digestible. (*See also* CALCIUM.)

LINCTUS. Any thick syrupy medicine which has to be licked off the spoon is described as a linctus. Most of these medicines have honey or molasses as a basis and they are generally given as cough mixtures.

LINIMENT. Liniments, or embrocations, are preparations intended for application to the skin by rubbing. They are usually of an oily nature, which enables them to be absorbed, thus helping to remove pain and stiffness. One of the better known liniments for relieving pain is made up with aconite, belladonna and chloroform. It is known as chloroform liniment, and is popular for neuralgia, rheumatism, etc. Iodine liniment is applied to swollen joints, and opium liniment may be used to relieve various painful conditions. Liniment of ammonia, more popularly known as oil of hartshorn, is also good for painful conditions, and turpentine and the acetic liniment of turpentine, along with camphor, croton oil, ammoniated camphor, soap, are all excellent liniments for stimulating the skin.

LINSEED. The seeds of the common flax give us an oil known as linseed oil which is sometimes used in the treatment of burns. A linseed poultice may be applied to relieve pain, but the poultices should be smeared with oil to prevent their sticking to the skin. A mixture of equal parts of linseed oil and lime water forms carron oil, which is a favorite treatment for burns.

LINT. Lint is made from linen cloth which has been scraped on one side so that it presents a fluffy appearance. When applied to wounds, the smooth surface should always be next to the skin as it is less likely to stick. Boric lint is commonly used for dressing cuts and sores. Lint is also a useful way of applying ointments to the skin, and here again, the smooth side should be undermost.

LIPOMA. Lipoma is the name given

to tumors which are largely composed of fat. These tumors may be found in any part of the body, but they seldom give rise to any trouble beyond that connected with their size and position. (*See also* TUMORS.)

LIPS, DISEASE OF. Cheilitis glandularis, or inflammation of the red lips, is not a very common disease, but most troublesome when it occurs. The lower lip is the one chiefly affected, but both are involved. The mucous glands swell, and form small blisters, which vary in size from a pinhead to a rice-grain. When pricked they discharge mucus, or a mixture of mucus and pus. In the latter case, especially, the lips become much thickened and tend to turn out.

The disease is due to various causes. Sometimes, not very commonly, it seems to spread from a skin disease on the face, as in dermatitis of the upper lip due to chronic nasal catarrh; sometimes chronic pyorrhea (q.v.) will cause it; and sometimes a dentifrice, generally containing carbolic acid or salol, which happens not to suit that particular person, produces a preliminary irritation which merges into the disease.

Treatment. In these obvious cases the treatment is simple, but in other cases the cause cannot be found, and the local condition alone can be treated. Some recommend potassium iodide internally, frequent gargling with potassium chlorate, and a *mild* cauterizing of the lips with silver nitrate or the thermocautery. It is generally found, however, that cheilitis is most rebellious to treatment, and none but the most active and persistent measures seem to do any good. The most successful method, so far, appears to be to apply pure carbolic acid, twice weekly, to the lips, taking care not to allow the acid to touch other parts. This application should, of course, be made only by the doctor in charge of the case.

LIQUOR AMNII. More commonly known as "the waters," liquor amnii is the fluid which surrounds the child in the womb. The average amount of this fluid is about a quart, and it serves to protect the child from injury. (*See also* LABOR.)

LICORICE. Licorice is obtained from the root and underground stem of a plant which is grown extensively along the shores of the Mediterranean. Licorice powder is a popular laxative, and is very suitable for children or for women during pregnancy. Licorice also disguises the taste of other preparations, especially that of aloes, cascara, Epsom salts, and other bitter substances. It is very soothing for cases of sore throat, and many sweets are made containing licorice which are useful for relieving a cough.

LITHOTOMY. The operation known as lithotomy literally means cutting for stone. This operation is one of the oldest in medical history, and it appears that stone in the bladder must have been a very common condition a few centuries ago.

LITMUS. Litmus is a blue vegetable dye which is obtained from various species of lichen, and it is employed for determining the presence of acids and alkalis. Litmus paper when steeped in an alkaline solution becomes blue, and with acid fluids, turns red.

LIVER. The liver is the largest gland in the body, weighing somewhere around three and a half pounds, and measuring about twelve inches from side to side and six inches at its thickest part. It lies on the right side of the abdominal cavity and is dark brown in color and solid to the touch. The upper part, which is rounded in shape, fits in and fills up the dome of the diaphragm, and its weight is supported by the other organs in the abdomen upon which it rests. The liver may be looked upon as the great storehouse of the body where chemical substances derived from the food are stored to be liberated as the need arises. For example, when an increase of energy is required, the liver gets busy and manufactures energy-giving substances out of the digested food, especially any kind of sugary or starchy foods.

If the diet is excessive or ill-balanced, the storage power of the liver may become overtaxed, especially if no exercise is taken to allow the liver to use up the extra sugar, etc. The liver also manufactures bile, which is an important substance in aiding digestion. Disturbance of the workings of the bile ducts causes the condition known as jaundice, which is dealt with under its own heading. (*See also* CIRRHOSIS OF THE LIVER; DIGESTION; GALL BLADDER.)

LIVERISH FEELING. A popular term to describe the feeling of depression accompanied by headache which is very often the result of overeating or overdrinking.

Treatment. A good dose of salts first thing in the morning and plenty of fresh air and exercise will do much to get rid of the depressed feeling.

LOBE. A rounded part of an organ which is subdivided from the neighboring parts is termed a lobe, such as the lobes of the liver or of the brain. The lowest part of the ear, which is soft and rounded, is known as the lobe or lobule of the ear.

LOBECTOMY. Removal of a lobe of a lung is being done successfully for disease confined to one part of the lung, such as chronic lung abscess, early cancer of the lung, and bronchiectasis. (*See also* BRONCHIECTASIS; LUNG.)

LOCHIA. The discharge which takes place from the womb during the first week or two after childbirth is known as lochia. During the first four days the discharge is usually composed of blood. On the fifth day it becomes brownish in color, and later it changes until it becomes almost whitish in appearance. If the red blood continues for any length of time or if there is any putrid odor connected with the discharge, medical advice should be sought, as it is usually the result of infection or a retained fragment of afterbirth. (*See also* LABOR.)

LOCKJAW. Lockjaw is the popular name for tetanus, which is a serious disease caused by infection with a germ found in contaminated soil. (*See also* TETANUS.)

LOCOMOTOR ATAXIA. *See* TABES DORSALIS.

LOIN. The loin is the part of the back which lies between the last rib and the top of the pelvis. Pain is felt in this part of the body during an attack of lumbago and in some forms of kidney disease.

LONG SIGHT. Medically known as hypermetropia, this condition is discussed under that heading.

LORDOSIS. When the spine is unnaturally curved forward the condition is known as lordosis. This condition may be due to poor muscular development or to weakness of the back caused by disease. It is present in a slight degree during pregnancy. (*See also* SPINAL CURVATURE.)

LOTION. Preparations which are used on the skin or for bathing wounds, etc., are known as lotions. The drugs are usually mixed with water or alcohol, and those of an oily nature are known as liniments. The most important type of lotion is the antiseptic one which may be made up from various drugs. Solutions of boric acid or carbolic acid are very commonly used. Lotions containing zinc or calamine are excellent for bathing all sorts of raw surfaces and ulcers, and it is a good application for many varieties of eczema and other skin diseases. Astringent lotions which draw the tissues together are much used nowadays in beauty preparations.

The best way to apply antiseptic lotions is to use a piece of lint. The lint should be wrung out of the lotion and applied with the smooth side next to the skin; and in order to prevent the antiseptic lotion from evaporating, the lint should be covered with a piece of oiled silk and a wad of cotton wool and the whole kept in place with a bandage or sticking plaster. Lotions such as hydrogen peroxide, etc., which are used to cleanse wounds, should be gently squeezed over the parts by means of cotton wool or lint. Gentle wiping with the lint or cotton wool dipped in the lotion is excellent for removing clots of blood or pus from a wound. Soothing lotions and cooling lotions are applied to inflamed and irritated parts, and it is best to use a piece of lint for the purpose. A very soothing eye lotion is made from weak zinc sulphate or boric acid and it should be applied by means of a proper eye bath. (*See also* BORIC ACID; EYE BATH.)

LOUSE. *See* HEAD LOUSE.

LOZENGE. Lozenges, also known as troches or cough-drops, are solid tablets containing drugs mixed with sugar and gum and flavored with some sort of fruit-paste such as blackcurrant. They are popular for the treatment of affectations of the mouth and throat, and as they are gently sucked the drug which they contain comes in contact with the affected parts. This method of treatment is especially good for children, as it is very difficult for them to gargle properly. Some of the substances most commonly used in lozenges for this purpose are penicillin, potassium chlorate, menthol, and carbolic acid. Lozenges made up with bicarbonate of soda and peppermint are convenient for carrying about in cases of indigestion.

LUMBAGO. In this affection, pain and stiffness are felt in the muscles of the small of the back. Men are more liable to attacks than women, and the condition may be brought on by exposure to wet and cold. Any bending or turning may be extremely painful; in fact, some patients may find that to sneeze or cough is a disastrous experience. Lumbago may also be caused by strain or injury or it may be due to a "slipped disc."

Treatment. If the pain is at all severe, the patient should remain in bed and be kept as warm as possible with hot water bottles placed near the back. Massage or vigorous rubbing with a liniment will help to relieve the pain. Turkish baths are good in slight cases, and aspirin tablets, not more than two at a time, will be found very soothing. The bowels should be kept open with suitable medicine. (*See also* RHEUMATISM.)

LUMBAR REGION. The part of the body which is most commonly called the small of the back is medically known as the lumber region.

LUMINAL. This is a proprietary name for the well-known sedative phenobarbital, which requires a doctor's prescription.

LUNGS. The lungs are structures which are among the most essential to life. There is a left lung and a right lung, situated in the thorax with the heart between them, and they are protected by the ribs. The function of the lungs is breathing or respiration, which means the interchange of the gases between the body and the atmosphere in which it lives. Air passes down the throat to the trachea or windpipe into the lungs, along the tubes called bronchi; these divide and subdivide into little bronchioles, the smallest of which

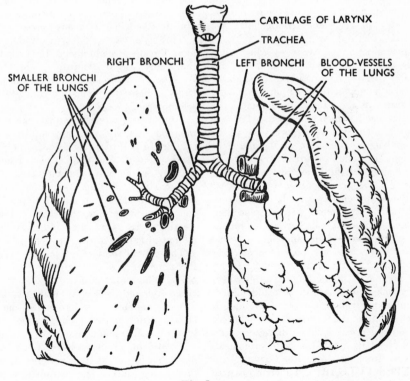

CARTILAGE OF LARYNX

TRACHEA

RIGHT BRONCHI   LEFT BRONCHI   BLOOD-VESSELS OF THE LUNGS

SMALLER BRONCHI OF THE LUNGS

The Lungs.

are tiny tubes less than a hundredth of an inch wide, and ending in little air sacs called "alveoli;" these alveoli are made of a delicate membrane covered by blood capillaries (the smallest blood-vessels), and so delicate are the microscopic walls of the alveoli and the capillaries that the blood can take up oxygen from the air in the avleoli and the air can take up carbonic acid gas and other impurities from the blood.

The lungs have a special blood circulation of their own, quite distinct from the circulation of the blood in the other parts of the body. From the right ventricle of the heart goes the pulmonary artery, filled with dark venous blood, and divides into two branches, one of which goes to each lung. The blood goes all over the lung in smaller and smaller blood vessels, until it reaches the microscopically small capillaries; then occurs the exchange of gases with the air already described.

The right lung is in three divisions, or lobes, and the left one (which is smaller, because of the heart being more on the left side) in two lobes. Both lungs are covered with a delicate moist membrane, the pleura, and the cavity in which they lie is also covered with a similar membrane, so that when the lung expands or contracts it moves freely within this cavity.

Diseases of the Lungs. Inflammation of the lung itself, which is caused by two or three different kinds of germs, is called *pneumonia;* inflammation of the lining of the lung is called *pleurisy; bronchitis* is inflammation of the lining of the air tubes or bronchi; *bronchopneumonia* is a kind of pneumonia which has spread from a bronchitis and is of a more "patchy" type than a *lobar* pneumonia, which is an inflammation of the lung tissue affecting a whole lobe or more than one lobe; *bronchiectasis* is a disorder of the smaller bronchi found most commonly at the lung bases in which the bronchial walls are dilated and subject to repeated infection. *Cancer* of the lung is more common than used to be believed, and modern research shows that there is no doubt about its association with prolonged, excessive smoking. (*See also* CANCER.)

LUPUS VULGARIS. Tuberculosis may attack the skin in various ways, producing

several distinct varieties of the disease.

Lupus vulgaris is the most common type. It is characterized by reddish-brown patches, composed of tiny nodules (called "apple-jelly" from their appearance) embedded in inflamed skin. The disease is destructive, causing ulceration and scarring. It tends to heal at one place and spread at another.

It usually begins in childhood, especially on the face and neck. In clean people, the disease may remain at this simple stage for years, only very slowly spreading. In the great majority of cases, however, the patches become infected with other organisms, and a crusted discharging eruption then results.

Later, ulceration takes place, with underlying infection of the lymph-glands, bones and other parts. The ulcers are irregular, deep, and do not heal. The nose and the lobes of the ears are commonly attacked by the disease and gradually "nibbled away." On the hands and feet, and about the genitals, deformities are likewise caused. The mucous membranes are also attacked in very many cases.

This type, when neglected, produces the most terrible disfigurement. It is supposed that many cases of "leprosy" of the Middle Ages were in reality lupus. Nowadays, badly disfigured patients are comparatively seldom seen.

Fibroid and *warty lupus* are also common varieties, and their appearance is very similar. In both there is a hard overgrowth of tissue, with few nodules, occurring especially on the limbs and buttocks.

Lupus Cancer is an occasional and very serious complication of simple lupus. It is caused by the prolonged use of X-rays in treatment. Its appearance and treatment is as that of cancer of the skin (q.v.).

The general outlook of lupus is exactly the same as that of tuberculosis of other parts. Where the patient lives a healthy, clean life and perseveres with treatment, which must often be prolonged, he has an excellent chance of cure, though some scarring will remain.

Treatment. Preliminary treatment varies somewhat in the different varieties. Crusted discharging ulcers are scraped with a "sharp spoon," followed by the constant use of an antiseptic ointment. Fibroid lupus is removed by blistering fluid and other caustics. Warty lupus is treated as warts (q.v.). After this, the aim of treatment is to destroy the tubercle organism.

Ultraviolet ray treatment by "sunlight lamps," the Finsen and Kromayer light methods, and radium and carbon dioxide snow for small areas are all excellent, the first especially so.

Remarkable cures have been effected in many cases by giving massive doses of calciferol or Vitamin D by mouth or by injection. But on the whole this has now been superseded by the usual specific treatment for tuberculosis elsewhere—i.e., streptomycin with PAS and isoniazid. Even without local treatment, the disease usually becomes arrested in a short time.

LUPUS ERYTHEMATOSUS. This skin disorder bears a resemblance at first glance to the more serious condition lupus vulgaris, but they bear no causal relationship to each other. Both conditions nearly always start on the face and there the resemblance ends.

The cause of lupus erythematosus is not known with certainty. It appears to be one of the allergic diseases in which the individual is unduly sensitive to some damaging agent which would not give rise to any reaction in a normal person. The agent to which these subjects are allergic is usually a bacterial toxin (a poison produced by disease germs) and the commonest infections to give rise to lupus erythematosus are tuberculosis and streptococcal infections. It is well known that the disease often appears for the first time after exposure to strong sunlight or the administration of sulphonamides or antibiotics, or to strong emotional stress.

The disease usually appears as a small red scaly patch on the face which extends slowly at the edges while healing at the center. It may affect the scalp, resulting in the loss of hair, and the fingers are frequently involved. Rarely the disease takes on an acute generalized form in which the patient is severely ill and may indeed die. Unlike lupus vulgaris there is no actual destruction of tissue in this disease.

Treatment is directed at the cause, if one can be found. Nowadays the treatment of choice are the steroids, especially large doses of prednisolone, even though this may give rise to side-effects.

LYMPH. The fluid which circulates through the lymphatic vessels of the body is known as lymph. This fluid is the watery portion of the blood which is filtered through the walls of the capillaries. The term lymph is also used to describe the serum obtained from the blood of calves which is used for vaccination. (*See also* DUCTLESS GLANDS; SERUM; VACCINATION.)

LYMPHATIC SYSTEM. The *lymph* is a clear fluid, derived from the blood, which nourishes the cells of the body and collects waste products from them. It circulates in the chinks between the microscopic cells which build up the different structures of the body, and these unite to form tiny vessels, which in turn unite to form larger vessels rather like small veins and, like them, have valves which prevent any back-flow. The lymph vessels pass through groups of lymph glands in different parts of the body, which act as filters to the lumpy circulation, and keep back germs and impurities from the blood-stream. Eventually the lymph vessels unite into larger vessels which discharge the lymph in the jugular veins at the root of the neck. Besides acting as filters the lymph glands manufacture lymph cells, which form part of the corpuscles of the blood. The *thoracic duct* is the largest lymph vessel in the body, which collects, in addition to lymph from the limbs and chest, the digested fluids absorbed from the stomach and intestines.

LYSIS. This means the gradual ending of a disease, especially of a fever. This gradual decline is typical of enteric fever or typhoid, in which the temperature falls each day until it reaches normal. The opposite of lysis is crisis, in which there is a sudden ending of the disease, the temperature returning to normal within a few hours.

LYSOL. Lysol is obtained from coal tar and it is a powerful antiseptic. Lotions made up with lysol are used for cleansing the skin or for vaginal douches. The usual strength is about a teaspoonful of lysol to a pint of warm water, but stronger solutions may be used if necessary. It is excellent for washing wounds or sores and can be used externally as an antiseptic whenever required. It should never be applied to the eyes or taken internally.

Should lysol be swallowed accidentally, the stomach should be washed out by a doctor and then white of egg or olive oil should be administered as an antidote. (*See also* CRESOL.)

McBURNEY'S POINT. This is a spot on the abdominal wall midway between the navel and the point of the haunch bone on the right side. In appendicitis, the point of tenderness usually lies directly underneath McBurney's point. (*See also* APPENDICITIS.)

MACULA. This term means a spot. A freckle, port-wine stain or any such spot may be called a macula. The *maula lutea* is the yellow spot in the retina of the eye. (*See also* BIRTHMARKS; EYE; FRECKLE.)

MADURA FOOT. Madura foot or fungus foot is a tropical disease, found in India and other hot countries, in which the foot swells, and cracks form in it. These discharge matter containing little black or white granules, which are really a species of fungus. The fungus probably gains an entrance into the foot through a sore or scratch.

MAGNESIUM. Magnesium is a silvery white metal which burns with a brilliant flame and is thus used for flashlight photography indoors. In medicine its various compounds are extensively used. Magnesium sulphate is the popular and powerful purgative known as *Epsom Salts.* Magnesium oxide, which is commonly called magnesia, is very useful in cases of stomach trouble where there is too much acidity. Milk of magnesia and magnesia cream are pleasant ways of taking it. A very favorite and useful mixture is the mixture of magnesium sulphate and magnesium carbonate called mistura alba or *white mixture.* Magnesium trisilicate is extensively used to neutralize excess of gastric acid in cases of dyspepsia and peptic ulceration.

MAGNET. Magnets are used in surgery to withdraw steel or iron splinters from wounds. They are especially useful for foreign bodies in the eye where they could not easily be reached without risk of damaging delicate tissues.

MALAISE. By malaise is meant a feeling of illness or physical discomfort. Most illnesses are heralded by a day or two of malaise before the acute stage is reached. (*See also* MIGRAINE.)

MALAR. The malar bone is the cheek bone, from the Latin *mala,* the cheek. (*See also* BONE.)

MALARIA. Malaria is a very common disease which is now largely confined to tropical regions. It is also known as marsh fever, jungle fever, or just "fever." During the second World War it was one of the chief causes of illness among troops in the Mediterranean campaign (especially in Sicily) and in India and Burma.

Malaria is a recurrent disease and is commonly divided into three groups, according to the periods at which the bouts of fever return: (1) *quotidian,* or daily; (2)*tertian,* or recurring every third day; and (3) *quartan,* recurring every fourth day.

Symptoms. A typical attack of malaria is divisible into three stages. The first stage is one of shivering and malaise. The patient feels tired with aching head and limbs, and cold with bouts of shivering. He may, describe himself "chilled to the bone," and his teeth may chatter uncontrollably. This stage is short, lasting only an hour. The second stage is the hot and feverish stage. The temperature rises very suddenly to great heights and the pulse and breathing become rapid. The aches continue and there is great restlessness and often delirium. Vomiting and diarrhea are common. This stage lasts several hours and patient's condition becomes more and more uncomfortable until the third stage, or stage of sweating, is reached. This stage is in the nature of a crisis. Sweating is profuse, the temperature comes down rapidly and the patient becomes much more comfortable. The trouble is not over, however, because unless it is energetically treated the attack will return in exactly the same way, after one to four days, according to the type, and each attack will leave the patient weaker.

Treatment. Malaria is one of the diseases for which there is a very definite line of treatment and for which several drugs are specific—that is, curative for that disease. For some three hundred years the treatment of malaria could be summed up in the word "quinine," but more recently other and more effective drugs have been introduced. At the beginning of World War II in 1939 quinine was replaced by mepacrine, which proved to be more generally useful, but this has since been replaced by newer drugs, especially Atabrine and Camoquin. These act very rapidly in the treatment of an acute attack of malaria, and in addition they have less toxic side-effects and do not stain the skin. Paludrine, which is also used, is slow-acting and therefore not so effective in the treatment of an acute attack. Atabrine and Camoquin are each given in a dose of four tablets followed by two more tablets in six hours, then two tablets daily for two days more.

In severe cases, which may go on to coma, the Atabrine or quinine should be given intravenously, repeated if necessary after four hours. In all cases of malaria, fluids should be given freely by the mouth, and the patient should be well fed once the fever has subsided.

In blackwater fever, blood transfusion may be necessary, and the steroids are often useful.

Relapses can be prevented by taking one of the antimalarial drugs in moderate doses over a period of several months. Atabrine acts by destroying the early stage of the malaria parasite and so give protection against the disease. On entering a malarial district one table should be taken daily (with suitably smaller doses for children), and it is usually free from side-effects. Atabrine or Camoquin, in a dose of two tablets per week, similarly gives protection. All of these drugs must be taken regularly. (*See also* MOSQUITO; QUININE.)

MALE FERN. The oily extract of the root of male fern (*filix mas*) is the chief remedy for destroying tapeworms. (*See also* FERN; WORM.)

MALIGNANT. By malignant is meant dangerous to life. A malignant growth usually means a cancer. The opposite of malignant in medicine is benign. Malignant forms of fevers are those in which the patient becomes dangerously ill in a few hours. Malignant pustule is a name for anthrax.

MALINGERING. Malingering is a deliberate attempt to appear to have a disease or disability for the purpose of evading a duty or gaining some financial or other advantage. Hysteria and hypochondriasis are not malingering.

MALNUTRITION. Malnutrition is the state of being undernourished owing to insufficient food, the wrong sort of food or some constitutional reason which prevents the food eaten from being utilized.

MALT. Malt is obtained from barley which has been allowed to sprout and has then been heated in a kiln to prevent furthergrowth. It contains a ferment or digestive substance called *diastase* which works of starch and turns it into malt sugar. In the form of extract of malt it is a valuable aid to a weak digestion, and is also nourishing and strengthening because of the malt sugar (maltose) it contains. It is therefore often prescribed for people suffering from wasting and weakening diseases. It mixes well with other substances, and is a useful vehicle for cod-liver oil, iron, etc. For commercial purposes malt is chiefly useful for beer-making. By adding yeast to malt, alcohol is formed, and with the addition of hops, beer is manufactured.

MALTA or UNDULANT FEVER. Malta fever, which is also called undulant fever, is a common complaint around the Mediterranean Sea and in other warm countries where goat's milk is used, due to infection by a germ first described by Col. Bruce in 1886. Occasional cases of it occur through infected cow's milk in other countries, too. Boiling the milk makes it safe. In Malta, where it is a serious problem, the government takes important steps to deal with its prevention and cure.

Symptoms. The illness is not a very severe one, although it may continue in a long-drawn-out form over a period of years. There is loss of appetite, headache, sleeplessness, and slight fever; in the evenings, neuralgic pains and swellings in the joints appear. The patient may become very much emaciated and exhausted.

Treatment. In an uncomplicated case tetracycline every six hours is usually effective; in chronic cases it should be given along with streptomycin and sulphadiazine.

MANDIBLE. The lower jaw is called the mandible. (*See also* JAW.)

MANGANESE. Manganese is a metal whose properties resemble those of iron. In medicine it is chiefly used in the form of potassium permanganate. Potassium permanganate takes the form of purple crystals which are very easily dissolved in water, forming a solution ranging from light pink to deep purple, according to the amount used. It is a powerful antiseptic, disinfectant, and deodorant. Taken internally it is used as an intestinal disinfectant and it is also a favorite solution for washing out the stomach or intestines. Solutions are also used for mouth or nose washing, especially in conditions where a deodorant is required. It may be used for vaginal douching and as an injection in gonorrhea.

MANIA. Insanity in which the patient becomes dangerously excited is called mania. (*See also* INSANITY; MEGALOMANIA; MENTAL DISEASE.)

MARASMUS. Wasting in a small child is called marasmus. (*See also* WASTING.)

MARCH FRACTURE. This term describes a fracture of the second or third metatarsal bones of the foot, due to the stress of unaccustomed physical strain, usually in the training of young soldiers.

MARMITE. Marmite is a proprietary preparation which contains yeast and is a useful way of supplying the vitamin known as Vitamin B or the antineuritic vitamin.

MARROW. Bone marrow is a substance found in the inner channels of the long bones. It is the site of manufacture of the red cells and granular white cells of the blood.

MASSAGE. The word massage is derived from the French "masser"—to knead. Scientifically administered, massage has beneficial effects upon the whole structure of the body.

The Circulatory System. Massage aids the circulation of the blood by direct pressure and by stimulating the nerves. Thus the blood flow is quickened, nutrition is increased, and the heart's action is strengthened. The quantity of red and white blood corpuscles is increased, especially in the parts under treatment.

The Nervous System. Massage has a profound effect upon the whole nervous system. This influence varies according to the methods used, which may be either stimulating or soothing. The stimulating movements increase the activity of the muscles, vessels and glands. The soothing movements relieve pain and nervous irritability.

The Lymphatic System. Massage quickens the activity of the lymphatic ducts and glands by direct pressure. Absorption is promoted by pressure on the tissues, thereby getting rid of harmful substances.

The Respiratory System. The improved local circulation causes more carbon dioxide to be formed in the tissues. The lungs respond to this call for extra activity by producing deeper breathing.

Digestion. Massage promotes movements of the bowels by exciting the reflex action of the nerves controlling the movements of the stomach and intestines.

Massage strengthens the muscular walls of the abdomen, improves circulation in the walls of the food tract, and thus aids absorption of the digested food substances by the blood and lymph capillaries.

Elimination. Massage aids elimination of waste products from the body by increasing the activity of the lungs, skin, and kindneys, by aiding absorption and oxidation, and by improving the circulation of blood and lymph.

The Muscular System. Massage aids muscle development by improving the circulation and nutrition of the parts treated.

Bone. The improved circulation of the blood and lymph in the muscles leads to improved circulation and nutrition of the underlying bones. Thus bone development is indirectly influenced by massage.

Rules to be Observed During Massage Treatment. The patient should be in a comfortable and restful position.

The masseur or masseuse should be in an easy position for working.

The room should be sufficiently warm and the patient covered except for the part actually under treatment at the time.

The masseur or masseuse should wash the hands before starting and see that they are warm before touching the patient.

At the beginning of a course of treatment the massage must be light. As the condition of the patient improves, the length and strength of the movements may be increased.

All the movements should be performed rhythmically.

A small blanket and pillow are useful to cover the patient and to support the part undergoing manipulation.

During the menstrual period it is better to suspend treatment or omit massage of the loins and abdomen.

General Massage. This means massage of the whole body. The patient must be undressed, but only the part under manipulation is exposed. One hour is needed for the treatment, the time being divided as follows: the legs, 20 minutes; the arms, 15 minutes; the chest, 5 minutes; the abdomen, 10 minutes; and the back, 10 minutes.

General massage should not be given within one and a half hours of a meal, and the patient should lie down quietly and rest for one hour after treatment.

Head massage is a useful means of relief in cases of neuralgia, headache, or insomnia.

Face massage is helpful in cases of facial paralysis, and relieves facial neuralgia.

Abdominal massage is useful in indigestion and constipation. It helps to remove superfluous fat and to tone up the abdominal walls.

Indirectly it increases the absorption of food substances, stimulates the secretion of gastric juices, and aids the expulsion of gases generated in the stomach and intestines. At least two hours should elapse after a meal before abdominal massage is commenced.

The patient lies down with the shoulders slightly raised and the knees drawn up, separated, and resting upon a pillow.

The bladder should be emptied before the treatment.

MASSETER. The masseters are a pair of muscles passing over the ends of the jaws in front of the ears. They are the chief muscles used in chewing. (*See also* JAW.)

MASTICATION. By mastication we mean the act of chewing. Chewing food is really quite a complicated process which is carried out by the combined action of the jaws, tongue, cheeks and the muscles which serve them. Good mastication is necessary in order to turn the food into the pulpy well-salivated mass which is suitable for swallowing into the stomach.

MASTITIS. Mastitis is another name for inflammation of the breast. It is fairly common in nursing mothers and is then usually due to the blocking of a milk duct with hardened milk, or to infection which has reached the interior of the breast through a crack in a nipple. (*See also* BREAST.)

MASTODYNIA. Any pain in the breast may be called mastodynia, though it is commonly used to refer to a neuralgic ache for which there is no discoverable cause. Very heavy and pendulous breasts often ache, and a loose support such as a well fitted brassière will give relief. Some women feel neuralgic pains in the breasts at period times or when they are tired and run down. It must never be forgotten, however, that a woman who is not used to having pain in the region of the breast should have herself examined by a doctor when such a pain appears, because it may be the beginning of some more serious condition. For fleeting attacks of mastodynia, warmth over the breast or a belladonna plaster will usually give relief. (*See also* BREAST.)

MASTOID. The mastoid process is part of the temporal bone of the skull; it is the rounded part that projects behind the ear. It contains numerous air cells, the purpose of which is to protect the delicate structures of the internal ear. The air gets into these air cells from the middle ear, behind the ear drum, to which air is brought from the throat through the eustachian tube. It will thus be seen that germs or inflammation can spread from the throat up to the middle ear and on to the mastoid cells.

MASTOIDITIS. This is an inflammation of the mastoid which was apt to spread to the brain and cause meningitis but is now usually prevented by the injection of penicillin in adequate dosages when the middle ear is inflamed, before mastoiditis develops. The *simple mastoid operation,* when necessary, is very effective when performed early and leaves no ill-effects. The *radical mastoid operation* is done in chronic cases and in brain complications; it brings about a degree of deafness, as the whole middle ear has to be cleared out.

MASTURBATION. This is also known as self-abuse and is a bad habit common among adolescents, and to which all kinds of serious nervous and mental diseases used to be attributed. It may be one of the symptoms, though not a cause, of mental disorder. In infants, masturbation may be due to the irritation of a tight foreskin or to intestinal worms, and is curable by attention to these. Most adolescents grow out of the habit, which, though not a healthy one, is not one to be taken too seriously. (*See also* SEX HYGLENE; PSYCHOTHERAPY.)

MATERIA MEDICA. Materia medica is the old name for the science of drugs. This is now called *pharmacology,* which includes the action of drugs upon the body.

MAXILLARY BONES. The maxillary bones are the pair of bones which form the upper jaw. They reach from the eye sockets to the mouth, and from the cheek bones to the side of the nose. Each maxillary bone, or maxilla as it is called, contains a hollowed-out cavity called the maxillary sinus or more commonly the antrum, which is filled with air. The air reaches the antrum through a small opening into the nose, and it is therefore liable to infection from a catarrhal cold or influenza. An infected antrum is very difficult to treat because drainage of pus and mucus is readily obstructed at the narrow opening. Operation is often necessary. (*See also* ANTRUM; JAW.)

MEASLES. This is a very infectious disease which is common among children in springtime. In most places it is notifiable to the Health Department authorities. The incubation period, or time it takes to develop after exposure to infection, is three weeks. It is worthy of note that measles is much more serious in children of under five years of age than in older children and theirs are always urgent cases. Gamma globulin given intramuscularly within five days of exposure to infection is an effective prophylactic.

Symptoms. The first sign the mother notices is that the child is off color for four or five days, and seems to have a bad cold in the head with running eyes and nose. If the mother looks inside the child's mouth at this period she may notice some little white patches the size of a pinhead on the inner side of the cheek, and the child will by this time have developed a hard, ticklish cough. On the fourth day of the illness the child becomes very feverish and a rash appears first behind the ears and round the mouth and spreads rapidly all over the body. The rash is red and blotchy and may last from three to five days. It is accompanied by fever, which disappears as the rash fades, and the cough becomes less troublesome.

Mothers do not, as a rule, realize the seriousness of measles, and sometimes allow the rest of the children to sleep in the same room, so that "they may all get it while they are at it." This is not advisable because of the complications arising from measles.

Complications: *Pneumonia.* This is the most usual and serious complication and is generally the result of letting the child get out of bed too soon. *Ear troubles.* These sometimes occur and require skilled attention. *Eye trouble.* Any discharge from the eyes or ear should be reported to the doctor at once, as careful attention is needed. Neglect of the right treatment under these circumstances has been known to lead to permanent deafness or blindness.

Treatment. The doctor should be in attendance on all cases and, wherever possible, the child should be isolated and treated at home. It is possible to "overtreat" measles, and the doctor will usually only give doses of penicillin to counteract any complications. Put the child to bed with lots of blankets in a warm room. A dose of opening medicine, preferably castor oil (one tablespoonful for a child of seven and two teaspoonfuls under that age), should be given, followed by a daily dose of milk of magnesia, unless there are signs of diarrhea.

All through the illness it is advisable to give the child as much fluid to drink as possible in the form of ordinary cold water, lemonade and orangeade made from fresh fruit, barley water (made by boiling and straining pearl barley), or imperial drink, made by mixing lemonade and barley water together. If the child is restless and hot it should be sponged down frequently with luke-warm water with a drop of disinfectant in it. The room should be kept darkened, as the light is irritating to the child's eyes. This can be accomplished by using dark blue or green curtains. The window should be kept open, but care must be taken that the bed is not in a draft; that is to say, it should not be placed between the window and the door or between two windows. If the room is built in such a way that the bed must be in one of these bad positions, then a screen must be used. A useful screen can be made by arranging a blanket or a rug over a clothes-horse, or by tying a rope from the top of one bedpost to the other and throwing a blanket over it.

The *eyes* should be bathed hourly with a piece of cotton-wool dipped in weak boric lotion, each piece being burned as soon as it has been used once. The *mouth* should be swabbed three times a day in the same way with glycerine and borax or hydrogen peroxide or glycothymoline. If the *ear* discharges or if there is pain behind the ear, the doctor should be informed at once. The *cough,* which is the most troublesome feature, is treated by medicine to loosen and soothe it. In cases where the cough remains hard and troublesome, kaolin (obtained from any druggist, with directions for use on the jar) should be applied on the back and front of the chest morning and evening. Kaolin is best applied on plain white lint, but if this is not obtainable, an old flannel shirt can be cut up for the purpose. It needs to be warmed before being put on, and to test the heat the mother should place it against her own cheek. After it is applied to the skin, the chest should be covered with cotton-wool back and front, made in the form of a pneumonia-jacket. If the child is likely to be ill for some days it is wise to make two jackets so that one can be aired while the other is in use. A steam tent is also of value in helping the child to breathe more easily. It can be rigged up by attaching four poles to the corners of the bed and throwing over a sheet, so that one side is left open, through which the steam comes from the boiling kettle. A teaspoonful of compound tincture of benzoin should be added to the water each time the kettle is filled.

The child should not be allowed to return to school in less than fourteen days from the date of the first appearance of the rash, and a child who has been exposed to infection should not return until sixteen days have elapsed. (*See also* DISINFECTION; GERMAN MEASLES; INFECTIOUS DISEASES.)

MEATUS. The word meatus refers to a passage or tunnel in the body. The passage in connection with which it is most generally used is the external auditory meatus or ear-hole. (*See also* EAR.)

MECKEL'S DIVERTICULUM. *See* DIVERTICULUM.

MECONIUM. For the first two days of an infant's life it frequently passes motions of a dark greenish-black sticky fluid. Thus substance is called meconium. After the first forty-eight hours of life the meconium disappears and the normal baby stools appear. (*See also* STOOLS.)

MEDIASTINUM. The space lying between the two lungs is called the mediastinum. It contains the heart, the windpipe and gullet, and the aorta and other great blood vessels of the chest.

Inflammation occurring in this region is known as *mediastinitis*. Such inflammation may spread from the neighboring organs and may be the result of some condition such as pleurisy. (*See also* PLEURISY.)

MEDICAL GYMNASTICS OR SWEDISH REMEDIAL EXERCISES. Remedial exercises consist of positions or movements of the body performed by the individual, either alone or with assistance, and by their aid many physical deformities, inherited or acquired, may be corrected either totally or in part.

General Principles for the Administration of Remedial Exercises.

1. The exercises and their strength should be adapted to the age, constitution, and strength of the patient.

2. Nervous and highly strung patients should be given slow, rhythmical, soothing exercises; lethargic patients need brisk, stimulating exercises, which demand attention and alertness.

3. The patient should never be allowed to get overtired or breathless.

4. Passive movements should precede active, which in turn are followed by resisted movements.

5. Breathing exercises should always commence and terminate the treatment, and they may also be freely interspersed throughout.

6. When resistance is given it should begin weak, wax to strong in the middle of the movement, and wane near the end. If trembling or jerks occur, either the exercise or the resistance is too strong for the patient.

7. The patient should not be tired at the beginning of a treatment and benefits more when the treatment is followed by a rest.

MEDITERRANEAN FEVER. This is a feverish disease caused by a milk infection and prevalent along the coasts of the Mediterranean Sea, especially on the island of Malta. It is described under its more common name of MALTA FEVER.

MEDULLA or BULB. This is the part of the nervous system which lies at the back of the head, occupying the lowest part of the skull and which joins the brain above to the spinal cord below. The medulla is about ¾-inch across and ¾-inch long, and within this tiny compass are contained all the means by which we are able to move our limbs; to feel such things as pain and temperature in every part of the body; and most important of all, by which we are able to breathe. The action of the lungs is controlled by nerves which have their endings in the medulla, and if these nerves are injured breathing stops at once and death results.

MEGALOMANIA. This term describes an exaggerated belief in one's own power or ability. Simple megalomania is fairly common in a mild form, but as a symptom of more serious mental trouble it is very common. One of the first symptoms of *general paralysis of the insane* (q.v.) is often megalomania.

MEGRIM. This condition is described under its more usual name of MIGRAINE.

MELENA. By melena is meant the dark-colored, almost black, stools which contain blood and are passed in conditions like ulceration of the bowels or stomach. The bleeding when the stools are black is usually from the lower part of the stomach, the duodenum, or the higher parts of the small intestine. Bleeding from the stomach proper is usually vomited and bleeding from the large intestine is more or less its normal color. It must be remembered that many mixtures which are taken as medicine will darken the stool, notably those containing iron and bismuth. (*See also* STOOLS.)

MELANCHOLIA. This is a disorder of the mind in which depression may be so marked that the patient seeks refuge in suicide. The bodily health is also affected in this disorder, and the patient looks and feels physically ill as well as being mentally sick. The mental picture in melancholia is one of utter and unrelieved misery.

Melancholia is a disorder that occurs mainly in middle life, and is rather more common in women that in men. It is especially common in women about the time of the change of life and many a mild case of melancholia goes unrecognized as such, the utter misery and depresson being put down to the "change of life." The outlook in melancholia is good if the patient is properly treated and is kept from committing suicide. These patients *are* physically ill; they become very thin, their complexions get muddy, and constipation is always marked. The digestion is poor, and this, together with the fact that many patients have delusions about being unable to eat, soon leads to what is practically starvation. For this reason, if for no other, it is advisable to have these patients under supervision in a mental hospital.

Remarkable cures can sometimes be effected by inducing convulsions electrically or by injections. Rest, and treatment of the physical state, is all important. Relapses may occur in melancholia, but provided that the patients weather the actual attacks, the outlook for ultimate recovery is good.

MELANOTIC CARCINOMA, or MELANOMA. (Greek, *melan,* black.) This is a tumor, occurring at all ages, which contains a great deal of melanin pigment, a dark brown or black coloring matter; this coloring matter is formed by some of the skin cells, whose particular work it is. Sometimes the pigment is increased in special areas, for some unknown reason, and a small pigmented patch called a pigmented mole results. This may remain very small, and never cause any trouble; on the other hand, it may be excited by some unknown irritant, when it grows rapidly, ulcerates, and spreads with extraordinary rapidity along the lymph channels. Indeed, quite often the first sign of anything wrong is the enlargement of the neighboring lymph glands, which frequently form tumors considerably larger than the original growth. This may, on the other hand, be sometimes so small as to be missed entirely.

In some cases the spread is universal throughout the body. The secondary growths are generally more deeply pigmented than the first; they may be quite coal-black. In recurrence of the diseases, which sometimes follows operation, the coloring matter may be absent. The urine may be darkened in color by the presence of pigment.

Treatment. The outlook in these cases is grave. The treatment is immediate removal of the growth. This is done very thoroughly; the mole, the tissues beneath it, the nearest lymph glands, and the subcutaneous fascia, or flattened tissue lying beneath the skin, between the growth and the glands, must all be removed. Radium and deep X-ray treatment are also employed. (*See also* CANCER; CANCER OF THE SKIN.)

MEMBRANE. A membrane is a thin sheet of tissue covering or lining any organ of the body. Membranes such as those lining the intestines, the nose, etc., which are moistened by the sticky fluid substance called mucus, are called the *mucous membranes.* In a state of ill health these mucous membranes are apt to develop an additional amount of mucus and catarrh is produced.

MEMORY. Memory may be defined as the result of storing up impressions in our minds by which we are able to recognize these impressions when they present themselves again.

Memory fails not only in old age, but also in many disorders of the mind. One of the earliest symptoms of *general paralysis of the insane* (q.v.) may be failure to recall at will impressions previously recorded. In such conditions as *senile dementia,* or *confusional insanity (see* IN-

SANITY), loss of memory is a striking feature, and it also occurs in certain forms of chronic alcoholism. In alcoholism the loss of memory is peculiar in that recent events are not remembered, but things which happened long ago can be remembered perfectly. If recovery takes place, memory returns, showing that the cause of this loss of memory is quite different to the cause of the loss of memory in old people.

MENDEL'S LAW. An Austrian naturalist, Johann Mendel, who lived from 1822–84, conceived a theory dealing with the inheritance of characteristics, by which he stated that when two individuals, each with a definite characteristic, mate, their offspring will have only one of their characteristics, known as the dominant, and the other characteristic will be recessive or undeveloped.

MENIERE'S DISEASE or SYNDROME. Ménière's disease is a chronic progressive disease in which there are attacks of giddiness, deafness on one side of the head only, noises in the head (tinnitus), and vomiting. It is called after the French physician who first described it in 1861. It is thought to be due to pressure disturbances in the fluid which fills the internal ear and semicircular canals.

Treatment. Sometimes the condition improves considerably of its own accord, with rest in bed, otherwise the recognized forms of treatment are to restrict the intake of fluids, take a salt-free diet, with ammonium chloride internally, and clear up any unhealthy condition in the nose or throat. Some doctors prescribe sedatives or antihistamines, and in suitable cases an operation is performed although it has the disadvantage of affecting the hearing. (*See also* EAR; TINNITUS.)

MENINGES. These are the coverings of the brain and spinal cord which protect the delicate nervous structures from injury and also serve to carry the blood away from the brain when all its oxygen has been used up by the tissues. There are three layers to these coverings; the outermost one is the *dura mater,* a thick, strong layer which lines the skull and the canal in which the spinal cord lies, being continuous through a hole in the bottom of the skull through which the spinal cord passes from the bulb. The *arachnoid,* which is the next innermost layer, is a much more delicate, filmy structure, while the *pia mater,* which lies in direct contact with the brain and dips into the folds of the brain, is even more fragile. In between the arachnoid and the pia mater there is a small space, filled with a fluid produced in a gland-like structure in the brain. This fluid, called cerebro-spinal fluid, circulates all over the brain substance and the spinal cord, and is the fluid that actually nourishes the brain, the gland-like structure extracting from the blood just those things which are required to nourish the brain and rejecting the remainder. Sometimes the pia mater and arachnoid get stuck together, so that the fluid is no longer able to circulate freely. When this happens, the fluid gets dammed back into certain parts of the brain, producing what is called a hydrocephalus or "water on the brain." (*See also* HYDROCEPHALUS.)

MENINGITIS. Meningitis is inflammation of the meninges (*see* MENINGES), and it may occur as a result of some general disease of the body, as tuberculosis, or it may be caused by the spread of some disease in the ear or nose through the skull into the meninges. One particular form of meningitis is called CEREBROSPINAL FEVER and has already been dealt with under that heading. The general symptoms of any form of meningitis are the same; they differ only in their severity. The forms caused by spread of germs from the ear or nose often recover, and even those due to tuberculosis need no longer be regarded as hopeless.

The symptoms of meningitis depend on two facts, one that the germs causing the condition irritate the delicate membranes and the brain tissue which lies under them; the other, that the skull is a closed box and any increase in the contents of that box, such as occurs in meningitis, gives rise to a certain pressure.

The meningitis of tuberculosis is always found with tuberculosis in some other part of the body. It occurs more commonly in children than in adults. The early signs are those of a general upset of health; the child becomes irritable, out of sorts, is frequently sick for no apparent reason, and is constipated. Then signs of irritation of the

meninges begin to appear: severe headache is complained of, the child may develop an obvious squint and may have a fit. By this time the child will be unwilling to be examined or questioned, but will lie curled up in bed, probably with its head buried in the pillow to avoid looking at the light. There may be some rise of temperature, and the temperature as a rule goes on rising until just before death. Pain is a most distressing feature of the disease and the child often gives rise to a plaintive cry which once heard is never forgotten. The head is held back with the chin tilted into the air. A certain sign, called "Kernig's sign," is nearly always present in these cases: if a child is placed on its back in bed so that one leg is resting on the bed and the other one is bent at the hip and knee, it is found that it is not possible to straighten out the bent leg at the knee joint without causing pain to the patient and pulling up the leg which rests on the bed. Without treatment the disease lasts only a few weeks. The condition is recognized and the type of germ causing the meningitis is determined by withdrawing some of the cerebrospinal (*see* MENINGES) fluid from the spinal canal with a needle. In cases of meningitis, the fluid drawn off consists of pus in which the germs can be seen under the microscope.

Treatment. The outlook on the treatment of meningitis has completely changed with the introduction of the sulphonamides and penicillin. Meningitis caused by the pneumococcus, or germ of pneumonia, can be controlled by full doses of a sulphonamide, especially sulphathiazole or sulphadiazine, or else by injections of penicillin either into the muscles or into the spinal canal. Sometimes surgical operation is carried out as well, especially in meningitis arising from the spread of mastoid inflammation. A diagnosis of tuberculous meningitis was formerly a certain death warrant, but this is no longer so. Treatment with an antibiotic known as streptomycin has so altered the picture that there are now many recorded cases of cure. This drug is given by injection into the muscles and into the spinal canal and may need to be given for as long as six months before all signs of the disease are finally eradicated. (*See also* SULPHONAMIDES; PENICILLIN.)

MENINGOCELE. This is a lump which may appear in the midline of the back of a newly born child at any place from the bottom of the skull to the lowermost part of the spine. This lump is made up of the meninges (q.v.) of the spinal cord and its appearance is due to an error of development in which the bony parts of the spine have not joined up as they should. When the baby coughs or cries, the lump gets larger and can be felt to be soft, with fluid contents. Meningocele is a very mild form of the errors in development which may happen to the spinal cord and its meninges. In the worst forms the whole spinal cord opens on to the skin, and this, of course, does not allow the child to live more than a few days. Meningocele may sometimes be treated by surgery, and the lump taken away without damage to the spinal cord underneath; but many cases are best left untouched, since the condition gives rise to little or no trouble, and the lump should then be protected by a suitable shield. The surgeon is the only person who can safely decide whether it is advisable to remove the meningocele.

MENOPAUSE. This is the change of life which occurs in women between the ages of forty-five and fifty. (*See also* CHANGE OF LIFE; MENSTRUATION.)

MENORRHAGIA. This is the name given to excessive loss of blood during ages of forty-five and fifty. (*See also* HEMORRHAGING; MENSTRUATION.)

MENSES. This is the name given to the monthly periods in a woman. (*See also* MENSTRUATION.)

MENSTRUATION. Menstruation is the medical name for the monthly loss of blood which occurs normally in adult women, and which is popularly called by such names as "the courses," "the periods," "being unwell," etc. It consists of a periodic discharge from the womb. Every woman differs both as regards the duration of the periods and the length of time between them; for example, bleeding may occur at intervals of three to five weeks and may last for as short a time as two days or as long a time as ten days. But each woman should be regular in the pattern which she normally follows from month to month. If she has a three or four days' flow

every twenty-eight days, which is the most usual period, she should be able to count on the period appearing every four weeks with great regularity and lasting the same number of days each time. Menstruation usually begins between twelve and fourteen years of age and lasts until the woman is forty-five to fifty-five years of age. The late forties are the most usual age for its cessation, which is called the menopause or climacteric, or more popularly is referred to as the change of life. Before the menstrual period a tiny egg, or ovum as it is called, which is so small that it can only be seen with the aid of a microscope, is set free from the ovary and passes down the *fallopian tubes* to the womb. If it meets the male fertilizing agent (spermatozoon), the menstrual flow does not take place and pregnancy begins; otherwise, it is discharged from the womb with the menstrual flow.

In addition to the inconvenience caused by the periods, most women experience slight feelings of discomfort before the period begins. They may feel languid, nervous, and irritable, and have pains in the abdomen or in the back. Some women are always constipated during a period, while others start the period with a attack of diarrhea; but unless there is some definite reason for it, menstruation must not be regarded as a period of ill health. It is a perfectly normal function, and for most women entails no interference with their usual activities. It may be as well to take a little extra care to avoid chills and overtiredness, but otherwise life should go on much as usual. Some women do not take a bath during the period, but for those who are used to a daily bath it may be safely continued so long as it is restricted to a short warm bath.

Abnormalities of Menstruation. Amenorrhea, Menorrhagia and Metrorrhagia.

Amenorrhea. This term is applied to the absence of the menstrual period. In some cases menstruation never begins owing to imperfect development of the womb or other internal organs. This may be rectified by a surgical operation, but not always. It is much more common for the menses to stop after having made an appearance. Chlorosis, or anemia, accounts for many cases of amenorrhea in young girls. There may be other causes, such as excitement, shock, mental strain, change of climate, or exposure to cold before or during the menstrual period. It is usual for the menses to make their reappearance after the cause has been removed, even in the case of amenorrhea resulting from disease. The natural causes of amenorrhea are pregnancy, the onset of the menopause or change of life, and usually lactation or nursing.

Menorrhagia and Metrorrhagia. Excessive bleeding at the menstrual period is called *menorrhagia,* while irregular bleeding at times between the period is called *metrorrhagia.* Anything over a week is excessive for a period, but many women have periods as long as a week, quite normally, and it is quite common in young girls who usually grow out of the tendency when the periods become established. Certain blood diseases such as anemia may cause profuse periods. The cause of metrorrhagia or irregular bleeding should always be investigated by a doctor, especially if it comes on in a woman whose periods have previously been regular. All the causes of profuse and irregular bleeding are discussed in the article on FLOODING, which is a general name for the condition. (*See also* CHANGE OF LIFE.)

MENTAL DEFICIENCY. This is a condition in which the mind has failed to reach a normal stage of development. It is one of the three groups into which all cases of abnormal minds can be divided, the other two being mental disease (q.v.), and mental decay or dementia (q.v.). Mental deficiency is the condition in which an individual is so undeveloped mentally from birth that he is unable to adapt himself to the ordinary requirements of society except under care, supervision and control. There are three grades of mental deficiency: idiocy, imbecility, and feeble-mindedness, of which the first and the last, being of most importance, are treated under their separate headings. Imbecility is the state of those persons in whom there exists from birth or from an early age mental defectiveness not amounting to idiocy, yet so pronounced that they are incapable of managing their affairs or themselves, or, in the case of children, of being taught to do so.

MENTAL DEPRESSION. Everyone is bound to feel a certain amount of depression at various times when things go wrong. At other times attacks of depression are to be expected such as the depression that so often follows influenza, but these are temporary phases and should wear off. Often gloom is simply a bad habit that the individual has fallen into and will take no trouble to rid himself or herself of. There are, however, unfortunate people in whom depression is a symptom of mental disease, such as anxiety, hysteria, melancholia, hypochondriasis, and general paralysis of the insane. For a description of these various states of mental disease, see under their own headings and *also* MENTAL DISEASE.

MENTAL DISEASE. This is one of the penalties of civilization, and there is no doubt that owing to the rush and hurry of modern life it is—at any rate in its milder forms—on the increase. The causes of mental disease may be divided into those which arise in the mind itself and have nothing to do with any bodily condition and those which may be traced to some disturbance of a physical nature, either in the brain or elsewhere in the body.

Physical Causes of Mental Disease. It is only within the last thirty years or so that it has been realized what a very great part infection by germs outside the brain may play in the production of mental disease. Poisons produced by these germs which live in the digestive organs, or in the throat or sometimes at the roots of the teeth, constantly get into the blood and are carried to the brain, and in some people whose nervous systems are not as strong as they might be severe mental breakdowns are caused in this way. There are many other bodily conditions which may cause mental disease, and of these the most important are syphilis, alcoholism, and disease of the blood vessels that occurs in old age. Reference to the types of mental disease which may be caused by these conditions will be found under the headings of ALCOHOLISM, DEMENTIA, and GENERAL PARALYSIS OF THE INSANE. Epilepsy, too (q.v.), may cause mental disease. In people in whom there is a family history of mental trouble, the too great crises of life, sometimes prove too much for the individuals and they escape, as it were, by developing mental troubles. Childbirth also can affect women in this way; but it is exceedingly rare for grave mental trouble to follow childbirth unless there is some definite history of it in the family.

Mental Disease Which has its Origin in the Mind. To the ordinary person, mental disease means insanity, but there are a very large number of minor forms of mental trouble which enable people to live among their fellows without being regarded as in any way different from them. The victims of these minor mental disorders are never happy people; life is always hard for them. But unless their difficulties are solved by the right treatment, they go on suffering in silence. These disorders are described under the separate headings of ANXIETY, HYPOCHONDRIASIS, NEURASTHENIA, and PSYCHONEUROSIS.

The Chief Forms of Mental Disease Not Associated with Physical Disease. 1. *Manic-Depressive Insanity.* In this form of mental trouble, periods of wild excitement alternate with periods in which the patient is plunged into gloom, like a typical case of melancholia (q.v.). In the depressed stage the condition of the patient is, to all intents and purposes, the same as in melancholia and the same treatment is adopted. The latest view on the subject of this form of insanity is that all cases of melancholia, except those which occur in women at the time of the change of life, go through a cheerful stage in which they are unusually happy and noisy. The alternating periods of happiness and gloom tend to be the same length in the same patient, and often the patient himself will be able to name the very day on which the particular period of happiness or despair begins. In the manic stage, these patients are very talkative, noisy, and restless. The interval between the manic and the depressed stage may be a long one, so long in fact that many of these patients are sent home from mental hospitals in between the attacks on the understanding that they return when the symptoms of either stage appear.

2. *Delusional Insanity.* This is one of the most important, because it is one of the most dangerous forms of mental trouble; dangerous, because the patient may come into contact with the law before it is realized that he is not responsible for his actions. In delusional insanity, delusions

(q.v.) are not only strongly held by the patient, but he justifies their existence and attempts to regulate his life to fit his delusions. It is essential that as soon as this type of insanity is recognized the patient should be put under supervision.

3. *Dementia Praecox.* This form of mental trouble occurs in young people and has been fully discussed under the heading SCHIZOPHRENIA.

4. *Melancholia.* This also is referred to under its separate heading.

5. *Acute Mania.* This type of mental disease best fulfills the popular idea of a "mental patient." Such a patient is unusually happy and a joyous sense of well-being possesses him. Nevertheless, he looks pale and ill and is nearly always thin and anxious looking.

Sleep is almost absent in these attacks—from one to three hours sleep may be all that is obtained without the use of drugs for several weeks.

As a result of this loss of sleep, and also of the extreme activity of the body while he is awake, the plight of the patient with acute mania who is not carefully treated becomes a bad one within a very short time. Unless a patient with acute mania can be given sleep, he will probably die; large doses of drugs may have to be given in order to procure for him the necessary rest. Another, and more recently introduced, method of treating acute mania is by putting the patient into a very warm bath, above body temperature, and keeping him in it for as long as the condition of his heart will allow. This treatment has a most extraordinary effect in quieting a restless and wholly unmanageable patient.

6. *Confusional Insanity.* This may occur either in association with bodily disease or without it. At all events, the patient is always examined for evidence of any bodily cause such as alcoholism, syphilis, or myxedema, before coming to the conclusion that the disorder has its origin in the mind alone. In a state of confusion the patient is lost to himself and his surroundings; he does not know who he is, how he is, or where he is. As a rule these patients look ill; their complexions are muddy and they have coated tongues.

Confusional insanity is one of the more hopeful of the disorders of the mind, since a large proportion of the patients recover.

The Modern Treatment of Mental Disease. In no branch of medicine has so much progress been made during the last fifty years as in the treatment of mental disease. Less than a hundred years ago, the insane were treated like animals; kept alive and fed, but no more. Today, the modern mental hospital offers every chance of recovery to a patient who enters its doors. Early treatment in such a hospital holds out the very best chance of recovery a patient can be given.

MENTAL HYGIENE. This is a matter of education in order to secure that "healthy mind in a healthy body" which makes for happiness. The training of a child in his relationship to the outside world and to his fellow men must be begun at a very early age, and often it is this lack of training of the only child that makes him such an unbearable personality in adult life.

The question of the mating of the mentally unfit is too large a question to discuss in detail, but it may be said that whereas mental trouble on one side of a family may or may not give rise to mental trouble in the next generation, the occurrence of mental trouble on both sides most certainly will. In general, there is very good evidence for the inheritance of at least some forms of mental trouble; thus it would be wiser for those in whose families there is a history of mental disorder to seek medical advice before deciding to start a family of their own.

MENTHOL. Menthol is a substance in the form of white crystals which is obtained from certain varieties of peppermint. It is useful as a local anesthetic and is made up in various ointments to relieve itching in disorders of the skin. The crystals themselves are a favorite inhalation for colds in the head, sore throats, etc. Put a pinch of the crystals in a bowl and pour boiling water over them. Throw a towel over the head and the steaming bowl and inhale the steam. The eyes should be protected or they may smart.

MERCURIAL POISONING. Poisoning by mercury may be the result of an attempt at suicide through swallowing one of the many preparations of it, or occasionally it is found among persons who work with mercury in the course of making mirrors, thermometers, barometers, etc. In cases where substances containing mercury have been swallowed, the mouth will be burnt and the patient will be in great pain; there will also be vomiting and collapse. An ordinary emetic such as salt in water may be given, and restoratives in the shape of brandy in milk to treat the collapse. A doctor will have to be sent for at once. (*See also* FIRST AID SUPPLEMENT.)

MERCURY. Mercury, or hydrargyrum as it is called in Latin, is a liquid metal substance and is very useful in medicine. It is very easily expanded by heat, and this property is used to measure temperatures. A small amount is placed in a bulb in an enclosed tube to form the thermometer.

The favorite powder for infants, known as gray powder, is a mercury preparation, and so is calomel which has such a powerful effect on the liver. Mercury is a very powerful antiseptic (perchloride of mercury), and it forms the basis of many useful ointments widely employed today.

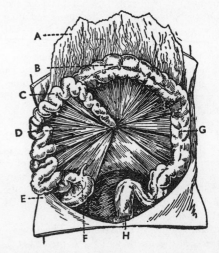

Mesentery: A. *Omentum;* B. *Transverse Colon;* C. *Jejunum.* D. *Mesentery;* E. *Ileum;* F. *Caecum, with Appendix;* G. *Descending Colon;* H. *Rectum.*

MESENTERY. The organs of the stomach are enclosed in a large bag of membrane called the peritoneum. In the peritoneum there are folds called mesenteries which attach the various parts of the food tube to the back wall of the abdomen.

There are three of them. One attaching the lower part of the colon (large bowel), one the upper part of the colon, and the other the small intestine. This latter is the most important of the mesenteries. (*See also* ABDOMEN; INTESTINE.)

MESMERISM. Mesmerism is an older name for hypnotism, which is the term generally used now. (*See also* HYPNOTISM.)

METABOLISM. By metabolism we mean the various processes by which our food is transformed into substances which are absorbed into the bloodstream for the purpose of nourishing and building up the body. In this process the various organs of the digestive tract play a large part. The utilization of absorbed food substances by the tissues is to some extent controlled by the secretions of the ductless glands. Certain diseases are called disorders of metabolism, such as diabetes, gout, myxedema, and obesity. (*See also* BLOOD; DIGESTION; DUCTLESS GLANDS.)

METACARPUS. The metacarpal bones are the five bones in the palm of each hand to which the fingers are attached. When the hand is closed the ends of the metacarpal bones can be felt as the knuckles. The metacarpal bone of the thumb is shorter than the other metacarpals, but has a much larger range of movement. (*See also* FINGER; HAND.)

METASTASIS. By metastasis is meant the spread of disease from one organ to another. Cancer spreads by metastasis.

METATARSUS. The metatarsus is composed of the five metatarsal bones of the foot. (*See* diagram on page 293.) The metatarsal bones are the bones in the main part of the foot to which the five toes are attached. The ends of the metatarsal bones form the ball of the foot. (*See also* FOOT.)

METHYL SALICYLATE. Methyl salicylate, or oil of wintergreen, is of the greatest use for the treatment of rheumatic and other pains. It is easily absorbed through the skin, and can be used either as a liniment or more frequently as an ointment for rubbing in. It has a very pungent and characteristic odor.

METHYL ALCOHOL. A mixture of nearly pure alcohol and wood alcohol, is not now allowed to be sold in a pure form because of the use that was being made of it as an intoxicant. In the mineralized form in which it is now sold for domestic purposes it is very unpalatable and not so likely to lead to people becoming addicted to the drinking of it. The effects of drunkeness from methyl alcohol are of much longer duration and more quickly serious than those of ordinary alcohol. It gives rise to a form of blindness which often develops within twenty-four hours of drinking methyl alcohol and may be permanent. Methyl alcohol, in the form known as surgical spirit, is of the greatest use in surgery for the disinfection of instruments, avoidance of bedsores, etc.

METRITIS. Inflammation of the wall of the womb is known as metritis. It has many causes. Too-frequent pregnancies, childbirth late in life, the condition known as subinvolution of the womb, gonorrhea, or any other infection of the womb may cause metritis. It is one of the commonest causes of the condition known as flooding in which there is severe loss at the period. In its early stages, rest in bed may cure it, together with hot douching and the appropriate medicines which would be prescribed by a doctor.

METRORRHAGIA. This means irregular bleeding from the womb. (*See also* FLOODING; MENSTRUATION.)

MICROBE. A microbe is a germ. The word microbe literally means a small living thing. Microorganisms, bacteria, and bacilli are other names for microbes. (*See also* GERM.)

MICROSCOPE. A microscope is an instrument which magnifies small objects very greatly. Without the microscope we would know nothing about the germs of disease, blood cells, and many other minute things which are of the utmost importance to our health. They can only be seen by high-powered microscopes, and scientists are led to believe that there are many other germs which have not been discovered yet simply because no sufficiently powerful microscope has yet been invented to see them. The germ of measles, which almost certainly exists but has not yet been seen, may be one of these ultramicroscopic germs.

MICTURITION. By micturition is meant the act of passing urine. The surplus water from the body is withdrawn from the system by the kidneys and is then passed on to the bladder, where it is stored up for some hours until such a time as the bladder is full. Then the nerves in the wall of the bladder send a signal to the muscle of the bladder which contracts and expels the urine. In babyhood the action is purely reflex; that is, when the bladder is full it automatically empties itself, but as this would be very inconvenient in later life we train ourselves to make the action of emptying the bladder a voluntary one. If the call to empty the bladder is received at an inconvenient time we can wait our own time to perform the act of micturition. Certain diseases may upset control temporarily. Some children are very backward in learning control, and mentally deficient people may have little control. (*See also* BEDWETTING; BLADDER, DISEASES OF.)

MIDDLE EAR. The part of the ear between the drum and the passage leading to the nose is called the middle ear. This is not to be confused with the outer ear, and the internal ear (which contains the essential organ of hearing, the cochlea). Inflammation of the middle ear is called *otitis media*. For a full description of the ear, *see* EAR.

MIDRIFF. This is an old-fashioned name for the diaphragm, and it is described under that name.

MIGRAINE. This is a form of nervous headache (q.v.) which occurs periodically. There is some evidence that it runs in families, and if a mother is subject to these headaches then it is likely that her children will also suffer from them. The word "migraine" comes from a French word meaning "one side of the head" and in many of the attacks of migraine the headache is felt either on one side or the other, though this is not an invariable rule. Every person who suffers from migraine has his or her own particular form, but generally speaking the sufferer awakes in the morning feeling as if he is "in for it." The headache is often the last thing to occur, and the unfortunate victim may wonder what is the matter with him until he realizes that his trouble is only migraine.

After a period, which may vary from half an hour to a day or more, the headache stops, either after the patient has been sick or after he has slept. Most people who suffer in this way find that if they can sleep they wake free from headache, though feeling weak and "washed out," as though they had had a sleepless night. It is important to state here, that while migraine itself is a common, annoying, but harmless disorder of the nervous system, there are grave disorders of that system—one being tumor of the brain, which may mimic the symptoms of migraine very closely—and it is necessary to have expert advice before saying that any severe headache which occurs with sickness is "just migraine." Most cases of true migraine start at a very early age; the subjects of it are liable to "bilious attacks" in childhood and after puberty the headaches seem to take their place.

No one cause has been found for this disorder. Many things are known which will bring on an attack in anyone who is subject to the attacks. Excessive tiredness, either bodily or mental, is a well-known cause. Certain articles of diet such as chocolate, sweets, rich pastry, or fruit will bring on an attack in others. Eyestrain, infection of the back of the nose and of the tonsils has been known to produce frequent attacks which were lessened on removal of these causes. Certain emotions, especially rage or humiliation which the subject could not at the time express for fear of the consequences, have often been known to bring on attacks.

Treatment. Prevention of the attacks amounts to discovery of the particular cause in a particular case and the treatment thereof. In the attack itself little can be done for the victim except to leave him, or her, in a darkened room which has been selected for its quietness and to let him lie or sit in whichever position gives the most relief until sickness or sleep relieves his pain. No one drug had been found to suit every case of migraine, but ergometrine tartrate gives immediate relief in many cases. Some cases seem to be allergic in origin and are helped by an antihistamine, and some cases respond to ovarian extract. In general, it is easier to ward off the attacks by small doses of a sedative than to relieve an attack once it has started. (*See also* HEADACHE.)

MILIARIA. Miliaria is the very common condition known as sweat rash or heat rash. It is also called sudamina. A description is given under the heading SWEAT RASH.

MILIARY TUBERCULOSIS. This is a severe form of the disease in which the tuberculosis spreads rapidly throughout one or more organs of the body and tiny hard lumps which are said to resemble millet seed (whence comes the name) are found in the various organs affected, most commonly the lungs. (*See also* TUBERCULOSIS.)

MILK. There is only one food so far as we know on which it is possible to live solely for any length of time—milk. An adult doing hard work would need, it is said, over a gallon daily; it is not therefore a convenient form of sustenance.

Milk is regarded as the only form of animal food containing all the constituents necessary to the perfect food—protein, fat, carbohydrate, mineral salts and vitamins in sufficient quantity.

Mother and Baby. The principal differences between cow's milk and and human milk are that there is too much casein in cow's milk and not enough milk sugar; this is one reason why the mother's milk is the perfect food for her baby. The curd of cow's milk forms larger lumps than the natural milk, and the infant's stomach cannot deal with it. Diarrhea and other digestive disturbances may easily result from undiluted cow's milk.

Milk is the natural food of babies. As every mother knows now—for doctors and nurses have preached it for years—it is the mother's duty to feed her baby herself if she can do so, and personal convenience should never be allowed to stand in the way.

The Baby's Bottle. If it is necessary to feed by bottle, and later, when the teeth begin to appear and when weaning becomes due, the question of the milk used is of vital importance. It is usual to give cow's milk with water and a little cream and sugar; to start with, about twice as much water as milk is used, the proportions being altered gradually until all milk is given. Some recommend similac, dextromaltose or powdered lactum.

Milk for Children. For the growing child, milk continues to be a necessary food unless for some reason it cannot be taken and some substitute has to be found. Especially when signs of rickets show themselves, as they do in some children, generally about the sixth month or a little later, the question of milk becomes of supreme importance. While it is true that fresh air and sunshine play an important part in preventing this disease, the amount of fat and the presence of vitamins in the child's food are of great importance also.

Milk in Illness. Just as milk is the best food for children while their stomachs are weak and their digestion easily upset, so it is of great value when the adult's digestion is disturbed by illness. But not everyone can take milk alone; in such cases it may be found useful to add a little sugar, or a pinch of salt, while soda water or lime water often prevents indigestion. A little citrate of soda may help to avoid acidity. Plain water is too apt to produce diarrhea and other digestive troubles.

Milk as a Disease Carrier. Milk is perhaps the most important disease carrier we have, hence the great importance of ensuring that the daily supply comes from healthy cows cleanly milked, and that it is conveyed in properly sterilized bottles.

The officially recognized grades of milk are:

(1) *Certified Milk.* The cows must be inspected every six months for tuberculin, milked under clean conditions, the milk cooled immediately and put into bottles closed by a cap which forms a seal; the cap has on it the address of the farm, the date of milking, and the words "Certified Milk." It is delivered direct from the farm, which is responsible for its purity.

(2) *Grade A (tuberculin tested) Milk.* The conditions are the same as above; but the milk is sent to the dairies to be bottled and delivered to the consumer.

(3) *Grade A Milk.* From a herd which is examined every three months by a veterinary surgeon, but not necessarily tested for tuberculin, and not delivered to the consumer sealed.

(4) *Pasteurized Milk.* The milk raised to a temperature below boiling point, kept at this heat for half an hour, and immediately cooled.

Other forms of milk preparation are

drying, condensing, peptonizing, and humanizing. Dried cow's milk diluted with water forms a curd in the infant's stomach more like that formed by the mother's milk than that formed by untreated cow's milk, being in smaller lumps, doubtless for this reason some infant welfare centers provide it for mothers who cannot nurse their infants, or to supplement the mother's milk. Condensed milk is also sometimes used for infants where the mother cannot nurse; great care should be taken in choosing the right brand; some must, by regulation, be marked as unfit for babies. By peptonization the milk is partly digested before being given, thus making the process of digestion easier. Humanized milk is treated so as to make it as much like the mother's milk as possible.

MILK FEVER. Milk fever is the popular name for an attack of feverishness coming on in the mother about the second or third day after the birth of a child. It used to be very common, and was usually put down to nervous and constitutional upset caused by the first coming of the milk to the breasts, hence the name. It is now known that these fevers are really caused by infection in the genital tract or breasts. Milk fever has become much rarer since aseptic methods have been used at the time of labor and since women have been taught to prepare and harden the breasts beforehand so that cracked nipple does not occur. (*See also* PREGNANCY.)

MIND. This may be defined as the result of our thoughts and feelings which have been built up by our training and experience. The higher development of the mind is, of course, what distinguishes man from the highest of animals, the apes. At birth only one primitive instinct is present in the human child, as in all other young, namely, the instinct to preserve its life by acquiring food, which it does by the process of sucking. Later, the selfishness of the child, whose only interest if left untrained would be in himself, is replaced as a result of education and training by more desirable qualities which make the individual a fit member of society as it exists today. But all memories of every experience which have affected a person during his life are stored up in the mind.

Some of these memories consist of thoughts which can be recalled at any given time; these thoughts form the conscious mind. Other experiences are forgotten, either owing to lack of interest or because they were painful and unpleasant. The former may be recalled to the conscious mind easily, but the painful or unpleasant memories and ideas are "locked up," as it were, and can only be recalled with the greatest of difficulty and usually only by the help of pscyhoanalysis (q.v.)

Normal people direct the energy, which is caused by the primitive instincts in the unconscious mind struggling to make themselves felt, in a useful way; most of the arts, such as music, painting, and literature, provide an outlet, as it were, for this unwanted energy. Games also, especially in the young boy or girl, are excellent means by which this energy can be side-tracked into useful channels. There is much to be done in the treatment of nervous and mental disorder along the lines of providing some kind of outlet or means of utilizing this stored up energy. If this happy result of transforming the energy of the primitive, socially objectionable instincts into useful activities is not attained in normal people, then what is called a "conflict" is caused, and this gives rise to much mental trouble of a more or less serious nature, according to the particular individual in whom it occurs. The influence of the bodily health on the mind in such cases is of great importance, and it is absolutely necessary that in any case which shows signs of nervous or mental trouble the physician should be consulted before a person condemns himself as a victim of "nerves" and becomes more and more wretched in consequence. The majority of physicians now practice psychotherapy and are therefore in a position to treat not only the bodies but the minds of their patients. (*See also* MEMORY; MENTAL DISEASE; MENTAL HYGIENE.)

MINERAL WATERS. Practically any water can be described quite accurately as a mineral water; but, as a general rule, the term is used to apply to waters specially bottled at some health resort because of the extra amount of some mineral they contain. Some waters have extra amount of iron, sulphur, arsenic, or calcium in them which makes them specially suitable for different complaints.

MINER'S ELBOW. Constant friction or pressure on the little bag of fluid called the bursa at the back of the elbow causes a chronic swelling of bursitis. This is popularly called "miner's elbow." A similar condition on the knee is called "housemaid's knee." (*See also* BURSITIS.)

MINER'S NYSTAGMUS. A condition sometimes found in miners in which the eyeballs jerk from side to side. It is thought that the dim light in which the miner works may be the cause. (*See also* NYSTAGMUS.)

MISCARRIAGE. If a pregnancy terminates before the baby is old enough to have a separate life—that is, before the 27th week of the pregnancy—there is said to have been a miscarriage. (*See also* ABORTION; CHILDBIRTH; PREGNANCY.)

MITRAL VALVE. The mitral valve is the valve between the two left chambers of the heart. It is supposed to resemble the shape of a bishop's miter. The mitral valve may become narrowed or may not work properly, in which case there is said to be mitral disease of the heart. (*See also* HEART.)

MIXTURE. Any two or more liquids added together and well mixed for the purpose of being swallowed as medicine can be called a mixture, or mistura. The typical mixture as prescribed by a doctor will consist of two or more drugs, with a quantity of water to dilute them to a strength at which they can be safely swallowed, and a flavoring matter. Sometimes a coloring matter is added as well.

MOLAR. The molars are the back teeth with which we grind our food. (*See also* TEETH.)

MOLE. A mole is a tumor in the skin containing the brown coloring matter of the skin in excessive quantity. Sometimes the mole will be covered with hair as well. It is one form of birthmark. (*See also* BIRTHMARK; SKIN.)

MONGOLISM. This is an unfortunate severe type of mental deficiency with which a child is occasionally born. It is called Mongolism because the child has the square face and upward-slanting eyes which are characteristic of the Mongolian race. It is not known what causes Mongolism; but the child is usually the last of a large family, and it is surmised that the mother's powers of reproduction have become impaired. It is important to distinguish Mongols from cretins, because the cretinous child can be turned into a normal human being by suitable medical treatment, whereas there is nothing much to be done for the little Mongol child beyond caring for it in as kindly and sympathetic manner as possible. Their mentality remains that of a young child; but they are usually happy, cheerful, and affectionate people and easy to get on with. (*See also* MENTAL DEFICIENCY.)

MONTHLY SICKNESS. Monthly sickness, periods, or courses are all ways of alluding to the natural process of menstruation, under which heading the process is described.

MORBUS. Morbus is a Latin word meaning disease. It used to be the habit to call all disease, drugs, and medical things in general by Latin names; heart disease, for instance, would be called morbus cordis. The adjective from morbus is morbid, which is still used sometimes to mean diseased.

MORNING SICKNESS. One of the very earliest signs of pregnancy is morning sickness, which is a feeling of nausea or actual sickness on first rising from bed in the morning. The degree of sickness varies from case to case. Some women feel nauseated and sick all day; others have such disturbances as constipation, flatulence, profuse watering at the mouth, etc. The condition lasts until about the end of the third month of the pregnancy. It is supposed to be nothing more than the reaction of the nervous system to the new order of things, and needs no treatment or special consideration as things adjust themselves in due course. If the nausea should be bad, however, and it is certain that it is not the result of nervousness, it is obvious that a doctor should be consulted, for he can often help it with hormone and other treatment. (*See also* CHILDBIRTH; PREGNANCY.)

MORON. A moron is a person of little sense. In the U.S. it is used to denote the highest grade of mental defective, equivalent to the word feeble-minded. (*See also* IDIOCY; MENTAL DEFICIENCY; MENTAL DISEASE.)

MORPHIA. The name morphia is applied popularly to morphine and the drugs derived from it. It is an alkaloid obtained from the opium poppy.

Morphia, used properly, is one of the greatest blessings that have been granted to the human race. It is the greatest of all pain-killers. It is usually given by hypodermic injection. The chief characteristics of morphia are that it speedily relieves pain and produces drowsiness or sleep, it acts on the nerves of the intestines, produces constipation, and it soothes the respiratory system. It is used in order to allay severe pain, to aid in arresting severe bleeding by keeping the patient quiet, to control severe diarrhea; also, various derivatives from it such as heroin or chlorodyne, are used to soothe coughing.

Although the uses of morphia are so many and when properly used it is so beneficial, it is unfortunate that it is very much abused. The taking of morphia very soon becomes a habit and craving is developed for it which the victim will go to any lengths to satisfy. (*See also* DRUG HABITS; OPIUM.)

MORPHINE. *See* MORPHIA.

MORPHINISM. Chronic poisoning by morphia and the development of a craving for morphia are known as morphinism. (*See also* DRUG HABITS; MORPHIA.)

MORTIFICATION. The mortification of a part of the body means the death of that part by gangrene. (*See also* GANGRENE.)

MORTON'S DISEASE. This is the name given to a condition in which there are severe neuralgic pains shooting down from the ball of the foot into the toes. It is caused by the dropping and flattening of the arch of the foot, which results in pressure being put on the nerves where they pass into the toes. The condition is also known as metatarsalgia from the fact that the pain is in the region of the metatarsal bones of the foot. The treatment for this pain is to obtain proper support for the transverse arch of the foot by specially fitted shoes which are wide enough at the toes and have low and broad heels.

Exercises and massage may be helpful in restoring the arch of the foot. (*See also* FOOT.)

MOSQUITO. There are more than a thousand different species of mosquitoes, but only a certain number of these are responsible for carrying the germs of malaria. The female insect is the bloodsucker, as the digestion of blood helps her eggs to mature. Mosquitoes cannot become dangerous unless they themselves become infected by biting a patient suffering from malaria. In this way we are comparatively free from the disease in this country, though there are many mosquitoes which are able to carry malaria.

Mosquitoes can be destroyed in houses and camps by using a spray of D.D.T. in kerosene. They can be discouraged from alighting on the skin by the use of an insect repellant like dimethyl pithollatn. Oil of citronella is also used for this purpose. In the tropics, certain precautions must be taken to guard against their bite. It is important to see that all possible inlets to a house are adequately covered with screens. (*See also* BLACKWATER FEVER; FILARIASIS; MALARIA.)

MOTIONS. It is usual to talk of the evacuations of the bowels as motions or movements. (*See also* STOOLS.)

MOTOR AREAS. Our movements which we perform deliberately are caused by discharges of energy from cells in a region of the brain which is known as the motor area, meaning the area which deals with movement. For a full description of the mechanism of the brain, *see* BRAIN.

MOUNTAIN SICKNESS. People who go from a lower altitude into the mountains are liable at first to be overcome by attacks which are called mountain sickness. There may be a feeling of great muscular weakness, headache, and a necessity to gasp for air. Sickness or nausea are often present. Mountain sickness is caused by the diminution of the quantity of oxygen in the air at higher altitudes, and it is therefore common among airmen who go up to great heights. People who go to live in the ordinary inhabited mountainous regions such as Switzerland often feel the mountain sickness at first, but they become acclimatized after two or three weeks. It is the lack of air suitable for human beings to breathe that has made it so difficult to reach the summit of such mountains as Everest. Special respirators have been invented to make breathing possible at great heights.

MOUTH. The mouth is generally considered in two parts. The *vestibule* or space between the lips and cheeks and the teeth and gums, and the mouth proper, which is the large cavity between the teeth and the throat. Above, the mouth is bounded by the hard palate, which merges into the soft palate at the back of the mouth. The tongue lies on the floor of the mouth, which contains the blood vessels and glands which pour the saliva into the mouth. The whole of the mouth is lined by mucous membrane. The various parts of the structure of the mouth—the teeth, tongue, lips, jaws, etc.—are described under their own headings.

Inflammation of the mouth is called *stomatitis;* inflammation of the tongue is *glossitis,* and inflammation of the gums is *gingivitis.* The mouth is subject to ulceration from such causes as a jagged tooth, neglected stomatitis, etc. Various diseases such as measles and chicken pox can be diagnosed by the appearance of rashes in the mouth.

As the whole food supply of the body passes through the mouth, it is obvious that it should be kept clean and in good health.

A septic condition in the mouth, either from the teeth or the tonsils, will often cause trouble further down in the digestive tract.

MOUTHWASH. It is useful to have a mouthwash handy and occasionally to give the mouth a good rinse out and gargle in addition to the usual teeth-cleaning operations. Common salt, bicarbonate of soda, boric acid, glycerine of thymol, potassium chlorate, or hydrogen peroxide are all very useful mouthwashes, and there are many variations put up in handy form in tablets for dissolving in water. Tablets containing penicillin or other antibiotics must be used with caution and only under medical or dental advice.

MUCO-PURULENT. This is an adjective meaning a mixture of mucus and pus

(matter). The discharge from the nose in the later stages of a bad cold is often muco-purulent, as will be seen from its yellowish color.

MUCOUS MEMBRANE. The linings of various organs of the body are moistened with the sticky substance called mucus and are called mucous membranes. The organs of the digestive system, of the breathing apparatus, and the genitourinary passages are the chief regions lined with mucous membrane. Any inflammation of a mucous membrane increases the flow of mucus and causes the condition known as catarrh. (*See also* CATARRH; MEMBRANE.)

MUCUS. Mucus is a sticky, slimy substance which is poured out over the mucous membranes which line various organs of the body. It protects these organs against friction and attacks by germs. Thus when anything irritates the mucous membrane a greater flow of mucus than usual is poured forth. The saliva contains a large amount of mucus which serves to bind together the food into a mass ready to be swallowed. In the stomach and the intestines the mucus also serves this purpose of binding the contents in order that they may be more easily propelled along the digestive tract. (*See also* CATARRH; COLITIS; MUCOUS MEMBRANE.)

MULTIPARA. A woman who has had more than one child is called a multipara.

MULTIPLE NEURITIS. Neuritis occurring in more than one nerve at the same time is called multiple neuritis. It is of course an extremely painful condition, and is usually the result of some poison which is circulating in the blood, or of a chronic disease such as diabetes. Chronic alcoholism is often accompanied by multiple neuritis, which is relieved by injections of Vitamin B_1. (*See also* NEURITIS.)

MUMPS. Mumps is one of the commonest of the acute infectious diseases caused by a virus. It is more common in childhood than among adults, but is apt to cause more distress to adults. It is very infectious, and the danger of infection is not over for two to three weeks after the symptoms appear; then the *incubation period* is also up to three weeks, so no household that has had a case of mumps is safe from it until nearly six weeks have elapsed. As it is extremely difficult to get people, especially children, to remain in isolation for that length of time, it is often found that a second case occurs in the same household when it has been thought that all danger was past.

Symptoms. The usual fever symptoms are present, raised temperature, up to 100 deg. or higher, being the rule. The most characteristic symptom, however, is the swelling of the glands of the neck under the ear and perhaps under the chin. These are the parotid glands and the submaxillary glands. The swelling and soreness begin on one side and after a few days usually spread to the other side of the face as well. The worst points of tenderness are about the ear and under the edge of the jaw. The swelling may be immense and there may be a great deal of pain, though as a rule the patient does not become as sick and feverish as in some of the other fevers. Sometimes the patient may become delirious, and in rare cases he may pass into a comatose state.

Treatment. The patient must, of course, be put to bed and isolated with all the usual precautions against the spread of infectious disease. Fluid diet and sponging will keep the fever in check. The mouth must be rinsed at intervals with an antiseptic mouthwash such as potassium permanganate, and hot or sometimes cold fomentation should be applied over the swollen glands. It may be necessary for a doctor to prescribe something for the relief of pain. After the patient recovers, remember that the period of quarantine is three weeks. The germ of mumps does not live for very long, so drastic measures of disinfection are not usually necessary.

Complications. Although simple mumps is not a dangerous disease, there are several complications which may be serious. The worst of these complications is inflammation of the pancreas, called *pancreatitis*. This requires careful treatment, as in some cases diabetes has followed upon inflammation of the pancreas during an attack of mumps. In males, the testicle sometimes becomes inflamed, a condition which is known as *orchitis,* and requires immediate treatment lest the gland should become weakened. Less commonly, inflammation of the ovaries and breasts may occur in females. Eye, ear, and brain complications are fortunately rare with mumps, but they do occur sometimes, and incurable deafness is not very uncommon. Inflammation of the kidney (nephritis) may also arise after mumps.

MURMUR. Any unusual sound, other than the ordinary heart sounds, which is heard when listening to the heart is called a mumur, or a bruit, which is a French word meaning noise. Some murmurs are evidence of heart disease, but some have no special significance. This was well shown during both wars, when many men with "heart murmurs" performed striking feats of endurance. (*See also* HEART.)

MUSCLES. The muscles of the body are composed of cells which have the power of changing their shape, and it is by this power that the movements of the body are carried out.

Muscles are divided into three classes; striped muscle, which is also called skeletal or voluntary muscle; unstriped involuntary muscle, and the heart muscle. *Striped muscle* is so-called because when it is examined under a microscope its fibers show cross-striping. *Voluntary muscle* is one which can be controlled by the will of the individual, whereas *involuntary muscle* works without the conscious knowledge of the individual. The muscles of the arm are voluntary muscles, but the muscles of the bowel are involuntary. *Skeletal muscle* is the muscle tissue which covers our bones. It is voluntary muscle, and it forms the greater part of the entire muscular tissue of the body. A skeletal muscle has an origin and an attachment. For instance, the origin of the biceps muscle of the arm is on the shoulder bone, and its insertion is into the radius, one of the bones of the forearm. As well as a beginning and end, there is the more bulky and fleshy main part of the muscle, which is usually called the belly of the muscle. Muscles vary in shape: there are ribbon-shaped muscles, spindle-shaped muscles thicker in the middle than at the ends, and muscles like those in the abdominal walls which are in the form of thin sheets of muscular tissue.

Each muscle is composed of bundles of fibers separated by connective tissue and wrapped round in a sheath. Muscles are

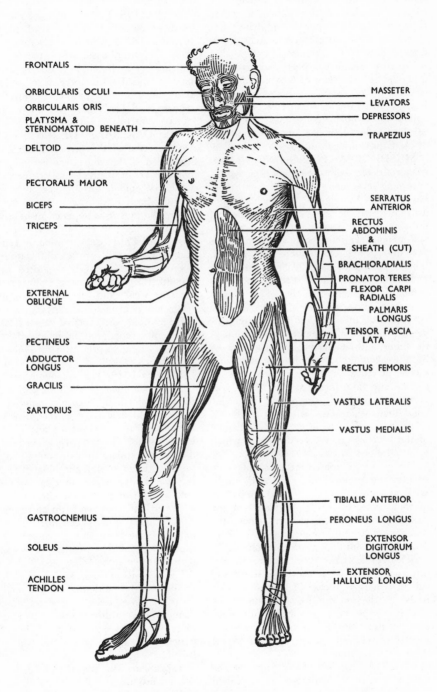

FRONTALIS

ORBICULARIS OCULI

ORBICULARIS ORIS

PLATYSMA &
STERNOMASTOID BENEATH

DELTOID

PECTORALIS MAJOR

BICEPS

TRICEPS

EXTERNAL
OBLIQUE

PECTINEUS

ADDUCTOR
LONGUS

GRACILIS

SARTORIUS

GASTROCNEMIUS

SOLEUS

ACHILLES
TENDON

MASSETER

LEVATORS

DEPRESSORS

TRAPEZIUS

SERRATUS
ANTERIOR

RECTUS
ABDOMINIS
&
SHEATH (CUT)

BRACHIORADIALIS

PRONATOR TERES

FLEXOR CARPI
RADIALIS

PALMARIS
LONGUS

TENSOR FASCIA
LATA

RECTUS FEMORIS

VASTUS LATERALIS

VASTUS MEDIALIS

TIBIALIS ANTERIOR

PERONEUS LONGUS

EXTENSOR
DIGITORUM
LONGUS

EXTENSOR
HALLUCIS LONGUS

The Muscular System.

417

dependent on the nerves which are attached to them. These nerves provide the stimulus which puts the muscle in action. If, therefore, the nerve supplying any muscle is paralyzed or severed, the muscle loses its power of movement.

When a muscle has been over-stretched it is said to be *strained*. A typical case of strain is when the ankle turns over suddenly and the muscle is sharply stretched. There is pain, and stiffness develops. Strained muscles should be rested and hot or cold applications put on to relieve pain.

MUSHROOM POISONING. Mushrooms are classed as *poisonous* or *edible,* according to species. The word "toadstool" has no scientific significance, being popularly used to decribe various species of poisonous mushrooms.

Poisonous varieties can be fatal. The two most dangerous poisons are *phallin,* found in the Death Angel (*Amanita phalloides*) and related species, and *muscarine,* contained in the *Fly Agaric* (*Amanita muscaria*). In the former, first symptoms occur about ten hours after eating, with severe abdominal pains, cramp in the limbs, and convulsions. This is followed by a weakening pulse, with vomiting and severe diarrhea. The victim may die in two to four days. In the case of Fly Agaric, vomiting, diarrhea, suppression of urine, and dizziness appear within two hours. Drowsiness, cold sweating, and weakening of the heart's action precede death, which usually follows in two or three days.

Treatment for muscarine poisoning consists of the removal of undigested mushroom as soon as possible, and the injection of some powerful heart stimulant. In the case of phallin poisoning again remove the remains of the mushroom promptly. There is no known antidote to the poison.

MYASTHENIA. Myasthenia or myasthenia gravis, as it is more frequently called, is a rare disease of the muscles. It is due to the too rapid destruction of the chemical substances responsible for muscular contraction. The symptoms are immediately relieved by an injection of the drug physostigmine.

MYDRIATIC. When the pupil of the eye is excessively enlarged it is called mydriasis. Drugs such as atropine, which are used to increase the size of the pupil,

are called mydriatics. (*See also* ATROPINE; EYE PUPIL.)

MYELITIS. Inflammation of the spinal cord or softening of the cord is called myelitis. The condition is a serious one if it is due to disease, when paralysis and wasting occur, but if it is due to pressure on the spinal cord there is a possibility that the pressure may be removed and recovery effected. (*See also* PARAPLEGIA; POLIOMYELITIS; SPINAL CORD.)

MYOCARDIAL DEGENERATION. Degeneration of the myocardium or heart muscle may be due to different causes, but the result is the same, namely heart weakness and failure. A common cause of myocardial degeneration is fibrosis, where the muscle is impeded in its working by an over-growth of the fibers which surround it. Fatty degeneration is another common cause of myocardial failure. In obese people the fat is deposited in and around the heart muscle, causing it to become weak and degenerated. Another form of degeneration, known as waxy degeneration, also occurs, usually as the result of a condition in which there has been a long septic illness. (*See also* HEART.)

MYXEDEMA. This is a condition which is fairly common in middle-aged women, though it occurs in men and children also. It is due to deficiency in the juice which is produced by the thyroid gland.

Symptoms. The typical patient is a middle-aged woman who becomes fat and puffy, with coarse skin and bloated features. She has pudgy hands, muddy complexion with a slight flush over the cheekbones, and a loss of hair from the scalp and eyebrows. The intellect usually becomes duller, the patient being heavier and clumsier in her speech and slower in her understanding than she used to be.

Fat deposits occur in such regions as the shoulders, the abdominal wall and the breasts. A well-developed case of myxedema is easy to distinguish, but the condition may creep on gradually without the patient noticing it until it is well established.

Treatment. As the disease is due to thyroid insufficiency the results of administering thyroid extract appear almost miraculous. In a very short time the woman regains her health and will retain it as long as the takes the thyroid extract. A word of warning is due here. Thyroid extract has a marked effect on the heart and must never be taken except on a doctor's advice, and while the patient is on it she should be kept under observation from time to time and should report at once any untoward symptoms such as palpitations or breathlessness. (*See also* DUCTLESS GLANDS; THYROID GLAND.)

NAILS, DISEASES OF. *Abscess* of the nail is very often the result of a splinter entering the tissues under the nail. Pus, or matter, collects, and there is always a great deal of throbbing pain owing to the pressure of the tight, firm nail upon the sensitive nail-bed. In order to allow the pus to discharge the nail may have to be cut or split, otherwise the pain may be almost unendurable, and there is always the possibility that the inflammation may spread and cause damage to the whole nail. As soon as there is any hint of inflammation occurring in the nail, hot fomentations or kaolin should be applied. (*See also* WHITLOW.)

Ingrowing nail is a condition which occurs in the nail of the big toe. The main cause of this condition is trimming the nail in the wrong way, and in addition, when too-tight shoes are worn, the nail is pressed into the flesh at the side, causing inflammation. The nails should be cut straight across and not trimmed down in the corners, or they may be cut in a concave manner, thus: ⌣ (*See also* INGROWING TOE-NAIL.)

Injuries to the nails cause them to turn black owing to the presence of blood beneath them. If the injury has been severe, the nail is almost sure to come off; but a new one should grow unless the injury has damaged the nail-bed very severely. A new nail takes, as a rule, about six months to grow again, and during this period it should be protected by a bandage.

The appearance of the nails very often indicates the general state of health; for example, white spots usually make their appearance when the health is a bit below par and grooves indicate the presence of rheumatism.

NAPHTHOL. A coal-tar product, naphthol is used as an antiseptic in cases of diarrhea, typhoid fever, etc. It is used as an ointment on the skin in the treatment of pediculosis, scabies, and other skin disorders. It is of great use as an insecticide (a substance which kills insects), and as such it is used in mothballs for preventing moths from living in and destroying furs and clothes.

NARCOSIS. This is a state of unconsciousness closely resembling deep sleep. The drugs which produce this condition are known as narcotics. (*See also* ANESTHETICS.)

NARCOTICS. The most important narcotics or sleep-producing drugs are opium, hyoscine, and veronal. Alcohol, chloroform, and the other anesthetics are also included. (*See also* ANESTHETICS; DRUGS.)

NASAL CATARRH. See CATARRH, NASAL.

NASAL FEEDING. See FORCIBLE FEEDING.

NASO-PHARYNX. The naso-pharynx is the name given to the part of the throat which lies between the nasal passages and the back of the mouth.

NAUSEA. A feeling of sickness, or the feeling that vomiting is about to take place is known as nausea. (*See also* MORNING SICKNESS; PREGNANCY; SEA-SICKNESS; VOMITING.)

NAVEL. This is a small wrinkled cavity in the middle of the abdomen known also as the umbilicus. It marks the spot where the umbilical cord unites the child to the mother before birth. (*See also* CORD; UMBILICUS.)

NECROSIS. Necrosis means the death of a part of the body, but the word is used with special reference to the death of bone. This state is usually caused by stoppage of the blood supply.

When the blood supply is cut off from a part of a bone it becomes necrosed, and the vessels surrounding it form what is known as a layer of granulations. This granulation tissue gradually eats away the dead bone from the living so that it becomes loose, and it is then known as a sequestrum. If this is very small it may be discharged with the pus which is given off from the granulations. The cavity will rapidly heal once the irritation caused by the dead bone is removed. This happy state of affairs, however, does not always come about spontaneously, and the sequestrum often has to be removed by surgical operation. (*See also* BONE; EROSION; GANGRENE.)

NEPHRITIS. Nephritis, or Bright's disease, is a condition in which there is inflammation of the kidneys.

There are several forms of this disease, but the chief varieties may be classified as acute and chronic.

Acute nephritis is frequently caused by exposure to cold or wet, or it may arise as a complication of some other disease such as scarlet fever, erysipelas, or sore throat. Adequate treatment of such diseases with penicillin or other antibiotics will help to prevent kidney complications. Infected tonsils are known to cause nephritis sometimes, and should be removed after an attack. It mainly affects young people.

Symptoms. In some cases the onset of the disease may be insidious and the first symptoms to be noticed are redness of the urine and a certain amount of puffiness around the eyes. Dropsy, or body swelling, with puffiness of the eyes, face and ankles, is almost always present in varying degrees. Vomiting and nausea frequently occur early on in the condition, and this leads to loss of appetite and disturbance of the digestive system. The temperature is commonly raised to about 100 deg. or 101 deg. F., though in adults there may be no fever. The skin is dry and the tongue furred, and headache is common. There is frequently pain in the back and loins, and diarrhea may develop. Changes take place in the urine from the very beginning of the disease. It is greatly reduced in quantity and the color becomes dark and smoky from the presence of blood. When tested, a large amount of albumin is found to be present and it also contains enormous numbers of blood cells.

Treatment. As soon as a patient shows the slightest sign of nephritis he must be put to bed and kept as warm as possible. Blankets should be used instead of sheets, and flannel should be worn next to the skin. The temperature of the bedroom should be moderately warm and all drafts avoided. The bowels must be kept open daily in order to help the elimination of waste matters from the body and so ease the work of the kidneys. It used to be thought that by restricting the intake of fluids and foodstuffs the acutely affected kidneys would be spared work. Nowadays it is usual to give fluids from the very beginning in amounts equal to the volume of the previous day's output of urine. It is usual also to give penicilin for four or five days. In severe cases of acute nephritis it is true that the patient may not be able to take anything for a few days except fluids, sweetened fruit juices or diluted milk, not more than two pints a day. In other cases, however, the diet should consist of thirty ounces of milk in a day, with starch and fat foods, but very small amounts of protein.

No salt should be added in cooking as long as there is any swelling present in the body. The patient must be kept in bed until all traces of blood have disappeared from the urine, the swelling has gone, and the temperature is normal. Iron tonics should be given during convalescence to deal with the anemia which usually makes its appearance in connection with nephritis; these tonics will help to improve the appetite. The patient must guard against chills, wear warm clothes, and avoid overfatigue.

Chronic Nephritis may follow an attack of acute nephritis, but in some cases the acute attack may have passed unnoticed.

Treatment. Special care must be taken to avoid chills and the diet must be regulated by a doctor. The bowels should be kept open and no alcohol should be taken. It is now recognized that restriction of protein may be harmful in chronic nephritis, but the high protein diet now advised should not be given when the activity of the kidney is impaired. (*See also* KIDNEY; EDEMA.)

NERVOUS BREAKDOWN. This results from disturbance of balance between a person and his circumstances. Either the person is himself unable to adapt himself to his circumstances or the difficulties to be overcome are very great.

Treatment. The treatment of such a nervous breakdown varies, but nearly always begins with prolonged rest in bed and as much sleep as the patient can be made to obtain.

NERVOUS HEADACHE. This may mean one of two things: either true migraine, or a means of escape from some unpleasant situation which the victim does not, unconsciously, want to face. The prospect of a long railway journey, or a visit to a disliked relative, will in many people produce the most violent headache. This headache is nearly always said to be a "pressure," rather than an ache, and is mostly situated on the top of the head. The scalp is tender, and any slight noise, or even a whisper, will irritate the victim beyond measure. Drugs may, or may not, give relief; but as the underlying cause of the headache is in the mind, only by getting to the real source of mental conflict and bringing it into consciousness is there hope of permanent cure. (*See also* MI-GRAINE.)

NERVOUS SYSTEM. This is the means by which each part of our body is made aware of what the condition is at any particular moment of every other part, and also is the means by which we communicate with the outside world.

In man, the nervous system is generally divided into the central nervous system, which consists of the brain and the spinal cord, and the peripheral nervous system, which consists of all the nerves in the body other than those attached to the brain itself. The brain is described under a separate heading, and under this heading also will be found an account of the peculiar structure of nervous tissue. Here it will only be mentioned that the nervous system consists essentially of nerve cells and a supporting tissue.

A nerve cell has a body and processes. Processes which take impulses away from the cell (like an electric charge along an electric wire), are called *axons;* while those which take the impulses to the cell are called *dendrites*. There are countless numbers of these nerve cells and their processes in the nervous system, but their function is the same, that of conducting

impulses. Each cell with its processes is one unit, and many units are bound up together according to the various kinds of impulses they conduct, rather like a number of coaches being joined up to form one long train going to a certain place. Some of these bundles of units control the movements of the body; others are responsible for telling us where our limbs are in space, or whether we are touching something hot or cold. Some bundles of units run from the brain, down through the spinal cord and out into the nerves, right into the skin. Others do not run throughout the nervous system in that way, but run only in the nerves and into the spinal cord.

The *spinal cord* is a nervous tissue which runs from the bottom of the skull, inside the backbone, down to the level of the top of the haunch bones. It contains all those conducting paths whereby we move, feel, and know where our limbs are when our eyes are shut. If the spinal cord is cut across by a broken backbone, for example, the body below the injury is completely paralyzed; and if the injury occurs above a certain level, death is bound to follow almost immediately because the chest muscles become paralyzed, so that the lungs can no longer expand and breathing stops.

From the spinal cord, nerves are given off in pairs all the way down the spinal cord to travel outwards through a space in the bony backbone to supply all the muscles of the limbs, internal organs, and skin of the body. These nerves are like long pearl-gray cords when they first leave the spinal cord, but they split up into smaller and smaller branches as they pass on their way, until it is almost impossible to see their small branches to the skin with the naked eye. These nerves carry different bundles of nerve units also.

There are units which run to the muscles and cause them to contract; these are called *motor* units. Then there are the units by which we feel touch or pain or temperature; these are called the *sensory* units. If a nerve is damaged, usually both these systems of units are injured, but certain diseases seem to pick out certain units. For example, in lead poisoning the "motor" units are mainly affected, and weakness of the limbs is especially noticed.

In neuritis caused by alcohol poisoning the "sensory" units are chiefly picked upon and pain is the outstanding feature of this condition.

The internal organs, such as the heart and digestive organs, have a special nerve supply called the *autonomic* nervous system which governs activities outside our conscious control. It is divided into two anatomical groups—the sympathetic and the parasympathetic nervous systems. When there is a need for sudden action on the part of the whole body, as, for example, to run for one's life from a wild beast, the sympathetic system takes charge and enables all the energy of the body to be concentrated on the act of running. The muscles get an extra blood supply because the sympathetic system tells the blood vessels to the muscles to enlarge; the heart pumps more forcibly to send the utmost amount of blood as quickly as possible through the body; all digestion stops so that as little blood as possible is taken up by the digestive organs, and lungs expand and contract more strongly than normal to get as much oxygen into the blood in as short a time as possible. In some people the sympathetic system is more irritable than in others, and in them, a very slight fright will produce all the symptoms which we associate with a state of terror. The parasympathetic system has the opposite effect and its stimulation causes slowing of the heart, increased movement of the intestine and secretion of the digestive glands. (*See also* BRAIN; NEURITIS.)

NERVOUSNESS. This is also one of the features of the condition of anxiety and must then be looked upon as part of that affliction.

In children, nervousness is very common, especially in only children upon whom too much attention is lavished. The family doctor is the right person to try to gain the child's confidence to find out the cause of the nervousness. Often the child is too frightened of its parents to confide in them. A child who suffers from nervousness, if untreated, becomes an adult who suffers from a neurosis, and nervous disease in adults is much more difficult to cure than it is in children, in whom fewer paths of memory have been established. (*See also* ANXIETY; NEUROSIS.)

NETTLE-RASH. An eruption of the skin, similar to the effect produced by the sting of a nettle, is known as nettle-rash, or urticaria. It is often allergic in origin and may be relieved by injection of a few drops of adrenalin. The itching is soothed by the application of bicarbonate of soda solution. (*See also* URTICARIA.)

NEURALGIA. This is the name for pain felt along a nerve. There are very many different causes for neuralgia as well as many different positions where the pain may be felt, but the character of the pain is nearly always the same. It is of a severe shooting or throbbing nature and the skin, along which tiny branches of the nerves run, is often very tender to touch. Another curious feature of the pain of neuralgia is that it is not continuous but occurs in little bouts, which are made worse by exposing the skin to the cold. Neuralgia may be the result of changes in the nerves, when the pain is said to be due to neuritis; or the nerves themselves may be healthy, the pain being caused by pressure on the nerves by other structures; or the nerves may be irritated by some disease of structures with which they are in contact. In some cases it is not possible to find out why neuralgia occurs, and this, unfortunately, is the fact in one of the most painful forms of neuralgia—the kind known as *tic douleureux*.

This is felt on the face, usually on one side only, all over the one side, or round the eye only, or rarely, round the nose and chin only. The pain is exceedingly sharp and is always felt worst in a draft or in cold weather. The skin of the part of the face on which the pain is felt is so tender that patients dread washing their faces, and if asked to show where the pain is situated they do not touch the face, but carefully keep their pointing finger a half an inch away from the painful area when indicating its extent. The lightest touch in severe cases will bring on an attack of this tic douleureux, and the pain may become so bad that these unhappy patients will even think of suicide rather than endure it. Fortunately, we can relieve this pain by means of an injection of alcohol into a nerve of the face. The result is that the patient loses the pain, but is left with a numb feeling on that side of the face. It may be necessary to repeat this injection in a year or eighteen months, but the relief afforded by the injection can really only be appreciated by those who have suffered from this pain of tic douleureux.

In a few cases it would seem that some kind of irritation causes the pain, not in the nerve itself, but in a collection of nerve cells called a ganglion, connected with this nerve inside the skull. In these cases, injecting the nerve has no effect; but, luckily, it is possible to inject alcohol into this ganglion and usually, when this operation—which in skilled hands is a slight but tricky one—is carried out, the relief is permanent.

But not every pain on the face is due to tic douleureux. Much more often is neuralgia of the face caused by decaying teeth, the nerves of which are connected with those of the face. And even a plug of wax in the ear has been known to give rise to very bad neuralgia of the temple. Neuralgia of the back of the head is very common after sitting in a draft, and this is due to a slight thickening of the covering of the muscles of the back of the neck which presses on the sensitive nerves.

One form of neuralgia may puzzle many doctors before the spots of "shingles" appear. Perhaps four or five days before a crop of "shingles" shows itself, a patient may complain of neuralgia on one side of the chest, abdomen, or face. Nothing can be found to account for this pain until the spots appear.

Other causes of neuralgia may be such general diseases as diabetes or arteriosclerosis, while the early pains of tabes dorsalis are often taken for a simple neuralgia. *Sciatica,* which is one of the forms of neuritis and is described under that heading, always starts as a neuralgia.

Treatment. The cure of any type of neuralgia depends entirely on the cause, but the pain itself is dealt with in three main ways. These are by means of heat, warmth, and the use of drugs which make the whole nervous system less sensitive to pain. Heat and warmth are best applied by hot-water bottles, or kaolin. The drugs which "damp down" the sensitiveness of the nervous system to pain are many, and the choice of a suitable drug for this purpose depends on the individual. The coal tar group of drugs such as aspirin, phenacetin, and pyramidon are often helpful,

while in other instances the bromides or tincture of gelsemium afford relief. Rarely, if ever, is the use of morphia required or justified in neuralgia, since the habit of taking morphia is soon acquired, and many a morphia addict first learned the effects of the drug through being given it to deaden the pain of a severe neuralgic attack. (*See also* ARTERIOSCLERIOSIS; NEURITIS; TABES DORSALIS.)

NEURASTHENIA. This is a state of chronic mental and physical weariness for which there is no obvious cause. People who suffer from this very common complaint feel bodily and mentally tired as soon as they attempt to undertake the ordinary tasks of life.

This tiredness, which is so characteristic of neurasthenia, may be accompanied by many other symptoms which suggest bodily illness. Thus, mental effort may produce a violent headache, or more commonly a feeling of pressure on top of the head. Reading makes the eyes ache or produces the sensation of spots in front of the eyes. Walking makes the patient with neurasthenia desperately weary; food makes him feel sick or gives him indigestion, while any special excitement gives him violent palpitation or pain over the heart. All these complaints may be made in the course of a single interview by a patient with neurasthenia, and such a case may need the most careful examination to exclude any true bodily illness.

Treatment. The treatment of neurasthenia is both mental and physical. At first rest in bed free from all worry is essential. Daily routine exercises which are graded according to the doctor's estimate of what the patient can comfortably do are an important part of the treatment. These exercises are daily increased so that the whole physical system is built up. Usually there is constipation and this should be thoroughly treated. Any sources of sepsis, such as bad teeth, must be attended to. On the mental side encouragement and help must be given.

Traumatic Neurasthenia. This is a state of fear combined with pain which follows on some direct injury or shock. It is very common after train accidents in which the patient has not himself actually been hurt, but has seen others hurt. It very seldom follows serious injury. After a slight injury in an accident the pain persists long after the injury has healed and the patient suffers from general nervousness and, as in ordinary neurasthenia, is unable to concentrate on his work. Traumatic neurasthenia has been the subject of much discussion in the law courts. There is little doubt that the possibility of earning compensation does much to perpetuate this disorder. Often the patient labors under a sense of grievance yet the mechanism of his symptoms is not consciously understood. (*See also* NERVOUSNESS.)

NEURITIS. Neuritis is the name given to the inflammation of a nerve, and the changes in the nerve are those of swelling and redness which are associated with that process. Consequently the work of the nerve cannot be carried on normally.

The causes of neuritis are many; but, generally speaking, the chief causes are poisons, whether simple chemical poisons, or the poisons produced by diseases in the body, or by such germs as that which causes diphtheria.

Alcoholic neuritis is the result of drinking spirits in large quantities over a long period. It is one of the most painful forms of neuritis known, and attacks both the arms and legs.

In diphtheria, neuritis of a particular type occurs: the nerves which control the movements of the eyes and of the palate are damaged by the poison made by the germ of diphtheria and so the patient is unable to read, as he cannot fix his eyes on the print; and food, instead of going down the gullet, is brought back through the nose. The outlook for this form of neuritis is good, as it nearly always gets better within a few weeks.

Treatment. The first thing is to discover the cause and to remove it at once. In the first stage of treatment, after the cause has been removed, the patient must rest in bed. When the pains are severe, application of heat and liniments containing belladonna often give relief. Massage, at first very gentle and then more energetic, is very helpful. (*See also* NERVOUS SYSTEM.)

NEUROLOGY. This name is applied to branch of medicine which deals with the nervous system and its diseases.

NEUROMA. Neuroma means a tumour connected with a nerve. They are usually composed of nerve tissue and may be exceedingly painful. (*See also* TUMOR.)

NEURON. A neuron is one of the countless number of units of which the nervous system is composed. Each neuron consists of a cell and its various processes. (*See also* NERVOUS SYSTEM.)

NEUROSIS. Neurosis is a mild form of mental disorder in which the troubled mind draws attention to itself by causing some bodily symptoms. There are many different kinds of neurosis, and the more important ones are discussed under the headings of ANXIETY, HYSTERIA and NEURASTHENIA. Broadly speaking, a neurosis is the result of a battle between the conscious mind, which has been trained to adapt itself to our present social code, and the unconscious mind, which is for ever striving to obtain for the individual that pleasant, selfish and wholly irresponsible life which he enjoyed as a baby, and which is forever beyond his reach. (*See* MIND.)

Normally people manage to balance their lives so as to satisfy their primitive instincts without much conflict between the conscious and unconscious minds, but when the conflict is at all severe a neurosis develops to hide the real cause of the conflict.

One particular kind of neurosis is known as *occupation neurosis*. It is not yet certain exactly how this type of neurosis is related to the common types. An occupation neurosis may occur in any occupation in which there is a constant repetition of similar movements. The most familiar example is *writers' cramp*. Telegraphists and violinists are also very liable to suffer from the same complaint. The hand cannot perform the required movements: cramp in the small muscles of the hand produces stiff fingers which cannot hold a pen or draw a bow once across a violin.

Often there is discomfort or actual pain in the affected hand. Any other movements, except those connected with the occupation, are, nevertheless, well performed. The outlook for people with an occupation neurosis is not very good, since, although one attack may be cured by the rest from the particular occupation combined with *psychotherapy*, yet the condition often returns when the occupation is resumed. In writers' cramp, very often devices can be made to overcome the spasm of the muscles: other fingers may be used to hold the pen, or a larger or smaller pen may be used. The detailed treatment of the neuroses will be found under separate headings, but in general the treatment of all types of neurosis consists in psychotherapy together with treatment of such bodily conditions as overtiredness and sleeplessness. (*See also* PSYCHOTHERAPY.)

NEUROTIC. Anyone of a very temperamental nature whose actions are influenced by the emotions is said to be neurotic.

NEVUS. This is the name applied to moles, or birth-marks, especially those marks known as port-wine stains, strawberry marks, etc. (*See also* BIRTHMARKS.)

NIGHT BLINDNESS. In this condition the eye does not possess the normal power of rapid adaptation to a dim light. A patient so affected gets along quite well in daylight, but when the sun goes down he is practically blind. If he leaves a brightly lighted room for a dark one, he gropes along helplessly. Many night-blind people cannot see the stars, their light being insufficient to affect the eye.

Night blindness is due to lack of Vitamin A, which is the "mother substance" of visual purple, and sufferers from it nearly always become normal after adequate treatment with Vitamin A. It is sometimes associated with beriberi, which is due to lack of Vitamin B₁.

NIGHTMARE. This is a terrifying dream in which the sleeper undergoes horrible experiences. The victim of a nightmare awakes either with a cry, or in a cold sweat, and always with a feeling of suffocation. Formerly it was supposed that a nightmare was due to indigestion following a heavy meal late at night, but recently it has been shown by Freud that a nightmare must be explained in the same way as any other dream (*see* DREAMS): that is, as a disguised expression of a childish wish. (*See also* PSYCHOTHERAPY.)

NIGHT TERRORS. These occur in highly strung nervous children who are permitted too much excitement and indigestible articles of food last thing at night. While not serious, the attacks are alarming, the child waking up after an hour or two in bed, screaming and in a state of terror. The child is soon soothed however by a few comforting and reassuring words. A routine of regular meals, exercise in the open air, and an avoidance of excitement or fatigue should be practised and strictly adhered to.

NIPPLES, CRACKED. Women are apt to suffer from cracks at the apex or base of the nipple during the nursing period. This is specially liable to happen with the first baby when the milk may be scanty and the infant thus compelled to suck vigorously. Cracks usually heal rapidly and spontaneously, but they may become infected, giving rise to painful fissures which make suckling difficult and predispose to breast abscess. If a crack does appear, it is advisable to stop feeding from the affected breast until it is healed. The milk from the damaged breast should be expressed by hand and fed to the infant by spoon. The crack itself should be kept scrupulously clean and be dressed with compound tincture of benzoin, whereupon healing should not be very long delayed.

When the nipples are at all flat or indrawn it is necessary to prepare them carefully during the last few months of pregnancy, especially with the first baby. They should be gently massaged between the finger and thumb and drawn out using a little lanolin as a lubricant. Alcohol should not be used to harden the nipples, as it forms cracks.

NIPPLE, PAGET'S DISEASE OF. This is a serious disease of the nipple which begins with a peculiar hardness of the skin and goes on to intractable ulceration. It is a form of cancer which commences in the milk ducts or tubes on the surface of the nipple.

The surface of the nipple and areola becomes raw, dark red, granular or roughened, and moist.

The disease nearly always attacks women of middle age. It often happens that the patient "knows there is something wrong," but lets the condition run on from day to day, and month after month, until at last, frightened by increasing pain, she seeks medical advice. Pain in the breast should always have the opinion of a doctor, even if it does turn out to be only a comparatively harmless neuralgia.

Treatment. This consists in the removal of the whole breast. This may sound rather drastic as a cure for what appears to be merely a patch of raw skin, which in its earlier stages might be covered by a penny; but attempts at removing a part of the breast are found to give very unsatisfactory results. (*See also* CANCER; DERMATITIS; PAGET'S DISEASE.)

NITRATE. A salt formed by nitric acid. In medicine the nitrates in common use are nitrate of potassium and nitrate of silver.

NITRITE. Nitrites are salts which have a powerful effect on the blood-vessels and they are used to check spasms of all sorts. The most commonly used nitrites are nitrite of amyl, of potassium and of sodium. (*See also* AMYL NITRITE.)

NITROGEN. About two-thirds of the atmosphere is made up of nitrogen, a colorless, odorless gas necessary to all animal and plant life. (*See also* AIR; OXYGEN.)

NITROGLYCERINE. This oil, which is well known in other circumstances as an explosive, has the same action as amyl nitrite and it is frequently taken by people who suffer from angina of effort. Occasionally it is given to relieve asthma. It has also been used in the treatment of seasickness and conditions in which there is excessive blood pressure. (*See also* AMYL NITRITE; ASTHMA.)

NITROUS OXIDE. This is also known as laughing gas and it is given as an anesthetic for short operations. (*See also* ANESTHETICS.)

NOCTURNAL EMISSIONS. Emissions of the seminal fluid during the night should be looked upon as natural and quite harmless unless they occur too frequently and are followed by depression next morning. The length of time between each emission varies with each individual; but, as a rule, an interval of ten days or two weeks may be looked upon as normal. Plenty of exercise, a cold tub in the morning and good plain food are helpful in reducing their frequency. (*See also* SEX HYGIENE.)

NODE. A node is a lump or swelling, usually upon the surface of a bone. The term nodule means a small swelling.

NORMAL. Generally speaking, the term normal is used in connection with anything that conforms to regular and established order. *Normal saline solution* is common salt dissolved in distilled water, so-called because the concentration is similar to that in the body fluids.

NOSE. The nose contains the sense organ of smell. It also forms the upper end of the air passages, and its most important function is to warm and moisten the air before it descends to the lungs. The nose may be divided into two parts, the projecting or external part, and the internal or nasal cavities. The external part of the nose is formed by bone and cartilage and at the lower part are two openings, the nostrils, which form passages into the internal cavities. When the nose is injured, some of the cartilage is liable to become dislocated, thus altering the shape of the nose and the whole expression of the face.

The interior of the nose is divided into two narrow cavities by a thin partition known as the septum, and these cavities run directly backwards for about two inches. On each side three delicate bones, the turbinates, project into the nasal passage; they come from the ethmoid bone, which has air cells in it connected with the nose, similar to the frontal sinus and the maxillary sinus or antrum. The inner parts of the nose are lined with mucous membrane beneath which lies what is known as erectile tissue, that is, tissue which is capable of being engorged with blood. When cold air is drawn into the nose this engorgement takes place, so that the air is warmed before it descends into the more delicate air tubes. Besides being warmed the air is also moistened, and the little hairs which project from the cavities serve as filters for particles of dust. (For diseases of the nose *see also* ADENOIDS; ANTRUM; CATARRH, NASAL; FOREIGN BODIES; POLYPI; SINUS.)

NOTIFICATION OF DISEASE. The diseases a medical practitioner is compelled by law to notify are the following: Smallpox, scarlet fever, typhus fever, typhoid fever, poliomyelitis relapsing fever, puerperal fever, puerperal pyrexia, diph-

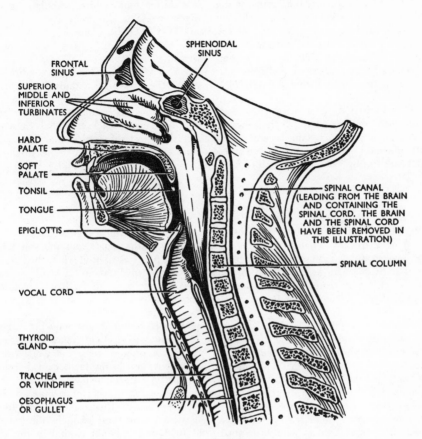

The Nose and Throat.

theria, erysipelas and tuberculosis. Others are notifiable at the option of the local authority.

NOVOCAINE. Novocaine was introduced as a substitute for cocaine and it has entirely taken the place of that drug as a local anesthtic. When injected it is just as efficient as cocaine and it has the advantage of being much less poisonous. (*See also* ANESTHETICS; COCAINE.)

NUCLEUS. The central part of a cell which controls its activities is called the nucleus.

NUCLEUS PULPOSUS HERNIATION. This term describes the protrusion of an intervertebral disc (the cartilage between the vertebrae), and is recognized as a common cause of sciatica and pains in the back. It is usually relieved by rest in bed or in a plaster jacket, but may sometimes require surgical removal. (*See also* DISC, SLIPPED.)

NUMBNESS. Apart from being a symptom of a disease, numbness or loss of sensation may occur in a limb by pressure on a nerve. Such a condition is sometimes noted in the hands when pressure has been put on the elbows. In many diseases of the nervous system, numbness may occur in various parts of the body, especially in the hands and feet. This is frequently found in those who suffer from hysteria. Limbs may go numb if they are left too long in one position, and patients who are bedridden should be moved from time to time in order to allow the blood to circulate freely. (*See also* HYSTERIA; NERVOUS SYSTEM.)

NURSING, DOMESTIC. *See* SICK NURSING.

NUTMEG. Nutmeg is the kernel of the seed of a plant which grows in the East and West Indies. The covering of the nutmeg is mace. The oil of nutmeg as well as the nutmeg itself is much used in cookery because of its aromatic flavour. The oil is sometimes included in sleeping draughts.

NUX VOMICA. The dried ripe seeds of the nux vomica plant, which grows in India and Ceylon, contain several alkaloids, the most important being strychnine and brucine. Nux vomica, in small doses, is a bitter tonic which stimulates gastric digestion. (*See also* STRYCHNINE.)

NYCTALOPIA. This is another name for night-blindness. (*See also* NIGHT-BLINDNESS.)

NYSTAGMUS. This is a condition in which the eyes are continually moving in a jerky manner, either from side to side, up and down, or round about. Nystagmus usually affects both eyes and is caused by disturbance of the semicircular canals (organs of balance), or by some disease of the nervous system. (*See also* EYE.)

OBESITY. Obesity is either a disgrace or a disease. That is a crude but accurate way of stating the plain fact that people who are too fat have become so either by reason of overeating or because there is something wrong with them.

There are two different kinds of fat people: one called *exogenous,* that is, coming from outside; and the other *endogenous,* that is, coming from inside. This means just that in the one case too much is taken in, which is simple overeating, and in the other case the control of what is taken in, whether too much or too little, is out of gear and deals with the intake in an unusual way.

Exogenous Obesity. Too much fat, whether from one reason or another, is a very real danger, so much so that no insurance company will take people who weigh much outside the average limit. Why? Because they know from experience that fat people seldom live to a good old age. And worse than merely shortening life, the fat person gets ill more easily, and has less capacity to fight the infections he catches so readily.

Certain foods are much more fattening than others. But, curiously enough, it is not the fats that are fattening, it is the starchy foods; bread, cakes, potatoes, sugar, plums, prunes, bananas, puddings. And it is just these that form the basis of all meals and are so convenient at odd times. Sugar, bread, and potatoes are the chief offenders. It is these that should be restricted, and it will be noticed that in the diets included, these are carefully regulated. It is the purpose of the sugars and the starches to provide physical energy; when they are not actually needed, as in lack of sufficient pyhsical exercise and fresh air, then they are carefully stored up by the body in the form of fat.

Diet is essential in reducing weight. The amount of food taken has to be strictly in proportion to the work (physical) done, and in the fat person the intake should be reduced below that level. This is done so as to get fat people to draw on the reserves they have stored up—in short, to spend some of their spare capital of food. But it is not capital in the sense of an asset; it is a dangerous overdraft on the bank of health.

Fat reduction is a very personal and often a very difficult thing. It requires exact knowledge of the case and exact and careful dieting.

Although it is true that thyroid extract can bring about fat reduction, and amphetamine and preludin have had similar results, all such drugs must be taken with caution and only under medical advice.

Endogenous Obesity. This type of obesity is due to certain diseases involving the internal glands of the body: the thyroid, the pituitary, the ovaries, the testicles, the suprarenal, etc. Disturbance of the ovarian function at the menopause or change of life often leads to abnormal deposits of fat in women. Most young people who get fat do so by reason of some defect of the glands. There are, of course, many types and conditions, but it is important

DESIRABLE WEIGHTS FOR
WOMEN OF AGES 25 AND OVER*

Weight in Pounds According to Frame (In Indoor Clothing)
*(For girls between 18 and 25, subtract 1 pound
for each year under 25.)*

Height (with shoes on) 2-inch heels		Small Frame	Medium Frame	Large Frame
Feet	Inches			
4	10	92–98	96–107	104–119
4	11	94–101	98–110	106–122
5	0	96–104	101–113	109–125
5	1	99–107	104–116	112–128
5	2	102–110	107–119	115–131
5	3	105–113	110–122	118–134
5	4	108–116	113–126	121–138
5	5	111–119	116–130	125–142
5	6	114–123	120–135	129–146
5	7	118–127	124–139	133–150
5	8	122–131	128–143	137–154
5	9	126–135	132–147	141–158
5	10	130–140	136–151	145–163
5	11	134–144	140–155	149–168
6	0	138–148	144–159	153–173

*Courtesy of Metropolitan Life Insurance Company.

DESIRABLE WEIGHTS FOR
MEN OF AGES 25 AND OVER*

Weight in Pounds According to Frame (In Indoor Clothing)

Weight (with shoes on) 1-inch heels		Small Frame	Medium Frame	Large Frame
Feet	Inches			
5	2	112–120	118–129	126–141
5	3	115–123	121–133	129–144
5	4	118–126	124–136	132–148
5	5	121–129	127–139	135–152
5	6	124–133	130–143	138–156
5	7	128–137	134–147	142–161
5	8	132–141	138–152	147–166
5	9	136–145	142–156	151–170
5	10	140–150	146–160	155–174
5	11	144–154	150–165	159–179
6	0	148–158	154–170	164–184
6	1	152–162	158–175	168–189
6	2	156–167	162–180	173–194
6	3	160–171	167–185	178–199
6	4	164–175	172–190	182–204

*Courtesy of Metropolitan Life Insurance Company.

to observe that such cases are often due to diesase. The disease may be encouraged and assisted by overfeeding; but that is not the primary error, though it may be an accompanying factor. These cases are difficult and require skilled and careful attention, not only to remove the fat but to correct the other symptoms of disease that are unfortunately commonly present.

No such case should be allowed to experiment with diets or medicines or drugs; they require very careful treatment.

The Banting Diet. Banting suffered from an extreme degree of obesity. Under the advice of a medical friend named Harvey, he adopted a special régime with such success as to lose 35 lb. in thirty-eight weeks. He subsequently published the system in 1863 and it is well known under his name. By contemporary standards, it contains an excessive amount of protein. Banting did, however, point the way, and the diet which follows is the natural outcome of his method.

A Useful Reducing Diet. The following is a simplified form of a reducing diet freely used by the writer. It will be noted that it reduces the fluid intake as well as food. The total calorie value is about 1,400.

On Waking.—½ cup of hot water or tea.
Breakfast.—½ cup of tea or coffee; one tablespoonful of milk. No sugar.
   1 oz. toast Ry-krisp. Limit butter.
   1–2 oz. fish, if desired.
   Grapefruit, or an apple, or an orange.
Lunch.—A small portion of meat, fish or fowl.
   4–6 oz. cooked green vegetable; i.e., a large helping.
   1 oz. Ry-krisp or toast. Limit butter.
   Up to 1 oz. cheese (cream), if desired.
   2–3 oz. stewed fruit (cooked without sugar) sweetened with saccharine.
   ½ cup of any fluid.
Mid-afternoon.—1 cup of tea or coffee with milk only.
Dinner.—(Soup ½ cup).
   Meat, fish, fowl, or egg dish.
   4–6 oz. green vegetables.
   Stewed fruit; no sugar.
   Junket or baked custard (small helping).
   1 oz. Ry-krisp or toast.

It is important that the diet should be followed exactly, nothing being taken beyond it, and nothing omitted from it.

OBSESSION. This may be defined as a thought, feeling or impulse, which in spite of the efforts of the will of a person, forces itself upon the mind. Obsessions are of three kinds:

Obsessions of Indecision. These occur in normal people to a mild degree. We have all experienced the feeling of doubt sometimes as to whether we have locked the door at night, or have remembered to switch off a light, and have gone back to make sure. One return and we are satisfied that all is in order; not so the patient with an obsession of indecision. He will go back again and again to reassure himself that all is dark and safe. Even repeated assurances fail to remove from his mind the doubt that something remains to be done. Anything which serves to raise a doubt in his mind will serve to produce an obsession of indecision in one disposed to this disorder. Intense mental distress accompanies the period of indecision.

Obsessions of Fear. *See* PHOBIAS.

Obsessions of Impulse. These cause their victims to have irresistible impulses to commit certain acts, which only too often bring them into contact with the law. For this reason, for their own protection as well as for that of others, those who suffer from such obsessions are safer in institutions. Examples of common obsessions of impulse will illustrate this point: *pyromania* is the impulse to set things on fire. It does not matter to the culprit whether he burns a haystack or a palace; it is all the same to him, and he has no feeling of guilt about it. *Kleptomania* is the impulse to steal, and is a real obsesssion when the article stolen is of little value compared with the patient's means. It is important to realize that although at the time the impulse is uncontrollable and the stealing of something worthless or the setting fire to a building is attempted, yet once the period of the impulse is over for the time being, the culprit is overcome with shame and terror. It is obvious that such people cannot be treated as criminals, but may be judged insane and treated accordingly.

OBSTETRICS. The branch of medicine which deals with pregnancy and childbirth is known as obstetrics.

OBSTRUCTION. When the term obstruction is used it generally refers to obstruction of the bowels; but obstruction may also occur in the bile ducts or the urinary tract. The causes of obstruction of the bowel are various. There may be a gallstone embedded in the intestine or there may be a kink in the gut due to adhesions. Tumors are a very common cause; also intussusception, a condition in which one part of the intestine slips into the part beyond. Obstruction immediately takes place in cases of strangulated hernia and there is absolute constipation accompanied by distention of the abdomen. In cases of obstruction where there is interference with the blood supply, the need for operation is usually urgent, for an intestine thus left without its blood supply rapidly dies.

Symptoms. The patient is suddenly seized with severe pain in the abdomen which as a rule, causes vomiting to take place. The colicky pains gradually get worse and the patient usually looks extremely ill. The doctor should be sent for immediately and no purgatives should be given in the meantime, otherwise damage may be caused. (*See also* BOWELS; CALCULUS; INTUSSUSCEPTION.)

OCCIPUT. The back part of the head is called the occiput. (*See also* HEAD.)

OCCUPATIONAL DISEASES. Most occupations have some features which may interfere with good health yet not seriously damage it. On the other hand, there are occupations or trades which definitely predispose to certain diseases and forms of poisoning. Workers in lead, which is used in many trades, have to be specially protected against poisoning, also workers who handle arsenic, phosphorus, mercury, and those who are exposed to the fumes of india rubber.

Wool-sorters are liable to suffer from a condition known as anthrax, which is caused by a germ getting into cuts or abrasions in the hands due to working with fleeces. Coal miners suffer from the variety of chronic lung disease, called silicosis. Stonecutters, steelgrinders, cotton workers, and flourmillers are liable to respiratory disease through inhaling irritating particles. Divers, and those who work under compressed air, may suffer from pains in the limbs which sometimes lead to paralysis. Occupational cramp is due to a spasm of a group of muscles which are excessively used in the daily work; some such occupa-tions include writing, type-writing, type-setting and telegraphy, and others. Skin complaints play an important part in occupational diseases, and the following article deals with the matter quite fully. (*See also* ANTHRACOSIS; ANTHRAX; CAISSON DISEASE; LEAD POISONING; NEURITIS.)

OCCUPATIONAL SKIN DISEASE (Dermatitis). This is one of the commonest forms of dermatitis or skin disease (q.v.), and since it is so frequently found, and is of such enormous practical importance—not only to the individual, but to the various trades concerned—it is considered separately.

It is due to contact with any irritating dust or liquid with which the patient comes into contact at his work.

Some substances are far more liable to produce dermatitis than others. Some, on the other hand, seem only to cause irritation when the worker is in a low state of health, as after influenza, or if anemic. These have the effect of lowering his resistance and rendering him liable to infection. He may have been exposed to the particular form of irritant for many years before he became "sensitized," but after a first attack, recurrences are very probable.

It is a very important and unfortunate characteristic of the disease that the worker may stay away from his work and undergo treatment for some time, and the skin may become almost completely healed, and then —for no apparent reason, perhaps a lowering of the general health, perhaps a little carelessness—it breaks out again as badly as at first. It is impossible, moreover, to give any estimate of the length of time the trouble may last; it may be one month or it may be twelve; and recurrences are very likely. In many cases it is advisable for the patient to change his occupation. This may seem rather hard advice, especially to a man who has spent years at training for his particular trade, but it often saves time, trouble, and expense in the end. It is as well, however, always to have the advice of a specialist on the matter, as on the surface it may appear that an eruption is due to some irritant at work, but it has been found that this is not always the case. "Not every eruption from which a baker suffers is baker's itch."

Treatment. This differs in no way from

the usual methods of dealing with dermatitis, except that the worker should not be exposed to the irritant during the time of treatment. If, however, he cannot give up or change his occupation immediately, he must endeavor to protect the affected skin as far as possible. This is done by the use of an oily application, which is not easily dissolved off. The hands should be washed only once a day, preferably at night, and very well rinsed to remove every trace of soap, which often adds to the irritation. They are then dressed with a bland oil or ointment, as is described under DERMATITIS (q.v.). In the morning the hands are rubbed over with dry cotton-wool, and a mixture of wax and lanolin massaged in. This may be reapplied as desired during the day. Housewives should, as far as possible, do all their "dirty work" at once, then thoroughly wash and rinse the hands, dress them as directed, and endeavor to keep on the dressings for the rest of the twenty-four hours.

Dermatitis Among Coal Miners. The subject is very wide, and it is impossible here to give more than a brief summary. It may, however, be of interest to consider one trade—that of coal mining—in more detail, as an example of the varieties of dermatitis that may occur in *susceptible* workers. Not every coal miner is attacked by this disease.

"Water-rash" is fairly frequent among coal miners. Water, on filtering through the earth into the pit, dissolves many irritating substances. Sulphuretted hydrogen and sulphur dioxide, both irritating gases, are present in the air of the mine, and are also dissolved. With constant wetting from this water, an itching, moist dermatitis develops on the parts exposed to it.

Another form of dermatitis, which is not a true occupational dermatitis, may be included here as an example of irritation occurring as a result of dirty, heating work, but not directly due to a *special* irritant. It occurs in hewers, i.e. the men who "pick down" the coal. The armpits, and any other places where one part of the skin rubs against another, are affected. Right-handed hewers rest the right forearm inside the right thigh, and left-handed

hewers the left, as they work; these surfaces are very commonly affected. The genital region is also frequently affected, as many of the men leave this area uncleansed in their daily wash.

The skin is first chafed, and feels hot and sore, then the surface becomes rubbed off and fluid is poured out upon it. If the condition goes on, softening of the skin occurs, so that it peels off in large flakes, and has a very offensive odor. If still neglected, it may become general over the whole body. It may be noted, however, that no case of cancer from coal-dust irritation has been recorded, though the soot cancer of chimney sweeps was well known. This form of dermatitis may be prevented by cleanliness, and may be cured by the same means, i.e., by strict attention to personal hygiene and a thorough wash all over each day.

OINTMENTS. A fatty substance, rather like butter, to which drugs have been added and which is used for application on the skin is called an ointment. Lard, benzoated lard, paraffin, vaseline, and lanolin (a fat obtained from sheep's wool) are the usual substances used as a base. Ointments are only intended for external use, and it is unwise to put any on a wound or sore from which there is much discharge as this will tend to prevent proper drainage.

OLD AGE. *See* AGE CHANGES.

OLFACTORY NERVE. The first cranial nerve, the nerve of smell, is also known as the olfactory nerve. (*See also* NOSE.)

OLIVE OIL. The oil obtained from ripe olives which is pale greenish-yellow in color, is one of the most commonly used oils we have. It is much used as an article of food and can provide nourishment if vigorously rubbed into the skin. This is an excellent way of providing babies with extra nourishment and it also helps to keep the skin smooth. It is given freely by mouth in certain cases of poisoning as it is very soothing to the mucous membranes. It is a mild laxative, and for this purpose it can be given with food such as salads, etc. An enema of warm olive oil may be injected into the bowel in order to relieve severe constipation. It often gives relief to patients who have gallstones, and is used in the treatment of colitis. It serves as an ingredient of liniments, ointments, and plasters.

OMENTUM. A long fold of the peritoneum which hangs down over the intestine is known as the omentum. It is more or less loaded with fat, and it is the increasing deposit of fat in this structure that causes middle-aged spread. (*See also* Obesity.)

OMPHALUS. This is another name for the navel or umbilicus.

ONYCHIA. A disease in which inflammation takes place in the nail bed is known as onychia. The nail usually becomes discolored and is thrown off, but is replaced by the growth of a new one. (*See also* Nails.)

OPHTHALMIA. This is inflammation of the eye. The term ophthalmia is often used in place of conjunctivitis. (*See also* Conjunctivitis; Eye.)

OPHTHALMOSCOPE. An instrument for examining the interior of the eye is called an ophthalmoscope. It consists of a mirror with a hole in it through which the doctor looks and light is thrown into the eye from the mirror. (*See also* Eye.)

OPIUM. Opium is perhaps the best known of all the narcotic (sleep-producing) drugs and it is the oldest and most effective remedy for pain. It is the dried juice of the unripe seed-capsules of the white poppy, and it contains a large number of alkaloid substances, at least eighteen in number, of which the following are the most important: morphine, codeine, narcotine, and thebaine.

Although opium is used a great deal in medicine, its sale is restricted because it is a very harmful drug and a craving for it is readily established. Large doses in a person unaccustomed to the drug are liable to cause death. There are many preparations made from opium including such well-known ones as laudanum, and paregoric.

In its action, opium at first causes mental excitement, but this is soon followed by sleep which may be accompanied by pleasant dreams. It is excellent for giving immediate relief from pain, but it is not advisable to give it in cases of acute abdominal pain as it may mask the symptoms of a condition requiring emergency operation. Looseness of the bowel is often treated by laudanum, as it arrests diarrhea and dysentery. Cough mixtures frequently contain codeine as it tends to lessen cough. (*See also* Drug Habits.)

OPIUM POISONING. Poisonous doses of opium may cause slight excitability at first, but very soon a feeling of intense drowsiness sets in. This is rapidly followed by loss of movement and sleep, and finally unconsciousness from which it is impossible to rouse the patient. The face becomes blue and the skin cold, although there may be a great deal of perspiration. The pupils of the eye contract until they are almost pinpoints. The breathing gradually becomes slower and more irregular and, without treatment, the patient may die.

Treatment. It is sometimes difficult to tell the difference between opium and alcohol poisoning, but the pupils are more contracted in poisoning by opium and the patient is more easily roused in alcohol poisoning. An emetic should be given as soon as possible, and in addition the stomach should be washed out with a solution of permanganate of potassium. The patient must be roused and kept awake by walking him up and down, pinching him, or flapping him with a wet towel. Strong coffee should be given, and if he is unable to swallow it, it should be injected into the rectum. If necessary, artificial respiration should be employed.

Those who are in the habit of taking opium or morphia may suffer from a state of chronic poisoning. There is loss of appetite, indigestion, sluggish bowels, and anemia. These people rapidly degenerate and lose all sense of right and wrong. They should be kept under constant care and watched to see that no drug is obtained. Such treatment is best carried out in a mental hospital. (*See also* Drug Habits.)

OPTIC NERVE. The second pair of cranial nerves are called the optic nerves and they connect the eye with the brain. (*See also* Eye; Field of Vision.)

ORBIT. The bony cavity which contains the eye is called the orbit. (*See also* Eye.)

ORCHITIS. Inflammation of the testicle is known as orchitis. When the infection spreads along the cord it is known as epididymitis. (*See also* Epididymitis; Testicle.)

433

ORGANIC DISEASE. Disease of an organ which causes an alteration in the workings of the body is said to be an organic disease. A disease in which no such changes can be found is said to be functional.

ORTHOPEDICS. This is the term given to a branch of surgery which deals with the treatment of fractures and joint affections and the correction of deformities.

OSMOSIS. The passage of fluids through a membrane is known as osmosis. Osmotic pressure is the term applied to the pressure exerted by the fluid to pass through the membrane.

OSSIFICATION. The formation of bone is called ossification. Very early in life the bones are represented by cartilage and fibrous tissue and from these the true bones gradually develop. While the child is still in the mother's womb, ossification is going on all the time, and at birth considerable progress has been accomplished, but it is not until about the age of twenty that the bones are completely developed. (*See also* BONE.)

OSTEITIS. A chronic disease of the bones which does not commence until late in life is known as osteitis deformans, or Paget's disease of the bones. The bones show signs of softening which alters their shape to a certain extent, but subsequently they harden, leaving them deformed. Such cases develop curvature of the spine, curvature of the bones of the leg, and enlargement of the head. The condition develops very slowly and as the health is not in any way affected, the patient may not notice any change in himself other than requiring a larger size in hats. Gradually the bones of the legs alter in shape and the other bones of the body may alter accordingly to meet the new situation.

In rare cases these are limited to a single bone, but even in severe cases the hands and feet remain unaffected. The cause of the disease is not known, but a patient may live for twenty to thirty years after the onset of the condition. There is no special treatment, but aspirin will be found helpful in relieving any pains. (*See also* BONE; OSTEOMYELITIS.)

OSTEOARTHRITIS. This is a painful inflammation in the joints during which changes take place in the bones. (*See also* RHEUMATOID ARTHRITIS.)

OSTEOMALACIA. This is a condition of the bones in which they become softened and are liable to break. It may be due to a lack of Vitamin D in the diet, or to a lack of sunshine, and is accompanied by deficiency of calcium in th blood. It occurs usually in women, and as the bones of the pelvis and spine are the ones most commonly affected, it naturally follows that this condition interferes very seriously with childbirth.

Treatment. The patient should be given cod-liver oil and put on a diet rich in calcium and phosphorus obtained from eggs, milk fish, and vegetables. As much sunshine as possible should be obtained, and unhygienic surroundings should be avoided. (*See also* BONE.)

OSTEOMYELITIS. This condition is most commonly met with in children between the ages of three and fourteen, but it may occur in adults. The term osteomyelitis means inflammation in the marrow of a bone, and it is caused by germs called staphylococci. They are carried to the affected bone by the blood stream from trivial septic places on the skin.

Symptoms. Severe pain is usually felt in the bone (usually a leg bone) and the neighboring joints may feel painful and tender. Very shortly after the first symptom of pain, the patient begins to feel ill, and there may be high temperature and swelling of the affected limb. Without treatment an abscess will form, which will gradually make its way through the tissues of the skin. In some cases the abscess may burst or spread into a neighboring joint.

Treatment. In the first place it is usual to give large doses of penicillin or other antibiotics in the hope that the infection will be overcome. This treatment nearly always succeeds in localizing the infection so that operation to let out pus or dead bone, when this is needed, becomes a simpler and safer procedure.

OTITIS. Inflammation of the ear, internally or externally, is called otitis. (*See also* EAR.)

OTORRHEA. A discharge from the ear

is known as otorrhea. (*See also* EAR; MASTOID.)

OTOSCLEROSIS. This is a type of deafness in which changes occur in the bony walls of the labyrinth or internal ear. These changes result in fixation of the mobile stapes, the innermost of the tiny bones of the middle ear. There are usually noises in the ears and deafness gradually becomes worse as time goes on, though it seldom goes on to stone deafness. An ear specialist should be consulted early, and he will advise either a hearing aid, or the delicate operation called stapedectomy, which is successful in over 90 per cent of cases. (*See also* EAR.)

OVARIES. There are two ovaries in the female, one on each side within the pelvis, each about an inch in length and oval in shape. Each ovary is joined to the womb (uterus) by a broad band which contains within its folds a tube known as the Fallopian tube, along which the tiny ovum (the microscopic egg, or female sexual element) is conveyed from the ovary to the womb. The period of menstruation takes place when an ovum is set free (at regular intervals of about four weeks) from the ovary and travels down to the womb. If it is not impregnated it escapes from the womb with the blood which comes away. Each menstruation resembles a slight pregnancy which has not been made complete through the ovum not having been impregnated. (*See also* MENSTRUATION.)

OVEREATING. The danger of overeating, especially after middle age has been reached, cannot be too strongly emphasized. Many of the ills of later years could be avoided if the right sort of diet were taken after the age of thirty. Up until about the age of thirty the digestive organs may be in a fit state to stand up to a little extra work, but after that age, any strain begins to weaken them considerably, so it is necessary to avoid overworking them as much as possible. (*See also* FORCIBLE FEEDING; OBESITY.)

OVUM. An ovum is the single cell which comes from the ovary of the female, and after it has become impregnated by the male, it is capable of developing into an individual. (*See also* EMBRYO.)

OXALIC ACID POISONING. Oxalic acid poisoning is usually the result of taking salts of lemon in mistake for Epsom salts or a like substance. Oxalic acid, or salts of lemon, is very often used for domestic cleaning purposes and, as it is similar in appearance to bicarbonate of soda and other harmless white powders, it should never be bought in larger quantity than can be used immediately, and should never be beft lying around. It is a very corrosive poison, and it destroys any tissue it comes into contact with. It causes intense burning in the mouth, throat, and stomach, followed by vomiting and collapse.

Treatment. On no account should an emetic be given as this will only cause further irritation to the throat and stomach. Lime, chalk, or whiting mixed with a little water are the best remedies, and if these substances are not at hand, strip some plaster off a wall or ceiling. Follow with a dose of castor oil, and keep the patient for three or four days on nothing but milk and lime water.

OXYGEN. A colorless gas, odorless and tasteless, oxygen forms rather more than one-fifth of the bulk of the atmosphere. It is necessary to life, and every time we breathe we give the blood a fresh supply.

Oxygen is prepared in large quantities for commercial purposes and it is stored in steel cylinders from which it can be obtained at any desired rate by turning a stop-cock. In many conditions the blood is not capable of carrying its normal amount of oxygen, and in such cases the administration of the gas gives great relief. Pure oxygen is supplied by means of inhalation in the cases of asphyxia, especially in pneumonia, valvular disease of the heart, and anemia.

OZONE. Ozone is a specially concentrated form of oxygen and it is erroneously supposed to be produced near the seaside and in the air of pine-clad mountains more patricularly than in other districts. It has a slightly peculiar smell which may be noticed when standing near an electrical machine or dynamo, as ozone is produced by the passage through the air of electric sparks; it is produced in large quantities during a thunderstorm. (*See also* OXYGEN.)

PAGET'S DISEASE. Paget's disease of the nipple is a serious condition and is discussed under the heading NIPPLE. Paget's disease of bone is a chronic disease described under OSTEITIS.

PAIN. Different types of pain may be felt in various conditions; for example, the feeling of pain may be described as gnawing, throbbing, stabbing, burning, and so on. Pain felt in a certain part of the body may lead to diagnosis of some disease, but it must be remembered that disease in a certain organ often causes pain in a different part of the body owing to the distribution of nerves. An inflamed gall bladder may give rise to pain in the right shoulder, or disease of the hip may manifest itself as a painful knee on that side.

Relief should always be given when possible, as it is undoubtedly very bad for the nervous system and very wearing to the patient to be continually under the strain of bearing pain. Hence morphia is given to people suffering from shock, after severe injuries. Drugs which afford relief are called anodynes or analgesics. The expression labor pain is used in connection with the pain felt before childbirth owing to the contraction of the womb. (*See also* LABOR; NERVOUS SYSTEM.)

PLATE. The arch which forms the roof of the mouth is known as the hard palate. At the back of the mouth the fleshy part which hangs down is called the soft palate, and from the middle of the soft palate hangs the narrow projection known as the uvula. (*See also* CLEFT PALATE; MOUTH.)

PALLIATIVE. Any treatment which is given to relieve symptoms but which does not cure the condition is said to be palliative.

PALPITATION. Although our hearts continue beating day in and day out throughout our lives, we normally remain unaware of it. When a person becomes aware that his heart is beating against his chest wall, he is said to be suffering from palpitation. This symptom is rarely due to heart disease: it is more commonly due to an oversensitive nervous system. Treatment is usually directed to the sleeplessness and anxiety which so often accompany this symptom.

PALSY. This is another name for paralysis.

PALUDRINE. This is a drug which has proved most successful in the treatment of malaria.

PANCREAS. The gland known as the pancreas is one of the most important organs of the body. It is about six or eight inches in length, and lies across the back of the abdomen, directly behind the lower part of the stomach. A duct or channel runs through the whole gland and joins up with the bile-duct from the liver, which eventually opens out into the small intestine. Through this duct an essential fluid known as the pancreatic juice passes into the small intestine. This juice contains ferments and salts which are necessary for the proper digestion of our food. Insulin is manufactured by groups of cells known as the "islands of Langerhans," which are to be found in the pancreas, and when these cells are damaged in any way the loss of insulin causes the condition known as diabetes mellitus. The pancreas of animals is known as the sweetbread. (*See also* DIABETES; DIGESTION; DUCTLESS GLANDS; INSULIN.)

PANDEMIC. A wide-spread epidemic (q.v.) covering a whole area or population is called a pandemic.

PAPILLOMA. Papilloma is a growth on the skin or mucous membrane, such as a wart. These growths are usually simple in nature, but there is the possibility that some may become malignant. (*See also* WART.)

PAPULE. A small, solid raised spot on the skin is called a papule. (*See also* PIMPLE.)

PARACENTESIS. In this operation the wall of a cavity is punctured in order to allow fluid to escape. The term is commonly used for the incision of an inflamed ear drum. (*See also* EAR; MASTOIDITIS.)

PARAFFIN. The paraffins used in medicine are either hard, soft, or liquid, and they are obtained by distillation from shale. White and yellow Vaselines are prepara-

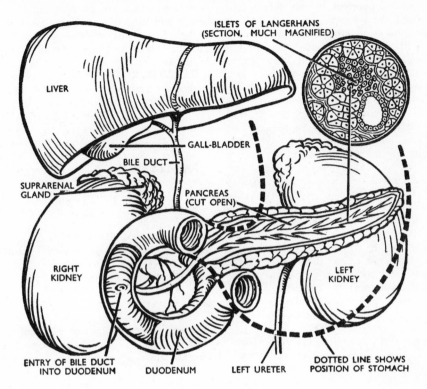

ISLETS OF LANGERHANS
(SECTION, MUCH MAGNIFIED)

LIVER

GALL-BLADDER

BILE DUCT

SUPRARENAL
GLAND

PANCREAS
(CUT OPEN)

RIGHT
KIDNEY

LEFT
KIDNEY

ENTRY OF BILE DUCT
INTO DUODENUM   DUODENUM   LEFT URETER

DOTTED LINE SHOWS
POSITION OF STOMACH

The Pancreas.

tions made from soft paraffin, which is also known petroleum jelly. Hard and soft paraffins are used as a basis for many ointments which are used to protect wounds or sores. Liquid paraffin is an excellent substance for producing an easy motion of the bowels without any griping. It is said to inhibit the absorption of the fat soluble vitamins from the intestine, and should not be used continually.

Many other preparations are obtained from the distillation of shale oil, such as benzine, kerosene, and gasoline. Kerosene is used for destroying lice, fleas, flies, etc., and for preventing their further attack.

PARALDEHYDE. This is a sleep-producing drug which is very safe to give, because it is unlikely to give rise to addiction owing to its unpleasant taste and smell. (*See also* ANESTHETICS.)

PARALYSIS. This is a term used to describe loss of power of movement in a part of the body and is due to some injury to, or disease of, the nervous system. This damage to the nervous system may be either in the central nervous system, which consists of the brain and spinal cord, or in the limbs and face. (*See* NERVOUS SYSTEM.) The extent of any paralysis depends entirely on which part of the nervous system is damaged and to what the damage is due. Sometimes the damage is only temporary and by removing the cause of it the nerves will recover and so will the paralysis. This happens, for example, in various forms of neuritis. In infantile paralysis, which is caused by a germ attacking the central nervous system, the paralysis is greatest during the initial stage of the illness because much of the paralysis is due to swelling of the spinal cord, which later passes off leaving a certain number of dead nerve cells. It is only the movements formerly controlled by these killed nerve cells which become permanently paralysed.

In adults, paralysis of one side of the body and the corresponding arm and leg is the most common paralysis, and this is discussed under hemiplegia. One of the diseases of old age is paralysis agitans, or the 'shaking palsy," in which there is a stiffness of the muscles of the limbs, especially of the arms with tremor first of the fingers, and later, of the whole arm. The face shares in the stiffness, being mask-like, and the patient walks stiffly with little running steps, as if constantly trying to catch up with his center of gravity. This disease runs a very long course and may take years to develop all the symytoms described above. Weakness of the muscle may appear long after the stiffness and the trembling have made recognition of the disease possible. There is no curative treatment, but much can be done to relieve the rigidity and troublesome salivation (so often a symptom) by the use of drugs. The patient must be encouraged to remain up and about as long as possible.

Certain forms of paralysis are due, not to organic disease of the nervous system, but to that curious condition called hysteria in which bodily weakness and paralysis of the limbs is caused by mental trouble. Only when the mental trouble is dealt with can the "paralysis" be cured. Partial paralysis of the ankle muscles, giving rise to "foot drop" is often due to alcoholic neuritis. Similarly, "wrist drop" is a common manifestation of lead poisoning. (See also DISSEMINATED SCLEROSIS; ENCEPHALITIS LETHARGICA; HYSTERIA; NEURITIS; ST. VITUS'S DANCE; TABES DORSALIS.)

PARANOIA. Paranoia is the term applied to a mental disorder in which there are delusions, usually of persecution. (See also DELUSIONS; INSANITY; MENTAL DISEASE.)

PARAPLEGIA. Paralysis of the lower half of the body or of the lower limbs is known medically as paraplegia. (See also PARALYSIS.)

PARASITE. An animal or vegetable which lives upon or within another creature is known as a parasite. The creature that harbors the parasite is termed the "host." The vegetable parasites include bacteria and various fungi. The lowest of the animal parasites is the ameba, of which several varieties exist. There are many varieties

of worms which are parasitic on human beings and animals, causing a great deal of damage and disease. (See also BED BUG; FILARIA; GUINEA WORM; HEAD LOUSE; ITCH; JIGGER; LIVER FLUKE; WORM.)

PARATHYROID. Two pairs of small glands are embedded in the back of the thyroid gland in the neck are known as the parathyroids. When these glands become damaged or removed the nervous disorder known as tetany commonly results soon after. (See also TETANY.)

PARATYPHOID. A type of fever which closely resembles typhoid fever, though milder, is known as paratyphoid.

PAREGORIC. This is a soothing tincture of camphor and opium once used as a cough mixture. Paregoric should never be given to children without medical advice. (See also CAMPHOR; OPIUM.)

PARESIS. This term is applied to a state of slight or temporary paralysis. (See also PARALYSIS.)

PARESTHESIA. Unusual feeling in the skin such as tingling, numbness, burning or chilliness, apart from that produced by obvious causes, is referred to as a paresthesia. Formication is the term used for the sensation of ants running under the skin, and is a common experience of the cocaine addict. Paresthesia is common in some nervous diseases, and in anemia. (See also NERVOUS DISEASES.)

PARIETAL. The term parietal is used in connection with the walls of a body cavity. For example, the layer of pleura covering the wall of the chest is called the parietal layer. The term is also used in connection with the bones which form the central part of the roof of the skull.

PARKINSON'S DISEASE. This is another name for paralysis agitans. (See also PARALYSIS.)

PAROTID GLAND. One of the most important salivary glands, the parotid gland lies just in front of the ear and its duct or channel (called Stenson's duct) runs across the cheek and opens out into the mouth opposite the second upper molar tooth. Inflammation of this gland is known as parotitis, and epidemic parotitis is more commonly known as mumps. (See also MUMPS.)

PAROXYSM. This term is frequently used in connection with a spasm, convul-

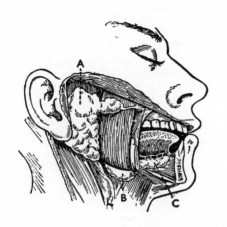

A. *Parotid Gland;* B. *Submaxillary Gland;*
C. *Sublingual Gland.*

sion, or fit. It is also used to describe the sudden onset of symptoms. For example, there may be a sudden paroxysm of coughing.

PARTURITION. The act of giving birth to a child is known as parturition. (*See also* LABOR.)

PASTEURIZATION. Pasteurization is a method of sterilizing milk without actually boiling it. The milk should be heated to a temperature of 167 deg. F. for twenty minutes; this is sufficient to destroy or render harmless the germs that cause disease such as scarlet fever, enteric, summer diarrhea, and most important of all, tuberculosis. A low-temperature pasteurization may be carried out in which the milk is heated for at least half an hour at a temperature between 145 deg. and 150 deg. F. This is sufficient greatly to reduce the number of bacteria or germs and delays the souring of the milk. (*See also* MILK.)

PATELLA. The small rounded bone projecting from the knee joint is known as the patella or kneecap. Swellings on the kneecap occur in housemaid's knee, and the condition is described under bursitis. (*See also* KNEE.)

PATHOLOGY. Pathology is the science which deals with the causes of and the changes produced in the body by disease.

PEDIATRICS. The branch of medicine which deals with the diseases of children is termed pediatrics.

PEDICULOSIS. A state of lousiness

caused by pediculi or lice is known as pediculosis. (*See also* HEAD LOUSE.)

PELLAGRA. A curious disease which occurs usually in tropical and subtropical countries, pellagra is characterized by eruptions on the skin accompanied by disorders of the digestive and nervous systems. It is a deficiency disease due to improper diet and lack of the Vitamin B_2 complex.

PELVIS. The pelvis is the space contained within the hip bones. It contains the lower part of the large intestine, that is the pelvic colon and rectum, the urinary bladder, and in the female, the womb and ovaries. Deformity of the bones of the pelvis, caused by rickets or other disorders, may interfere greatly with childbirth.

PEMPHIGUS. A disease of the skin in which blisters or large blebs appear is called pemphigus. (*See also* DERMATITIS; SKIN.)

PENICILLIN. The story of the discovery of penicillin is in three stages. First, Sir Alexander Fleming found in 1929 that a mold, *penicillium notatum,* prevented the growth on laboratory cultures of staphylococci and other bacteria which caused important diseases in human beings; he applied a solution of the mold to a number of cases of skin infections and found the effect superior to that of antiseptic dressings; but he also found that it was very unstable (it did not keep) and difficult to concentrate. He named the active principle of the mold "penicillin" and used it in his laboratory for bacteriological research, though not for the treatment of disease.

Secondly, Sir Howard Florey, by improved methods, was able to isolate and concentrate penicillin from the mold, and on February 12 1941, the first patient was treated (a case of inflammation of the mastoid)—though, after dramatic improvement, the patient eventually died because the penicillin supply became exhausted. At first, as was natural, only desperately ill patients were given the new drug.

The third stage was the development of the supply of penicillin. It was impossible, in the middle of 1941, to divert chemical factories in England to the experimental manufacture of this new drug, and Professor Florey, under the auspices of the Rockefeller Foundation, came to the

United States—not yet at war—and persuaded first of all the laboratories of the Department of Agriculture to develop the production of the mold. In a few months, enterprising American drug firms started large-scale production.

At first it was necessary to give the penicillin by injection every three hours in order to keep up a sufficient concentration in the blood to kill the germs, but now a single massive dose of procaine penicillin may be given once a day or even less frequently. Additional developments in this direction may be confidently expected. Although it is so deadly to most germs, penicillin has very few ill effects upon the patient, although there are some people who develop skin rashes or allergic reactions. Not all germs are killed by penicillin, and it is often necessary to make sure that the germs are "penicillin sensitive" before starting treatment, for example, in cases of septicaemia, pneumonia or meningitis. Penicillin has been particularly successful in the treatment of venereal disease and for wounds and burns.

A whole series of antibacterial compounds, or "antibiotics," have been and are still being obtained from different molds and bacteria, but only a few have been proved suitable for use in medical treatment, notably streptomycin, aureomycin, and terramycin.

PENIS. The penis is the male organ of generation. It is through the urethra, or tube of the penis, that the contents of the urinary bladder as well as those of the seminal vesicles escape. (*See also* Sex Hygiene.)

PENTOTHAL. This is a barbiturate preparation, given into a vein as an anesthetic.

PEPSIN. This term is applied to one of the ferments found in the juices produced by the stomach. Pepsin is capable of converting proteins into simpler peptone bodies so as to aid digestion. Pepsin is sometimes given along with other prepared ferments in cases where the digestive powers have become enfeebled owing to old age or illness. (*See also* Digestion; Ferment.)

PEPTONIZED FOOD. A peptonized food is one which has been artificially digested or predigested by means of various ferments before it is taken into the body.

Peptonized milk is very often used for children who find it difficult to digest ordinary milk.

PERCHLORIDE OF MERCURY. Perchloride of mercury is commonly referred to as corrosive sublimate. It is a powerful antiseptic, but it is an extremely dangerous poison. For cases of poisoning by this substance, the white of an egg is the best treatment until medical help is obtained. (*See also* Corrosive Sublimate; Mercury.)

PERCUSSION. This is a method of examination used by the doctor when he strikes one finger upon another over certain organs of the body (usually the lungs). The note obtained helps him in diagnosing disease in that particular organ. (*See also* Auscultation.)

PERICARDITIS. Inflammation of the pericardium, the bag in which the heart lies, is called pericarditis. This bag, or sac, is lubricated inside so that the heart, while it is beating, can move up and down with ease. As soon as the pericardium becomes inflamed, the two surfaces become roughened and scratch against each other, producing a "rubbing" sound. This friction, however, soon produces an outflow of fluid and a condition is set up known as pericardial effusion. The condition is a serious one and requires the early attention of a doctor. (*See also* Heart.)

PERICARDIUM. The pericardium is the membrane or bag that surrounds the heart. (*See also* Heart; Pericarditis.)

PERINEUM. The area situated between the opening of the bowel behind and the genital organs in front is termed the perineum. During labor it is common for this area to become torn and a stitch or two is often necessary.

PERIOD. This is a common term referring to the period during which menstruation occurs.

PERIOSTEUM. The membrane covering the surface of the bones is known as the periosteum. This membrane is well supplied with blood-vessels and nerves which help in the nutrition and development of the bones. Disease of the periosteum may lead to necrosis or death of the underlying bone. (*See also* Bone; Necrosis.)

PERIOSTITIS. Inflammation on the surface of a bone which affects the periosteum is known as periostitis. Any knock or injury to a limb may bring about this condition and cause swelling and tenderness. The severer forms of periostitis are due to germs; these are found in the pus which subsequently forms in the bone marrow.

Treatment. The mild cases require only rest and hot fomentations and injections of penicillin. Severe cases require immediate operation so that the pus can be removed from the bone, otherwise the inflammation may spread and involve neighboring joints. (*See also* BONE; NECROSIS; OSTEITIS.)

PERIPHERAL NEURITIS. This is a bilateral disease of the peripheral nerves, chiefly those serving the limbs, characterized by interference with both motor and sensory functions. There are many causes, among them being alcoholism, diphtheria and arsenic poisoning. (*See also* NEURITIS.)

PERISTALSIS. The peculiar wave-like movement by which the contents of the stomach and bowels are propelled forward is known as peristalsis. This is produced by a series of contractions of the muscles. Obstruction in the intestines causes a severe form of pain known as colic due to the muscle going into spasms in an endeavor to overcome the obstruction. (*See also* COLIC.)

PERITONEUM. The membrane which lines the abdominal cavity is known as the peritoneum. It also forms a covering for most of the organs contained within the abdominal cavity and as it passes from one organ to another the peritoneum forms numerous folds. (*See also* ABDOMEN; MESENTERY; OMENTUM.)

PERITONITIS. Peritonitis means inflammation of the peritoneum. Inflammation of this membrane varies a great deal in its severity and, as can be readily understood, it can be caused by a variety of conditions. The inflammation may be localized in one spot or it may spread over a large area and involve many of the abdominal organs. Appendicitis is the commonest cause, but a perforated peptic ulcer or tuberculosis may be responsible.

Symptoms. The symptoms usually bgein with severe pain in the abdomen accompanied by vomiting. The temperature may rise as high as 104 deg. or 105 deg. F. There may be a certain amount of diarrhea at first, but the bowels soon become constipated. The patient is found to lie on his back with the knees drawn up and the breathing is very shallow. The abdomen becomes distended and is very tender to the slightest touch. The tongue becomes furred and dry and the facial expression is drawn and anxious. The outlook is very serious, especially in the puerperal form which sometimes comes on a few days after childbirth.

Treatment. Immediately upon diagnosis, the question of operation must be considered. In cases due to perforation, operation is usually carried out immediately, because it is necessary to remove any septic material from the abdomen as soon as possible. Peritonitis due to tuberculosis is usually treated medically and not surgically. The patient should be kept in bed, preferably in the open air, and the diet should be good and nourishing. (*See also* PERITONEUM.)

PERNICIOUS ANEMIA. This is a serious disease of the blood sometimes affecting men in middle life and usually manifesting itself in a gradually increasing weakness and a yellow color of the skin. The diagnosis, suspected on clinical grounds, can be clinched only after examination of a blood film, which will show marked changes in the blood cells.

Pernicious anemia is different from the ordinary anemia that responds to treatment with iron and also from the anemia due to loss of blood. Normally an intrinsic factor produced by the stomach combines with an extrinsic factor (present in the Vit. B group), to produce an antianemic factor, which is stored in the liver. In pernicious anemia, the stomach does not produce this intrinsic factor.

Pernicious anemia causes degenerative changes in the spinal cord, and invariably proves fatal unless treatment is instituted. Drs. Minot and Murphy, working in Boston, first realized the beneficial effects of large doses of liver by the mouth (a patient would eat as much as 1 lb. per day). Such a diet soon became intolerable and intramuscular injections of liver extracts were next tried, soon to be followed by injections of Vitamin B_{12}.

Pernicious anemia is really a vitamin deficiency disease, and the primary cause of pernicious anemia is to be found in a defect in the mucous lining of the stomach, the lack of an enzyme (not yet identified) normally present which is essential for the absorption of the important Vitamin B$_{12}$. Injections of Vitamin B$_{12}$ (cyanocobalamin) should be started at once and given regularly; concentrated liver extract is effective but troublesome, and is no longer used. Folic acid, which used to be recommended, is no longer used as it has no effect on the spinal cord changes and may even be harmful to them. Iron, in the form of ferrous sulphate, is sometimes also necessary.

With this treatment, improvement in the patient's condition is immediate, though if spinal cord changes are present the treatment may have to be continued for as long as six months and the patient will require to have maintenance doses of cyanocobalamin all his life. Regular blood examinations should be carried out at least every six months.

PEROXIDE OF HYDROGEN. This is an antiseptic fluid, H$_2$O$_2$. (see HYDROGEN PEROXIDE.)

PERSONALITY. This term describes the sum total of an individual's response to life. It is quite distinct from character, which is to a large extent dependent upon training and teaching.

There are in general two types of mental personality: one is the "hail fellow well met" type, who is sociable, friendly, much affected by his surroundings and very adaptable to them; the other is the quiet, retiring, rather shy individual, who is hard to understand and who shows his feelings only in a sympathetic atmosphere, being very hard to "draw out."

PERSPIRATION. Moisture which is given off from the skin is known as perspiration or sweat. (See also SWEAT.)

PERTUSSIS. Pertussis is another name for whooping cough. (See also WHOOPING COUGH.)

PESSARIES. An instrument for supporting the womb when it is displaced is called a pessary. The term is also used for medicated suppositories which are introduced into the vagina.

PETECHIA. A small round spot caused by bleeding into the skin is called a petechia. (See also PURPURA.)

PETIT MAL. This is a transient clouding over of consciousness. The person may stop what he is doing for a minute, a vacant expression will come over his face, but no convulsion occurs and he recovers in a few seconds. (See EPILEPSY.)

PHAGOCYTE. A cell which is able to destroy germs and other harmful particles in the blood is termed a phagocyte. (See also LEUCOCYTE.)

PHALANGES. The bones in the fingers and toes are known as the phalanges. There are three of these, in each finger and toe, the proximal, the middle and the distal; but the thumb and the big toe have each only two.

PHARMACOLOGY. The part of medical science dealing with the knowledge of the action of drugs about the body is called pharmacology. It was formerly known as materia medica.

PHARMACOPOEIA. The official publication dealing with the recognized drugs and their doses is known as the pharmacopoeia. Most countries have a pharmacopoeia of their own.

PHARMACY. Pharmacy is the term applied to the preparing of drugs and medicines.

PHARYNGITIS. This condition is an inflammation of the part of the throat immediately beyond the mouth. A simple iodine paint such as Mandl's paint is usually sufficient to clear up the condition. (See also LARYNGITIS; TONSILLITIS.)

PHARYNX. The pharynx can be seen at the back of the mouth. The term throat is popularly applied to this part, but strictly speaking the pharynx is the cavity into which the nose opens above and from which the larynx and gullet open below. The part which lies behind the nose is called the naso-pharynx. (See also PHARYNGITIS.)

PHENACETIN. This drug is commonly used to give relief in headaches and neuralgia as it is particularly good for deadening pain, but it should not be taken in quantity as it has a very depressing effect.

PHENOBARBITAL. Phenobarbital is one of the most powerful of the group of barbiturate drugs used for their sleep-inducing properties. It takes rather longer to produce its effects than other members of the group and its action continues for a longer time. It is one of the doctor's most valuable drugs and is without harmful effects in normal doses. Its most important use is in controlling the frequency and severity of fits in epilepsy, and in diminishing the convulsive movements in chorea and tetanus. In smaller doses it is very generally used to diminish the sense of mental tension which accompanies states of anxiety.

PHENOL. Phenol is a derivative of benzine and it is more commonly known as carbolic acid. (*See also* CARBOLIC ACID.)

PHIMOSIS. A condition in which the foreskin cannot be drawn back to uncover the glans of the penis is called phimosis. In many cases the opening may be so small as to prevent the passage of urine, and this, along with the accumulation of secretion, causes great irritation. The only satisfactory treatment is by circumcision, which consists in removing a part of the foreskin so that it can be easily drawn back. The operation should be carried out as early as possible, because in very young children it is a slight affair, while the longer it is postponed the more troublesome it becomes. (*See also* BALANITIS; PENIS.)

PHLEBITIS. Inflammation of the veins, usually accompanied by clotting of the blood in the veins, is known as phlebitis. It may occur after childbirth, typhoid fever, or a surgical operation, and is frequently a complication of varicose veins. The affected limb is tender and subject to aching and shooting pains. The part surrounding the vein becomes swollen and there may be bad cramps in the limb. It is treated by rest and soothing applications, such as belladonna in glycerine. Phlebitis is chiefly dangerous because of the risk of a clot becoming detached and traveling to some vital organ such as the heart, when it may cause sudden death. The patient, therefore, must be kept in bed until all inflammation has disappeared. It may be necessary to wear an elastic bandage or stocking for support if the limb is inclined to swell. Drugs which tend to prevent the blood clotting, namely heparin and dicoumarol, are now used in the treatment of phlebitis. (*See also* THROMBOSIS.)

PHLEGM. The material which is brought up after coughing is popularly called phlegm. It is also medically known as sputum or expectoration. (*See also* EXPECTORATION.)

PHOBIAS. Phobias are obsessions (q.v.) of fear. They are very persistent and may become so chronic that they overwhelm the mentality of the individual and eventually leave him with one fixed idea, the fear of something. These phobias may take many shapes. The most common ones are fear of places, such as fear of being shut in a room, or in the subway, fear of heights or of rivers. Fear of certain animals is very common also, such as fear of rats and mice, or of cats. Fear of certain diseases may produce real nervous or mental breakdowns in those unfortunate enough to be afflicted with such phobias. The case of the doctor who committed suicide because he was afraid he had cancer is a typical example of what such a phobia may lead to. Fear of cancer tuberculosis, or syphilis are perhaps the most usual phobias of disease. Treatment of these fears depends on the power of the medical adviser to secure the trust of the patient, and in some cases on psychoanalysis. (*See also* CLAUSTROPHOBIA; OBSESSION.)

PHOSGENE. Phosgene, also known as carbonyl chloride, was one of the chief poison gases used during the 1914–18 War.

PHOSPHORUS POISONING. In cases of phosphorus poisoning an emetic should be given at once and after the stomach has been emptied, some white of egg should be administered. Small doses of sulphate of copper in water should be given at frequent intervals. (*See also* POISONING in FIRST AID SUPPLEMENT at end of book.)

PHOTOPHOBIA. A condition in which a person is afraid of letting a bright light shine upon the eyes is known as photophobia. It is one of the symptoms of inflammation of the eye, and is also a common feature of meningitis. (*See also* CONJUNCTIVITIS; EYE.)

PHTHISIS. Any disease in which there is much wasting away of the body, especially as in tuberculosis, is known as phthisis. (*See also* TUBERCULOSIS.)

PHYSICIAN. A physician is a doctor who treats the diseases by drugs and non-surgical methods.

PHYSIOLOGY. The branch of medicin in which the normal workings of the body are studied is known as physiology.

PHYSOSTIGMINE. This drug is obtained from the calabar bean and is used in eye work and in the treatment of myasthenia gravis (q.v.) (*See also* CALABAR BEAN; PROSTIGMINE.)

PIA MATER. This name is given to the inner of the three membranes surrounding the brain and spinal cord. (*See also* BRAIN.)

PIGEON BREAST. A deformity of the breast in which the breastbone sticks out in front giving a pointed appearance to the chest. It is usually due to rickets, but may also be caused by frequent attacks of bronchitis in infancy. (*See also* RICKETS.)

PIGMENTATION. Pigment is the term applied to the coloring matter of various substances in the body, particularly in the blood. The absence of this coloring matter leads to albinism. In various diseases (e.g., Addison's disease) there is an increase of pigmentation, and in jaundice the discoloration that takes place in the skin is due to increased bile pigment in the blood. (*See also* ALBINISM; JAUNDICE.)

PILES. Medically known as hemorrhoids, piles is a varicose condition of the veins of the lower part of the rectum. The expression "an attack of piles" means an inflammation of one or more of them. Any sign of bleeding when the bowels move should lead one to suspect the presence of piles and medical advice should be sought on the matter, especially in an elderly person.

Piles may be external or internal. External piles appear as tags of skin outside the opening of the rectum and do not cause much irritation unless they become chafed or infected, when they cause great pain and discomfort for several days. Internal piles have no very marked symptoms until they begin to bleed, but they may protrude from the opening and if not pushed back, they may become strangulated and acutely painful.

Chronic constipation, alcoholic excess

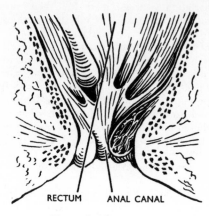

Hemorrhoids or Piles.

and pregnancy are the most usual causes of piles. To cure them, the constipation must be treated by diet and drugs if necessary. The parts around the opening should be kept scrupulously clean, using absorbent cotton instead of toilet paper, and a soothing ointment containing local anesthetic may be applied at intervals. If the piles do not disappear with improved habits and hygiene, they should be injected with a sclerosing solution by a doctor. Operation is only advised in the more severe cases. (*See also* FISSURE.)

PILL. Pills are round masses containing drugs held together by syrup, gum, or some other adhesive extract. They are usually coated with sugar or gelatine, but pills that are intended to act upon the bowels only are coated with keratin a substance which does not dissolve in the stomach. If any difficulty is experienced in swallowing a pill, it should be taken with a mouthful of water or inside a piece of bread.

PIMPLES. Small raised and inflamed spots on the skin are called pimples or papules. (*See also* ACNE; DERMATITIS.)

PINEAL BODY. A small structure situated on the upper part of the brain is known as the pineal body. Its function is unknown. (*See also* BRAIN.)

PINK EYE. This popular term is often used to describe the condition known as conjunctivitis (inflammation of the eye). The eyeball is very red and irritable, and a doctor should be called. (*See also* CONJUCTIVITIS.)

PINS AND NEEDLES. The sensation popularly referred to as pins and needles may occur after a limb has been "asleep." It is a form of paresthesia, this being the term applied to any abnormal sensation produced in the skin. (*See also* PARESTHESIA.)

PITTING. When pressure on the skin leaves a depression which takes some time to disappear, the phenomenon is termed pitting. The tissues in such a case are waterlogged and are said to be edematous. A patient's legs are often edematous in heart failure and acute nephritis: the face is often puffy in the latter condition. (*See also* TEDEMA.)

PITUITARY GLAND. Attached by a stalk to the underside of the brain, but well protected from possible injury by a bony case of its own, lies a very wonderful part of the nervous system, the pituitary gland. This organ, which is only partly composed of nervous tissue, the other part having developed from the same tissue as the inside of the mouth, controls not only our height, our weight and our width, but also our mental powers ·and physical energy.

The front part of the pituitary is mainly concerned with controlling growth. In it are formed some 10 or more hormones. These substances are poured into the blood and upon the amount of them depends our rate of growth. If *too much* hormone is formed in early life, every part of the body, but especially the bones, grows at too fast a rate, so that people so affected become giants.

Too little of this hormone formed in the front part of the pituitary gland produces different effects according as to whether the patient is a child or an adult. In a child, one of two things may happen: growth in every sense may be stopped; the child remains a child, but grows enormously fat and the reproductive organs do not develop beyond the childish stage. The mind, too, remains that of a rather stupid child. This picture is that of one type of dwarf. The other type is quite different: the child becomes a "man in miniature." The body is small, but not the round fat body of a child, the body having undergone the normal changes from an infant to that of an adult. The sexual organs are well-developed and the intelligence is often above normal.

The action of the back part of the pituitary is a very complicated one. One definite substance called "pituitrin" has been prepared in a pure state from it and this has a real value in saving life. This substance causes certain types of muscle to contract strongly, and has saved many mothers from dying from hemorrhage after the birth of their children, and has shortened the time of their labor by making the womb contract more strongly. Other substances formed in this amazing little structure, which is only the size of a small cherry, control the use and storage of sugar in the body and the output of water. The pituitary is said to be the "leader of the endocrine orchestra," as it controls the activity of the other ductless glands, (i.e. thyroid, pancreas, adrenals, etc.) (*See also* DUCTLESS GLANDS.)

PLACENTA. The placenta is a structure planted on the wall of the pregnant womb which connects the blood supply of the mother with the circulation of the developing baby (or fetus) by means of the umbilical cord containing important blood vessels. When the baby is born the placenta comes away a few minutes afterwards and so is called the "afterbirth." (*See also* AFTERBIRTH.)

PLAGUE. (*See Bubonic plague.*)

PLANTS, POISONOUS. Although most plants are perfectly harmless, there are a few which contain dangerous poisons. The most common wild species in this category are poison ivy, poison sumac, foxglove (*Digitalis purpurea*), laburnum (*Laburnum vulgare*), and deadly nightshade (*Atropa belladonna*). These highly-colored plants contain irritant poisons, and are unfortunately attractive to children. For symptoms and treatment *see* **Poisons and Poisoning** in FIRST AID SUPPLEMENT.

PLASTER OF PARIS. Dried calcium sulphate is used to make plaster of Paris splints. Bandages impregnated with the powder are called plaster of Paris bandages, and are used when the limbs must be immobilized.

PLEURA. This is the membrane that covers the lungs and also lines the cavity— in which the lungs lie—called the pleural cavity. The pleura secretes a fluid which allows the expanding or contracting lung to slide smoothly up and down in the pleural cavity. (*See also* under LUNG.)

PLEURISY. This is inflammation of the pleura, or covering membrane of the lung. Usually only one lung is affected, and often only part of its surface. It is generally caused by exposure to cold and wet; but it may be a manifestation of tuberculosis or a complication of pneumonia, or fractured ribs, and of course the cause must be treated.

In Dry Pleurisy there is a sticky exudate in the pleural membrane and the two surfaces stick together, causing severe pain on breathing. The temperature is usually a little raised, 99 deg. F. or 100 deg. F., the breathing is shallow (to avoid expanding the lung over-much), the pulse quickened and the patient complains chiefly of a severe "stitch in his side," worse on breathing. Conditions that may be confused with dry pleurisy are intercostal neuralgia (neuralgia of the nerves that run between the ribs), and herpes, or shingles, before the eruption appears.

Treatment. The treatment of pleurisy includes rest in bed, fluid diet, the application of tincture of iodine or of antiphlogistine to the affected side; strapping the ribs firmly with adhesive tape almost right round. If the iodine or antiphlogistine is not enough to relieve the pain, a sedative cough mixture and ten grains of aspirin or something similar at bedtime. After pleurisy the chest should always be X-rayed to make sure that the lung is healthy once again.

Wet Pleurisy or Pleurisy with Effusion. This is the second type of pleurisy, when the inflammation of the pleural membrane is followed by an outpouring of fluid between the wall of the chest and the surface of the lung. The symptoms are much the same as in dry pleurisy, but the patient may be more blue and short of breath, and complains less of a stitch in his side.

Treatment. The doctor, when he examines the chest, finds marked dullness over the affected lung, and may have to draw off the fluid with a syringe, especially when it shows signs of pressing on the heart. Convalescence must be prolonged, the chest X-rayed, and breathing exercises carried out regularly. Pleurisy with effusion often indicates tuberculosis of the underlying lung.

PLEXUS. A network of nerves or vessels is called a plexus. The most well-known network of nerves, etc., is the solar plexus which supplies branches to all the organs in the abdomen. (*See also* NERVOUS SYSTEM.)

PLUMBISM. The Latin word for lead is plumbum, so lead poisoning is often referred to as plumbism. (*See* LEAD POISONING.)

PNEUMOCONIOSIS. Diseases of the lungs which are brought about by the inhalation of dust are known as pneumoconiosis. (*See also* ANTHRACOSIS; OCCUPATIONAL DISEASES; SILICOSIS; TUBERCULOSIS.)

PNEUMONIA. This is an inflammation of the lungs, and is of two types called broncho-pneumonia and lobar pneumonia.

Bronchopneumonia is an extension, patchy in distribution, of bronchitis (inflammation of the lining of the little tubes that lead air into the lungs) into the tissue of the lung. It is more common in children than in adults, and frequently complicates measles or whooping cough. It often follows an attack of bronchitis in the elderly, however, and tends to be a tedious illness, requiring prolonged convalescence.

Treatment. The treatment is similar to that of bronchitis. Careful nursing and plenty of fresh air are the essentials, with light nourishing foods to keep up the strength. Steam kettles, menthol and benzoin inhalations and oxygen (*not* when the patient is at the point of death, but when the complexion is bluish), are all useful.

Lobar Pneumonia is the variety commonly meant when the term "pneumonia" is used.

It is so called because an entire lobe or division of the lung is affected by the inflammation and may be "solid" with the thick secretion that is poured into the air vesicles. The lower lobes are those that are generally affected. Men get pneumonia more often than women.

Symptoms. It is usually not difficult to tell when a person has pneumonia. Pain in the side of the chest, shivering, a high temperature—from 101 deg. F. up to 104 deg. F. or more, a quick pulse, rapid breathing, "rusty" sputum, and a flushed face are all features of pneumonia. Sometimes, however, the pain is low down and appendicitis may be diagnosed, but it usually soon becomes clear that the chest and not the abdomen is affected. The disease is caused by a germ called the pneumococcus of which there are several types.

Treatment. The course of the disease and the treatment of pneumonia have completely altered with the discovery of the sulphonamide group of drugs and the antibiotics. Formerly the temperature and pulse-rate would keep up until the eighth day, when a "crisis" used to occur, with sudden fall of temperature and pulse rate. Today, in all cases of pneumonia, the patient is put on full doses of sulphadiazine or penicillin. With these drugs the temperature usually begins to fall after forty-eight hours and the patient makes a rapid recovery; in some cases the temperature falls almost at once. Sulphadiazine is less expensive and sometimes better tolerated than the antibiotics; in severe pneumonia it is better to give large doses of penicillin by injection than synthetic penicillin by the mouth. A patient on a course of any sulphadiazine must drink plenty of fluids in order to prevent the rare complication—renal damage.

In addition to chemotherapy the chief treatment is careful nursing. Fresh air and adequate sleep are essential to the patient with pneumonia. When pain is severe, morphia may be necessary to aid sleep. Kaolin poultices are also helpful. During convalescence the patient should be instructed in breathing exercises.

PNEUMOTHORAX. A condition in which air is present in the pleural cavity is known as pneumothorax. In modern treatment of tuberculosis of the lung, it is introduced artificially by a needle to collapse the lung and so rest and heal it. (*See also* EMPHYSEMA; LUNG; PLEURISY.)

POISONS AND POISONING. These headings are discussed fully in the FIRST AID SUPPLEMENT at the end of the book. Poisonous drugs will be found under their own headings.

POLIOENCEPHALITIS. Inflammation of the brain in which the gray matter is particularly affected is called polioencephalitis. (*See also* BRAIN; ENCEPHALITIS.)

POLIOMYELITIS. Inflammation affecting parts of the spinal cord which control the muscles responsible for the movement of the arms and legs is known as poliomyelitis. This condition is most common in children and was for long better known under the name infantile paralysis, under which it is discussed in this volume. This disease is caused by a virus and is much more prevalent during the summer months. It is apparently spread by "droplet" infection in the nose and throat. (*See also* INFANTILE PARALYSIS; IMMUNIZATION.)

POLYDACTYLISM. This term is used to describe the condition in which there are more than the normal number of fingers or toes on each hand or foot. The condition is usually present at birth. (*See also* CHILDBIRTH; HEREDITY.)

POLYNEURITIS. Polyneuritis, or multiple neuritis, is a disease due to inflammation of the nerves in various parts of the body. (*See also* NEURITIS.)

POLYPUS, NASAL. Growths which occur on one or both sides of the nose are called polypi (plural of polypus). They are really not true growths, but water-logged lining membrane from the nasal sinuses. Breathing is very often impaired and there may be a watery discharge from the nose. Removal of the polypi, which is a simple matter, may make a great difference to the patient's health. A polypus may also occur in the ear or in the womb. (*See also* EAR; NOSE; WOMB.)

POLYURIA. The passing of an excessive amount of urine is known as polyuria. The average amount passed in one day is about two and a half pints. Excess may be due to nervous causes when no treatment is required, or to some serious disease such as diabetes or inflammation of the kidney. There may be a temporary state of polyuria after fever. (*See also* DIABETES; NEPHRITIS; URINE.)

PORTAL VEIN. This is the large vein which enters the liver bringing the blood from the abdominal organs. It is peculiar among veins for it starts and ends in capillaries without going towards the heart.

PORT WINE STAINS. Red birthmarks are referred to as port wine stains. (*See also* BIRTHMARKS.)

POST MORTEM. This term, meaning

after death, is used in connection with an examination of the body following death, when the cause is uncertain or unknown.

POTASSIUM. Potassium is a metal belonging to the alkaline group and many of its salts are used in medicine. Potassium citrate is used as an alkali and is often given with sodium bicarbonate during a course of sulphonamide. It is also a useful diuretic.

Potassium bromide is a depressant and is used to control epileptic and troublesome senile elements. (*See also* BROMIDE; IODINE.)

POTT'S DISEASE. This term is frequently applied to curvature of the spine which results from tuberculous disease. Percival Pott (1713–1788), a famous English surgeon, was the first to describe the condition. (*See also* SPINAL CURVATURE; TUBERCULOSIS.)

POULTICES. Home-made poultices are not so much used now as they were formerly, because kaolin and similar preparations are available. But as this is not always at hand, poultices have still frequently to be made. The commonest in use are made of bread, linseed, starch, and mustard.

Bread Poultice. Stir some bread-crumbs into boiling water, beating well all the time. Cover bowl and place in boiling water until the bread is swollen. Drain off the water and spread evenly over a piece of linen or cotton. Turn the edges neatly in, spread the side to be placed next to the skin with olive oil or cold cream, then apply to the part. Try a corner first, in case it is too hot for the patient to bear. Cover with oiled silk and a bandage.

Mustard Poultices are linseed poultices with the addition of two tablespoonfuls of mustard.

PREDNISONE and PREDNISOLONE. Synthetic (laboratory-made) steroids analogous to cortisone and hydrocortisone. (*See also* CORTISONE.)

PREFRONTAL LEUCOTOMY. *See* LEUCOTOMY.

PREGNANCY. Pregnancy is the state of being with child. The earliest symptom is the stoppage of the monthly periods, and the child's birth may be expected approximately nine months and one week from the first day of the last period. There is usually no doubt, however, after quickening has been observed. Quickening is when the movements of the child in the womb become so strong that the mother feels them; this usually occurs at four and a half months. After cessation of the periods, the next symptom to be noticed is "morning sickness." A small quantity of clear tasteless fluid may be vomited each morning on rising. If there is a persistent vomiting or if the condition continues after the fourth month, a doctor's advice should be sought.

After one or two months, the breasts enlarge, distended veins are visible on their surface, the nipples become more prominent and the area around them becomes darker in color with raised pimple-like bodies on the areola. During the first three months there may be a frequent desire to pass water, but this feeling disappears for a few months. When it returns, it usually signifies that the end of the pregnancy is very near. In the later stages of pregnancy there is a brown line running downwards from the navel, and there are lines of stretching on the abdominal wall which may remain as faint white scars after childbirth. These are called striae. (They may be caused by any disease which produces distension of the abdomen.)

During pregnancy there is often constipation, and there may be heartburn. There may sometimes be a dislike for certain articles of food and a longing for others. The weight of the abdomen may cause swollen legs with varicose veins. There may be great irritation of the genital organs, and some women have a heavy white discharge. All these symptoms should be treated and a little care will help to lighten any inconveniences. The danger signals which must be referred to a doctor at the earliest possible moment are bleeding, fits, albuminuria (the presence of albumin in the urine), and the stopping of the movements of the child in the womb. Bleeding may be the sign of a miscarriage. Albumin in the urine, or a sudden fit, may be symptoms of the condition known as eclampsia, as may swelling of the ankles. (*See also* CHILDBIRTH; ECLAMPSIA; LABOR; PUERPERIUM.)

PREPARATION OF NIPPLES. Prepa-

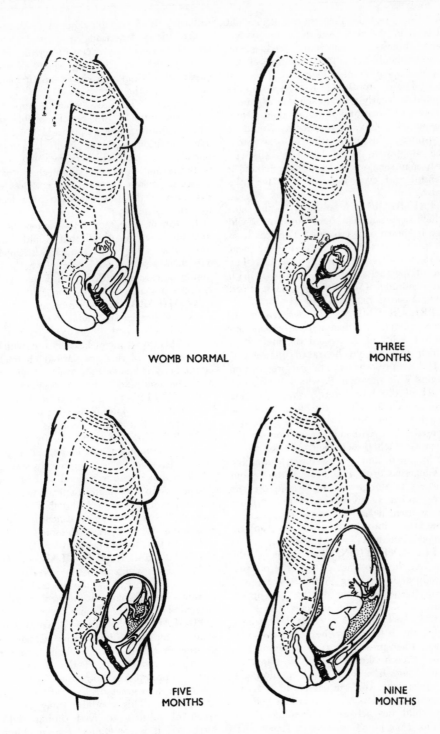

WOMB NORMAL

THREE MONTHS

FIVE MONTHS

NINE MONTHS

Pregnancy: Development of Child.

tion for breast-feeding should begin not later than the sixth month of pregnancy. Small breasts do not make feeding any more difficult but an examination of the nipples is important. These should be well shaped and protruding. Retracted nipples should be gently pulled each day and massaged with soap and water. If they cannot be pulled out at all, the doctor should be consulted. This preparation is to accustom the nipples to being handled, otherwise they may soon soften and crack, making it painful and even impossible to feed the baby.

PRESBYOPIA. A condition of the sight which occurs as a natural outcome of old age is known as presbyopia. The lens loses its power of focusing properly, and near work becomes increasingly difficult. The use of spectacles is necessary to deal with the condition. (*See also* ACCOMMODATION; EYE; VISION, ERRORS IN.)

PRESCRIPTION. The written directions ordered by a doctor for a patient containing a list of drugs and the method in which they should be taken or used, is called a prescription. Every prescription begins with the sign R which is the first letter of the Latin word *recipe,* meaning "take." Then follow the names of the drugs and the quantity of each to be dispensed, along with any instructions to the chemist. Each prescription must be signed or initialled, and a prescription containing a dangerous drug must bear the name and address of the person for whose use the prescription is given. Some prescriptions are written in Latin, though the custom is now falling into disuse. (*See also* APOTHECARIES' WEIGHTS AND MEASURES.)

PRESENTATION. The part of the child in the womb which is in the position to appear first during childbirth is referred to as the presentation. In the most favorable cases the child presents the head, with its back directed towards the mother's front; this is known as the vertex presentation. Other presentations are described as brow, breech, shoulder, foot, or transverse and so on. In a breech presentation, the child presents the buttocks, and a transverse presentation means that the body of the child lies across the opening of the womb. (*See also* CHILDBIRTH; LABOR.)

PRICKLY HEAT. Prickly heat, or miliaria, is a troublesome skin disease which affects Americans in tropical countries. It is caused by excessive perspiration, which blocks up the tiny ducts of the sweat glands and produces an irritable condition of the skin.

Symptoms. The rash, when it appears, takes the form of tiny vesicles or blisters which cause extreme itching and pricking. The condition is not in itself dangerous, but the scratching which follows may lead to the formation of boils or infected areas. In weak persons the irritation and loss of sleep caused by this condition may lead to serious consequences.

Treatment. The most important point is to avoid anything at all that would tend to cause sweating. After the bath, in which only a mild soap should be used, the body should be carefully dried, then dusted with an antiseptic powder. (*See also* MILIARIA.)

PRIMIPARA. This term is applied to a woman bearing or giving birth to her first child.

PROBE. A slender, flexible rod which is used for exploring the various channels of the body is known as a probe. It should never be used except in expert hands.

PROCTITIS. Inflammation of the rectum or anus is known as proctitis. (*See also* ANUS; RECTUM.)

PROGNOSIS. An opinion or forecast of the course, duration and ending of a disease is described as a prognosis. In stating whether the prognosis is good or bad, the doctor has to take many factors into consideration. The health and habits of the patient, the response to treatment and the reputation of the disease are some of the chief points. (*See also* DIAGNOSIS.)

PROGRESSIVE MUSCULAR ATROPHY. This is a disease of the nervous system which occurs in middle life and which is much more common in men than in women. Its cause is obscure.

PROLAPSE. The falling downward of some organ of the body from its normal position is called prolapse. Falling of the womb is perhaps one of the commonest forms of prolapse in women and it can be the cause of a great deal of suffering and unhappiness. This condition may be the result of injuries received during childbirth, but it is sometimes seen in elderly women owing to atrophy of the uterine ligaments following the menopause. Satisfactory results can be obtained by operation, but if an operation is not advisable, the condition can be remedied by wearing a suitably shaped pessary. Wearing a pessary does not cure the condition but only holds the parts together as long as it is worn. (*See also* ANUS; WOMB.)

PROPHYLAXIS. The prevention of disease is known as prophylaxis, and any measures taken to prevent disease are known as prophylactic measures. Examples are vaccination and immunization, which are carried out to prevent smallpox and diphtheria, respectively. (*See also* INOCULATION.)

PROSTIGMINE. This is a synthetic preparation of physostigmine which has been found valuable in the treatment of myasthenia gravis. It is also used to relieve distention of the bowel and retention of urine after operation.

PROSTATE GLAND. The organ surrounding the neck of the bladder and the beginning of the urethra in the male is known as the prostate gland. It is rather like a chestnut in shape and can be felt from the rectum behind. So far as is known its only purpose is to secrete a fluid that lubricates the urethra and is excreted with the semen. This gland is of importance, because in old age it often increases greatly in size, thus causing obstruction to the urinary outflow. There is difficulty in passing water, which can be overcome only by inserting an instrument known as a catheter to draw off the urine from the bladder. An operation known as prostatectomy can be carried out, in which all

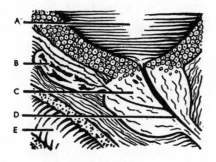

Prostate Gland:
A. *Bladder;* B. *Seminal Vesicle;*
C. *Prostate;* D. *Urethra;* E. *Rectum.*

or most of the enlarged prostate can be removed, so leaving a free passage for the urine. Inflammation of the prostate gland is known as prostatitis and is usually the result of gonorrhea, but it may also occur as a result of infection from the kidneys or bladder. The condition is a very painful one and the patient should consult a doctor as soon as possible. (*See also* GLEET; GONORRHEA.)

PROSTRATION. A feeling of extreme weakness is called prostration. One type of this condition is known as nervous prostration, which is much the same as neurasthenia. (*See also* LASSITUDE; NEURASTHENIA.)

PROTEIN. Protein is an organic substance found in various forms in vegetable and animal life. Albumin, or white of egg, meat, and gelatine are examples of protein substance.

PROTOPLASM. The sticky material which is an essential part of all living cells is described as protoplasm. It is composed mainly of proteins, and the whole working of the body depends upon its chemical activities. (*See also* CELL; EVOLUTION.)

PROTOZOA. Protozoa are the lowest form of life consisting of a simple cell (protozoon) or groups of cells. The protozoon, or ameba, is responsible for many diseases in man, e.g. amebic dysentery. (*See also* AMEBA; GERMS; PARASITES.)

PROUD FLESH. This is a popular name given to granulation tissue, which is formed during the healing of ulcers and gaping wounds. (*See also* GRANULATION TISSUE.)

PRURIGO (Besnier's). This is a skin eruption, affecting the forehead, neck, upper part of chest and back, front of elbows and back of knees. It is characterized by areas of thickened skin covered with isolated papules, and often follows infantile eczema. The eruption is very irritating, and scratching not only wears the patient out but may produce infection of the skin. The course of the disease is very long, and cure is usually only temporary. Like urticaria, it is regarded as being an allergic manifestation and often occurs along with asthma. People who develop it are usually nervous and highly strung.

Treatment is rest in bed, sedation and

the application of tar preparations. (*See also* SKIN.)

PRURITUS. The term pruritus is used for all forms of itching, and this unpleasant and irritable state of the skin can be brought about in a great many different ways. Itching may be a symptom of many skin diseases, such as dermatitis, lichen planus, prurigo and urticaria, etc., and the scratching which naturally follows may set up a serious state of affairs. Contact with rough or woolen clothes is a common cause of itching, especially in children. Parasites, such as lice, etc., may bring about the condition, and the bites and stings of insects are also liable to prove troublesome. The skin condition known as "the itch," or scabies, is caused by a tiny parasite which burrows under the skin, but once the mite is destroyed the condition very quickly clears up.

Itching may be brought on through handling various substances such as flour, sugar, detergents, etc., and these conditions are discussed under the heading OCCUPATIONAL SKIN DISEASES. The application of drugs to the skin may cause a rash or eruption, or exposure to sunlight may be the cause of much irritability. Some people are very sensitive to plants, and contact with the leaves or flowers, or even smelling the flowers, may bring on an attack of itching. Certain nervous diseases as well as diseases of the liver, when there is jaundice, may have pruritus as a symptom. Itching around the anus may be caused by piles, fistula, fissure, or the presence of threadworms, while itching around the genitals in women is commonly due to a discharge from the vagina. It should be remembered that itching is not a disease, but it may be the symptom of some diseases, and if it continues, the advice of a doctor should be sought. (*See also* DERMATITIS; OCCUPATIONAL SKIN DISEASES; LLCHEN PLANUS; PRURIGO; PSORIASIS.)

PRUSSIC ACID. Also known as hydrocyanic acid, prussic acid is contained in the oil of bitter almonds, but it can be manufactured by distillation of potassium ferrocyanide with dilute sulphuric acid. It is one of the most poisonous substances known, and its inhalation may cause death within half a minute. (*See also* HYDROCYANIC ACID.)

PSITTACOSIS. A contagious disease of parrots, which when communicated to man produces a pneumonia-like disease. Restriction of the importing of parrots has caused it to disappear.

PSOAS. This name is given to a powerful muscle which arises from the spinal column. It passes down through the pelvis and groin, and thus joins the inner side of the thigh bone. This muscle is brought into use in the act of bending the trunk forward or in flexing the thigh at the hip. Disease of the spine is very liable to lead to an abscess within this muscle and the pus may travel down the sheath, and finally work its way into the upper part of the thigh. Such an abscess is known as a psoas abscess and it is usually the result of tubercular infection of the spine. (*See also* ABSCESS; TUBERCULOSIS.)

PSORIASIS. Psoriasis is a common chronic inflammation of the skin, characterized by rounded reddened patches of various sizes, which are covered with dry silvery scales. The eruption may be widespread, and appear as suddenly as a fever-rash, or there may be a few chronic patches. The scalp, ears, elbows, knees, and the back below the waist are the parts commonly affected; but psoriasis has been known to attack all parts, including the nails. Both sexes and all ages are affected; it is most common in young adults. The eruption appears in many varieties, and one of its chief features is its tendency to recur. The cause is unknown.

Treatment. As internal treatment, very many drugs have been tried. Gold injections have a favorable influence, especially in those cases associated with arthritis. Arsenic, used cautiously, and thyroid in elderly cases, are also in general use.

Externally, chrysarobin in petroleum jelly is by far the best treatment. It is rubbed in twice daily, baths being taken regularly to remove the scales. (The face and eyes are protected, as chrysarobin is irritating.) About two weeks suffice for a cure. The disadvantages are a temporary inflammation of the sensitive parts of the skin, and a permanent purple staining of the clothes. Tar in any form is very safe; common coaltar, though unsightly, is a good though slow remedy.

Hot sea-water baths and X-rays are good

in some cases. Very widespread inflamed cases should be treated as dermatitis. The diet must be plain, and alcohol entirely avoided. Derangements of the general health should receive attention. Lastly, the patient should always be on the lookout for recurrences, especially on the scalp. In all cases, the disease should be compared with the inconvenience of treatment, as the latter may prove a greater hindrance to the patient than would the symptoms of a mild case of psoriasis. (*See also* DERMATITIS.)

PSYCHOLOGY. This is the name given to the study of the mind and of behavior. It has become of increasing importance during the past thirty years, since events like the two wars have shown that the mind and the body work together so intimately that the mind may actually cause bodily illness, and only when the condition of the mind is investigated and treated will the bodily illness get better. Another important aspect of psychology is the study of the development of the mind of the child. Formerly a naughty child was punished; nowadays an attempt is made to discover why the naughtiness occurs. Such causes as jealousy of a newborn brother or sister, or an unhappy home atmosphere, when removed, may transform such a child into a perfectly normal one. (*See also* MIND; PERSONALITY.)

PSYCHONEUROSIS. This is a mental disorder which is akin to a neurosis but which is more difficult to cure, because the root of the trouble lies away back in childhood and it is only by the aid of prolonged psychotherapy that it can be traced. A psychoneurosis is said to be caused by incidents, or wishes which occurred in childhood and which, owing to their conflicting with the training of the individual, have been banished from consciousness to the unconscious mind, from which they are ever trying to escape. The battle between the "censored" wish or thought and the conscious mind may manifest itself as a psychoneurosis, of which the best example is one form of hysteria. (*See also* HYSTERIA; NEUROSIS; PSYCHOTHERAPY.)

PSYCHOSIS. Psychosis means a disorder of the mind, but in actual practice the term is restricted to the more severe forms of mental disorders, which will be found discussed under the heading of INSANITY.

PSYCHOTHERAPY. This is an essential part of the treatment of all disorders of the mind, but it must be combined with the necessary bodily treatment of the patient to achieve a perfect result. The basis of all psychotherapy is to explore the patient's mind; to find out the origin of the mental symptoms; to recognize the source of the trouble and to help the patient to rearrange his ideas for a better adaptation to the events of daily life. There are three main methods used in psychotherapy, though in any particular case, more than one may have to be employed.

Suggestion is the power that some people have of impressing their views, and their will, on others. Some individuals are able to suggest by their very presence that all will be well with a patient, and it is such as these who become famous physicians. Suggestion is of value in psychotherapy only in so far as the patient is consciously aware of his mental difficulties; it is of no value in the psychoneurosis, in which the trouble is in the unconscious mind.

Hypnotism has already been fully discussed under its own heading and can therefore be dismissed here with the note that it is a procedure bringing about a mental state in which suggestion is more easily accepted than normally. It is of value in curing the bodily symptoms of hysteria as a preliminary measure to discovering the true cause of the hysteria. It is also of value in curing imaginary pains and in producing sleep.

Psychoanalysis is an attempt to bring long-forgotten experiences of the patient's childhood to light and to associate them with his consequent experiences and troubles. By this means such buried (or repressed) incidents assume their rightful proportions among the events of a person's life and no longer lie seething in his unconscious mind. They therefore cease to be the source of the mental distress which has given rise to his particular symptoms.

So much nonsense has been written in recent years about the method of psychoanalysis, that a brief description of the way the method is carried out will be given.

The patient is first physically examined thoroughly and the full history of his mental trouble and symptoms are recorded. He is then asked to lie down on a couch and to relax as much as possible. The analyst sits behind the top of the couch so that the patient does not see him at all. The patient is then requested to speak any words which come into his head, however unimportant they may appear to him. The analyst suggests nothing to the patient; the patient does all the work; the analyst only asks such questions as are needed to link up the words the patient uses. Often a patient will lie silent for some time, and then will disclose some vital fact which has hitherto been concealed under the mask of shyness or of fear. Especially in that condition known as "anxiety" is it found that ideas concerning sex, often not very far removed from consciousness, are the true cause of the fear.

It is the duty of the physician who practises psychoanalysis to overcome his own prejudices on this subject and to allow the patient to discuss with him the mental aspect of sex as naturally as he would discuss a pain in his stomach. As sex is one of the primitive instincts which has to be controlled by the dictates of modern civilization, it is not surprising that, on analysis, only too often is it found that sexual problems are the essential cause of the mental trouble. Once the fact has been realized, it is necessary to direct the patient's energies so that social activities provide suitable substitutes for individual selfishness. The method of psychoanalysis is, of necessity, a slow form of psychotherapy, and many interviews may be required before the real cause of the patient's symptoms is unearthed. No single interview can last longer than one hour; it would be too much strain on both patient and physician. The other criticism that has been leveled at this method is that the female patient is liable to "fall in love" with the psychoanalyst. As a matter of fact, many women patients are analyzed by women doctors, and of those who are treated by men, nearly all take a strong dislike to the doctor after about the second interview, because they are afraid they have "given themselves away." This attitude of dislike sometimes persists up to the end of the treatment, but is usually replaced eventually by a neutral attitude.

Freudism. This is the name of the theory formulated by the eminent psychologist, Sigmund Freud, to throw light upon the way in which certain disorders of the mind are caused. According to Freud it is possible in many cases to trace the various steps by which a given cause gives rise to the symptoms of mental disorder, and by retracing these steps it is possible to cure the mental trouble. The method by which these steps are traced and retraced is the often-quoted but seldom understood method of psychoanalysis.

The principles of Freud's doctrine are as follows: there are present in all of us, from infancy onwards, certain wishes and instincts. Many of these wishes and instincts have to be restrained by social laws and conventions. For example, the sight of a pearl necklace in a shop window may arouse an impulse to possess it, but social laws and customs prevent us from attempting to obtain it by unlawful means. Whenever there is opposition between these instincts and wishes and the social laws which prevent their fulfilment a *conflict* is said to be present. Briefly, the conflict is between pleasure impulses and social impulses. In the present state of our civilization the instinct with which our social impulses are most in conflict is the sexual instinct. Freud uses the word "sexual" in a very wide sense and not merely in the limited physical sense in which it is commonly understood.

Treatment. These conflicts must be dealt with; and the process of dealing with them is called "resolving" them. The best method, and the one on which successful treatment depends, is by recognizing them as conflicts, meeting them and choosing the line of conduct to be followed. If this method were always possible and were always adopted, much nervous and mental trouble would be prevented; but many people do not recognize their mental conflicts and so cannot resolve them.

The wish which it is impossible to fulfil is banished from consciousness and then forms part of the unconscious mind. The conflict is forgotten and cannot be recalled by any effort of the will, but it remains in the unconscious mind and influences thought and action. Such an unconscious wish is called a "complex," and the mental process by which it is banished from consciousness is called "repression." The way in which these unconscious wishes or "complexes" influence conscious thought and action depends on the particular mental make-up of the individual. Most complexes arise in early life, when the child first learns what he may and may not do in civilized society.

The next best way of resolving conflicts is by what Freud terms "sublimation," in which the primitive, repressed wishes are translated into a useful form of energy. Art, music, hobbies are common examples of sublimation which are of great social value. Most of the finest charitable work in the world is done by those to whom such work is a sublimation, but only too often such a desirable result is not attained and the complex, with the unconscious wish seething underneath, is translated into a form of mental disorder. Anxiety, hysteria, and other nervous states are all the results of complexes which have not been allowed the social outlet of sublimation. It is the business of the psychiatrist to discover these hidden complexes and, by enabling the patient to recognize their existence, to get rid of them.

Helpful in this connection is a discussion of the patient's dreams with a psychiatrist; for during sleep the repressions are weakened, and the unconscious wishes of the sleeper rise into consciousness as *dreams*. In the child, in whom repressions have not yet taken place, dreams are a true reflection of the child's wishes; but in the adult the repressions are still present during sleep, although much weakened, and so the dreams are distorted. By discussing them with a psychiatrist, the patients themselves manage to find out exactly what their dreams mean and how they are linked up with their mental troubles. Such an analysis of dreams forms one of the chief ways in which Freudism differs from other methods of treatment of mental disorder.

It must be emphasized that the patient himself reveals his repressions, by analyzing his dreams himself. Much discredit has been brought on the method of treatment by psychoanalysis by people who, themselves not trained in dealing with disorders of the mind, attempt to treat patients by what they call psychoanalysis. In true analysis nothing is suggested to the patient and he has, in fact, to work out his own salvation. The analyst is there only to point the way, not to lead him along it. Once the complexes have been recognized and faced by the patient, the energy that was spent in repressing the complexes is available for use in more profitable directions: sublimation takes place and the neurosis or hysteria disappears. (*See also* DREAMS; PSYCHOANALYSIS.)

PTOMAINE. A form of poisoning due to eating decomposed food is known as ptomaine poisoning. (*See also* BOTULISM; FOOD POISONING.)

PTOSIS. Drooping of the upper eyelid is known as ptosis. (*See also* EYE; EYELID.)

PTYALIN. Ptyalin is the name of the ferment contained in the saliva by which starchy foods are turned into sugar in order to aid digestion. (*See also* FERMENTS.)

PUBERTY. The period in which the child gradually passes into manhood or womanhood is called puberty. It occurs between the ages of 13 and 15 and tends to be earlier in girls than in boys. (*See also* ADOLESCENCE.)

PUBIS. The bone that forms the front part of the pelvis is called the pubis or pubic bone. (*See also* BONE.)

PUBLIC HEALTH. This term is used for the department of medicine which concerns itself with preventive medicine and the health of the community.

PUERPERAL FEVER. This is a highly infectious fever occurring during the period immediately after childbirth, due to infection by the germ called the streptococcus. Formerly frequently fatal, although now usually responding well to penicillin or other antibiotics, it still remains one of the chief causes of maternal mortality. (*See also* CHILDBIRTH.)

PUERPERIUM. This is the time between the birth of a child and the restoration of the mother to perfect health, and usually lasts about a month. During this time the womb, from being big enough to hold an infant, has to regain its normal size of a pear, and the discharge from it, bloodstained at first, gradually becomes clear and then stops altogether. The breasts, which are of course enlarged in pregnancy, begin to secrete milk, generally beginning two or three days after the child has been born. It is usual for a mother to remain in bed for the first five days of the puerperium, though some specialists nowadays say that this is quite unnecessary and allow the patient up almost at once.

PULMONARY. Anything pertaining to or affecting the lungs is described as pulmonary. (*See also* LUNGS.)

PULSATION. The throbbing caused by the beating of the heart is called pulsation and it can be felt, and sometimes seen, on the left side between the fourth and fifth ribs. Pulsation may also be felt where an artery lies close beneath the skin, but abnormal pulsation or beating may be a sign of aneurism (swelling of an artery). Pulsation can often be felt in the upper part of the abdomen, especially in thin people, due to the throbbing of the abdominal aorta.

PULSE. The pumping of the blood through the heart causes changes to take place in the blood vessels, and each time blood is pumped through, the arteries swell and then contract again; this is known as the pulse. At each heartbeat, from four to six ounces of blood are pumped into the aorta, the largest artery of the body, and the wave of this fluid is carried along to all the other arteries. The pulse can be felt in any artery that lies near the surface; but the radial artery which runs over the bones of the wrist is chosen for this purpose. The examination of the pulse affords valuable information to the doctor. He is able to find out the state of the artery as regards its hardness, etc., and the rate of the pulse tells him much about the action of the heart. The pulse rate is usually about 72 beats per minute, but it varies a great deal in different people. Some people may have a quick pulse normally, while in others it may be habitually slow. To take the pulse, hold a watch with a second hand in the left hand, and place the three fingers of the right hand on the front of the forearm, about one inch above the furrows of the wrist and about half an inch from the outer edge. The pulse beats are counted for one minute. A rapid pulse occurs in fevers,

certain diseases of the heart, and nervous disorders. In typhoid fever, the pulse becomes very slow, and this is recognized as one of the symptoms of the disease. There is a type of irregular pulse common in young people, and also people recovering from infectious diseases, in which the pulse rate is affected by the breathing. (*See also* BRADYCARDIA; HEART.)

PUPIL. The pupil is simply a hole in the iris of the eye, which is composed of two layers of muscle. One layer is arranged in circular fashion, and on contracting diminishes the size of the pupil; the other is arranged radially and its contraction causes the pupil to dilate.

The pupil is *contracted* in old age, bright light, near work, and sleep. It is *dilated* in emotional upsets, such as anger, pain, and fear, and in dim light. Certain drugs have the power of altering its size; and in some diseases its size is a help in diagnosis. (*See also* EYE.)

PURGATIVE. Drugs or other methods which are used to produce an action of the bowels are known as cathartics or purgatives. A large number of substances act as purgatives and they are grouped according to the nature of their effects. The mildest types are known as *aperients* or *laxatives,* and they gently stimulate the bowels and render the motions slightly more frequent without causing any griping. *Simple purgatives* such as cascara sagrada, castor oil, aloes, etc., produce more copious and more liquid movements often accompanied, or preceded by, griping pains. *Drastic purgatives* cause a violent action of the bowels accompanied by considerable griping, and since they remove a considerable quantity of water from the system, they are also known as *hydragogues.* These should not be used unless prescribed by a doctor. Most of the important drugs are dealt with under their own titles. (*See also* APERIENT; CONSTIPATION; DIARRHEA; LAXATIVE.)

PURPURA. Small capillary hemorrhages into the skin or a mucous membrane are called purpura. It is not a disease, but a symptom of many diseases. It may occur in the course of many of the acute infectious fevers: the commonest of these are measles, scarlet fever, smallpox, typhus, and cerebrospinal fever or meningitis. It may occur as a result of poisoning of the bone marrow by heavy doses of X-rays, or by drugs, particularly gold and arsenic. The commonest type of purpura is associated with deficiency of platelets in the blood and is called thrombocytopaenic purpura. Its cause is still unknown.

Schonlein's purpura is the name given to a condition in which reddish-purple spots appear in the skin accompanied by swelling and pain in the joints.

Henoch's purpura is a similar condition accompanied by pain in the belly due to bleeding into the wall of the bowel. A purpuric rash on the skin is one of the characteristic features of scurvy, a disease which is due to deficiency of Vitamins C and P in the diet.

The treatment of purpura is to remove the cause where this is known. Where the cause is unknown, and therefore irremovable, and the disease is associated with a shortage of platelets in the circulating blood, the spleen is sometimes removed instead. Though this is by no means always necessary, it may be a lifesaving operation in thrombocytopaenic purpura. Iron, calcium, and vitamins are often prescribed and blood transfusion may also be necessary.

PUS. Pus, or matter, is a thick fluid which is found in abscesses, ulcers, and on any inflamed surface. It consists mainly of white blood cells destroyed by the bacteria responsible for the infection. The color may vary from white to greenish-yellow according to the type of germ causing the condition. The odor, too, may vary a great deal for the same reason, while much depends on which part of the body is affected. A discharge containing pus is spoken of as a purulent discharge. (*See also* ABSCESS; BOIL; CARBUNCLE.)

PUSTULES. Small abscesses appearing on the skin or mucous membranes are called pustules. They almost always appear as a feature of some disease, the most common, perhaps, being acne vulgaris. Smallpox and anthrax also are diseases characterized by the appearance of pustules. When the pustules eventually dry up there is always a certain amount of scarring left; this is particularly noticeable after smallpox. (*See also* ACNE; ANTHRAX; SMALLPOX.)

PUTREFACTION. The decomposition

that takes place in dead animal and vegetable matter is called putrefaction. It is due to the action of bacteria or germs, and in the course of the process various poisonous and offensive substances are formed. (*See also* DECOMPOSITION.)

PYELITIS. The pelvis of the kidney joins the kidney and the upper part of the ureter. Inflammation of the pelvis is known as pyelitis.

There is always a degree of concomitant nephritis, and cystitis is frequently present in addition. The infection is usually carried to the kidneys from the bladder, or germs may be present in the blood and carried directly to the kidney from the bloodstream. Pyelitis is fairly common in children, and the condition is more frequent in females than in males.

Symptoms. There is fever, pain in the region of the loins, vomiting and headache, and there is usually a desire to pass water at frequent intervals. Nervous symptoms may be present.

The urine is cloudy in appearance and, on examination, a large number of pus cells will be found.

Treatment. The patient should be confined to bed and the bowels cleared by means of a laxative. The administration of citrate of potash or other alkalis in large doses gives relief from the symptoms and is the most effective way of clearing up the inflammation. Urinary antiseptics may have to be given, e.g. hexamine or one of the sulphonamide group. (*See also* BACILLURIA; KIDNEY; NEPHRITIS.)

PYEMIA. This is a severe illness in which abscesses appear in various parts of the body due to spread of infection via the bloodstream. The symptoms of the disease resemble those of septicemia. (*See also* SEPTICEMIA.)

PYLORIC STENOSIS. This is a disease of early infancy and is four times as common in boys as in girls. The cause is unknown, but there is a great thickening of the pylorus (the exit valve of the stomach) and the child produces violent "projectile" vomits, loses weight rapidly, and becomes constipated. The condition is one that must not be allowed to continue and if it does not clear up soon on medical treatment, or is very severe, an operation has to be performed.

PYLORUS. The tube-like part of the stomach through which the partially digested food passes on into the duodenum is known as the pylorus. The duodenum is the first part of the small intestine. (*See also* DUODENUM; STOMACH.)

PYOGENIC BACTERIA. Germs which cause the formation of pus and so lead to abscesses and boils, etc., are known as pyogenic. There are many types of germs included in this group, but by far the most common are the staphylococci and streptococci. (*See also* GERMS; PUS.)

PYONEPHROSIS. This is a condition in which the kidney is converted into a bag of pus. (*See also* HYDRONEPHROSIS; KIDNEY.)

PYORRHEA. Pyorrhea is a disease of the gums which may cause serious upset to the general health. It is due to a germ (or, more accurately, an ameba) and it attacks people of all ages but those in good general health with carefully tended mouths will not be so liable to it as others. The teeth should be put in order by a dentist and antiseptic paints, toothpastes, or mouthwashes used freely until the condition is cleared up. (*See also* DENTAL DRILL; GINGIVITIS; GUMS, DISEASE OF.)

PYRETHRUM. The tincture of pyrethrum, prepared from the flowers, is used for killing household pests such as fleas and bugs and it can safely be dabbed on the hands and legs to keep off insects.

PYREXIA. Pyrexia, or fever, is the elevation of the temperature above the normal (98.4 deg. F.) due to disease. (*See also* FEVER.)

PYURIA. This term is used to describe any condition in which there is pus in the urine. There may be various causes. (*See also* URINE.)

QUARANTINE. The term quarantine is used in connection with the length of time which a person who has been exposed to an infectious disease must be separated from other people. The length of time depends on the type of disease. The importance of quarantine is obvious in connection with school children. The term quarantine is also used in connection with the length of time in which a ship that is carrying an infectious person on board must be kept free from personal contact with the shore. In the old days if a ship put into port with an infectious case on board, the crew and passengers were quarantined, or detained, for about forty days. This state of affairs proved to be too irksome to travelers and trade, and nowadays arrangements are made for a special mooring-place where passengers from a ship which is unable to present a "clean" bill of health can be landed. All passengers must undergo a medical examination before they are allowed to land, and all actual and suspected cases are taken to hospital. Names and addresses of all the passengers who land are taken and forwarded to the medical officers of health of their various districts, so that everyone can be kept under observation until any danger of an outbreak of the disease is over. (*See also* INCUBATION PERIOD; INFECTIOUS DISEASES.)

QUARTAN FEVER. This is a particular type of malaria characterized by severe bouts of fever, sometimes accompanied by delirium, occuring every fourth day. (*See also* MALARIA.)

QUASSIA. Quassia is a bitter, stimulating tonic which is obtained from the wood of a tall tree which grows in South America and the West Indies. Quassia is often given as an anthelmintic, the name used for a drug which has the power of killing intestinal worms, and is mainly used to get rid of threadworms which inhabit the lower part of the bowel. (*See also* APPETITE; BITTERS; DIGESTION.)

QUICKENING. This term is used to describe the feeling of movement inside the womb caused by the unborn child. (*See also* CHILDBIRTH; LABOR; PREGNANCY.)

QUICKSILVER. This is the popular name for mercury, which is a fluid, silvery metal of great mobility. The salts and other preparations of mercury are most important drugs. (*See also* MERCURY.)

QUINIDINE. This drug is obtained from cinchona bark and it is closely related to quinine. Besides being of use in the treatment of malaria, it is a very valuable drug in cases of auricular fibrillation, a heart disease in which the beats are tremulous and irregular. (*See also* CINCHONA; QUININE.)

QUININE. Quinine is a very important alkaloid drug obtained from several species of cinchona bark. The best-known use of the drug is in the treatment of malaria, and it is usually taken by the mouth. Quinine will not only cut short an attack of malaria, but it is capable of preventing one if taken about three hours before the attack is due. There are many preparations of quinine, but it is generally used in the form of one of its salts, such as the sulphate of quinine, hydrochloride of quinine, or tannate of qinine.

As a tonic, small doses may be taken after meals either liquid or in tablets, or it is more commonly taken with other tonic substances such as iron and strychnine. (*See also* MALARIA.)

QUINSY. This is an abscess in or around the tonsil. (*See also* TONSIL; TONSILLITIS.)

RABIES. This is an illness caused by a bite or lick from an animal suffering from a serious infective disease. Dogs, cats, horses, cattle, etc., may be afflicted with this complaint. In man it is known as hydrophobia. (*See also* HYDROPHOBIA.)

RADIAL NERVE. The radial nerve comes from the armpit, winds round the humerus, and controls the muscles extending to the elbow, wrist, and fingers. It is affected in the conditions known as *crutch paralysis* and *wrist drop*.

RADIOACTIVE ISOTOPES. A great advance in our understanding of the working of the human body has been brought about by the discovery that certain chemical substances can be made "radioactive." These substances, though behaving to all intents like the real thing, have a minute physical alteration in the structure of their atoms which make them detectable by special methods. Thus physiologists have been able to follow the absorption, distribution and fate in the body of many chemical elements. Radioactive iodine has been shown to accumulate rapidly in the thyroid gland, and use has been made of this fact in the treatment of Graves' disease. Radioactive gold is taken up by the liver, kidneys, and in the joints of patients suffering from rheumatoid arthritis which has been held to explain the beneficial effect sometimes observed from the use of gold in this disease. Use has been made of radioactive phosphorus in a rare disease of the red blood cell forming elements of the bone marrow (polycythaemia). (*See also* RADIUM.)

RADIOGRAPHY or SKIAGRAPHY. This describes a photograph taken by means of X-rays. Other names given to this form of photography include photography by Röntgen-rays, skotography, skiagraphy, electrography, etc. A skiagram is not an actual photograph, but is really a silhouette of an object which is denser than its surroundings. (*See also* X-RAY.)

RADIOTHERAPY. It is generally recognized that the rays given off by radium have a close physical, chemical, and biological similarity to those possessed by X-rays. From the point of view of treatment, however, the rays of radium are much superior. There is also a far greater advantage in the fact that the radium rays can be applied to parts of the body which cannot be reached by X-rays.

Radium treatment of extreme activity should not produce any irritating effect if the duration of the application is sufficiently short; e.g., not longer than three minutes. The general principle is to use rays with a feeble penetrating power for slight skin troubles, and the rays with more penetrating power for deep-seated growths. By this last method it is possible to have a great effect on the deeper tumors without irritating the skin.

Radium is used more and more in the treatment of cancer, either by the insertion of radium or radon "seeds" into and around a growth, or at a distance, as in a "bomb" containing several grams. Fewer cases of cancer are now being treated by surgery alone than by radium alone. Radium is particularly useful in the treatment of cancer of the tongue, breast, and womb. (*See also* RADIUM.)

RADIUM. This is a white metallic element belonging to the group of alkaline earths which also include barium, calcium, magnesium, and strontium. It is found in pitchblende together with uranium. For medical purposes a salt of radium is usually employed. The bromide of radium is a soluble salt, while the sulphate is an insoluble one.

The element radium, without appearing to receive any energy from surrounding substances, gives off in a constant fashion a large quantity of energy in the form of gas emanation, heat, and electricity. In spite of this, pieces of the element have been kept for several years and have not apparently lost any weight. These are facts which appear to be contrary to certain fundamental laws of physical science. The gas given off is known as an *emanation* and is called *radon*. It is used for medical purposes. It follows the laws common to all gases. It can give surrounding substances a temporary radioactivity—induced radioactivity. (*See also* RADIOACTIVE ISOTOPES.)

It is now known that radium is derived from uranium by a gradual splitting up of the uranium atom. In a similar way the energy which radium possesses is derived from a splitting of its atomic structure, and the ultimate product is lead.

The emanations of radium are subdivided into what are known as α (alpha) and β (beta) rays—definite particles which are given out at a very great speed. The discharge of the α and β rays causes waves in the ether which in turn give rise to γ (gamma) rays, which are similar to X-rays.

The α-rays are relatively few in number and have a poor power of penetration. The β-rays are emitted in large numbers and are mixed from the point of view of their powers of penetration, some being nearly as weak as the α-rays, and others being able to penetrate one millimeter of lead. The β-rays seem to play the principal part in medical treatment, because of their direct action and also because of their production of secondary X-rays. Each time a γ-ray passes through a substance, the emission of a β-ray has been produced. A theory based on this fact is that the γ-rays have an effect on the tisues of the body chiefly by the secondary production of β-rays which transmit heat and negative electricity. The γ-rays are much fewer and have a very great power of penetration (up to 10 centimeters of lead). (*See also* RADIOTHERAPY; X-RAYS.)

RADIUS. The radius is one of the two bones of the forearm. The radius is slender at the top, and has a shallow, cup-like end which moves freely over a rounded surface on the lower end of the humerus, the bone which joins the elbow with the shoulder.

The radius is much bigger at the lower end, and joins with the two bones of the wrist. If we rest the forearm flat on the table, with the palm of the hand upper most, this is called "supination;" the radius and the other bone of the forearm, the ulna, are now parallel with each other. If we now turn the hand round till its back is uppermost ("pronation") the ulna does not change its position, but the lower end of the radius has turned round this bone, crossing it, and carrying the hand with it. Thus the upper slender end of the radius rotates on a pivot formed by the rounded portion of the lower end of the humerus, and is held in this position by means of a circular ligament, while its lower end revolves round the ulna. This ability to pronate and supinate is one of the reasons for man's supremacy over the lower animals.

The most powerful muscle of the arm, the *biceps,* is inserted into the radius, and when this muscle is contracted with the elbow flexed, it causes supination.

Fractures of the Radius. One of the commonest fractures through the lower end of the radius is known as a *colles' fracture.* It occurs through falling on the palm of the hand with the arm stretched out. The deformity caused by the fracture is often referred to as a "dinner-fork" deformity; the hand is drawn towards the thumb side, and there is a swelling on the back of the wrist and another on the front, below which there is a noticeable depression. In a young person the growing end or epiphysis may be separated by a fall of this type and give the typical appearance of a Colles' fracture.

The anatomical position of the arm is assumed to be with the arm hanging down by the side and the palm facing forwards, so that the radius is on the outer side. All descriptions are made on the assumption that the arm is in this attitude. In this way the adjective "radial" means anything on the outer or "radial" side of the arm. The radial artery is the outer of the two branches into which the main artery of the arm (the brachial) divides. At the wrist it lies just under the skin and to the radial side or outer side of the outer of the two prominent tendons of the front surface of the wrist. It is here that the pulse can easily be felt. The name of the radial nerve used to be applied only to the nerve supplying the skin on the radial side of the back of the hand, but it is now applied as well to the whole of the musculospiral nerve. (*See also* ARM; COLLES' FRACTURE; FOREARM.)

RAMUS. This is a branch, especially of a vein, artery or nerve. It is a term also applied to a piece of bone which projects like a twig or branch from a larger piece, as for instance a part of the lower jaw.

RANULA. A cystic swelling under the the tongue. It is generally due to the blocking of one of the ducts of the sublingual salivary glands. The obstruction is usually due to a stone or calculus. It grows slowly without giving any signs of its presence at first, till it becomes awkward on account of its size and interference with speech or swallowing. The tongue may be bitten during mastication. The swelling disappears if the wall is punctured and the contents are allowed to escape. The treatment is by removal of the cyst, walls and all, otherwise it is liable to recur. (*See also* CALCULUS; SALIVARY GLANDS.)

RAYNAUD'S DISEASE. The disorder described by the famous French physician, Raynaud, is characterized by disturbance of the circulation in various parts, especially the fingers. There is apparently no organic disease of the arteries, and the interference with the blood supply is due to temporary spasm of the blood vessels. The condition is comparatively rare. It is more common in damp and in cold weather, and is practically unknown in warm climates. There is a widespread spasm of the arteries and smaller blood vessels so that not a drop of blood enters the part affected. Sometime later the blood vessels open out widely and the dead white fingers become bright pink. There is often a stage in which the part is blue for a time between the white and the pink stages.

Curiously enough, in frostbite the order of events is reversed. In frost-bite the part becomes pink, then blue, and finally white; whereas in Raynaud's disease the part becomes white, blue, and then pink. In moderate grades of the blue stage some little blood trickles through the sluice gates; but in the deep purple skin of a typical example the circulation has ceased entirely.

Treatment. The tendency of this should be countered, if possible, by warm clothing in the winter. The gloves, shoes, etc., must be sufficiently loose not to cause any constriction of the circulation. A tight glove will often cause a very cold feeling, which it is worn to prevent. The mild attacks require no treatment. In the more severe forms the parts affected should be wrapped in absorbent cotton and kept at rest. The use of calcium lactate, nitroglycerine, etc., proves helpful in some cases. Galvanism and ultraviolet light are additional forms of treatment. If gangrene occurs, the parts affected must be kept covered with antiseptic dressings.

An elastic bandage, or better, a pneumatic tourniquet, should be applied to the part sufficiently tightly to shut off the blood supply for a few minutes. On releasing the constriction the arm or leg flushes brightly, owing to relaxation of the blood vessels. This may have to be repeated several times in cases of severe spasm. Section of the sympathetic nerves around the main blood vessels to the limb affected is now being done, with successful results in many cases. (*See also* CHILBLAIN; SYMPATHECTOMY.)

REACTION. This term is used in medicine in many different senses. A chemical reaction is a process in which original chemical substances are changed into others. Chemical reactions are always going on in the body and are very complicated in character.

Reaction also applies to the response

of some tissue to a stimulus. For instance, a bright light shining into the eye will make the pupil contract. There is always a definite period of time between the application of the stimulus and the response; this is known as the reaction time. The quality of the mental powers of attention and decision may be tested by directing a person to do something on being given a certain signal, his powers being judged according to the length of his "reaction time."

Reaction is also used to denote an opposite and contrary state: for instance a person who is at first unduly excited and elated and then becomes depressed is said to suffer from reaction.

The reaction of degeneration is one shown by muscles cut off from connection with the nerve centers when stimulated by an electric or other source of energy. (*See also* ELECTRICITY, MEDICAL.)

RECTAL FEEDING. A certain amount of fluid is absorbed from the large bowel under normal conditions, and it is this process which renders the motions, or stools, more solid than they are at the end of the small intestine (*see* DIGESTION). There is also a certain amount of muscular contraction which pushes the contents backwards (antiperistalsis). Solutions of glucose are partially absorbed into the blood-stream. Milk which has been peptonized or digested for 24 hours is absorbed to some extent from the larger bowel; if peptonized for a shorter time it is quite useless. The fluid must be at body temperature when it is introduced into the bowel, and should be about 100 deg. F. in the vessel containing it. It is best given by means of the tube-and-funnel method. The rubber tube is most satisfactory when shaped at the end like a catheter, e.g. has a blind end and an opening at the side near the end.

RECTIFIED SPIRIT (Spiritus Vini Rectificatus). This preparation, consists of 90 per cent, by volume, of alcohol. The spirit is a very powerful solvent for drugs and is used to make tinctures and other medical preparations. Owing to the tax on alcohol, however, it is expensive and substitutes are used wherever possible. For instance, methylated spirit is used for lotions and liniments which are applied externally only.

RECTOCELE. This term describes a weakness of the wall of the rectum which shows itself as a protusion, in a woman, of the front wall of the rectum through the back wall of the vagina which lies immediately in front. It is most liable to occur after the birth of a child when the structure between the back portion of the vagina and the anal orifice, known as the perineum, is damaged, and no longer offers a support to the walls of the rectum. It rarely occurs by itself but is usually associated with a general looseness of all the structures, and if of a mild degree can be treated with a support, such as a pessary; but if severe a repair operation is indicated.

RECTUM. This is the end part of the bowel, extending from an S-shaped bend, known as the sigmoid flexure, down to the anus, where it opens to the exterior. It is over six inches in length. It lies in the cavity of the lower portion of the backbone, the sacrum and coccyx. Just before reaching the exterior the walls are more distended and the cavity is known as the ampulla. This can vary greatly in size and is able to contain large quantities of fecal material. The anal portion is surrounded by two sets of muscle; the inner one is a thickening of the bowel and is under involuntary control. It is known as the internal sphincter. Outside this is a voluntary muscle under the direct control of the conscious mind and it is known as the external sphincter.

There is a network of blood vessels in the lower portion of the rectum. Some of the blood from the veins forming this plexus goes direct to the heart, and the rest to the liver. Any congestion of the liver is thus likely to lead to a swelling of these veins and hence to the formation of piles. It is the entrance of feces or stools into the rectum which gives rise to the desire to evacuate them. A reflex action tends to relax the internal sphincter, but sensory impulses also pass to the cerebrum (the conscious portion of the mind) and this enables one to control the external sphincter, and overcome the natural desire to go to stool when circumstances are not suitable.

Diseases of the Rectum. Foreign bodies include solid accumulations of fecal matter. This occurs usually in old men, paralytics, and the insane. Sometimes there is a core consisting of a stone, fruit stone, or intestinal worm. These foreign bodies produce a sensation of discomfort and heaviness, colic, and pains in the loins and legs. There is also a constant and frequent desire to go to stool usually without any result except a few drops of mucus due to the straining. The treatment is to give a rectal douche to soften the mass and then a suitable aperient. If there is complete paralysis of the muscle of the bowel it may be necessary to remove the foreign body with a curette.

Cancer of the Rectum. This is not common before the age of 50. At first there are very few signs. Thin streaks of blood may be noticed. If the growth is fairly high up the rectum any hemorrhage may show itself by the passing of tarry stools, as the red coloring matter of the blood has become altered during its passage to the exterior. There may be pain and difficulty in passing the motions, alternating diarrhea and constipation. The motions are sometimes narrow or ribbon-like in character if the growth is circular in the wall of the bowel and narrows the passage markedly. Straining may produce the passage of mucus; and the growth will interfere with the return flow of blood in the veins and give rise to piles. General symptoms are anemia and wasting. The growth may ulcerate into the neighboring structures, such as the bladder or vagina. The condition lasts from one to two years and causes death by progressive poisoning, uremia, or other diseases.

Treatment. The only treatment which offers any hope is complete surgical removal. The result of this depends on the stage at which the operation is carried out. If too far advanced for surgical removal, radium and X-rays are useful in relieving symptoms.

A polyp. This is a simple, nonmalignant growth which grows from the wall of the rectum and is attached to it by means of a stalk or pedicle. It is more common in children and grows very slowly. Its presence is indicated by the passage of blood from the rectum, straining at stool without effect, and the presence of a tumor inside. This simple growth is readily removed by the simple operation of burning or cutting though the stalk.

Rectal prolapse. This is a term used to describe the passage through the anus of some portion of the wall of the intestine. It is common in infants when the external muscles are weak. It is aggravated by diarrhea. In old people, piles and polypi cause much straining and chronic diarrhea, which eventually weakens the muscles at the opening of the rectum.

When rectal prolapse is marked there is a long rounded tumor which is red and moist. In the child, attention to the consistency of the motions and injection of the bowel with astringent lotions will usually result in a cure. It may be necessary in the case of elderly persons, if the condition is at all severe, to cut out the loose mucous membrane. In certain cases the wearing of an apparatus to retain the rectal walls will be necessary.

Inflammation of the rectum. This is known medically as *proctitis,* and usually follows inflammation of the large intestine. If it is due to local trouble, the cause is usually inflamed piles, venereal infections, eczema, foreign bodies, immoral practices, drastic purgatives, etc. There is much pain and straining. The condition may heal or become chronic. Abscess formation, ulceration, the development of a fistula and stricture are all possible complications.

Stricture of the rectum. This may result, apart from a new growth, from any previous inflammation. The symptoms are those of chronic obstruction. The original cause of the condition must be treated and dilation of the stricture by the passage of instruments, or even a cutting operation, will be needed. (*See also* COLITIS; INTESTINE.)

REDNESS OF THE SKIN. This is due to the small blood vessels or capillaries in the skin becoming filled with blood. (*See also* BLUSHING; DERMATITIS; ERYTHEMA; RASH.)

REDUCTION. This means to put a thing back into its proper place. In surgery, the replacement of a broken or dislocated bone into its correct position is known as reduction. Emptying the contents of a hernial sac or rupture is another form of reduction. It is also a term applied to chemical changes. (*See also* DISLOCATION; FRACTURE; HERNIA.)

REFLEX ACTION. An unconscious act which is controlled by the spinal cord without the intervention of the will. When the skin of the soles of the feet is tickled the feet are drawn away. In a frog, for instance, this will take place even when the *cerebrum* is completely destroyed. The stimulus passes to the spinal cord (afferent impulses) and these cause further stimuli (efferent impulses) to pass the muscles of the leg and so draw it away.

A more delicate reflex of the soles of the feet is obtained by stroking the outer side of the sole, when the big toe, and the others as well, will become flexed so that the sole of the foot becomes more concave. In some diseases of the nervous system such tickling will result in extension of the toes instead of flexion.

A reflex action of a mucous membrane is well illustrated by the effect produced by tickling the back of the throat with a feather, when retching or even vomiting will occur.

The knee-jerk is an example of a deep reflex or tendon reflex as opposed to a superficial reflex, which is caused by irritation of the skin. It is obtained by making the patient sit on a chair and crossing one leg over the other. The one which is crossed should be hanging loosely, and the tendon should be tapped smartly just below the kneecap. In a normal individual the leg below the knee will jump forward due to the contraction of the muscle which ends in the tendon tapped—the quadriceps extensor. This jerk is exaggerated if the path from the brain to the spinal cord is damaged, thus cutting off control by the will. It is absent entirely if there is any disease of the reflex path, as occurs in tabes, etc. (*See also* KNEE-JERKS.)

REGENERATION. This describes the restoration of diseased or injured tissues to their original state. When damage to a tissue is so marked as to cause definite destruction, regeneration is rare. Repair then takes place by the formation of scar or fibrous tissue. A nerve can, in favorable circumstances, regenerate by means of a fresh growth from the healthy end, but it may be as long as six to nine months before the new portion works normally.

RELAPSE. The recurrence of a disease after convalescence has apparently begun is described as a relapse. As a rule the symptoms of the relapse are like those of the original attack, but milder in character.

RELAPSING FEVER. This is an infectious illness due to a germ of the spirochaetal type.

RELAXED THROAT. This term is often used to indicate a chronic inflammation of the throat, or chronic pharyngitis. This state of affairs is often due to external causes, such as excessive smoking, eating or drinking food which is too hot, or the irritation caused by chronic nasal catarrh. These causes should be remedied, and locally Mandl's solution (which contains iodine) or astringent gargles can be used. Tonics are useful, and a few days' vacation at the seashore will often effect a cure. (*See also* PHARYNGITIS; TONSILLITIS.)

REMITTENT. When the temperature fluctuates considerably, but does not drop down to normal limits, the fever is said to be of the "remittent type." One form of malaria is often referred to as *remittent fever*.

RENAL. This means something belonging to the kidney. Renal function means the duties of the kidney; renal calculus, a stone in the kidney, etc. The paroxysm of pain caused by the passage of a stone down from the kidney to the bladder along the ureter is known as renal colic. Renal insufficiency means that the kidney is not doing its work properly. (*See also* KIDNEY.)

RENNET. There is a substance present in the normal digestive juice found in the stomach which has the property of clotting milk. It is known as rennin. It can be obtained from the stomach of the calf and is sold commercially under the name of rennet and is used in the making of junket.

These enzymes or ferments are most active at body temperatures, 37 deg. C. or 98.6 deg. F., and are destroyed by boiling. It is common knowledge that the preparation of rennet is not effective if the milk is allowed to boil. (*See also* FERMENTS.)

REPRODUCTIVE SYSTEM. In the

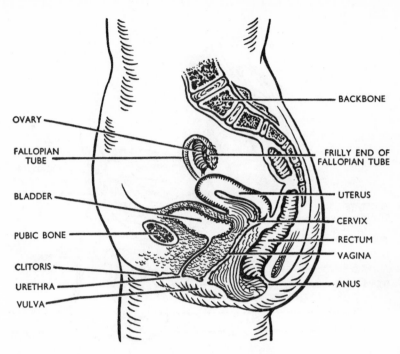

OVARY

FALLOPIAN
TUBE

BLADDER

PUBIC BONE

CLITORIS

URETHRA

VULVA

BACKBONE

FRILLY END OF
FALLOPIAN TUBE

UTERUS

CERVIX

RECTUM

VAGINA

ANUS

Female Reproductive System.

male the reproductive system consists of the testicles, which secrete the seminal fluid containing spermatozoa, the vas deferens or duct of the testicle, the seminal vesicles, in which the fluid is stored, the prostate gland, the urethra, and the penis. In the *female* the reproductive system consists of the ovaries, which give rise to the ova, the Fallopian tubes, which convey them to the womb, the womb or uterus, the vagina or passage up to the womb, and the genitals.

RESPIRATION. Respiration is the act of breathing by which the living animal, human and otherwise, exchanges the gases which it manufactures in itself for the gases in the air in which it lives. This exchange of gases is absolutely necessary for the maintenance of life, since the gases breathed out carry poisonous waste materials and the gases breathed in bring oxygen, which is food for the tissues of the body. In cases in which breathing has suddenly stopped as a result of an accident, such as drowning, efforts are made by *artificial respiration* to continue the action

of breathing until the lungs can take it up again of their own accord. This treatment very often saves the person's life. In certain very severe illnesses, such as pneumonia, where the patient is suffering because not enough oxygen can be taken in by breathing to keep him going, it is possible to give him additional oxygen to breathe by means of a cylinder of the pure gas.

Respiratory System. The respiratory system includes the larynx, the trachea, the two main bronchi and the two lungs; all of these are described elsewhere under their own headings. The nose (and in some cases the mouth) are the entrances by which air gains access to the body, but they can be dispensed with as far as the actual act of breathing is concerned unless they are impassably blocked up so that air cannot pass through. The larynx, or voice box, is the upper part of the respiratory tract. Its position in the front of the neck is recognizable by the jutting-out junction of two of the plates of cartilage which form the larynx, and which is popularly known as the *Adam's apple.* Its medical

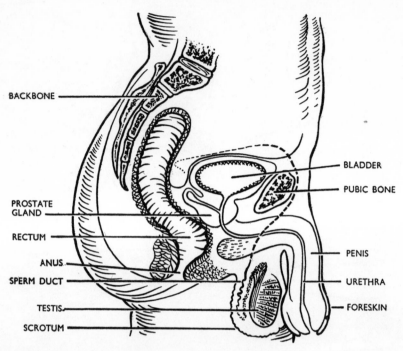

BACKBONE

BLADDER

PUBIC BONE

PROSTATE
GLAND

RECTUM

PENIS

ANUS

SPERM DUCT

URETHRA

TESTIS

FORESKIN

SCROTUM

Male Reproductive System.

name is the thyroid cartilage. Below the larynx comes the long passage of the *trachea,* or windpipe, which carries the air to and from the left and right *bronchi.* Immediately below the larynx the trachea is crossed by the narrow part of the thyroid gland joining its two lobes, which lie one on each side of the neck.

Below these the trachea enters the chest and divides into two branches, one going to the left lung and one to the right. These two branches are called the *bronchi* or bronchial tubes; these lead to the *lungs* and divide and subdivide into smaller and smaller tubes. The lungs are two in number, and fill the chest on each side of the breastbone below the shoulder. They act as the filters and machinery by which the oxygen is withdrawn from the air and passed into the bloodstream, and the impurities and waste materials which are to be discarded from the blood by way of the lungs are given off. The process by which this is accomplished is a very complicated one and is described in the articles

on the Bronchi and Circulation of the Blood.

Act of breathing. Respiration really consists of two separate actions, inspiration and expiration. *Inspiration* is brought about by the contraction of the muscles of the chest and the diaphragm. The chest muscles expand the ribs and the diaphragm presses down the organs in the abdomen; this results in a negative pressure or "pull" inside the lungs, which is relieved by air passing through the respiratory passages of the nose and throat. The lungs are lined by a membrane called the *pleura* between them and the chest wall, and the inner surfaces of the pleura are lubricated by a serous fluid which allows respiration to take place without undue friction.

Expiration takes place when the muscles relax and allow the ribs to contract by reason of their own elasticity. The abdominal organs then push the diaphragm up again to the chest, and air is driven out of the lungs until the pressure in the lungs is the same as in the surrounding atmosphere.

Then the process of inspiration begins again and is automatically followed by expiration. (*See also* ARTIFICIAL RESPIRATION.)

RESTLESSNESS. Restlessness may be described as an output of energy which fulfils no purpose, and is not under the control of the will. The causes of restlessness may be either bodily or mental. In most people any grave illness, like pneumonia, is accompanied by great restlessness. It is one of the chief features, therefore, in confusional insanity and acute mania. In children in whom the nervous system has not yet been brought under such control as it has in adults, slight digestive upsets, intestinal worms, or adenoids will produce a picture of a restless child who is always "on the go." Worry about schoolwork and overtiredness after strenuous games are also very common mental causes of such restlessness in children. When the cause is an obvious one care should be taken that the last hour of the waking day is spent pleasantly and not in doing homework. Exhausting games should be prohibited just before bedtime and a fairly substantial, but easily digested, meal should be given within a couple of hours of bedtime. If the cause of restlessness cannot easily be detected, such bodily ailments as worms, enlarged tonsils and adenoids, or a mild form of St. Vitus's dance must be considered. These, of course, need expert treatment.

RETINA. The innermost coat of the eyeball, which is sensitive to light, is called the retina. If the retina becomes inflamed the condition is called *retinitis*. (*See also* EYE.)

RHESUS FACTOR. For many years the cause of certain blood diseases occurring in newborn infants had evaded explanation in spite of much careful investigation. This state of affairs was brought to an end in 1940 when Landsteiner and Wiener discovered that the serum of rabbits which had previously been injected with the red cells of a rhesus monkey would bring about the clumping and solution of 85 per cent of human red blood cells. They referred to this group as Rh positive and to the remaining 15 per cent with no clumping as Rh negative. The importance of this discovery became

apparent when it was found that "hemolytic disease of the newborn" occurred only in the Rh positive babies of Rh negative mothers. This took place because the mother developed antibodies in her serum which would cross the barrier of the placenta and dissolve the red blood cells of her infant.

It was not long before some practical application was found for these purely theoretical discoveries. It became the practice to blood test mothers attending antenatal clinics to determine their Rh group. Only Rh negative mothers were liable to give birth to infants with this disease, and then only if the father was Rh positive, since it was found that the inheritance of these blood groups followed strict mendelian laws. Further, many Rh positive fathers transmitted to their offspring Rh negative and Rh positive genes in roughly equal proportions. Thus it became important often to determine the father's group in order to estimate the risk of an affected infant. It was also found by serial blood testing throughout pregnancy that the development of antibodies in the mother could be traced, so that the patient could be brought into labor at the time best calculated to give a live baby.

Since the discovery of the mechanism of hemolytic disease it has been the practice to tranfuse severely affected infants with Rh negative blood soon after birth. More recently the practice of "exchange transfusion" has been widely adopted. In this method the infant's blood is withdrawn while fresh Rh negative blood is transferred at the same time, and it seems probable that it will be followed by a fall in the mortality of hemolytic disease.

RHEUMATIC FEVER. *See* RHEUMATISM, ACUTE.

RHEUMATISM. This is an ill-defined term used popularly to describe various painful affections of muscles and points. There are several clear-cut forms of disease for which the use of the term should be reserved. Acute rheumatism is more often known as rheumatic fever. Chronic rheumatism is commonly called rheumatism. Muscular rheumatism or myalgia and rheumatoid arthritis are other forms.

Rheumatism, Acute. Acute rheumatism,

commonly called rheumatic fever, is a severe illness accompanied by fever which may have serious complications and should be treated with great care. It used to be supposed that it was caused by exposure to cold and damp, but during the war, when many people endured great hardships from cold and damp, rheumatic fever was not as prevalent as it might have been supposed. It is now believed that the disease is due to a widespread sensitivity to the toxins or harmful products of a germ known as the streptococcus.

Symptoms. A child may slip into an attack of rheumatic fever gradually without the beginnings of the attack being noticed. The child may be out of sorts, complaining of pains in the limbs, and if the temperature is taken it will be found to be slightly raised. "Growing pains" are now generally supposed to be rheumatic in origin and should be taken as a warning. One day the child will become acutely ill, with a temperature of 100 deg. F. or over, and there is acute pain and swelling in a joint, or several joints. Sometimes as one joint subsides another may swell. In most cases there is a good deal of sweating and the sweat has a characteristic sour smell. There may be sore throat. Sometimes rheumatic nodules or little lumps are found under the skin in such places as the back of the hands, chest, over the knees, at the elbows and so on. These nodules or swellings may come and go quite quickly. The temperature, with proper treatment, will usually return to normal in about a week or ten days, and the pain will fade out of the joints, although it may go from joint to joint for some time.

Treatment. Rheumatic children should have their throats and teeth well cared for and any unhealthy teeth or tonsils should be removed as they render the child more liable to an attack of rheumatic fever. Children subject to relapses of rheumatic fever can be protected by a small daily dose of one of the sulphonamide drugs.

When the attack occurs it is of the greatest importance to put the child to bed and keep it there, not allowing it to get up at all, or even to have more than one pillow. The bedpan should be brought to it. A doctor will be necessary, as the child is in danger if rheumatic fever is neglected. The salicylate drugs are of the greatest use in the treatment of all forms of rheumatism. The affected joints should be kept wrapped up in cotton-wool. A long convalescence will be required, which since it must take the form of almost complete rest, is easier to obtain at a convalescent home. The danger in all cases of rheumatic fever is that the heart will be damaged in some degree unless the greatest care is taken and there is very prolonged rest.

RHEUMATOID ARTHRITIS. This is a general progressive disease chiefly affecting the joints, which become swollen and painful. If untreated, the joints eventually become badly deformed. It occurs in two quite different forms. It attacks women more often than men and usually begins between the ages of 20 and 40. The one form is particularly common in women during the childbearing period of life and the cause of the condition is quite unknown, although measures which are effective in other forms of arthritis sometimes relieve, though they seldom cure, this particular one. Because the cause of this form of rheumatoid arthritis is unknown, it is called "primary" rheumatoid arthritis, to distinguish it from the other form, which occurs with equal frequency in men and women; the other form is due to long-continued infection, and is therefore called "secondary" rheumatoid arthritis.

"Primary" rheumatoid arthritis. There may be attacks of cramp or weakness in the muscles of the hand, or the hands may become unnaturally cold in mild weather. Sometimes the onset may be acute, with a rise of temperature, accompanied by a swelling of the joints of the fingers. It is characteristic that the muscles and joints of the fingers are first and most severely affected. Both sides are attacked and gradually the disease spreads to other joints, so that they become stiff and swollen. Wasting of the muscles is very marked, and in advanced stages the joints become deformed. In association with the changes in the joints, the patient's general health declines, and such symptoms as anemia, palpitation of the heart with a quick

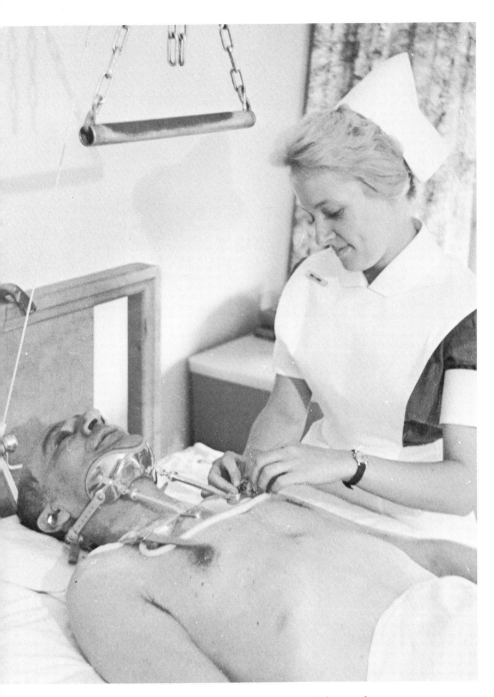

Neck traction provides necessary support during early re-
cuperation from a dangerous injury.

The results of daily medical checkups during hospitalization assure a more complete recovery.

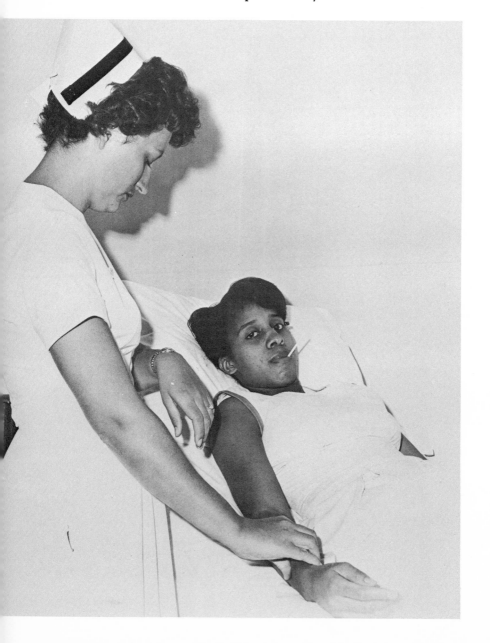

pulse, sweating, and extreme coldness of the hands and feet may arise. It was thought at one time that infection from such places as the teeth, tonsils, or air-sinuses of the nose was responsible for this form of arthritis, but in a very large number of cases no such infection could be found. If in any particular case, of course, such infection is present, it must be dealt with.

Treatment. When cortisone was isolated by Kendall in 1935 and introduced by Hench and his colleagues at the Mayo Clinic in 1949 for the treatment of rheumatoid arthritis it was hailed as a miracle-working drug. But it was soon found to have undesirable side-effects, such as hypertension, obesity, mental depression, bleeding gastric ulcers, and the activation of quiescent tuberculosis.

Controlled trials revealed that over two or three years cortisone was no more effective than aspirin, and its use in rheumatoid arthritis is no longer recommended. Its place has been taken by synthetic (laboratory-produced) steroids, especially prednisone and prednisolone.

"Secondary" or Infective Rheumatoid Arthritis. This may come on acutely, with a high temperature, when it may be mistaken for rheumatic fever, or it may arise rapidly with no signs of fever. The disease attacks both large and small joints, the fingers, wrists, elbows, toes, ankles, and knees being commonly attacked on both sides of the body. The usual signs of inflammation of a joint are present: the affected joints are swollen, "doughy" to the touch, tender on pressure, and very painful when moved. The muscles just above and below the affected joints are wasted. Sweating of the hands and feet, a feeble circulation leading to coldness of the limbs, and anemia are common.

Treatment. This is first, removal of the infection when this is traced. Next comes the building up of the general health by means of fresh air, sunshine, and a suitable diet, which need not exclude red meat. Aspirin is the best drug for alleviating painful symptoms; butazolidin relieves pain but has no curative effect. Where many joints are affected, baths of a certain type and of high temperature are often given.

After the swelling of the joints has gone down, movement at the affected joints must be encouraged. (*See also* BATHS; RHEUMATISM, ACUTE.)

RHINITIS. This is the medical name for inflammation of the mucous membrane of the nose such as is found in the common cold. It shows itself as catarrh. (*See also* NASAL CATARRH; NOSE.)

RHONCHI. This is a name used for the harsh wheezing sounds made by a person who is suffering from bronchitis. These sounds are heard through the stethoscope, or by applying the ear closely to the chest.

RHUBARB. The powder obtained from various forms of rhubarb stem or root has long been in use as a digestive agent and a purgative. For use in cases of indigestion it is usually made up with some such substances as bicarbonate of soda, bismuth, cinnamon, etc. Compound Powder of Rhubarb is a favorite way of taking it. It has a stimulating action on the digestive system and increases the flow of bile. As a purgative it is often followed by slight constipation which makes it especially valuable in the treatment of some forms of diarrhea.

RIBS. These are curved bones which enclose the chest cavity and serve to protect the heart and lungs from injury. There are twelve pairs of ribs, of which the upper seven are directly attached to the breast bone (or sternum) in front. Of the remaining lower five pairs of ribs, each of the upper three is attached in front, not to the breast bone, but to the most forward part of the rib above it, the part which is called the costal cartilage, as it is not made of bone, but of a softer material, gristle. The lowermost two ribs are not attached to other ribs in front; their most forward parts lie free, and these last two ribs are therefore called floating ribs. Behind, the ribs are all attached to the spinal column (backbone). They are attached by means of two joints so that they are able to turn on the spine, making a movement rather like that of a handle of a bucket.

Fracture of a rib is a very common accident. "A broken rib" is often taken very lightly, but if the broken piece is forced inwards instead of outwards, as unfortunately so often happens, then the injury may be very serious. A broken rib is more frequently the result of crushing of the chest, as when a vehicle runs over the body, than the result of a blow. The fracture usually occurs at the angle of the rib, and the broken pieces are displaced outwards. There may be little or no discomfort from such an injury except pain on breathing.

Treatment. Where there is outward displacement of the broken ends of the bone, strap the chest with adhesive tape well above and below the broken rib, so that the tape overlaps. As a rule, a broken rib heals very quickly and the victim of such an accident soon forgets his injury. But if the broken ends of the bone are displaced inwards, as sometimes happens when the fracture is the result of a direct blow on the chest, then there is a great danger that, unless carefully watched for, any sudden movement on the part of the patient may drive the broken ends of bone into the lung or into the covering to the lung—the pleura. If this happens, not only will the patient cough up blood from damage to the tissue of the lung, but there is also danger of infection reaching the lung through the skin if this has been torn by the blow causing the fracture. The first-aid treatment of fractures of the ribs is described under the heading of FRAC-TURES.

RICKETS. This is a disease of growing children and infants which occurs between the ninth month and third year. The disease is due to a lack of Vitamin D, either because this is not being supplied in sufficient amount in the diet, or because it is not being manufactured by the child in its body. Vitamin D is present to a large extent in most animal fats. It is abundant in normal human milk, but is most abundant in cod-liver oil.

RIGOR. Rigor describes a sudden severe shivering fit which occurs in certain fevers, particularly in malaria, and may occur at the commencement of an attack of pneumonia or septicemia. The patient first looks blue in the face and has a pinched expression. He then begins to shiver, and the movements are so violent that he may shake the bed and his teeth may chatter. The rigor may last from a few minutes up to an hour or so, after which the patient feels warm again. Although the patient feels cold, yet the temperature is actually above normal. It is essential that during the rigor the patient should be kept warm. This may be accomplished by the use of extra blankets, hot-water bottles, and by giving the patient hot drinks, such as hot lemonade.

RIGOR MORTIS. This is a stiffening of the muscles which occurs after death and is due to chemical changes in the composition of the muscles when blood ceases to flow through them. The degree of rigor mortis varies according to the time a person has been dead, and after allowing for certain errors it is possible for a doctor to estimate to within a few hours how long death has been present.

RINGWORM. Ringworm is a skin disease caused by a fungus. It attacks any part of the skin, and its manifestations vary greatly in different areas.

Ringworm of the scalp. In the adult this is exceedingly rare; most of the cases occurring between 5 and 12. One or more rounded spots, partially bald, are seen, in which the remaining hairs are short, dull, and twisted. The diseased spots are scaly, and often outlined with a reddish ring. The fungus can be seen in the hairs (and skin scrapings) under the microscope.

Ringworm of the beard appears in two forms: (1) As ringworm of the body; (2) resembling barber's itch. The affected parts are swollen, painful, and nodular.

Ringworm of the body. Here the "rings" to which the disease owes its name are chiefly seen. The patches are red and scaly. These cases spread rapidly, especially in the armpits and the groins, where heat and moisture are present. Ringworm of the groins is common in hot countries, where it is called by various names, such as dhobie itch, craw-craw, etc.

Ringworm of the palms, soles, and nails. This is far from uncommon. On the palms are found two forms: (1) The acute, which resembles an acute dermatitis; (2) the chronic, where the palm is dry, scaly, and slightly reddened. So little inconvenience is caused that the patient may go on for years without treatment. The soles may be similarly affected, but in the commonest form the skin between the toes is white and sodden, peels off in large flakes, and leaves an oozing red surface. Cracks at the base of the toes are common, and itching is troublesome. All these cases are very difficult to diagnose unless scrapings from the skin are examined microscopically.

The outlook in ringworm depends on various factors. Ringworm of the nails requires very persevering treatment, and the time taken to cure it on the palms and soles varies with its thoroughness.

Treatment. This is far from easy. It is simple enough to destroy the ringworm fungus itself; the difficulty in practice is to destroy the fungus without affecting the patient.

Ringworm of the scalp is treated by shaving the head, washing daily, and thoroughly rubbing in an antiseptic ointment. Care is taken in using brushes, towels, caps, etc., and the affected child must sleep alone. Other children should always be carefully examined for traces of the disease. X-rays, in expert hands, is one of the best and quickest methods, thousands of cases being treated successfully every year.

Ringworm of the beard is treated by removing the hairs with forceps and thoroughly rubbing in an antiseptic ointment.

Ringworm of the body is easily cured by antiseptic ointment such as Whitfield's ointment or by application of Castellani's paint. If the groins and armpits are affected, soothing remedies, such as zinc oxide paste, are applied as preliminary treatment.

Ringworm of the palms and soles is treated by antiseptics; a good plan is to have a daily 10 minutes' soak with dilute permanganate solution, and then apply antiseptic ointment.

Ringworm of the nails is by far the most obstinate of all forms. If untreated it remains for life. The best method is to apply a solution which softens the nails, such as Fehling's solution, so that they can be removed without pain. Antiseptic treatment is then applied to the nail-bed until no fungus remains.

RODENT ULCER (Latin *rodens,* gnawing). This is a surface cancer of the skin where ulceration is the chief feature.

ROMBERGISM. This is a term applied to the inability to stand without falling

over, when the eyes are shut. It is found as a symptom in some diseases of the nervous system, especially in tabes dorsalis.

RONGTEN RAYS. This is another name for X-rays, from the name of their discoverer.

ROSACEA. Rosacea, sometimes called acne rosacea, is a skin disease which appears only on the face. It starts as a slight flush or congestion of the nose and cheeks, sometimes of the chin and the middle part of the forehead. This redness, which is due to over fullness of the surface blood vessels, is apt to become chronic. Accompanying this, there is often an oily appearance of the skin, with red pimples and spots; the appearance is rather like that in ordinary acne but without blackheads.

Treatment. General health treatment is of special importance in this disease. Particular attention should be paid to regularity of the bowels. Extremes of temperature should be avoided as far as posssible, even to taking warm baths in preference to hot or cold.

As regards local treatment, seborrhea of the scalp, if present, must be treated. It is useless to try to cure rosacea without removing one of its chief causes. Sulphur in some form is applied to the face, either as a lotion or in the form of sulphur soap.

If the skin is very irritable, a calamine lotion should be used for a few days, before beginning the sulphur treatment.

In the more chronic cases the sulphur treatment will not produce much effect; it is then necessary to use something to make the skin peel, such as the resorcin paste method described for acne vulgaris. The soap massage and steaming methods, so useful in acne, are of course quite unsuitable here.

If the blood-vessels are very numerous and much dilated, treatment by light and X-rays is by far the most satisfactory. Very prominent vessels may be destroyed by the galvano-cautery.

ROSEOLA. This is a term applied to any rose-colored rash. (*See also* ERYTHEMA.)

ROUND LIGAMENT. A flat cord-like ligament that attaches the womb to the groin on each side of the body is called the round ligament. (*See also* CORD.)

RUBELLA. This is another name for german measles.

RUPTURE. Rupture, or hernia, usually refers to the protrusion of part of the abdominal contents through the abdominal wall. The weak places where ruptures are liable to occur are at the navel or in its immediate neighborhood (umbilical rupture), or in the groin (inguinal or femoral rupture). The chief surgical authorities assert that a rupture is always due to a congenital weakness in the wall of the abdomen, and that exertion or accident never play a really important part in the production of a rupture.

A hernia will be felt as a bulge in the abdominal wall, which is more noticeable when the patient strains in any way, as in coughing. If the swelling can be pushed back into the abdominal cavity, the hernia is said to be reducible; if the mass will not return, the hernia is irreducible, and if the circulation in the contents of the hernia becomes interfered with, it becomes strangulated. If a strangulated hernia cannot be reduced, immediate operation is necessary in order to prevent that portion of the bowel from becoming dead or gangrenous. The symptoms are acute pain, violent vomiting, and intestinal obstruction.

In children, the commonest form of hernia is the umbilical. A flat disk, or a coin, is strapped over the swelling and kept there night and day, with replacements only for the sake of cleanliness, until the muscles have fully developed and the weak area has disappeared.

Inguinal hernias (ruptures in the groin) are rather more common in boys. The rupture is usually easily reducible by placing the child on his back and pressing gently on the swelling, at the same time supporting the edges of the opening with the other hand. If the protrusion keeps returning, operative treatment must be considered, or a properly fitting truss must be worn all the time. (*See also* ABDOMINAL BELT; HERNIA.)

S ACCHARIN. Saccharin is an intensely sweet crystalline powder derived from toluol (methyl-benzol). It is chiefly employed as a sweetening substance, especially in cases of diabetes and obesity when sugar cannot be taken. (*See also* SUGAR.)

SACRUM. The lower part of the spinal column is composed of five vertebrae which are fused together to form a massive bone known as the sacrum, or sacred bone. This bone lies between the two haunch bones, and it forms the back wall of the pelvis, and in consequence, is slightly wider in women than in men. (*See also* PELVIS.)

ST. VITUS'S DANCE. This is a disease found mainly in children between the the ages of five and fifteen years, and it occurs more often in girls than in boys. Although the disease itself may appear trivial, it is one of the crippling diseases of childhood. St. Vitus's dance, or to give it its medical name, **chorea,** is one of the forms of that scourge of childhood, rheumatism. Every child who has had even a slight attack of chorea is a candidate for rheumatic heart disease unless every precaution is taken against it. For this reason it is of supreme importance that St. Vitus's dance should be recognized in its early stages and treated correctly.

Although the movements are the most striking symptoms of chorea, yet they may be very slight. In a considerable number of cases, the most obvious sign to the parents is a weakness or apparent paralysis of one arm or leg. This may be so pronounced that the child is taken to the doctor as a case of paralysis. The limb is not, however, truly paralyzed; the child is only unwilling to use it because it is difficult to use it properly. The other important symptom of chorea is the mental change. A child with chorea becomes nervous, rather inclined to cry easily, and often silent. Although the victims of chorea are usually the clever, bright children, during the attack they become dull, are unable to give their attention to their lessons, and may suffer from sleeplessness.

Treatment. There are three main lines of treatment in chorea, but only one is of real importance and that is, rest, mental and physical. It will be realized that the main fear in chorea is that the rheumatic agent, whatever it may be, attack the heart. Rest in bed, alone in a room, or at least behind a screen, is the only treatment that matters. The child must be kept in bed until all movements have ceased for at least a week, and until the doctor is satisfied that no further damage can be done to the heart by the attack the child has passed through.

In very severe cases in which the movements are so violent that the child is in danger of hurting itself in an ordinary bed, either a padded bed is required or mattresses can be placed on the floor and protected from drafts by careful screening.

Chorea may show itself in its most severe form either at the beginning of adolescence or during pregnancy. During these times of stress, the movements may be exceedingly violent and the mental changes may be so severe as to lead to the necessity for temporary institutional care. But with the recovery from the attack of chorea, the mind regains its normal state.

SAL AMMONIAC. This is the common name of ammonium chloride.

SALICYLATE. This is a chemical compound called a salt of salicylic acid. The salicylates are much used in all treatment of rheumatism both internally and externally. The one most used as a medicine is sodium salicylate, while methyl salicylate or oil of wintergreen has a great reputation for its effect on rheumatic joints when used as an external application. (*See also* SALT.)

SALICYLIC ACID. This is a colorless crystalline acid which is found naturally in wintergreen and in the sweet birch tree, but it is now more cheaply prepared from carbolic acid, a product of coal tar. Salicylic acid has many uses in medicine. It has the property of reducing fever and is also an antiseptic inhibiting the growth of germs. It is given internally in acute rheumatism and rheumatic fever, and also in sciatica and certain forms of neuralgia. For its antiseptic properties it is used in skin diseases, and because it assists in dissolving off the outermost thickened layers of the skin it forms the chief ingredient in many corn cures. (*See also* RHEUMATISM.)

SALINE. Saline means "salty," and is correctly used when speaking of a solution of common salt. However, such common purgatives as Glauber's salts and Epsom salts are usually described as salines. (*See also* NORMAL SALINE, under NORMAL.)

SALIVA. Saliva or spittle is a somewhat sticky liquid and consists mainly of the secretions of the salivary glands, but may also contain mucus, and cells which are shed by the lining of the mouth. The saliva serves to moisten and soften the food, and by dissolving substances in the mouth it assists the function of taste. It contains a ferment called ptyalin, which alters the indigestible starchy foods so that they are ready to be digested by the ferments in the stomach. Therefore, by bolting a meal the stomach is given more work to do as the first stages in digestion have not been carried out by the saliva.

SALIVARY GLANDS. These are the glands which produce the saliva. There are three pairs of these glands: the parotid, which lies in the cheek, just in front of, and below the ear; the submaxillary, which is placed just below the body of the lower jaw; and the sublingual, which lies in the floor of the mouth, just underneath the front part of the tongue.

All these glands produce saliva which contains the ferment, Ptyalin. Ptyalin changes starch into sugar. The saliva produced by the submaxillary and sublingual glands is thick and sticky, while that from the parotid gland is thin and watery. There are several disorders of the salivary glands, of which the most uncomfortable for the patient is the formation of small stones in the glands. The pain caused by the movement of these stones along the passages or ducts of the glands leading into the mouth is often very distressing, being noticed most particularly when food is taken into the mouth, as the glands then attempt to discharge the saliva along the blocked ducts. Removal of these stones is a simple operation; but they may form again unless the infection of the teeth and gums which is always present is attended to. The parotid gland shares in the general enlargement of the glands due to mumps, and is nearly always the first symptom of that disorder. (*See also* MUMPS; PAROTID GLAND.)

SALPINGITIS. This is an inflammation of the tubes which lead from the ovaries to the womb (fallopian tubes). It occurs after infection of the womb in childbirth or after an abortion, and is also one of the chief complications of gonorrhea in women. (For the symptoms of the condition *see also* PERIMETRITIS; GENITAL SYSTEM; GONORRHEA.)

SALT. In chemistry this means a combination of an acid with a base. For example, Epsom salt (magnesium sulphate) is a combination of the metal magnesium with sulphuric acid. But, in everyday life, the term "salt" is applied to that combination of sodium and hydrochloric acid which is chemically called sodium chloride.

SALTS. In popular language these denote saline purgatives. They include Glauber's salt, which is sodium sulphate; Epsom salt, which is magnesium sulphate; Rochelle salt, which is potassium and sodium tartrate; "fruit salts," and others. Salts should be taken on an empty stomach, first thing in the morning, and are especially valuable for biliousness.

SALVARSAN. This drug, which was also known as "606," arsenobillon, arsphenamine, arsenobenzol, was a valuable one used in the treatment of syphilis, and in other diseases which are caused by similar coiled germs called spirochaetes.

SAL VOLATILE. This is ammonium carbonate, or aromatic spirit of ammonia, and it is a favorite remedy for faintness. About fifteen drops drunk in half a wineglassful of water usually serves the purpose. (*See also* AMMONIA.)

SAND-FLY FEVER. This fever is a disease of the tropics which is caused by an unknown germ conveyed by the bite of the sand-fly. It occurs in Egypt and India. The fever comes on suddenly, accompanied by headache and severe pain behind the eyes. The temperature usually reaches its highest level by the end of twenty-four hours and then gradually falls to normal by the end of three days. The disease is not fatal, though convalescence may be a long one. Treatment is mainly directed to the relief of headache, in which aspirin and phenacetin are as effective as most drugs.

SANITATION. Sanitation is one of the concerns of those responsible for the maintenance of the public health. It includes any measure taken to safeguard the health of the community, but more especially refers to the methods of disposal of refuse and sewage, the provision of public bathing facilities, the notification of infectious diseases and the proper disinfection of premises, and the inspection of houses and factories where defective drains are suspected. (*See also* DRAINS; HYGIENE.)

SANTONIN. This is a drug which is extracted from the dried flower-heads of the plant artemisia maritima. It is chiefly used in children to cure round-worms. The drug must be given on an empty stomach and a suitable purgative such as calomel must be given at the same time or just after. If too large a dose has been given, the child may complain that it "sees things yellow," as santonin has the property of sometimes producing yellow vision. Large doses produce vomiting and convulsions. (*See also* WORM.)

SARCOMA. This is a type of malignant growth. There are at least two important kinds of cancer. One arises from those tissues of the body which in the developing embryo formed the skin and gut; this kind of cancer is called a carcinoma. The different forms of carcinoma will be found under the heading CARCINOMA. The other important kind of cancer, sarcoma, arises from those tissue which in the embryo formed the connective tissue, that is, the muscles, and the supporting tissues of the body generally, including the bones. The malignancy of the sarcoma is greater as a rule than that of the carcinoma for two reasons; one is that true sarcomas consist of tissue that would be normal only in the developing embryo; they do not occur after embryonic life, while in the carcinoma an adult tissue may merely have "run riot."

The second reason why a sarcoma is so much more malignant than a carcinoma is because a sarcoma spreads through the bloodstream, and so the sarcoma cells may be carried throughout the body, while a carcinoma rarely spreads by this route, but mainly by the lymphatic stream (*see* LYMPHATICS). Both forms of cancer spread by eating into and destroying the healthy tissues around them; but sarcoma thus spreads more quickly than carcinoma because there is no barrier of connective tissue thrown out to resist its invasion.

One special type of sarcoma is called

the melanotic sarcoma; but there is much discussion as to whether this tumor should not be classed with the carcinomas. Its cells contain a dark coloring matter, melanin, which is found in the retina, in colored moles, and in the coloring matter of the deep layers of the skin. This type of sarcoma is a very deadly one. Another, much less malignant one, arises in the cells of the bone marrow and is called a myeloid sarcoma.

Symptoms. A sarcoma may arise in any part of the body and it may spread so rapidly that signs of spread of the growth to other organs may be present before the original growth is recognized. When a sarcoma arises in a place where it can be felt, it usually forms a swelling which is usually painless. It is often very difficult to say whether such a growth is a sarcoma or whether it is a harmless growth, or the result of inflammation. In such a case, removal of a small portion of the growth and examination under the microscope will decide the question. If left untreated, a sarcoma generally comes to the surface and bursts through the skin.

Treatment. If possible, the growth must be removed by operation, and if a limb is affected amputation is usually necessary to save life. When operation proves impossible, either owing to the situation of the growth or to involvement of other parts of the body, treatment by X-rays or radium must be tried. (*See also* CANCER; CARCINOMA.)

SASSAFRAS. This is the dried brown root of a tree which is found in North America. This root has valuable properties: it contains substances which promote sweating, and it is a gentle stimulant to the bowel muscle.

SCAB. A scab is a crust which forms over an ulcer or wound. It is composed mainly of blood clot, clotted lymph, or pus. It is difficult for healing to occur under an infected scab. Scabs may be softened and removed by soaking the part with a hot solution of bicarbonate of soda, or by means of a poultice composed of boracic acid or starch.

SCABIES. Scabies, or the itch, is a disease of the skin due to a tiny animal known as the arcus or sarcoptes scabiei. The female burrows into the skin in order to lay her eggs and this invasion is accompanied by a rash with intense itching. It is treated with sulphur ointment or painting the skin with benzyl benzoate. (*See also* ITCH.)

SCALD. This describes inflammation or damage to tissues by hot liquids or gases. It resembles a burn in every way except in its causation, and the treatment is that of a burn. (*See also* BURN.)

SCALP. The scalp consists of the covering to the top of the skull, or cranium. There are five layers covering the bone, viz. the skin, the fatty layer, a specialized sheet of muscle called an aponeurosis, a loose connective tissue layer, and a thick membrane called the epicranium. Owing to the looseness of the connective tissue layer under the muscle aponeurosis, the scalp can be moved fairly easily by pushing it with the fingers, and some people can move the muscle itself, so that they can move the scalp backwards and forwards at will. The fat underneath the skin of the scalp has a rather curious distribution. It is not packed loosely as in most parts of the body, but is disposed in more or less separate compartments. So that if an abscess or any other inflammation arises in the scalp it does not spread very far because of this curious distribution of the fat, which confines it to a small space. But if a wound is made into the scalp below the muscle aponeurosis, infection can easily travel along the loose connective tissue in this layer. Because of this danger, wounds of the scalp must be kept very clean and it is advisable to shave the scalp all round the wound.

Scales are often shed by the scalp, and these are described as dandruff. Cysts are fairly common on the scalp, caused by obstruction of the ducts of sebaceous glands. These cysts are called wens. (*See also* DANDRUFF; WEN.)

SCAPULA. This is commonly known as the shoulder blade. It is a broad, triangular bone which lies on the upper part of the back of the chest, to which it is firmly attached by strong muscles. If these muscles are paralyzed that part of the scapula facing the spine will be so turned that its edge can be seen when the arm is pushed forwards. This condition is called winged scapula. As the bone is triangular, it has three angles.

On the back of the scapula there is a

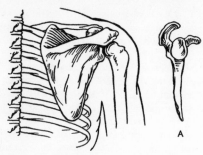

Scapula, viewed from behind: A. *Showing glenoid fossa at upper end, where the humerus articulates.*

thickening of bone called the spine of the scapula, which runs in an upward and outward direction. The hollow in which the ball-shaped head of the humerus fits is known as the glenoid fossa. Injuries of the scapula are not very common as it is well protected by muscles. Occasionally the coracoid process and the acromion may be broken off as a result of injury to the shoulder joint.

SCAPHOID. The scaphoid bone is one of the small bones of the wrist. It lies on the thumb side of the joint and is frequently broken in adults by falls on the outstretched hand. Pain is felt at the root of the thumb, but otherwise it may cause no signs and is often mistaken for a simple sprain. An X-ray is necessary to establish the diagnosis.

SCAR. A scar is the natural result of healing of tissue which has been damaged or destroyed by injury or disease. The space left by loss of tissue is gradually filled up and bridged by a mass of cells, some of which are newly formed in the tissues themselves, and others which have come from the blood vessels in the neighborhood of the damaged tissues. This mass of newly formed cells is called granulation tissue. At first, many blood vessels are formed in this granulation tissue; but later, as the granulation tissue becomes converted into ordinary connective or fibrous tissue, these blood vessels are squeezed out of existence, having served their purpose. So a recent scar is bright pink in color, while an old scar is white. Overgrowth of a scar is referred to as a keloid. (*See also* GRANULATION TISSUE; KELOID.)

SCARLET FEVER. This is an acute infectious disease caused by a certain variety of the germ known as the streptococcus, which enters the body through the nose and throat, and first produces its effects in a localized sore throat. Afterwards constitutional symptoms and a characteristic rash appear, the results of spread of the poisons produced by the germ in the throat and nose.

Scarlet fever is a disease of childhood, especially of the ages between five and ten years. But it is much more fatal in children up to the age of three years than in older children. The onset of the illness is usually abrupt: the incubation period is commonly two to three days, but may be anything from one to seven days. Sore throat, vomiting, headache, shivering fits, a rise of temperature up to 102 deg. to 103 deg. F. and a quick pulse are the usual symptoms. The throat and tonsils appear intensely red. The tongue is furred at the onset of the illness, and often has the appearance which gives rise to the term "white strawberry tongue." The surface is covered with a creamy white fur through which bright red spots project. Later, the fur strips off from the edges inwards, leaving a perfectly clean, bright red tongue, to which the name of "red strawberry tongue" has been applied.

On the second day the rash appears. This is seen first on the neck, then it spreads gradually over the body and limbs, but rarely appears on the face. The forehead and cheeks are flushed, and there is a pale area round the mouth which forms a striking contrast. The rash is composed of tiny red spots, each being surrounded by a paler pink area. These spots are so closely packed together as to give the appearance of intense redness to the skin. The rash fades in the same order in which it appeared, and this is followed by peeling of the skin. Peeling goes on for at least two to three weeks, and the skin peels off in fine flakes.

Even in a case of simple scarlet fever, without any complications, there is often some enlargement of the glands of the neck, but in the more severe type of the disease, this enlargement is marked, there is discharge of pus from the nose, sometimes sinusitis, sometimes acute ear inflammation. Scarlet fever must always be taken seriously because of its possible complications, and a rare case may still prove severe. (*See also* SEPTICEMIA.)

Complications of Scarlet Fever. The most common of all the complications is middle ear disease. Young children, especially those with enlarged adenoids and tonsils, are most liable to this complication. Rupture of the drum of the ear and the discharge of pus—which may continue for months or even years—is the usual sequel, unless the condition is recognized and suitable treatment given. Infection may travel backward from the middle ear and cause disease of the mastoid air cells, in which case an operation on the mastoid (simple mastoid operation) may be necessary, though this is seldom performed nowadays, with adequate dosage of penicillin.

Another serious complication of scarlet fever which occurs in the second or third week of the illness is inflammation of the kidneys. The amount of urine passed is greatly diminished and contains albumen and blood. Swelling of the feet, legs, and face occurs. This condition may become chronic and leave the victim with permanently damaged kidneys. In order to recognize the complication at the earliest possible moment, the urine should be examined at frequent intervals.

Inflammation may occur in the joints, the picture then resembling that of acute rheumatism, and sometimes the heart may be involved also.

Treatment of Scarlet Fever. Until quite recently the treatment of scarlet fever was simply that of an infectious disease, and of the condition of fever; but, since the discovery that the germ causing the disease is a variety of streptococcus, the antibiotic drugs which have a specific curative effect in streptococcal infections have been used in its treatment, in adequate doses, or synthetic penicillin can be given orally. The effects are commonly produced within twelve hours; the temperature and pulse rate fall, the general symptoms of germ poisoning are lessened or may even disappear, and the rash fades. There is ample evidence that the employment of antibiotics in full doses considerably reduces the liability to complications and shortens convalescence.

It is very important to prevent the spread of the germs causing the disease. Close contact with a person suffering from it is usually the way it is conveyed, but clothes from the patient, or things handled by the patient may also spread infection. Epidemics have been known to have been caused by infected milk. Patients who are convalescent may yet carry the germs of the disease in their throats and so infect others. That is why isolation of patients is insisted upon for at least four weeks. As long as there is any discharge from the nose, the patient can infect others by "droplet" infection. It is now recognized that the ordinary severe infectious sore throat occurring in an adult is caused by the same germ as that causing scarlet fever, and is liable to be followed by the same complications. When occurring in a household it should be treated as potentially dangerous and steps taken to prevent its spread, especially to children.

SCHICK REACTION. This reaction is a test which shows whether a person is liable to develop diphtheria or whether he has sufficient natural resistance to withstand the infection. The method was devised in 1913 by B. Schick, an Austrian physician.

In this test some of the poison obtained from the diphtheria germ is injected between the layers of the skin (intradermal). The poison is specially weakened so that it is harmless.

Some diphtheria toxin which has been heated to 75 deg. C. for 10 minutes is also required. With a suitable syringe the toxin is injected; this forms a small swelling or weal in the skin which lasts for a few minutes to half an hour. An equal amount of the heated toxin is injected in a similar manner into the opposite arm.

The resulting reactions are noted after 24, 72 hours, and ten days.

Positive Reaction. After 24–36 hours a dark raised swelling, about ½ to 1 inch in diameter, round or oval in shape, is seen at the place where the toxin was injected. The swelling reaches its maximum about the third day and then gradually fades away during the course of a week. The skin becomes dark and later will flake off up till the tenth day. This is a positive reaction and the person is liable to contract the disease. The other arm is used as a control in which the toxin which was inactivated by heat shows no reaction.

Immunization. This can be "passive" or "active." Passive immunization means that some ready-made antibody is injected into the body and will protect it from the diphtheria poison for a short time. Active immunization means that the body is made to manufacture its own antibody for any future occasion and will always be there to deal with a dose of diphtheria toxin.

Passive Immunization. This is done by giving diphtheria antitoxin, and is the best method available for treatment of an active infection of diphtheria.

SCHIZOPHRENIA. This is a mental disorder which causes, in its late stages, the most profound dementia. It begins as a rule in adolescence or early adult life, and mostly in persons who have a family history of established mental disease. Before the onset of schizophrenia, the patient nearly always shows some signs of mental peculiarity. Such a young person is unduly shy, very serious-minded, inclined to "withdraw into himself" and has unnaturally high ideals which he cannot share with his companions. Ambition is totally lacking. When the disease shows itself, all these characteristics become exaggerated. The patient "withdraws from the world." Life is long in these patients, mainly because they are well taken care of. There is no hope of a real cure; but in certain, and unfortunately, few cases, it is possible to train these patients to look after themselves and to carry out the simplest of domestic tasks.

SCIATICA. This is a symptom with many different causes. The symptoms of true sciatica are very characteristic and consist in pain along the course of the sciatic nerve from the buttock to the ankle. The nerve itself is tender to the touch and much pain is produced on stretching the nerve by bending the extending leg at the hip joint. When standing up, the victim of sciatica rests his body weight on the sound limb and holds the painful leg slightly bent at the hip and knee, turned slightly inwards and with the heel raised from the ground. In most cases the pain is most severe at the onset of the attack,

and if sufficient rest is given the pain gradually lessens to negligible proportions within the course of a few weeks.

In some cases, however, pain persists, though in a milder form, and the condition may become chronic with more sharp attacks occurring during the winter months. Sciatica often follows an unusual lifting strain. It is then very often due to a rupture of one of the intervertebral discs producing compression of a nerve root as it leaves the spinal column. It often occurs in osteoarthritis of the spine and in cases of spinal tumor. When no course can be found, it is usually attributed to inflammation of the supporting tissues of the nerve itself. Sciatica is a disease of early and middle adult life and it is most common in men.

In the very acute stages of the attack, when pain is intense, rest in bed is essential. The leg should be steadied by means of sandbags or in a light splint if this can be borne. Hot applications to the limb sometimes give relief. It may be necessary in the most painful stage to give drugs to ease the pain. After the severe pain has passed, massage and movements of the limb are useful. Severe cases require to be immobilized in plaster of paris. An operation to remove the disc protrusion sometimes gives relief when this is the cause. In chronic cases it is sometimes found that they are being kept up by poisons—from bad teeth or infected sinuses—which are circulating in the blood. In such cases, of course, these conditions must be attended to and cured. Sciatica is sometimes seen in diabetes, but in this disease it is rare for the sciatica to affect one nerve only; nearly always both sciatic nerves are painful. With suitable treatment of the diabetes, the sciatica disappears.

SCIATIC NERVE. This is the largest nerve in the body, being about the thickness of the little finger. It supplies all the muscles at the back of the thigh, the calf and the foot and in addition, it contains many fibers which convey sensation from the skin of the back of the leg and foot. Thus the sciatic nerve has a very wide distribution. At the back of the knee joint the nerve divides into two branches, the internal and external popliteal nerves. The external popliteal nerve lies very near the surface of the lower part of the back of the knee joint and may, in a thin person, actually be felt. Inflammation of the sheath of the sciatic nerve is called sciatica.

The small sciatic nerve is a nerve which only contains fibers conveying sensation from the skin. It supplies the skin of the buttock, the back of the thigh and the upper half of the skin of the calf. (*See also* SCIATICA.)

SCIRRHUS. This is a particular type of cancer which is characterized by its hardness and firmness. (*See also* CANCER.)

SCLERA. This is the name given to the hard white membrane which, with the cornea, forms the outermost coat of the eye. It is continuous with the cornea in front and with the sheath of the optic nerve behind. (*See also* EYE; CORNEA.)

SCLERODERMA (Hidebound Skin). This disease is characterized by a hardening of the skin, and is found in two forms, the diffuse and the circumscribed.

SCOLIOSIS. This term is applied to a certain form of curvature of the spine. (*See also* SPINAL CURVATURE.)

SCROFULA. This is the old name for tuberculosis of the lymphatic glands and bones. (*See also* TUBERCULOSIS.)

SCROTUM. The scrotum is the pouch which contains the testicles. It consists of two pocket-like compartments, lying side by side, the division between them being marked by a seam on the surface. The left compartment is usually larger and hangs lower down. Underneath the skin of the scrotum, which is thin and brown in color, is a layer called the dartos, which contains muscle fibers. When these fibers contract the skin of the scrotum is thrown into folds. Swelling of the scrotum may be due to an enlargement of the testicle itself, or to a hernia (q.v.), or to a collection of fluid, which is called a hydrocele, or to enlarged and congested veins, which is called a varicocele.

Eczema of the scrotum may be caused by irritation from chemicals and is often seen in paraffin workers and tar workers. In these occupations also, cancer of the scrotum is more common than it is in occupations which do not involve the handling of irritant particles. In order to reduce the risk of cancer, persons engaged in these trades should observe strict cleanliness.

SCURVY. This is due to lack of Vitamin C in the diet. For hundreds of years it has been recognized that seamen who were fed on salted meat with few or no fresh vegetables developed this condition, and that it could be prevented by fresh fruit juice. It is only recently that the active agent in fruit juice has been isolated and named ascorbic acid or Vitamin C.

Scurvy is rare in adults; in children, however, the condition is not uncommon in those who are fed only on boiled or preserved milk or unsuitable patent foods. Scurvy in adults comes on very gradually with progressive loss of weight and strength, while pallor of the face is very noticeable. The gums become soft and bleed easily, and the teeth loosen and may drop out. Bleeding also may occur from the nose, and blood may appear in the urine and stools. Numerous small areas of bleeding appear in the skin and a very slight injury, such as a knock, may be followed by bleeding underneath the skin. The patient is depressed and suffers from sickness and diarrhea.

In children the disease commonly arises about the end of their first year. The child looks pale and anemic, its gums bleed readily and any teeth present may drop out. The characteristic feature of scurvy in children is the pain and tenderness of the bones, especially near the joints. This tenderness is so great that the child does not wait to scream until the limb is touched; it yells as soon as anyone approaches and appears to be going to touch it. The cause of this tenderness is bleeding of the bones.

Treatment. Treatment of both the adult and infantile forms of scurvy consists in giving a diet which contains sufficient Vitamin C and the administration of adequate doses of ascorbic acid. (*See also* INFANTILE PARALYSIS.)

SEABATHING. For those whom it suits, sea bathing is an excellent "tonic" and a most wholesome exercise.

In debility. No doubt many of the benefits ascribed to sea bathing are due to the change of air, scene, and company; but it has definite additional advantages. People who are debilitated, especially children, are often very much benefited, but in these cases sea bathing should be indulged in with caution.

When to avoid. During pregnancy, though it has never been definitely proved that sea bathing is harmful, it should be avoided. If there seems to be a tendency to miscarriage, it should most certainly be forbidden. No harm is done by sea bathing during the period of menstruation, but it will sometimes be found that the discomfort commonly felt at this time is increased thereby. The individual must judge for herself. She should, of course, refrain from attending public baths during the period.

People who suffer from attacks of giddiness or faintness from any cause, palpitation, high blood pressure, or any heart condition, should not sea bathe without first consulting their medical adviser.

SEASICKNESS. Here are a few suggestions to assist those who are not experienced enough to have made their own individual rules:

An hour or two before going on board, take a little light food and a cup of strong coffee (this upsets some people but may suit others.)

Secure a good position on the boat, away from the sides, a deck chair; have a rug over your knees, close your eyes and sleep if possible.

If, after all precautions, sickness does come on, a hot drink (not alcoholic) from a thermos flask may help, or a saline effervescent drink. Chloretone in 5-grain capsules, one every hour, is sometimes effective in preventing sea sickness on short voyages. Hyoscine in doses of 1/200 grain every four hours for a maximum of 36 hours is often remarkably effective, as are also the new sedative drugs such as Dramamine.

SEBACEOUS GLAND. These are attached to the pits or follicles out of which the hairs grow. They pour forth an oil product called sebum, which keeps the hairs and outermost layers of the skin smooth, slightly greasy, and therefore watertight. Sometimes the passage or duct leading from the glands into the hair follicles and skin becomes blocked and the sebum collects behind the obstruction, pro-

ducing a cyst or wen. Overproduction of sebum gives rise to an oily condition of the skin and leads to seborrhea and acne. (*See also* ACNE; SEBORRHEA; WEN.)

SEBORRHEA (Greasy Skin). This term means excessive activity of the sebaceous glands of the skin, so that the skin and scalp tend to be oily. In itself, it is of little importance, though it may be unsightly. It does not affect the health in any way, the only complaint being of a sallow oily skin, sometimes with prominent "plugs" of cheesy matter, and greasy hair. Seborrhea is important, however, because a greasy skin predisposes to the growth of disease germs, and therefore to other and more serious skin complaints.

The condition is a very common one, being found most often in brunettes, and associated with a coarse, large-pored skin and superfluous hair.

Treatment. The head should be washed daily with soap spirit, or, if this is irritant, with a milder soap. Slight cases will be cured by this means alone, but as a rule seborrhea of the scalp is very resistant to treatment, and other measures will be required. A sulphur and salicylic ointment is the best, or a lotion may be used. For treatment of cases where a true dermatitis occurs, *see* DERMATITIS. Seborrhea of the face is treated in the same way as acne vulgaris.

SECRETION. This is a function some cells have of separating certain substances from the blood and elaborating them. When a secretion is poured straight back into the blood it is called an internal secretion. Such a secretion is produced by the cells of the thyroid gland, the suprarenal gland, the pituitary gland, and the genital glands. The cells of such glands as the salivary glands, the liver, and the pancreas, on the other hand, convey their secretion to the body cavities by means of ducts. Secretion is mainly under the control of the nerves; but some cells, notably the cells of the glands of internal secretion, are excited to action by means of hormones. (*See also* DUCTLESS GLANDS.)

SEDATIVE. A sedative is a remedy which lessens excitement and reduces excessive activity. Many drugs are general sedatives. Of these, the barbiturates and the bromides are the best known. Other sedatives are selective in their action, having an effect on one system or organ alone. Any drug which relieves pain or itching in the skin may be called a local sedative. Hot baths, especially if taken for a fairly long time, are excellent as a general sedative.

SEIDLITZ POWDER. This is a saline purgative which consists of a white paper containing 35 grains of tartaric acid and a blue paper containing 40 grains of sodium bicarbonate and 120 grains of sodium and potassium tartrate. The contents of the two papers are mixed in a glass of water and drunk while the mixture is still fizzing.

SEMEN. Semen is the fluid of the male which is secreted by the testicles and contains spermatozoa, the male generative element. It is referred to as the seminal fluid. (*See also* TESTICLE; SPERMATOZOA.)

SENILE DECAY. Senile decay is the result of age upon the various organs of the body. These are discussed under the heading of AGE CHANGES.

SENNA. This consists of the leaflets of a pea-like plant which is found in Egypt and the East Indies. It is one of the most popular of all purgatives, as apart from the official preparations the active agent in senna can be extracted by leaving the pods to soak in cold water overnight, the resulting liquid being drunk. One advantage of senna is that it does not produce constipation following its use. The griping effect is prevented in the official preparations by combining it with belladonna or some other drug which stops spasm.

SENSATION. This is the means by which we are made aware of our bodies and of the surrounding world. Sensation may be divided into various groups: (1) Sensations which arise within our bodies, in the heart and blood vessels, the lungs, the digestive system, and from the muscles, the joints, and the tendons; (2) "common" sensations, which arise very early in our mental development, and are the sensations of heat, cold, and pain, and the sense of coarse touch (as whether an object is large or small); (3) special sensations, which are sight, taste, hearing, and smell, and the sense of fine touch which enables us to appreciate, for example, the fact that

a hair has brushed over our skin. All sensation is conveyed along the nerves to the central nervous system, where, in the spinal cord, certain forms of sensation are gathered up into bundles of nervous units which run upwards into the brain.

One contains all those nervous units which enable us to say whether something we touch is hot or cold as well as those through which we recognize that something is hurting us. In another bundle are collected all those nervous units which tell us of our position in space, whether we are standing on our head or our heels, and also those which allow us to judge of the size, shape and form of objects around us without using our eyes. These bundles are packed quite closely together in the spinal cord, so that any disease or injury to the cord may easily damage the bundles which are conveying sensations to the brain. For example, in tabes dorsalis (q.v.) the bundle which tells us of our position in space is damaged, and so a patient who suffers from this disorder cannot tell where his nose is when his eyes are shut, and cannot even point with one finger to his nose with closed eyes.

SEPSIS. Sepsis is poisoning by the products of decomposition of tissues and is caused by the agency of germs. A wound invaded by germs which produce pus is called a septic wound and takes much longer to heal than one in which no such germs are present.

SEPTICEMIA. This is a condition in which germs gain entrance to the general bloodstream where they live and multiply. Although in many infectious diseases, such as typhoid or pneumonia, the germs causing these conditions may get into the general bloodstream, they are soon killed off by the resistance which the patient develops, and the disease process then remains localized in certain organs of the body. In true septicemia, on the other hand, once certain germs have got a hold (it may be some quite trivial infection or injury such as a prick, or a small wound in the skin), they are able to break through the barriers which separate them from the bloodstream. There are two kinds of germs which commonly produce this condition of septicemia. One kind forms long or short chains and is called the streptococcal group. The other kind, when grown outside the body, produces forms which resemble bunches of grapes. This kind is called the staphylococcal group.

Streptococcal Septicemia is a particularly important form because it is an important cause of death after childbirth. After confinement it is found that the womb easily becomes infected with germs of the streptococcal group. The onset of shivering attacks or rigors, associated with an irregular fever, diarrhea, and anemia are signs of developing septicemia. Even more often does streptococcal septicemia follow abortion, where often less care is taken to prevent germs from gaining admittance to the womb. Surgeons run the risk of streptococcal septicemia if they prick a finger during a septic operation. The condition is always a very dangerous one.

Treatment. The treatment nowadays is to give the patient at once adequate doses of an antibiotic such as penicillin, though sulphonamides are still often useful. The only other measures to be taken are those designed to make the patient more comfortable. Tepid sponging if the fever is high; large quantities of fluid to drink; and sometimes a transfusion of blood will enable her to retain her strength.

Staphylococcal Septicemia is usually the result of an infection of the skin, such as a common boil.

SEPTUM. This is a dividing wall between two parts of an organ or between two cavities. A septum may be of bone, of cartilage, of muscle, of connective tissue or of skin. For example, the septum between the two sides of the nose is mainly of cartilage; that between the two sides of the tongue is of a special kind of skin.

SEQUELA. Sequela is any abnormal condition which follows, and is caused by, an attack of a disease. For example, heart trouble is often a sequela of acute rheumatism. A sequela differs from a complication of a disease, in that it follows the disease and does not appear concurrently with it.

SEQUESTRUM. This term is applied to a piece of dead bone which remains within the body. (*See also* NECROSIS.)

SERUM. When the blood is taken from an animal and allowed to stand in a clean vessel it clots. This process consists first in the formation of a very fine net of fibrin crystals throughout the blood. After a time this network of fibrin shrinks and in doing so retains all the undissolved parts of the blood within its meshes, but squeezes out the remaining fluid. This is a clear, yellowish liquid called bloodserum.

It differs mainly from blood in that it contains no cells or fibrinogen from which the fibrin of the clot is formed.

Part of the defense mechanism of animals and man against disease due to germs and other poisons is found in the blood itself. All healthy bloods are able to antagonize, to some extent, many poisons and organisms. This power varies from individual to individual, and from species to species, and is to some extent inherited. The blood, however, possesses the remarkable power to form new antibodies against special germs, or poisons. This is accomplished in two main ways. The first is the creation of a substance which combines with the poison, so forming a neutral non-toxic substance. These antitoxins are antagonistic only to the particular toxin.

The second defense mechanism developed in the blood serum is the production of bodies which either destroy or inactivate organisms themselves. These substances are less well-defined than antitoxins, and in some cases appear to be an added property of the blood, rather than the production of a substance which one may isolate. They are, however, also specific to the particular organism involved.

Sera and Antitoxins used in Medicine. In those diseases where powerful sera or antitoxins are available they constitute the very best method of treating the disease, for it is the natural way by which the body normally conquers its enemy. To obtain the best results it is necessary to use these substances as early as possible so that the disease may be prevented from damaging the body. Diphtheria treated adequately on the first day of infection is practically non-fatal; on the sixth it kills about one in four persons. Furthermore, the use of these substances is also of the greatest value in preventing disease. (*See also* DIPHTHERIA.)

SERUM SICKNESS. The reactions which take place in the body after an injection of serum vary a great deal with each individual. In some people no reactions are felt at all; in many the effects are mild in nature; but there are a few cases in which the symptoms are very severe. Mild cases of serum sickness usually tend to clear up within a few days and no treatment is necessary apart from giving aperients and calcium salts. The symptoms in a severe case of serum sickness may take the form of fever, vomiting and diarrhea, urticaria or hives, and often the glands become swollen. The symptoms begin about eight or nine days after the injection has been given.

Treatment. An injection of adrenaline should be given, and if the breathing becomes difficult, artificial respiration must be carried out. Any previous attack of serum sickness or a history of asthma must be mentioned to the doctor before the injection of serum is given so that adequate precautions can be taken. (*See also* ANAPHYLAXIS.)

SEX HYGIENE. The education of children in sex has been much argued, but it is possible to make too much of teaching "the facts of life." Children who keep rabbits or a cat soon learn a good deal about the facts of life, and the prospective arrival of kittens, their birth, and their early feeding teach a child more, and in a far better way, than any lecture in the schoolroom. Pre-puberty is the best time for preliminary instruction.

No girl should be allowed to have the shock of a first menstruation without some knowledge of what it means. It is a mistake to treat menstruation as a disease and put a girl to bed because of it, and girls should be allowed to lead their ordinary routine of life and play games regardless of menstruation. In the same way emissions of semen at night in boys should be looked upon in the proper perspective. Seminal emissions are quite normal in boys at puberty, and any suggestion of "lost vitality" is simply nonsense. If they become too frequent a doctor should be consulted, and he will usually prescribe some simple sedative, such as phenobarbital.

In early married life other sex problems arise. Every family doctor has known cases of young people who have not consummated their marriage simply because their knowledge of how the sexual act should be performed was inexact. Nowadays there are plenty of authoritative textbooks that will serve as counsellor and guide to young people, and ignorance on this subject is less common than it was. Methods of birth control have been in vogue since the earliest civilization of mankind, for that is what primitive "sex taboos" and infanticide really mean. Even celibacy is essentially a method of birth control.

There are family planning societies and clinics operating in different parts of the country, and more and more family doctors are becoming interested in the subject. (*See also* BIRTH CONTROL; FAMILY PLANNING.)

SHINGLES (**Herpes Zoster**). These names were originally applied to that form of the disease in which herpes started about the middle of the back, and crept round towards the front in girdle form; but the disease may affect any part of the body.

Symptoms. The two main symptoms are pain, followed on the third or fourth day by crops of little blisters on a certain area. The pain may be severe, and many cases are thought to be "neuralgia," "lumbago," etc., at first. The cause is an acute inflammation of a nerve center, together with degeneration of the nerve fibers passing through it. Hence only that area of skin supplied by the affected fibers suffers.

Treatment. The only local treatment required is to prevent breaking and infection of the blisters, as by an antiseptic dusting powder, cotton-wool, and a bandage. The pain is treated by aspirin, phenacetin, etc., or in severe cases by morphia. Any case in which the face and eye are affected, or if the patient is elderly, needs special care. A course of tonics, and especially a change of air, are valuable in convalescence.

SHOCK. The sudden severe lowering of the vitality of the body, due to injuries, loss of blood, or profound emotion. The essential feature of shock is a fall of blood pressure.

Treatment. The patient is kept at rest, the foot of the bed is raised so that blood flows back into the brain, and hot-water bottles are put all round the patient (care being taken not to touch the patient with the hot bottle, as it may cause a severe burn). A broad bandage may also be put round the abdomen to clear the blood from the dilated abdominal veins, and hot coffee, tea or other drinks may be given; alcohol is not good, as a depressing effect follows the initial stimulation. Blood or plasma transfusion is essential to replace loss of blood volume.

SHORTNESS OF BREATH. Shortness of breath occurs in health after moderate exertion and its degree is a measure of physical fitness. When the physical effort necessary to produce shortness of breath is slight or less than the patient was formerly accustomed to, it is a symptom of disease of the heart, lungs or blood.

Shortness of breath is also known as dyspnea or breathlessness. (*See also* BREATHLESSNESS.)

SHOULDER. The shoulder is the part of the body where the arm joins on to the trunk. It is formed by the meeting of the humerus (bone of the upper arm) with the scapula (shoulder blade) and clavicle (collarbone). The shoulder joint is formed by a saucershaped hollow (glenoid fossa) on the shoulder blade, into which the rounded head of the humerus fits and rotates. This joint is covered by a fibrous capsule and is protected by projecting processes from the shoulder blade and collarbone, to which ligaments are attached. But the strength and mobility of the shoulder joint depend chiefly on the strong muscles—the biceps, triceps, deltoid, etc.—that join the arm to the trunk. The shoulder joint is easily dislocated, but the dislocation is usually easily reduced without leaving serious after-effects. (*See also* FIRST AID SUPPLEMENT.)

SICK HEADACHE. Intense headache, accompanied by a feeling of nausea, is called sick headache or migraine. (*See also* MIGRAINE.)

SICKROOM NURSING. In almost all cases of serious accident or disease the patient is either removed from his home or a professional nurse is called in; but in minor illnesses and accidents the task of attending the sick devolves upon some member of the household, by whom the following simple rules of sick nursing may be found useful.

The Sickroom. Ventilation is of prime importance, but drafts must be avoided. Windows, therefore, should be opened at the top and care taken when opening the door. The bed should not be placed in a direct line between the window and door or between two windows. An easily moved screen should be a part of the sickroom equipment and use made of it to protect the patient from drafts and glare.

The normal sickroom temperature is 68 deg. F. and in winter this should be maintained even though the window be slightly open.

All utensils should be covered with a cloth, emptied immediately after use, and brought back clean.

Changing Sheets. The easiest way to change sheets is as follows:

Get the patient over to one side of the bed and roll up the soiled sheet until it reaches the patient's side. Replace the rolled up portion with a clean sheet previously similarly rolled. Transfer the patient on to the clean portion. Roll off the rest of the soiled sheet and unroll the clean one to replace it. Restore the patient to the middle of the bed.

A draw sheet is made by folding a large sheet lengthwise to one yard in width. It is then laid across the middle of the bed above a waterproof sheet and with one end reaching just to the side, where it is securely pinned. The surplus sheet is formed into a roll at the other side and can be unfolded as the sheet is drawn over. This sheet must be very firmly pinned in place so as not to wrinkle and bother the patient.

Isolation. When one member of the family falls ill with any contagious disease, care must be taken to prevent the disease spreading.

The patient should be placed in a room that can best be isolated from the rest of the house and where the ventilation is good. Curtain, carpets, superfluous furniture and draperies should be removed, and a bath containing 1 pint of carbolic acid to 5 gallons of water be provided to receive all soiled personal or bed linen immediately as it is changed.

Disinfection. To disinfect the room after the illness scrub the walls, floor, and furniture with carbolic soap. Then paste strips of paper over the windows, put a kettle on to boil on a small stove or use a vaporizer to supply steam, and light some stick sulphur—allowing 1 lb. of sulphur for every 1,000 cubic feet of room space. Close and seal up the door. Methylated spirits may be used to start the sulphur burning and the room should be left unopened for at least 24 hours. Any brass fittings in the room which cannot be removed should be thoroughly disinfected and then covered with tissue paper or wax, as the sulphur fumes will badly tarnish them if left exposed.

Formalin is a more suitable disinfectant than sulphur, but its use calls for special apparatus.

Enema. It is sometimes necessary to cause an evacuation by introducing medicine into the lower bowel. The procedure is as follows:—

The patient lies on his left side with the buttocks overhanging the edge of the bed. The pillow is withdrawn so that the head may lie low and is doubled up underneath the hips to give these the necessary height. A waterproof sheet should be laid over the bedding. A three-inch nozzle, which is first smeared with petroleum jelly is gently introduced into the rectum, and the soapy water—or other enema—is made to enter slowly. If it flows back the buttocks must be held against the nozzle. There is a natural tendency to expel the solution at once, so the patient should be warned of this and told to try to retain the enema as long as possible. A suitable pan must be close at hand for the evacuation.

Poultices. Like a fomentation, the object of a poultice is to relieve pain and reduce inflammation. A poultice should always be larger that the affected area and should be an even thickness of ½–1 inch throughout.

Bread Poultice. This is an old-fashioned, but effective, remedy for a festered finger or any other "gathered" sore.

Soak 2 oz. stale bread-crumbs into ¼-pint of boiling water for 2 minutes. Lightly press out the excess of water and spread the bread pulp on a piece of muslin or old linen. Cover with a piece of gauze, apply hot, and wrap in a clean outer cloth. (*See also* BEDSORE; ENEMA; FOMENTATION; POULTICES.)

SIDEROSIS. This is a type of lung disease due to the inhalation of tiny particles of metal by metal workers. (*See also* ANTHRACOSIS; LUNG.)

SIGHT, ERRORS IN, or ASTHENOPIA. In general the word is only used to mean lack of power to use the eyes for any sustained effort of vision. Any attempt to gaze fixedly at anything is accompanied by more or less wobbling or dimness of the sight. It is especially noticeable in using the eyes for close work. Complaints made by sufferers vary so very much that no attempt can be made to give them in detail.

The causes of weak eyesight are chiefly: (1) Errors in sight, especially long-sightedness; (2) muscular, which are probably due to fatigue of the nerves controlling the muscles of the eyes; (3) nervous, in which the greatest variety of symptoms is found, and which may render the slightest and most ordinary use of the eyes painful or troublesome in some way. Frequently one or more of these causes are combined, but in any case of weak sight the nervous elements should be borne in mind.

Treatment. The treatment of asthenopia is to treat the cause. Glasses should be prescribed if they are found necessary; alcohol, tobacco, tea, and coffee may have to be forbidden; the general health should be regulated with tonics, if necessary.

The headache so often complained of generally disappears with the above treatment.

Astigmatism. This is a common error of eyesight due to some imperfection in the shape of the lens or of the cornea, which may be unequally curved in different directions, so that rays of light cannot be brought to focus on the retina except by continued and irregular strain of the muscle. The condition causes objects to seem distorted and out of place; a ball, for instance, will be egg-shaped.

It is rare to find an eye that shows no sign of astigmatism, but slight degrees cause so little discomfort that they are generally disregarded. In more severe cases the distress caused by the continued strain may be readily understood. Astigmatism may be remedied by suitable spectacles, in which one surface forms part of cylinder. (*See also* EYE; SPECTACLES.)

Short Sight (Myopia). In this condition,

sometimes called long-eye, the distance from the lens to the retina is too great, so that distant objects are focused in front of the retina and seem blurred. Near objects, however, can be seen more clearly and easily than with normal eyes. The handwriting and sewing of short-sighted people tend to be exceptionally small and neat. The condition is uncommon in young children, but sometimes comes on at school, especially if the books are in small print and the light bad. (*See also* EYES; SPECTACLES; SQUINT.)

SILICOSIS. This disease is a form of fibrosis of the lungs and is due to the inhalation of particles of silica dust. (*See also* ANTHRACOSIS; FIBROSIS; OCCUPATIONAL DISEASES.)

SILVER. The most common preparation of silver used in medicine is nitrate of silver, or lunar caustic, which is chiefly used to destroy warts or small growths, etc.

Lunar caustic is the solid form of silver nitrate and it is usually prepared in the form of a short stick and fitted into a holder with a screw-on cover. (*See also* ARGYRIA; LUNAR CAUSTIC.)

SINEW. This is another name for a tendon. (*See also* TENDON.)

SINUS. A sinus is a hollow or cavity, and the term is applied medically (1) to a suppurating tract (such as a sinus leading from an abscess to the skin), (2) to large channels containing blood (especially the venous sinuses of the brain, such as the lateral sinus), and (3) to cavities within a bone (such as the maxillary and frontal accessory sinuses of the nose).

Sinus disease is a term which is popularly applied to infection of one or more of the accessory sinuses of the nose (maxillary sinus or antrum, frontal sinus, ethmoid sinus, and sphenoid sinus). These are situated in the bones adjacent to the nose and communicate with it, containing air. Sinusitis commonly follows influenza, though maxillary sinus infection may sometimes be caused by a tooth abscess. The treatment is usually surgical. It is often possible to control sinus infection by inhaling some suitable antiseptic in the form of a fine spray. Penicillin dust inhaled into the nostrils gets widely distributed through the nasal passages; some

gets absorbed into the blood and may exert a beneficial effect in this way.

SKELETON. The skeleton is the bony framework that supports the soft parts of the body; in some parts of the body, such as the larynx and the ends of the ribs next to the breast-bone, the framework is of cartilage, not bone; but all of the bones originally developed from cartilage in early life. There are over 200 bones in the human skeleton, which is divided into the *axial skeleton,* including the skull, spinal column, ribs, and breast-bone, and the *appendicular skeleton,* including the bones of the arms and the legs. (*See Frontispiece.*)

SKIN. The skin is made up of two layers, the epidermis, which covers the surface, and the dermis, or "true skin," underneath. Below the true skin is the subcutaneous or "underskin" layer, which is a loose tissue containing fat, blood vessels, and nerves, and serves to protect the deeper structures underneath, and to give roundness to the body.

The *epidermis* is composed of closely-packed cells. The deeper layers are soft, and are constantly increasing in number and size. The cells thus formed are gradually pushed up to the surface by other new ones forming below. They are gradually cut off from their source of nourishment, shrivel, become dry and horny, and are shed or rubbed off when they reach the surface. This horny layer is especially thick on the palms and soles.

The *dermis* or true skin is composed of a dense tough material called connective tissue. It contains many elastic fibers, tiny blood vessels, and nerves. None of the blood vessels actually reaches the epidermis, but they allow nourishment to soak through, as it were, to supply its growing layer. The outer surface of the dermis is not flat, but has a "hill and valley" arrangement. Each "hill" is called a papilla, and contains a little hoop of tiny blood vessels, called capillaries, which supply the epidermis, hairs, and nails, with nourishment. Some of the papillae also contain a tiny oval body attached to a nerve fiber; these provide the sense of touch. Some of the nerve fibers enter the epidermis.

The surface of the epidermis is raised

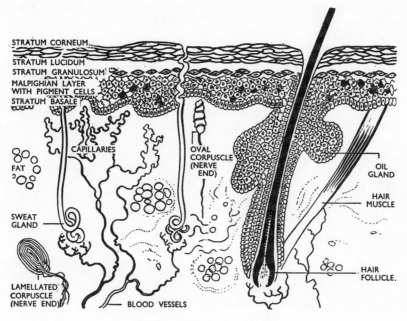

STRATUM CORNEUM
STRATUM LUCIDUM
STRATUM GRANULOSUM
MALPIGHIAN LAYER
WITH PIGMENT CELLS
STRATUM BASALE

CAPILLARIES

FAT

SWEAT
GLAND

LAMELLATED
CORPUSCLE
(NERVE END)

BLOOD VESSELS

OVAL
CORPUSCLE
(NERVE
END)

OIL
GLAND

HAIR
MUSCLE

HAIR
FOLLICLE.

Section through the Skin.

up into ridges. These are especially well seen in the tips of the fingers, where they are arranged in arches, circles, or loops. It is common knowledge that no two people have the same pattern, so that finger-prints, as they are called, are largely used for purposes of identification. If the ridges are magnified it will be seen that they are perforated by a large number of tiny holes. Each of these is the mouth of a *sweat gland* or coil gland.

The duct or "drain" passes in a twisting manner—rather like a corkscrew—back into the true skin, where it rolls up into a little coil, which is the sweat-gland itself. They are found on the skin all over the body, including the scalp, but are most numerous on certain parts of the body, the palms, the soles, the armpits, and the space between the buttocks. It has been calculated that, allowing ¼-inch for each gland and its duct, the skin contains something over two million glands, the length of which would be about eight miles!

Sebaceous glands, which are always in close relation to a hair, produce an oil which lubricates the hair and keeps it glossy; they also lubricate the surrounding skin. They are found wherever there is hair, i.e. all over the body, except on the palms and soles. Their action is seen especially on the scalp. If they produce too much oil, the hair becomes greasy and scurfy; if too little, it is dull and dry.

Hairs are made up of horny matter formed in the epidermis. Each hair grows from a little pit in the horny layer of the skin called a hair follicle, into the base of which enters a papilla of blood vessels, which nourishes the root of the hair. Hair is of two varieties: the coarser kind that grows on the scalp and in other situations, and the lanugo or downy growth which forms an almost complete though practically invisible covering for the body.

The *nails* also grow from the epidermis, by some of the horny cells in certain situations called "nail-beds," not falling off, but becoming closely pressed together. The nail-bed itself is formed by the true skin, and is nourished by the blood vessels there. It has no concern in the growth of the nail. The cells grow quickly, and the nail is simply pushed along the nail bed by its growth from behind. (For Inflammation of the skin *see also* DERMATITIS *and* SKIN, DISEASES OF.)

**SKIN, DISEASES OF. Inflammation of
the skin** (*dermatitis*) may attack any part
of the body, and it exists in many different
forms. Certain forms, have a fondness for
certain regions, and these are discussed
under separate headings. (*See also*
Rosacea; Cheilitis; Dermatitis; Eczema;
Frostbite; Head Louse; Intertrigo;
Lupus; Paget's Disease; Pellagra;
Psoriasis; Ringworm; Scabies; Seborrhea; Summer Prurigo; Xeroderma.)

SKULL. The skull is the bony framework of the head, and is divided into
two parts—the cranium and the face. The
cranium encloses the brain and is made up
of the occipital, frontal, two parietal, two
temporal, and ethmoid and sphenoid
bones. The bones of the face comprise the
two upper jawbones (superior maxillae)
and one lower jawbone (inferior maxilla),
two malar, two nasal, two lachrymal, two
turbinal, two palate bones, and the vomer.

SLEEP. Work and sleep are the natural
occupations of day and night in turn.
Healthy babies sleep most of the time,
only waking for food. Little children
should be put to bed once or twice during
the day. Older children, at school, need
ten hours' sleep. The quality of sleep is
of at least as great importance as its quantity. In later life the amount of sleep required depends largely on the individual.
Some quite old people doze a good deal,
though merely elderly ones often take only
a few hours' sleep. Sleeplessness—insomnia
—should not be allowed to continue; medical advice should be obtained. Sleep-
walking—somnambulism—when only part
of the brain is asleep, needs special care.
Children who walk in their sleep are
probably highly sensitive, and of excitable
temperament. Never make fun of a child
who walks in its sleep. If possible, lead it
gently back to bed without waking it; if
it must be wakened, the process should be
a quiet and gradual as possible. (*See also*
Insomnia; Sleepwalking.)

SLEEPWALKING. This is also called
somnambulism and is really the acting of
a dream. It occurs most commonly in
people who are the victims of hysteria and
is looked upon as one of the symptoms of
that disorder. It may also be produced
during hypnosis (*see also* Hypnotism) in
which state the patient can be asked to

dream and to act his dream, which he will
do with remarkable dramatic powers. As
a rule, sleepwalkers do not wander very
far and they are usually able to take care
of themselves. The case of a sleepwalker
having a fatal fall is exceptionally rare.
(*See also* Hysteria.)

SLEEPING SICKNESS. This disease is
also known as trypanosomiasis, and it is
caused by the bite of the tsetse fly. It
occurs amongst the natives of Africa, and
it is often described as African lethargy.
The term is also applied to *encephalitis
lethargica*.

Treatment. The best form of treatment
is the drug known as suramin, especially
when this is used in conjunction with the
arsenical drug, tryparsamide. It has recently been shown that a single dose of the
chemotherapeutic agent known as antry-
cide will cure the diseases in animals, and
large-scale experiments are at present in
progress in Africa.

SLEEPLESSNESS. Insomnia is another
term for sleeplessness. (*See also* Insomnia.)

SLING. A bandage for the support of a
limb is known as a sling. (*See also* Bandage.)

SLOUGH. Sloughing of the tissue occurs when a dead part becomes separated
from the living tissue. For example, the
"core" which appears in the center of a
boil or abscess is known as a slough. (*See
also* Gangrene; Necrosis.)

SMALLPOX. Smallpox, or variola as it
is also called, is an infectious disease, the
chief symptoms of which are fever and an
eruption of the skin. The cause of the
disease is a tiny germ known as a virus.
Smallpox is one of the most contagious
of all diseases. The infection is spread by
the breath of the patient and by contact
with him or his personal belongings. The
infection can also be carried by the clothes
of third persons not themselves infected,
and it is believed that the germs can be
carried through the air for some distance.

Symptoms. About twelve days after the
infection, the disease begins with an attack
of shivering, headache, pains in the back,
and vomiting. In children there may be
convulsions. On the third day, the fever
declines a little as a rash, somewhat resembling that of scarlet fever, makes its ap-

pearance. It commences on the face and head, spreads to the arms and trunk, and lastly appears on the legs. The distribution of the rash is important to the doctor in making his diagnosis. During the period between the third and sixth day the rash undergoes a change in appearance. Raised "pocks" appear and become filled with a clear fluid and in the center there is a slight depression. On about the eighth day these vesicles or blebs become larger in size and the fluid inside them changes into pus or yellow matter. The skin surrounding each "pustule" is inflamed and swollen, and as the eruption is more thickly spread on the face, it becomes very disfigured indeed.

The eruption is present on the mucous membranes as well, particularly in the mouth and throat, and the inflammation and swelling which takes place is often a serious matter to the patient as there is great danger of obstruction of the air passages. The fever which had somewhat declined after the first two days now makes its appearance again (secondary or suppurative fever), and the patient is extremely restless from the irritation caused by the rash. On the eleventh or twelfth day the pustules either break or dry up and blackish crusts form. The temperature usually drops at this stage, but there is great itching of the skin where a scab has formed over each pustule. The scabs gradually fall off leaving a scar or "pit" which is one of the characteristic marks of smallpox.

The symptoms just described are those met with in an ordinary case of smallpox, but in some outbreaks the type of the disease is much more severe. The course may be interrupted by dangerous complications, the chief of which affect the lungs, throat, eyes and ears. In the type of the disease known as *confluent smallpox* the symptoms are much more severe from the very onset, and the rash, instead of showing itself in isolated spots, appears in large patches, and the pocks are so numerous that they run into one another. Many of these cases prove fatal, while in those that survive, convalescence is a very prolonged affair and the scars left on the face are extremely disfiguring. An even more severe type of the disease is the *hemorrhagic* type in which bleeding takes

place into the pocks after they are formed. *Discrete smallpox* is the term used to describe mild cases, and *varioloid* cases are those in which the symptoms are very slight. This last type may occur in persons who have had a previous attack of smallpox or who have been vaccinated against it.

Treatment. The general treatment of smallpox is conducted along the same lines as for any other infectious disease. The patient is removed to an isolation hospital. All those who have been in contact with the patient are vaccinated, and the public health authorities keep a very strict watch in order to check any spread of the infection. The house and clothing must be thoroughly disinfected Recently penicillin has been employed locally and by injections, with marked success in avoiding the disfigurement usually caused by the pustules. There is no specific treatment for this disease and careful nursing is of paramount importance. It can be prevented or at least modified by protective vaccination. (*See also* INFECTIOUS DISEASES.)

SMELL. The organ of smell is in the specialized lining membrane of the nose and it is more highly developed in the lower animals than in man. The loss of the sense of smell is termed anosmia, and it may be due to a variety of diseases or injuries. The sense of smell is important to man because of its esthetic value; the flavor of food is really a compound of taste and smell and the smell stimulates the gastric juices and aids digestion more than most people imagine. (*See also* APPETITE; NOSE.)

SMELLING SALTS. These are usually made up of strong ammonia with various perfumes added to make the preparation more agreeable. It is used for reviving people who are faint or have fainted, or for those suffering from shock or collapse. (*See also* AMMONIA.)

SMOKING. *See* TOBACCO.

SNAKE BITE. *See* BITES AND STINGS.

SNEEZING. Any irritation in the nose may cause a fit of sneezing, as this is nature's way of getting rid of the irritation and infection. Sneezing is one of the symptoms of cold in the head, influenza, hay fever, etc. Unguarded sneezing is a highly antisocial practice which disseminates the germs of many respiratory diseases far and wide. (*See also* CATARRH, NASAL; HAY FEVER; INFLUENZA.)

SNORING. Snoring results from sleeping with the mouth open which causes the soft palate at the back of the throat to vibrate. Snoring in children is almost always due to the presence of adenoids. (*See also* ADENOIDS.)

SNUFFLES. Noisy breathing through the nose is a frequent accompaniment of a common cold, and occurs often in children who have adenoids. When this noisy breathing is heard in children of a few weeks old it may be due to congenital syphilis. (*See also* ADENOIDS; SYPHILIS.)

SOAP. Soap is a substance made up of a combination of a fat or oil and an alkali such as caustic soda. Some laundry soaps are made with ammonia instead of soda. Yellow soap—which is used for general household purposes—is prepared by mixing hard fatty soap with resin soap. In soft soap, or green soap, caustic potash is used instead of soda, while curd soap has tallow for its fat. Marine soap is made with coconut oil, and it is specially prepared so that it can be used with sea water for washing purposes. Transparent soap is made by dissolving ordinary soap in alcohol which is distilled off and the soap is then allowed to cool and harden in the usual way. Glycerine added to melted hard soap forms a transparent soap with a very lasting lather.

SODA. This term is generally applied to bicarbonate of soda (baking soda) or to the carbonate of soda (washing soda). Soda water consists of water charged with carbonic acid gas and it contains a very small amount of sodium bicarbonate.

SOFT PALATE. The soft palate is the roof of the mouth at the back of the throat, which is a muscular continuation of the bony arch forming the hard palate; it ends at the uvula. (*See also* PLATE.)

SOFT SORE. Soft sore, or chancroid, is a venereal ulceration which forms on the external genital organs. It is nonsyphilitic, but it is often mistaken for the syphilitic hard chancre. (*See also* SYPHILIS.)

SOMNAMBULISM. This is another name for sleep-walking. (*See also* SLEEP-WALKING.)

SOPORIFIC. Any drug which tends to induce sleep is known as a soporific. *See also* DRUGS; HYPNOTIC; NARCOTIC.)

SORE. This is a popular term for ulcer. (*See also* ULCER.)

SORE THROAT. The majority of cases are due to infection with the common cold or influenza, or to septic tonsils. Diphtheria may be mistaken for simple tonsillitis and on this account a thorough examination should be made when a child complains of a sore throat; if there is any suspicion a doctor will always take a swab from the throat and will usually inject antitoxin as a safety measure, without waiting for the result of the bacteriological examination. An injection of penicillin, followed by penicillin by the mouth, often helps.

A troublesome cold may start off with a feeling of soreness and rawness in the throat, and pharyngitis and laryngitis may be exceedingly painful; the best treatment is two aspirin tablets every three hours and inhalations of compound tincture of benzoin. A relaxed throat is a source of a good deal of discomfort, and it is quite common in people who are run down and need a holiday. Relief is best obtained by gargling with a hot solution of bicarbonate of soda or chlorate of potash and by painting the throat with a suitable paint such as the well-known Mandl's paint, which contains iodine in glycerine. (*See also* DIPHTHERIA; LARYNGITIS; PHARYNGITIS; TONSILLITIS.)

SOUTHEY'S TUBES. These are very fine tubes used for drawing off water from the body in cases of edema. (*See also* EDEMA.)

SPANISH FLY. This is a dried beetle which possesses strong blistering properties, and is frequently used as a counter-irritant in cases of rheumatism, pleurisy, etc.

SPASM. A convulsive movement or a painful contraction of the muscles is described as a spasm. Spasm may affect muscles in any part of the body, and it is not unusual to have a spasm of the muscles of the leg ("cramp"), especially when varicose veins are present. A spasm may be only temporary or it may be more or less constant. It may come in waves (clonic) or without any relaxed periods (tonic). There are general spasms of the whole body in such disorders as epilepsy, tetanus (lockjaw), strychnine poisoning, and hysteria. Some people suffer from facial spasm ("tic") in which the eye may be seen to twitch or other contortions may take place at intervals. These symptoms are usually due to some disorder of the nervous system. (*See also* HYSTERIA; NERVOUS SYSTEM; ST. VITUS'S DANCE.)

SPECIFIC. A remedy which has the power to cure a disease is said to be specific for that disease. For example, quinine is a specific for malaria, digitalis for certain conditions of the heart, and salvarsan for syphilis. The term is also used as a description of a definite disease, and commonly as a euphemism for syphilis.

SPECTACLES. In perfect eyes, images of external objects are focused exactly upon the retina. The eye has the power to accommodate itself for near and distant objects. In many cases, however, the eyes are in some way defective; in *long sight* the image is focused beyond, and *short sight* before the retina. In **astigmatism,** a distorted image is produced. In middle life, **presbyopia** occurs, and it becomes increasingly difficult to focus near objects. The ill-effects of these conditions may be removed by the use of suitable spectacles. Protective spectacles may be of colored glass, which protects the eyes against excessive light: e.g., the sun or high-power electric lights; or motor-goggles, which protect from dust and wind; or wire spectacles, which are used in such work as stone-breaking, hedge-cutting, etc., to protect from flying chips.

Contact Lens. This may take the place of the lens of spectacles, to correct an error of refraction, and consists of a carefully adjusted plastic lens applied directly to the surface of the eye, with the aid of a saline solution. It requires a good deal of practice to get properly adjusted and the eye accustomed to its use.

SPEECH. For the perfect performance of speech a most complicated series of happenings must take place. First of all, those parts of the brain which control speech must be healthy. The development of these parts of the brain in the child and the loss of speech caused by their damage or destruction is fully dealt with under APHASIA. The rest of the speech-producing apparatus consists of the tongue, the lips, the vocal cords, which are in the throat,

and the palate. If the nerves to any of these structures are damaged, either by pressure from other structures or by disease of the nerves themselves, then speech is altered in character or may be entirely lost. Loss of speech in such a case differs from a loss of speech due to damage to the central brain apparatus in that intelligent sounds can be whispered, a condition which is called *aphonia* to distinguish it from *aphasia*, where it is evident that the central apparatus itself is damaged.

There are a large number of different causes of aphonia. The most important is due to hysteria, and this form of aphonia rapidly recovers when the hysteria is treated. Treatment of the aphonia alone is of no value. Pressure on the nerves which control the movements of the vocal cords is a common cause of aphonia. The pressure may be either from a tumor in the upper part of the chest, or from an aneurism or from an enlarged thyroid gland in the neck. In any of these conditions, before the voice is lost, there is a period in which the voice alters and becomes somewhat harsh, and there may be a harsh "brassy" cough as well. (*See also* ANEURISM; APHASIA; DISSEMINATED SCLEROSIS; G.P.I.; HYSTERIA; NEURITIS; PROGRESSIVE MUSCULAR ATROPHY.)

SPERMATIC CORD. This structure is made up of arteries, veins, nerves, etc., leading to the testicle. Twisting of this cord causes strangulation of the blood vessels, and, if immediate treatment is not carried out, gangrene usually sets in and the testicle and cord may have to be removed by operation. The veins of the spermatic cord may become varicose and the condition is called a varicocele.

SPERMATORRHEA. This term is applied to the involuntary discharge of semen from the urethra in the male without any sexual excitement. People who live a continent life are liable to become worried and depressed over these discharges. The condition is normal if the discharges are not too frequent, otherwise a doctor should be consulted, who will probably prescribe a sedative mixture.

SPERMATOZOON. The human male germ which is able to fertilize the female ovum, or egg, is known as a spermatozoon. It is microscopic in size and consists of a head, a neck, a body and a tail. The tail is by far the longest part and acts as a powerful propeller which makes the tiny cell capable of active movement. These cells are able to live for quite a few days if kept at body temperature, but they soon die if exposed to the cold. (*See also* SEMEN.)

SPHINCTER. This term is applied to any ring of muscle which encircles the opening of a hollow organ. There are many such structures in the body, but the three chief ones are the sphincter of the anus, that of the bladder, and the one that surrounds the opening of the stomach into the duodenum. Certain nerves control the movements of these muscles causing them to contract, thus preventing the escape of the contents of the organ. In some diseases of the nervous system this action is interfered with, so that the power to relax or contract is lost, and escape or retention of the contents may have troublesome results. (*See also* ANUS; BLADDER; DUODENUM.)

SPHYGMOGRAPH. This is an instrument for recording the movements of the pulse. The name sphygmomanometer is given to an instrument which is used to measure the blood-pressure in arteries. (*See also* articles on BLOOD-PRESSURE; PULSE.)

SPICA BANDAGE. *See* BANDAGE.

SPINA BIFIDA. This term means literally a cleft spine and it aptly describes the condition. In the early days of growth, the spinal cord is represented by a groove along the back of the child while it is still in the mother's womb. The borders of this groove grow together and form a tube which is the central canal of the spinal cord. It is easy to see that if this tube fails to develop, the child will be born with the spinal cord open to the surface of the back. In such a case the child will probably be stillborn. Sometimes the neural tube has closed and the spinal cord is more or less perfectly formed but the outer covering of tissue may have failed to grow and enclose it, and the child is said to be born with split spine, or spina bifida. The usual appearance in this condition is a swelling in the lower part of the spine which contains cerebrospinal fluid. The treatment of the condition is surgical and many cases have been successfully operated upon. (*See also* SPINAL CORD.)

SPINAL COLUMN. The spinal column is also known as the spine, the backbone, or the vertebral column and it forms a very important part of the skeleton. (*See also* BACKBONE.)

SPINAL CORD. This is a part of the nervous system which is directly continuous above with the medulla (q.v.) and extends downwards as far as the lower part of the loins. It is contained in a bony canal—the spinal canal, which is enclosed by the vertebral column. The spinal cord is enclosed by the same three membranes as envelop the brain. It gives off the spinal nerves, which pass out through spaces in the vertebral column to form the nerves to the limbs, trunk and internal organs. The spinal cord is divided into five regions, the cervical (neck), the dorsal (trunk), the lumbar (loin), the sacral, and the coccygeal regions. There is an enlargement of the cord in the cervical region where the nerves to the arms are given off, and another in the lumbar region where those to the legs leave the cord.

The internal structure of the spinal cord is very complicated. It is divided into two lateral halves by a bridge of tissue. Each lateral half is made up of a central portion of gray matter, enclosed by an outer portion of white matter. The gray matter contains areas which are called anterior and posterior horns. In the anterior born are very large important nerve cells, which are motor nerve cells and are concerned with movement of groups of muscles. In the white matter are the nerve fibers which conduct messages to the brain from the muscles and skin, and those which carry messages from the brain to these parts. In fact, the white matter is the pathway to and from the brain. In addition, certain involuntary movements called reflexes result from nervous action in the spinal cord without any intervention of the brain and without an individual being conscious that they have occurred. (*See also* BRAIN; NERVOUS SYSTEM; REFLEXES.)

SPINAL CURVATURE. Deformity of the backbone consists of an exaggeration of its normal curves, or a new curve may form in a lateral or sideways direction. *Kyphosis,* commonly known as round shoulders, is described under its own heading, and *lordosis,* which is an increase of

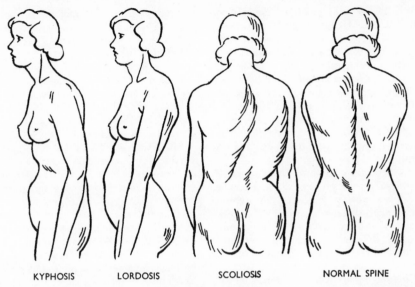

KYPHOSIS   LORDOSIS   SCOLIOSIS   NORMAL SPINE

Spinal Curvature.

the forward curve in the small of the back, is also described under its own heading. *Scoliosis,* which is the name given to a sideways curve of the spine, may be due to rickets in early childhood, to tuberculosis of the hip, or to great muscular weakness. In young growing children the habit of standing badly is very liable to lead to curvature of the spine.

The treatment of these conditions consists in keeping the general health in as good condition as possible by means of fresh air, suitable exercise, good food, and tonics if necessary. Special exercises should be practised daily, and any habit of standing or sitting badly should be avoided. Growing children should never be allowed to carry heavy weights. It is only in extremely marked cases that special mechanical supports are necessary, but massage is good as it helps to strengthen the muscles of the back.

Angular curvature of the spine, which is also known as *Pott's disease,* is a much more serious condition, and it is almost always caused by tuberculosis. The deformity in this case is caused by caries or rotting of the vertebrae, and, as the bone is destroyed, the spine gives way at the site of the disease thus causing a sharp bend forward.

Treatment. This is the same as for any other tuberculous condition: that is, rest, fresh air and good food. Early treatment may be successful in preventing deformity, and good results are often obtained by sunlight treatment and the application of suitable plaster casts. (*See also* BACKBONE; TUBERCULOSIS.)

SPIRITS. Substances such as whisky, brandy, rum, and gin are classed as spirits and they usually contain about 50 per cent of alcohol. Spirits of various drugs are used in medicine and among the most common are spirit of chloroform, sweet spirit of niter, aromatic spirit of ammonia (which is better known as sal volatile), spirit of ether, spirit of camphor, and spirits of various volatile oils such as peppermint, juniper, lavender and rosemary. Plain spirit (alcohol) or eau-de-Cologne are often used on the skin for their soothing effect and they are also used to harden the skin to prevent bedsores and foot soreness. (*See also* ALCOHOL.)

SPIROCHETE. The term spirochete is applied to a group of tiny germs or organisms which have a spiral structure. They are capable of wriggling their way through the blood or tissues, and they are the cause of several important diseases in human beings, especially syphilis and Vincent's angina. (*See also* GERMS.)

SPITTING. *See* EXPECTORATION.

SPITTING OF BLOOD. *See* Blood Spitting, *also* Hemoptysis.

SPLEEN. The spleen is an organ about 5 in. long, situated behind the stomach in the upper left corner of the abdomen. It is connected with the rest of the body only by its nerves, lymphatics, and comparatively large blood-vessels. Its function was for long a mystery and is not yet fully understood. The spleen can be completely removed surgically without affecting the health of the body.

Diseases of the Spleen. *Enlargement of the spleen* is an important sign in a number of diseases, especially malaria and typhoid fever; other diseases in which it may be enlarged are streptococcal septicemia, syphilis, tuberculosis, rickets, pernicious anemia, leukemia, splenic anemia, and the tropical disease kala azar.

Rupture of the spleen is a not uncommon result of an accident, especially when a vehicle has passed over the abdomen. The injured person has severe abdominal pain and shows signs (pallor, faintness) of internal hemorrhage. A surgical operation is necessary to save life.

Splenic anemia (Banti's disease) is a disease the cause of which is unknown. It occurs chiefly in young men, and is characterized by anemia, bleeding from the nose, stomach, or bowel, and enlargement of the spleen; it usually requires an expert physician to recognize the disease. If untreated, it is usually fatal, but surgical removal of the spleen, if done early in the course of the disease, gives good results.

SPLINTS. Splints are most commonly made of wood and padded with wool or some other soft material. They are used for keeping the ends of a fractured bone at rest and for maintaining the shape of a limb. In rendering first aid, splints extending beyond the joints above and below the fracture must be applied before the patient is moved. In an emergency splints may be made out of walking-sticks, broomhandles, branches, thick newspaper and, in fact, anything of suitable length and stiffness. (*See also* First Aid Supplement; Fractures.)

SPONDYLITIS DEFORMANS. This condition has in the past been classed with infective or atrophic arthritis (chronic rheumatism) but is now believed to be a separate disease, of a metabolic type (i.e. due to a chemical upset of the body.) (*See also* Rheumatoid Arthritis.)

SPORADIC. A disease is said to be sporadic if cases develop here and there. The term is used as opposed to epidemic outbreaks. (*See also* Epidemic.)

SPOTTED FEVER. This is a popular term for *cerebrospinal fever.* (*See also* Cerebrospinal Fever.)

SPRAINS AND STRAINS. A sprain is a joint injury with a stretching or tearing of ligaments. A strain is the wrenching of muscles or tendons. In a sprain, one or more of the ligaments of a joint are torn so that there is bleeding and weakness of the joint. The blood is usually seen under the skin in the form of a bruise. The membrane which forms the lining of the joint becomes inflamed and pours out a certain amount of fluid so that the joint swells and becomes stiff and painful to move. If possible, a firm bandage should be applied immediately so as to prevent the swelling becoming too large and also to prevent bleeding. It is the absorption of blood from the tissues which makes the cure of a sprain such a lengthy business. The parts surrounding the sprain should be gently massaged so as to keep the blood circulating at its best, and a suitable support such as adhesive strapping may be used to rest the part. The patient should be encouraged to exercise the joint gently as soon as he is able, otherwise adhesions may form. An X-ray examination may be necessary to exclude doing injury. (*See also* First-Aid Supplement.)

SPRUE. Sprue is a tropical disease, confined mainly to Ceylon, Southern India, China, the Straits Settlements, and the West Indies. Treatment consists mainly in dieting the patient with restriction of fats.

SPUTUM. This term is applied to the material spat out of the mouth. It may consist of saliva from the mouth or of secretions from the lungs, back of the throat, or nose. Examination of the sputum is useful in many cases, as it may reveal the presence of certain diseases in the lungs. In those who suffer from chronic bronchitis, it will be found that, on rising in the morning, a certain amount of sputum is always present. This is usually quite inoffensive, but should it acquire an offensive odor, it is characteristic of abscess or gangrene of the lungs. Sputum is normally of a grayish shade, but in those who smoke a great deal or who work in coal mines, etc., the expectoration may be black. In lobar pneumonia the sputum is often tinged with blood, and for this reason it is termed rusty sputum. In some cases of cancer of the lungs the sputum is said to resemble prune juice owing to the presence of blood. (*See also* EXPECTORATION; TUBERCULOSIS.)

SQUAMOUS. Derived from a Latin word meaning scale, the term squamous is used to describe several structures in the body to indicate that they are thin or flattened, or scale-like. (*See also* DESQUAMATION.)

SQUILL. This popular drug is obtained from the large round bulbs of a plant which grows along the shores of the Mediterranean. It has a very bitter taste, and owes its medicinal properties to a substance known as scillitoxin. This drug is classed as an expectorant, which means that it is capable of increasing the flow of saliva.

SQUINT (Strabismus). Squint or strabismus is caused by a number of conditions: (1) by an error in development; (2) by injury to one of the muscles which move the eye; (3) by injury, disease, or overstimulation of one of the nerves supplying these muscles, which causes paralysis and lengthening, or overcontraction and shortening, of the muscles; (4) by the presence of some defect in the eye, such as long- or short-sight. This is called *concomitant*, since it is (almost) equal whether the eyes be looking to right or left. *Divergent* squint occurs when one or both eyes turns outwards; *convergent* when one or both turns inwards. The former is sometimes found when there is constant excessive strain in short-sight, the latter in long-sight. The *treatment* of "muscular" squint is that of the injury or disease which has caused the trouble. Prismatic lenses may have to be used to correct the double vision that sometimes occurs. If all treatment fails, and only then, operative measures are attempted. The treatment of concomitant squint, in both long- and short-sight, is to wear suitable spectacles, which in most cases relieves the condition.

Exercises, prescribed by an ophthalmic specialist, are proving successful.

Two objections to spectacles are sometimes made by parents: (1) "The child will grow out of squinting." He may, rarely, but in the meantime weakening of the sight will occur. (2) "The child is too young to wear glasses." This is entirely mistaken; even a tiny child will be quite happy, and far from refusing to wear glasses, will ask to have them put on each day.

STAMMERING. This is a disturbance of speech in which, owing to faulty nervous control of the muscles used in speaking, there is a sudden check to the utterance of words, or the sounds with which the difficulty arises are repeated over and over again. It is the difficulty of performing the necessary movements of the tongue and lips with at the same time producing the sounds in the voice-box or larynx that causes a person to stammer. As a rule, the difficulty only arises with certain letters of the alphabet, most commonly with the consonants p, b, t, d, g, k, and is experienced generally only when these letters occur at the beginnings of words, no difficulty being shown when the same letters occur in the middle of words.

Treatment. The treatment of stammering consists mainly in re-educating the child in the use of his voice sounds, and encouraging him to persevere in breathing exercises.

STAPEDECTOMY. A delicate operation performed on the ear with the aid of the operating microscope, to relieve deafness due to otosclerosis. (*See also* DEAFNESS.)

STAPHYLOCOCCUS. This is the name given to a particular type of germ which is responsible for various pusforming diseases. (*See also* GERM.)

STARCH. Starch is a very important member of the group of foods known as carbohydrates and it is found to a great extent in vegetables and cereals. Starch is used as an ingredient in many dusting powders for application to chafed and inflamed areas of skin. A starch enema is often used to soothe an inflamed bowel and to check diarrhea. (*See also* ENEMA.)

STATUS LYMPHATICUS. A condition in which all the lymphatic tissues, the thymus, the spleen, and the bone marrow, etc., are markedly overgrown.

STENOSIS. The term is used to describe the narrowing of any of the natural openings of the body. This may be caused by disease, such as inflammation or the growth of a tumor, or it may be due to pressure from outside.

STENSON'S DUCT. The parotid glands, the largest pair of salivary glands, have tubes which convey the saliva to the mouth and are known as Stenson's ducts. (*See also* SALIVARY GLANDS.)

STERILITY. Barrenness or sterility means the inability to produce offspring. Sterility in the female may be due to some malformation (sometimes quite slight) of the generative organs, to a lack of healthy activity in the ovaries such as is often met with in cases of obesity, to thyroid deficiency, to displacement of the womb, or to inflammatory conditions of the genital organs. Many cases of sterility can be cured by treatment, operative and otherwise. In the male there may be nondevelopment of the testicles, but chronic inflammation of the male genital organs is the most frequent cause. When a marriage appears to be fruitless, it is advisable that both the wife and the husband should be examined by a specialist, and if living spermatozoa from the male can be seen by immediate examination under the microscope the wife is obviously the infertile partner. But it would be useless to treat her, surgically or otherwise, if it is the husband who is infertile.

STERILIZATION. The process by which substances, including foods, etc., are freed from germs is known as sterilization. (*See also* ASEPSIS; PASTEURIZATION.)

STERNUM. This is another name for the breastbone. (*See also* BREAST.)

STETHOSCOPE. An instrument used for listening to the sounds produced anywhere within the body is called a stethoscope. (*See also* AUSCULTATION.)

STICKING-PLASTER. *See* ADHESIVE PLASTER.

STIFF NECK. The commonest cause of stiff neck is muscular rheumatism or fibrositis, usually the result of exposure to cold, damp, or a draft. (*See also* FIBROSITIS; RHEUMATISM.)

STILBOESTROL. This is a synthetic estrogen (ovarian hormone) used in the treatment of cancer of the prostate and in menopausal conditions.

STILLBIRTH. A child which measures over thirteen inches in length and which shows no sign of life after it has been born is termed a stillborn child. (*See also* ABORTION; CHILDBIRTH.)

STILL'S DISEASE. This is a rare form of arthritis, called after the London children's specialist who described it. (*See also* ARTHRITIS.)

STIMULANT. Any drug or other agent which is capable of increasing the activity of the body is described as a stimulant. A stimulant may be given to produce an immediate effect on any part of the body, whereas a tonic is given when a more lasting effect is required. Alcohol in small doses acts as a stimulant, but in larger quantities it depresses the brain centers. Strong coffee and tea are well known stimulants. The application of heat will stimulate the action of the skin and cause increased sweating to take place. Stimulants are grouped according to the part of the body on which they have effect. For example, there are heart, lung, digestive, kidney, brain, spinal cord, skin, and other stimulants. (*See also* ALCOHOL; AMMONIA; CAFFEINE.)

STING. *See* BITES AND STINGS.

STITCH. A sudden spasm of pain in the side usually due to cramp in the muscles is popularly referred to as stitch. The pain may go as suddenly as it comes, and rubbing may give some relief if the part still feels tender. (*See also* CRAMP.)

STOKES-ADAMS DISEASE. This is the name (after the two Irish physicians who first described it) given to a condition in which the heart stops beating for a short period. The condition is a serious one, and requires the advice of an expert physician. (*See also* HEART.)

STOMACH. The stomach is a large, more or less pear-shaped dilatation of the digestive canal, about one foot in length and four or five inches in breadth, holding normally about two or three pints of fluid; it communicates at its upper end with the gullet (esophagus) and at its lower end with the first part of the small intestine (duodenum) through a valve-like opening called the pylorus. It is situated in the upper part of the left side of the abdomen, and when dilated may press through the diaphragm upon the heart (which lies above it) so as to give rise to palpitations and other symptoms that a nervous person may attribute to heart disease. The shape of the stomach naturally varies with the amount of food it contains and with the stage to which digestion has progressed.

The walls of the stomach contract in rhythmic waves, which take about half a minute each to pass along its whole length. Food reaching it is already masticated and mixed with saliva and mucus, and the business of the stomach is to continue the process of digestion that has been begun. The stomach wall has four layers, an outer layer of peritoneum, next a muscular layer, then a submucous layer, and last an internal layer of mucous membrane, in the folds of which are innumerable microscopic glands, some of which secrete mucus and some the gastric (digestive) juice. This juice contains two ferments, (1) pepsin, which softens and dissolves the fibrous part of meat; and (2) rennin, which digests and coagulates milk. It also contains hydrochloric acid, which facilitates the digestive action of pepsin and also helps to prevent putrefaction.

Food is not absorbed in the stomach— alcohol is an exception—but is mixed thoroughly there and converted into a milky semifluid substance called "chyme," and then squirted periodically through the small pyloric opening into the duodenum, where more important processes of digestion take place; absorption into the body takes place in the small intestine.

Diseases of the Stomach. With the exception of cancer of the stomach—which follows herewith—the diseases of the stomach are dealt with under separate headings. (*See also* DYSPEPSIA; GASTRIC ULCER; GASTRITIS.)

Cancer of the stomach most usually occurs in men over the age of 40, and, contrary to what used to be said, does *not* commonly result from a gastric ulcer. The symptoms are often like those of ulcer of the stomach, and it will need a specialist to make an accurate diagnosis, with the aid of testmeals and X-ray examinations; as the symptoms are sometimes like those of pernicious anemia (q.v.), a blood ex-

amination may also be necessary. A middle-aged person (especially about the middle fifties) who *suddenly* develops symptoms of dyspepsia, having never had them before, should seek the advice of his doctor.

The *treatment* is an operation for removal of the cancer, and the outlook is always hopeful if this is carried out early.

STOMACH TUBE. A soft rubber tube, usually about thirty inches in length, is used for drawing off the contents of the stomach or for washing out the stomach when it contains some poisonous material. (*See also* FORCIBLE FEEDING; IRRIGATION.)

STOMATITIS. Inflammation of the mouth is called stomatitis. It is treated by alkaline mouthwashes, such as warm bicarbonate of soda solution or glycothymoline, and attention to the teeth or other cause.

STONE. *See* CALCULUS; GALLSTONES.

STOOLS. Feces is the term applied to discharges from the bowel, but the terms stools or movements are more commonly used. These discharges naturally vary in color and amount in accordance with the state of the health and the quality of the diet, but normal feces are brown in color and the quantity discharged in one day by an adult should be approximately six ounces. The brown color is due to substances in the bile, the chief of which is a pigment called *stercobilin.*

Certain articles of food may change the color of the feces; for example, if the diet consists largely of meat, the discharges from the bowel will be darker in color, while milk and starchy foods tend to make them a light yellow color. Too much fat in the diet may produce stools of an almost milky whiteness, or this may be the result of some disease of the pancreas in which fat is not being properly digested. Pale, clay-colored stools usually indicate that the normal amount of bile is not entering into the intestines. This usually occurs in jaundice, and the odor of the stools may be particularly offensive. The motions of children suffering from diarrhea are commonly bright green in color.

Bright red blood mixed with the feces usually comes from the anus or rectum. When the stools are tarry-looking this is termed melena, and this condition is caused by the presence of blood which has altered in appearance in its passage through the intestines. This condition indicates that there is a hemorrhage high up in the bowel or in the stomach, usually from a gastric or duodenal ulcer. The color of the stools may vary as a result of taking certain drugs. For example, iron or bismuth may cause them to turn black; while rhubarb and senna may give them a bright color.

Incontinence of the bowel, or inability to hold the stools, is a symptom of certain diseases of the nervous system, or it may be due to laxness of the muscles surrounding the anus. Pain at stool is a very characteristic symptom of a fissure or it may be due to inflamed piles. (*See also* CONSTIPATION; DIARRHEA.)

STRABISMUS. This is another name for what is popularly known as squint. (*See also* SQUINT.)

STRAIN. Any part of the body may suffer harm by being taxed above its normal powers; and a continued strain, whether mental or physical, will eventually lead to harmful results. The main treatment for strain of any sort is rest, and, if the strain is muscular, massage should be given to the part in order to restore tone to the tissues. Cases of mental strain, caused by overwork or too much worry, should be treated by a complete change of surroundings, and tonics and fresh air will help to assist the cure.

STRAIT JACKET. A jacket used as a form of restraint when necessary for mentally diseased patients is referred to as a strait jacket. (*See also* JACKET.)

STRAMONIUM. This drug, which is used chiefly for asthma, is obtained from the leaves of the thorn-apple. Attacks of asthma may be relieved by smoking cigarettes made from stramonium leaves, or by inhaling the fumes given off from the burning powdered leaves. (*See also* ASTHMA; ATROPINE.)

STRANGULATION. The most popular use of this word is in connection with throttling or strangling which is caused by pressure on the windpipe, but the term is also used to describe a stoppage of the flow of blood due to pressure or constriction. The commonest condition in which this occurs is a strangulated hernia, an extremely dangerous condition. (*See also* HERNIA, RUPTURE.)

STRANGURY. This term is used to describe the condition in which there is a desire to pass urine, but the discharge is very slow and painful and only a few drops may come away. The causes of such a condition are numerous.

Treatment. This naturally depends upon the cause, but hot baths and large quantities of bland fluids will help to relieve the immediate pain. (*See also* URINE.)

STRAWBERRY MARK. This is one form of birthmark which shows on the skin as a red or bluish-red stain. (*See also* BIRTHMARK.)

STREPTOCOCCUS. A special variety of germ which, when seen under the microscope, has the appearance of a string of beads. It is responsible for a very wide range of diseases, including tonsillitis, scarlet fever, and erysipelas. (*See also* GERMS.)

STREPTOMYCIN. Work on the activity of antibiotic substances was stimulated by the discovery of penicillin and resulted in the isolation of streptomycin by Waksman and his associates in 1943. This remarkable drug is extracted from a mold known as actinomyces griseus which is found in soil. Streptomycin resembles penicillin in the way in which it interferes with the growth and reproduction of disease germs, but it is active against a different range of bacteria. Like penicillin it has to be given by injection, but it is more slowly excreted from the body and therefore needs to be given less frequently. Unlike penicillin it has unpleasant side-effects of which the commonest and most distressing is a disturbance of the sense of balance.

The most important disease against which this drug has been found effective is tuberculosis. It is the only form of treatment available against tuberculous meningitis, which was formerly regarded as invariably fatal. There are now many recorded cases of complete cure. In tuberculosis of the lung, the use of the drug is reserved for carefully selected cases of progressive disease; it is not used indiscriminately because it has been found that the germ of tuberculosis is able to develop resistance to the action of streptomycin which is therefore a trump card to be played at a carefully timed moment. In addition to all forms of tuberculosis, this drug has been found curative in cases of meningitis due to the germ found in influenza. It will cure tularemia and certain types of pneumonia and is very effective in most infections of the urinary tract.

The discovery that germs are able to breed strains resistant to the action of streptomycin during treatment raises a host of new problems and points the way to caution in the use of antibiotics for trivial infections or cases in which its usefulness would be uncertain. By giving a chemical substance "P.A.S." or para-amino salicylic acid by mouth, it has been found that the onset of streptomycin-resistance in tuberculosis can be delayed. In spite of this it is being realized that streptomycin is not a substitute for well-tried forms of treatment of tuberculosis but rather a new and powerful adjunct to these older methods.

STREPTOTHRIX. This name is given to a group of germs that are closely allied to fungus or mold and which occasionally produce diseases in man. Actinomycosis is such a disease. It is from solutions of this mold that streptomycin is obtained.

STRICTURE. The narrowing of any of the natural passages of the body, such as the urethra, the bowel or the gullet, is known as stricture. Most cases are caused by inflammation, but some are due to the growth of a tumor. In some situations a stricture is referred to as stenosis. (*See also* STENOSIS.)

STRIDOR. A peculiar harsh sound produced whilst breathing is known as stridor. It sometimes resembles a whistling noise, and it is due to obstruction in the larynx. (*See also* CROUP; CROWING; DIPHTHERIA; LARYNX.)

STROKE. A stroke is a sudden and severe attack of apoplexy or of paralysis, or it may be used to describe sunstroke. (*See also* APOPLEXY; PARALYSIS; SUNSTROKE.)

STROPHANTHUS. The drug known as strophanthus is a bitter, poisonous glucoside obtained from the seeds of an African plant from which the natives made the kombé arrow poison. In its action this drug is very similar to digitalis and it is used to strengthen the force of the heartbeat and to correct irregularities. (*See also* DIGITALIS.)

STRYCHNINE. Strychnine is an alkaloid drug which is prepared from the seeds of an Eastern plant known as nux vomica. Tincture of nux vomica is often given as a tonic in convalescence or in indigestion.

Strychnine is capable of increasing the tone of the muscles, and because of its stimulating effect it is included in many nerve tonics; as a hypodermic injection it is a powerful heart stimulant.

Poisoning by strychnine. Large doses are very poisonous indeed and may have fatal consequences. It causes the muscles all over the body to contract violently with the result that the patient is unable to breathe. The convulsion lasts a minute or two, then the muscles relax, and the patient feels exhausted and sweats all over. The convulsions soon come on again and increase in severity. The slightest noise or even a bright light will bring on the convulsions, and unless treatment is given the patient may die from exhaustion and asphyxia. The symptoms of strychnine poisoning are similar to tetanus.

Treatment. The patient should at once be anesthetised with chloroform or ether. The stomach should be washed out with a solution of permanganate of potash and large doses of chloral hydrate or bromethol should be injected into the rectum. Apply artificial respiration if necessary. (*See also* POISONS IN FIRST AID SUPPLEMENT.)

STUPOR. A mental and physical state in which the patient is unresponsive and indifferent to his surroundings. The condition varies from the mildest case in which the patient is little more depressed and indifferent to the world about him than are normal people suffering from a "fit of the blues" up to a state in which patient appears to be unconscious, lying in any position in which he is placed and not attempting to feed himself or attend to the calls of nature. If left alone, patients with severe stupor die of starvation, but if properly treated, and fed by a tube, they keep up their weight and may even improve in bodily condition during their illness. Recovery commences slowly but gradually, even though the stupor may persist for three to four months.

Stupor occurs in several different forms of mental disorder, but chiefly in manic-depressive insanity, during the depressed stage, and in melancholia. Stupor is also seen in certain diseases as an early stage of coma. (*See also* COMA; DIABETES.)

STUTTER. *See* STAMMERING.

STYE (Hordeolum). This consists in the formation of a boil in the "socket" of an eyelash. It may occur on either the upper or the lower lid; and styes often appear in crops, now on one lid, now on the other. Both eyes may be affected. The disease may occur at any time of life, but is especially common about puberty. In adults, it is often very painful, and the conjunctiva covering the eyeball may swell, causing much distress and alarm to the patient. A single stye may be caused by local infection; repeated styes, however, always indicate a poor condition of general health, or point to the need for glasses. Local treatment consists in removal of the eyelash, either by forceps or an incision, squeezing out the pus, and applying a warm boric acid fomentation (this is clear and easier to apply than a poultice). To prevent recurrence, the eyes should be bathed with warm boric lotion several times daily, and the lids then massaged

with yellow oxele of mercury ointment. If styes persist in spite of local treatment, tonics should be given, and glasses prescribed if these are necessary.

STYPTICS. Styptics are substances which check bleeding either by making the blood vessels contract or by causing the blood to clot. Drugs which are capable of arresting bleeding include adrenaline, ergot, hydrogen peroxide, perchloride of iron, sulphate of copper, nitrate of silver, tannic acid, and alum. (*See also* HEMORRHAGE.)

SUBCLAVIAN. The subclavian artery and vein are important blood vessels which pass to the upper arm between the collarbone and the first rib. (*See also* ARTERIES.)

SUBCONSCIOUS. Subconscious describes that state in which mental processes take place and objects and events are seen or experienced without the mind being completely aware of them. Although such subconscious events may be forgotten, yet they may have an influence over the mind or something may later arouse the mind to take notice of them. Nowadays a good deal of importance is attached to such subsconscious experiences, which are considered to be responsible for neurasthenic or neurotic conditions; these can then be

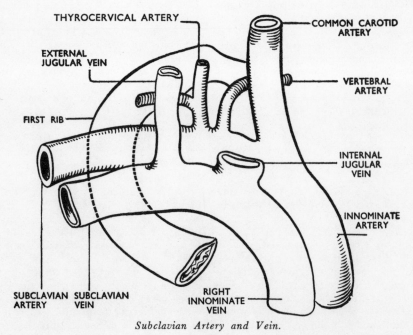

Subclavian Artery and Vein.

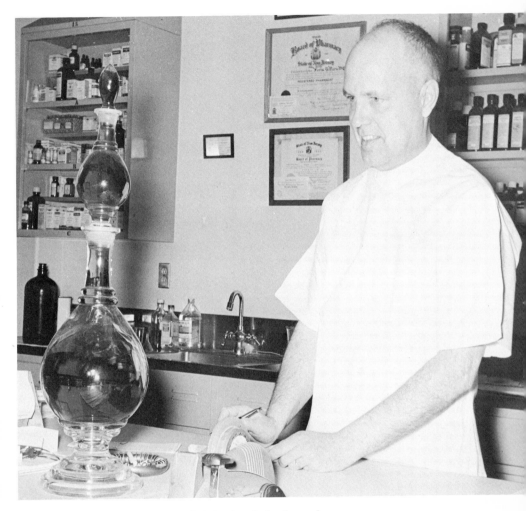

The pharmacist is an important link in the chain that safe-
guards your health.

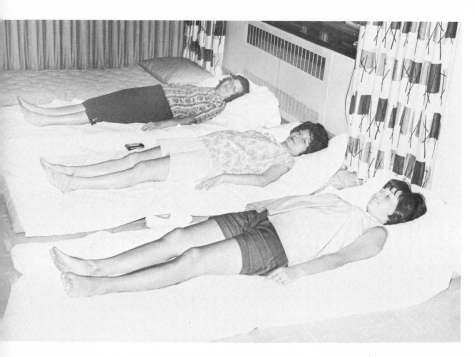

Many modern hospitals provide prenatal classes and exercises for women-in-waiting.

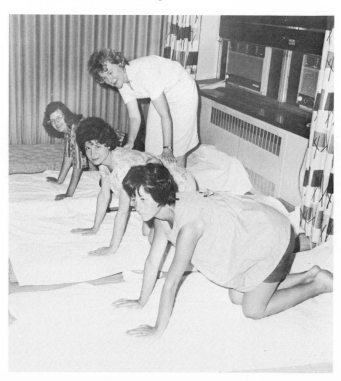

cured only by remembering fully the subconscious event or experience and getting the mind to look at it in its proper perspective.

SUBCUTANEOUS. An adjective meaning "beneath the skin." Thus hypodermic injections, or injections beneath the skin, are also described as subcutaneous injections. (*See also* INJECTION.)

SUBLIMATION. In chemistry this term is applied to the processes of converting a solid substance into a vapor and recondensing it. The term is also used in a mental sense for the process of converting instinctive sexual desires to other forms of activity. (*See also* SEX HYGIENE.)

SUBLINGUAL GLAND. The smallest of the salivary glands, the sublingual glands can be seen lying beneath the tongue. The ducts of the sublingual glands are eight or ten in number, but they are too small to be seen ordinarily. (*See also* SALIVARY GLAND.)

SUBMAXILLARY GLAND. A pair of salivary glands, lying one on each side of the tongue and between it and the lower jaw, are known as the submaxillary glands. (*See also* SALIVARY GLAND.)

SUCKLING. This term means the natural feeding of an infant at its mother's breast.

SUGAR. Sugar belongs to the carbohydrate class of food and it contains important chemical elements such as carbon, hydrogen, and oxygen. Grape sugar, or glucose, is found in various kinds of fruit, and it is sugar which is passed in the urine by patients suffering from diabetes mellitus. Cane sugar, or sucrose, is a valuable food and is supplies the body with heat and energy. It is also capable of producing fat, so an excess should be avoided by those who put on weight easily. (*See also* DIABETES.)

SUGGESTION. This term is applied to a mental process used in psychotherapy. The patient is led to accept facts without exercising his own will or judgment. (*See also* AUTO-SUGGESTION; PSYCHOTHERAPY.)

SULPHATE. A salt of sulphuric acid is called a sulphate. The sulphates of the heavy metals include iron, zinc, and copper, while those of the alkalis include magnesium sulphate, potassium sulphate, and the sulphates of sodium.

SULPHONAMIDES. The name given to a group of chemical substances which began a new era of chemotherapy, for these drugs could destroy germs throughout the body. The name "sulphonamide" covers all the drugs in the group, the best known of them being sulphanilamide, sulphapyridine, sulphathiazole, sulphadiazine, sulphaguanidine, sulphamezathine and sulphadimidine.

The story of these drugs dates back to 1908, when a German chemist made sulphanilamide, from which a whole series of dyes was developed; in 1935 Dr. Domagk, another German chemist, found by animal experiments that one of these dyes, a red chemical which he called prontosil, killed the virulent germs known as streptococci, which cause blood poisoning, puerperal fever, erysipelas, tonsillitis, and other serious diseases. Shortly afterwards other chemists and doctors proved that sulphanilamide, from which prontosil was derived, was quite as effective. Hundreds of different chemical substances are known to be derived from sulphanilamide, but only a few of them are of any use in curing disease, though others may yet be discovered.

The most dramatic effects were those of sulphapyridine in cases of pneumonia, meningitis, and gonorrhea; but it often had severe side-effects, and other sulphonamides or antibiotics are now used. The effect of sulphaguanadine in dysentery is just as dramatic and—in certain countries—as important. Many serious conditions are cured or at least alleviated by sulphonamides, and they are also used in the treatment of burns. But they are potent and poisonous drugs and must never be used casually like an occasional aspirin—they require the supervision of the doctor. Serious reactions from their use are not uncommon, such as cyanosis (blueing of the face and skin), nausea and vomiting, rashes, and sometimes fever. A doctor nowadays usually gives them for a few days only, starting with large doses and tailing off.

The idea that certain sulphonamides have a particular action against certain germs is inaccurate, though it is true that sulphanilamide is the most effective against streptococci, and sulphaguanidine against dysentery bacilli; but the different action merely depends on different strengths and on different rates of being absorbed and got rid of by the body. At one time it looked as if all bacterial infections might be brought under the control of one or other of the sulphonamides, but this hope has been disappointed. More recently, medical interest has switched to the still newer drugs called antibiotics, penicillin etc, which are effective in a rather different range of diseases.

SULPHUR. Sulphur, a yellow nonmetallic element, is used in medicine in two forms, the sublimated sulphur, or flowers of sulphur, and precipitated sulphur, also known as milk sulphur. Sulphur ointment rubbed into the skin is one of the best treatments for the itch, or scabies. The skin should be well scrubbed with soap and hot water before the ointment is rubbed in. The patient should do this before going to bed at night, and wash the ointment off the next morning. If this is done for three or four evenings the condition will probably be cured.

Mild sulphur preparations, especially a lotion made of the milk of sulphur, may be used for acne on the face. Sulphur is also used in baths in cases of skin diseases and for this purpose sulphurated potassium is generally used. Dandruff and seborrhea are also treated with sulphur, but as the drug is irritating to the skin great care must be taken not to prolong the treatment. Sulphur is a very good laxative, especially for children, and it is very commonly mixed with licorice powder. Lozenges containing sulphur are often taken at bedtime as a remedy for mild constipation. An old-fashioned treatment consists of sulphur and molasses mixed into a paste.

SULPHURIC ACID. Also known as oil of vitriol, sulphuric acid is a colorless, oily liquid which is very corrosive.

SUMMER DIARRHEA. This form of diarrhea is common in young children. It is highly infectious and carries an alarming mortality in infancy. (*See also* DIARRHEA.)

SUN-BATHING. By sun-bathing is meant the exposure of the body, with or without a minimum of dress, to the fresh air and the sun's rays. Sunlight is a stimulant, under certain conditions a powerful one, and it must be used in moderation,

if the effect is to be beneficial. Generally speaking, sturdy young adults, who bronze readily, tolerate the longest exposures. Red-haired, freckled, elderly, and infirm persons should exercise more caution, and no one suffering from an organic disease should indulge in sun-baths except on expert medical advice. (*See also* SUNLIGHT, ARTIFICIAL; ULTRAVIOLET RAYS.)

SUNLIGHT, ARTIFICIAL. The value of sun-bathing is due not to the heat rays but to what are called the *ultraviolet* or actinic rays, which are the shortest in the solar spectrum, and those of greatest therapeutic value. These rays are most intense in the clear air of mountains or by the sea, and are practically absent in the smoky atmosphere of a manufacturing town. Luckily, they can be obtained by other means than that from natural sunlight. All the "artificial sunlight" lamps are capable of producing ultraviolet rays, the mercury-vapor lamp being the "richest," but also the costliest. It can only be used by an expert, whereas some of the carbon arc lamps are simple enough for home use by careful people. These simpler lamps may prove of great benefit to health during the winter months.

SUNSTROKE. Sunstroke, or heatstroke, are the terms applied to the conditions produced by exposure to the strong rays of the sun or to overheated air without sufficient loss of the heat through the skin and its sweat glands. The symptoms may vary in severity from a headache to severe collapse, high fever, and delirium. Mild cases may occur in this country, especially at the beginning of a vacation, unless due precautions are taken to cover the head, neck and spine. Special care should be taken with children, otherwise they are liable to become irritable and feverish and may complain of sickness.

Treatment. The patient should be kept in a room and given plenty of cool drinks. Sponging the body with cold or tepid water at frequent intervals is very soothing and beneficial. In severe cases strong stimulants for the heart may be necessary, and such cases should not be allowed out under the direct rays of the sun for a long time. (*See also* SUN-BATHING.)

SUPPOSITORY. Suppositories are usually made of cocoa butter or oil of theobroma, and they are a convenient method of introducing drugs into the rectum, urethra, or vagina. Suitable suppositories may be inserted into the rectum in order to relieve pain or itching, or to act as a laxative. To produce a quick action of the bowels, a piece of ordinary soap may be shaped like a suppository and pushed into the bowel. Suppositories for the vagina are usually cone shaped, and are called pessaries.

SUPPURATION. This term is used to indicate the formation of pus or matter. (*See also* ABSCESS; INFLAMMATION; PUS.)

SUPRARENAL GLANDS. These are two small structures situated above the kidneys which belong to the group of ductless glands. They are also known as the adrenals, and the secretion of the glands is called adrenaline. (*See also* ADRENAL; ADRENALIN; DUCTLESS GLANDS.)

SURGEON. A surgeon is a member of the medical profession who specializes in surgery; in other words, who may be called upon to perform operations.

SUSPENSORY BANDAGE. A support for the scrotum or testicle is known as a suspensory belt. It consists of a waistband from which a bag is suspended. This form of support is necessary in diseases of the scrotum or testicle. (*See also* ABDOMINAL BELT.)

SUTURE. This term is used in two ways: it may mean the line of joining or closure between two bones, especially the bones of the skull, or it can be applied to the line of stitches used in closing a wound.

SWAB. A swab is a piece of cottonwool gauze, lint, or any similar material which is used for surgical purposes.

SWEATING, DISAGREEABLE. Bromidrosis is the term given to a condition in which the sweat becomes evil-smelling, and may be general or local. It occurs in some diseases in their acute stage, and may then, to the trained nose, be a guide to diagnosis. Diseases having a characteristic odor are rheumatic fever, diphtheria, smallpox, cholera, typhus, and severe diabetes. In some people not only the breath, but the perspiration, becomes odorous after taking such substances as onions, garlic, sulphur, and various others. Bromidrosis under the arms and on the soles of the feet is due to the decomposition of the sweat and of the softened upper layer of the skin by various bacterial organisms, and is equally irksome for the sufferer and for those near him.

Treatment. For the armpits frequent bathing with very hot water may suffice; together with the use of a dusting powder composed of boric acid, orris root and talc in equal parts (starch powders should *not* be used, as the starch forms a happy breeding-ground for the organisms). The use of dress-shields may aggravate the condition by damming back the sweat, and so helping on both the disagreeable decomposition and the softening of the skin; a form of eczema may follow.

For the feet there are many varieties of treatment, but all physicians are agreed that attention to cleanliness is the chief thing. The feet must be washed morning and evening, and, if necessary, during the day, after which an astringent lotion such as Eau-de-Cologne, or boric acid, ½ oz. to 1 pint water, should be used, followed by the powder mentioned above. Salicylic acid, grs. 20–48, to talc 1 oz., may be used as a powder; this helps to absorb the perspiration. A fresh pair of clean stockings should be worn daily, or, if there is much perspiration, as often as the feet are washed. The shoes should be easy-fitting; if possible, new ones should be bought, and changed as often as the stockings, each pair being well aired when not in use.

SWEETBREAD. The pancreatic gland (and sometimes the thymus) of animals is used for food and sold under the popular term sweetbread. The sweetbreads of young animals are very nutritious and digestible and, consequently, very suitable for invalids.

SYCOSIS. This is a skin disease in which the hair follicles, especially of the chin, are inflamed. The condition is described under the heading BARBER'S ITCH.

SYMPATHETIC NERVOUS SYSTEM. This is that part of the nervous system which sets energy free when it is most needed, that is, at a time when energy is wanted for bodily defense. In such a state of mind as fear, anger, or intense pain, the sympathetic nervous system comes into play and by its action the heart is enabled to beat more rapidly, the blood pressure rises, blood is sent in larger quantities than normal to the limbs, and certain substances such as sugar, which are normally stored in various organs of the body, are set free into the blood to enable the individual to act more quickly. The nervous units which make up the sympathetic system are mainly situated in little masses of nervous tissue alongside the backbone, through spaces in which they are connected with the spinal cord. More about the structure of the sympathetic system will be found under the heading of NERVOUS SYSTEM.

Symptoms of mild disturbances of the sympathetic nervous system are very common. Such symptoms include flushing of the face, blushing, slight attacks of giddiness, and curious attacks in which the patient thinks he is having a heart attack. The heart palpitates, beats very quickly, and the patient feels a sense of suffocation. It is sometimes difficult to reassure such a patient that there is nothing wrong with his heart, but the fact that there are other symptoms of mild disturbance of the sympathetic nervous system and no signs of real disease of the heart enables the condition to be recognized.

Recently a new advance has been made in surgery by operations on the sympathetic system for disorders of the blood vessels of the limbs.

SYMPATHECTOMY. The surgery of the sympathetic nervous system has made great progress of late, and cutting the sympathetic nerves surrounding the main blood vessels to the part affected is now the ordinary treatment of Raynaud's disease and other spastic conditions of the circulatory system. It is also useful in certain cases of chronic arterial obstruction, especially thromboangitis obliterans. Sometimes the ganglions of the sympathetic system along the vertebral column are operated upon and removed for the enormous dilatation of the bowel called Hirschsprung's disease. Similar operations are being done for the relief of anginal pain and for various affections of the pelvic organs. (*See* SYMPATHETIC NERVOUS SYSTEM.)

SYNCOPE. This is another name for fainting. (*See also* FAINTING.)

SYNDROME. A group of symptoms of a disease to which some particular name is given is known as a syndrome. For example, the Stokes-Adams syndrome is the occurrence of slow pulse and giddiness which occur in heartblock. There are other syndromes named after people who described them.

SYNOVIAL MEMBRANE. The membrane which lines the ligaments binding the bones of a joint together is known as the synovial membrane. Synovia or synovial fluid is secreted by this membrane, and in normal conditions it ensures easy movement of one bone on the other. (*See also* JOINT; TENDON.)

SYNOVITIS. Inflammation of the synovial membrane of a joint is known as synovitis. It is a very painful condition and is found in acute rheumatism and other inflammations of the joints. (*See also* RHEUMATISM.)

SYNTHETIC. Drugs which are produced by chemical processes in a laboratory are known as synthetic drugs. (*See also* DRUGS.)

SYPHILIS. This is a serious chronic disease which may be either "acquired" or "inherited." It is due to the entrance into the body of a special kind of germ, called a spirocheter. This germ was only discovered in the early part of this century, although the disease which it causes has been known since the Middle Ages. The germ is conveyed from one person to another most commonly through sexual intercourse. In congenital syphilis the children are infected before birth by the mother, and therefore syphilis is not— strictly speaking—an *inherited* disease, as it is acquired by the unborn child while in the mother's womb.

Symptoms. It is usual to describe the results of syphilitic infection in three stages. In the first stage, after infection has taken place about a month, a small, hard, painless sore appears at the place where the germ gained entry to the body. The bottom of the sore is very hard and the surrounding parts feel hard also. A slight colorless discharge accompanies the sore, in which the germ can be found. The glands in the neighborhood of this sore enlarge, though this enlargement may not be noticed by the patient as it is completely painless. If no treatment is carried out during the period when the sore is present, it gradually decreases in size, until at about the end of two months only a small scar remains. But during this time the germs have got into the blood and have been carried to all parts of the body. As soon as they are able to become active in the various organs of the body, the secondary stage of the disease may be said to have been reached. This usually happens between two to three months from the time of infection.

In the secondary stage, symptoms of a general nature appear. There is nearly always severe headache, usually worse at night; slight fever; pains in joints and bones; or there may be severe anemia. But the chief and most obvious feature of the secondary stage of syphilis is a rash. This rash may imitate nearly every known skin disease, and without certain tests it may be very difficult to tell if the rash is due to syphilis or not. During the secondary stage of the disease the germs get into the nervous system and, although at this time there may be no symptoms of any disease of the nervous system, examination of the fluid which surrounds the spinal cord, the cerebrospinal fluid (q.v.) will show whether or not the particular person in the secondary stage is likely to suffer later from either of the two severe diseases of the nervous system caused by syphilis, namely, general paralysis of the insane (q.v.) or tabes dorsalis (q.v.). In this stage too, the germs invade the heart and walls of the blood vessels, so that later on diseases of these important organs may occur, due to the effect of the activity of these germs.

It is hardly necessary to stress, in view of what has been said of the later results of syphilis (which are responsible for a greater number of deaths and lives of chronic invalidism than the mildness of the disease in its early stages would suggest), that no one should allow the secondary, or if possible the first stage of the disease to go untreated. But if left untreated, the secondary stage appears to clear up, and there is a period of freedom from symptoms which may last from two to twenty years; but, sooner or later, other symptoms arise and these form what is termed the tertiary or third stage of the disorder. During this period of freedom

from symptoms the resistance of the body prevents further activity on the part of the germs which are, however, lying hidden away in all the organs of the body. Many of these germs die out in the course of years, but some remain alive, and at any time they may re-awaken to activity.

There is no organ which may not be attacked in the third, or tertiary, stage of syphilis. Generally speaking, the disease in this stage takes the form of the production of tumor-like masses which become soft in the middle and then become ulcers. These tumor-like masses are called gummas, and they vary in size from a pinhead to an orange. The ulcers which replace them are slow to heal unless properly treated. The skin, the bones and joints, the liver, the palate, the tongue, the mouth, are all common places where this ulceration occurs. The ulceration of the tongue is particularly dangerous as it is apt to be followed by cancer of the tongue. Fortunately, with improved methods of treating syphilis, gummas and syphillitic ulcers are nowadays seldom seen. The end of the third stage of syphilis is often accompanied by disease of the large blood vessel, the aorta (q.v.), while later still the germs which have been allowed to remain undestroyed in the brain and spinal cord, where they settled down during the secondary stage, become active and give rise to obvious symptoms of disease of the nervous system.

Treatment of Syphilis in Adults. The importance of early treatment of the disease has already been stressed. But before treatment can be started, accurate recognition of the condition in its earliest stage is essential, and it should be the duty of everyone who notices a sore after exposure to infection to be examined by a doctor. If treatment is commenced early and prolonged by means of adequate doses of penicillin and the newer antibiotics (though long-acting procaine penicillin seems to be the most effective), before the germs have had time to get into the blood and spread themselves throughout the body, there is every reason to suppose that the disease may be really cured. Arsenic and bismuth preparations are still sometimes used as adjuvant treatment but are being superseded by the antibiotics. But once the secondary stage has been reached and germs have managed to get hidden away in the various organs, there is always a danger that however energetic treatment may be, many germs may not be reached, and later on they may resume their activity.

Fortunately there are certain kinds of blood tests, the Wassermann and Kahn reactions, which not only show the doctor whether or not syphilis is present in a particular patient, but also tells him how the treatment is affecting the course of the disease.

The question of marriage is often a problem to the patient who has suffered from syphilis. It can be stated that during the first and secondary stages the disease is highly infectious, and an individual who married, even while undergoing treatment, in either of these stages would be committing a crime against the human race. In the tertiary stage the chances of infection are less, but they are still probable. It is impossible to lay down any fixed period after infection when it would be absolutely safe for an individual who has suffered from untreated syphilis to marry. With regard to patients who have been energetically treated, the doctor who has treated them is the one who is best able to judge when the disease has been stamped out; the earlier treatment is begun, the more likely the chance of complete cure.

Congenital Syphilis. The children born of parents suffering from syphilis are liable to show the symptoms of the later stages of the disease. In these children the disease is always generalized, and any part of the body may suffer. The bones, the skin, the joints, and the liver are commonly affected. The eyes may be attacked if the children survive the infant period,

while a particularly complete form of deafness may occur in the early teens.

Treatment of Congenital Syphilis. The treatment of congenital syphilis really begins with the treatment of the mother while she is pregnant. If such treatment is thoroughly carried out, there is every chance that a healthy child will be born. Once the child is born, the treatment follows the same lines as those of adults. Penicillin in adequate dosage is as well tolerated by infants as it is by adults.

SYRINGE. Syringes are used for injecting fluids into the body or into its passages and cavities. There is a variety of shapes and sizes of syringe, which may be used for different purposes. A very useful form of syringe is that known as the bulb syringe, chiefly used for giving enemas or for using as a vaginal douche, though it is also useful for douching the nose or the ear. For douching the ears or nose there also are rubber syringes with a round or pear-shaped bulb attached, sometimes with a bone or vulcanite nozzle. Hypodermic syringes are made in many sizes, and they are used for injecting drugs directly into the body under the skin or into a vein. Syringes should be capable of being thoroughly sterilized.

SYRINGOMYELIA. This is a disease of the spinal cord in which there is a new growth in the gray matter around the central canal. The symptoms vary a great deal with the extent of the disease. There is loss of sensation to pain and an inability to feel heat or cold, so that such a patient may burn himself without knowing it. Another symptom is wasting of the muscles. The disease develops very slowly and is sometimes greatly relieved by deep X-ray treatment. (*See also* SPINAL CORD.)

TABES. This is an ancient Greek word which was used in medicine over two thousand years ago. It was used then to describe general wasting diseases, but it now means tabes dorsalis or locomotor ataxia, a nervous disorder caused by an old syphilitic infection of the spinal cord and brain.

TABES DORSALIS (LOCOMOTOR

ATAXIA.) This is a chronic disease of the nervous system which is one of the late results of syphilis. It is found in men at least ten times as commonly as in women, and the symptoms may first appear as long as twenty years after the infection. Fortunately it is nowadays much less common than it used to be.

Symptoms. The disease is due to destruction of the conducting paths in the spinal cord which carry certain forms of sensation to the brain from the nerves in the limbs. Consequently one of the features of the disorder is a loss of the sense of position in space. If a person with tabes dorsalis is asked to stand with his feet together and is then asked to shut his eyes, he sways from one side to the other, and may even fall, because no impressions as to where his feet are will reach his brain and so he cannot keep his balance without using his sense of sight. Similarly, if asked to point with his index finger to his nose, keeping his eyes shut, he will be unable to do so, but aided by his eyesight, he can do this perfectly. Changes in the coverings of the spinal cord (the meninges) produce pains, the character of which is peculiar to the disease.

These are called "lightning" pains, and they occur in bouts. They are felt as short stabs, rather as if red-hot needles were being pushed into the skin, through the limbs, not along them. These pains move about; at one time they are felt in the legs, at another time in the arms or in the back, but their character remains the same. They are especially liable to be felt at any spot where a bone comes to the surface, as at the ankle or wrist. This symptom of "lightning" pains may be present for many years before any other symptoms are complained of. In fact, it is not out of place to say here that tabes dorsalis has so altered its nature as a result of the early treatment of syphilis that twenty or more years may pass before a patient with this disorder suffers any more inconvenience from his trouble than occasional bouts of these pains.

But much depends on early treatment of the disease, and a patient in early middle life who suffers from what he thinks are bouts of "rheumatic" pains should at all events be examined to make sure that his pains are not the "lightning" pains of tabes dorsalis. By the time that pains are felt, certain signs are already present, such as changes in the normal reaction of the pupils of the eyes to light, which will enable the disease to be recognized. If it is not recognized at this stage, sooner or later unsteadiness in walking will appear, the patient noticing that this unsteadiness is greater in the dark. He will also notice

that he is apt to stagger when his eyes are covered, as when he washes his face. Sometimes, other pains are felt in the different organs of the body, and are commonly called "crises," because they are so severe that often they have led to unnecessary surgery.

The commonest of these "crises" is the stomach crisis. Every few weeks for months on end, the patient has attacks of intense pain and sickness, which for a time are bad enough to stop him working. These attacks last for a few days to a week, and then during the intervals between attacks, he has no pain or sickness whatever. There is also a crisis of the throat, in which the patient gets a spasm of the muscles of the throat accompanied by a barking, or crowing cough somewhat resembling whooping cough. These two are the commonest "crises," but there may be severe attacks of pain in the back passage, again occurring in bouts with intervals of freedom from pain. One other symptom which may arise quite early in the course of the disease is a mistiness of vision. This is rather serious, as it is due to a destruction of the nerve of sight itself.

Treatment. The treatment of tabes dorsalis is important, as by modern methods the disease can be so arrested that the stage at which a patient stages about and is stiff in his legs when walking is never reached. As a rule, the later the disease comes on, the better the outlook, whatever form of treatment is carried out. The course of the disease is much slower when it begins in people of from 50–55 years of age than when it attacks those of from 35–45; but the main thing is to have the trouble recognized early, so that the right treatment can be given. Penicillin is the most useful drug, given for a prolonged period or in repeated courses; bismuth and potassium iodide are still useful, usually given before the penicillin; fever therapy is now seldom used. In those patients who come under observation late in the course of the disorder, their most distressing symptom is difficulty in walking. Certain exercises have been devised by Frenkel to help these people to re-educate their muscles, so to speak. It has already been shown that the difficulty in walking is due to the fact that when a patient cannot see his limbs he is unaware of their position. Frenkel's exercises are directed towards improving the use of those nerve paths and fibers which are undamaged by the disease. The patient is taught to move his limbs quite accurately. For instance, he may be put on a couch and made to move his feet from square to square on a big wooden frame so that the heel is correctly placed on various marked spots, or he may be made to walk to a certain pattern laid out on the floor. These exercises not only make the best use of what undamaged nervous tissue is left, but what is even more important they give the patient confidence in himself. (*See also* SYPHILIS.)

TACHYCARDIA. Rapid action of the heart is described as tachycardia. (*See also* HEART; PULSE.)

TAENIA. This word means a band or ribbon, and the term taenia is applied to certain bands of nerve fibers in the brain. It is also the biological name for the tapeworm. (*See also* BRAIN; WORM.)

TALC. Talcum powder, or talc, consists chiefly of the silicate of magnesium. It is a very soothing dusting powder for the skin, and as it absorbs perspiration, it is especially useful for the feet and armpits. Sometimes an antiseptic, such as salicylic acid, is added to it. (*See also* MAGNESIUM.)

TALIPES. Clubfoot is a more popular name for this deformity. (*See* CLUBFOOT.)

TALUS. The talus, astragalus, or ankle bone, is the second largest bone of the foot. It rests on top of the heel bone and lies between it and the tibia or leg bone. (*See also* ANKLE.)

TAMPON. A wad of cotton wool rolled into a ball and used for plugging one of the cavities of the body, is described as a tampon. Drugs such as glycerine, tannin, and iodoform are often used along with the tampon. (*See also* SWAB.)

TANTALUM. This is a heavy but easily bent and molded metal, used chiefly in the repair of defects in the skull caused by injury.

TANNIN. Tannic acid, or tannin, is obtained from oak-galls and it is also present in several varieties of plants. When brought in contact with any tissue or mucous membrane, tannic acid dries it up, and because of this action is used in the treatment of ulcers, sores, and various moist eruptions. A solution of tannic acid sprayed over a burn will act as a protective covering. Tannin is also used as a styptic, which is the term used for any drug capable of stopping hemorrhage. In this way it is employed in cases of bleeding of the bowel, gums, fissures and ulcers and it is also used in tonsillitis, pharyngitis and diarrhea. Suppositories containing tannin are used for piles. (*See also* GALL.)

TAPEWORM. *See* WORM.

TAPPING. This term is used to signify the removal of fluid from a body cavity or from the tissues under the skin. Many inflammations cause the rapid effusion of watery fluid in one of the body cavities. Fluid accumulates, for example, in the pleural cavity in wet pleurisy, and the pressure so caused may interfere with the working of the heart and lungs. The fluid is removed by inserting a hollow needle attached to a syringe, or by a trocar and cannula, or by a special instrument called an aspirator.

TAR. Prepared coal tar is used medicinally in the form of liquor carbonis and liquor carbonis detergens. These preparations have antiseptic properties and, applied externally to the skin, have a stimulating action. They are mildly anesthetic and are valuable in relieving itching. In the treatment of psoriasis and chronic dermatitis, a tar ointment is often prescribed. Care must be taken in applying the ointments, as their excessive use may lead to irritation and blistering of the skin and in some cases to wart formation. (*See also* PINE.)

TARSUS. This is the collective name given to the seven bones which make up the ankle and adjacent part of the foot. (*See also* FOOT.)

TARTAR. The deposit which collects round the necks and adjoining parts of the teeth is described as dental tartar. It is hard, firmly adherent, light brown in color, and is derived from stagnating saliva or mucus on parts of the teeth not subject to friction. Tartar should be removed by scaling of the teeth. The eating of food requiring thorough chewing, and slightly acid in reaction—salad vegetables and fresh fruit—will help to prevent the formation of the deposits.

TARTAR EMETIC. *See* ANTIMONY.

TARTARIC ACID. Either in the form of free acid or of acid tartrate of potassium, tartaric acid is widely distributed in the vegetable kingdom, the most abundant source being the grape. It is chiefly used in combination with carbonates and bicarbonates for the production of effervescing and cooling drinks. The average of dose is from 5 to 20 grains. Larger doses produce stomach irritation.

TASTE. On the tongue are situated a number of fine nerve endings grouped together to form taste buds. To stimulate these nerves the substance must be in solution, and the sensations aroused fall into four groups sweet, sour, salt, and bitter. Sweetness is most appreciated by the tip of the tongue; sourness at the sides and bitterness at the back. It should be realized that the sense of smell is a powerful adjunct to the sense of taste. Flavors are often thought of as tastes, but actually they are really compound sensations of taste and smell. This explains why a "cold in the head" renders the food tasteless.

Loss of taste (*ageusia*) may arise if the tongue is too dry—or if its surface is disordered by the presence of furring. It will also occur if the nerve paths which convey the taste sensations to the brain are injured or the taste area in the brain is damaged. In the latter case, curious sensations of unpleasant tastes may result. Perversion of taste may occur in hysteria and in insanity. A bad taste in the mouth is most often a sequel to digestive disturbance, particularly constipation; more rarely it may arise when certain drugs such as mercury are taken. (*See also* SENSATION; SMELL; TONGUE.)

TATTOOING. The only method of removing tattoo marks is by cutting out the tattooed skin.

TEA. Tea has no actual food value, though the alkaloid extracted from it, theine, is practically the same as caffeine, which is extracted from coffee, and is a fairly harmless stimulant.

Tea poisoning is not unknown as a consequence of too much habitual tea drinking. Faintness, low spirits and attacks of nervousness are symptoms of this condition.

TEARS. These are the watery and slightly salty drops of fluid which moisten the eyes and which are produced abundantly during grief. They are secreted by the lachrymal glands, situated in the outer part of the orbit just above the eyeball. It is necessary for the cornea of the eye to be kept moist in order to preserve its transparency and the tears are carried across the eye by the blinking movements of the eyelids. The stream of tears also washes foreign bodies, e.g. dust, off the eyes, and has a slightly antiseptic action. Overflow of tears on the face (excepting during weeping) results when there is an obstruction to the tear passages leading to the nose. Children do not secrete tears at birth; this function is not established till three to four weeks of age. (*See also* EYE *and* LACHRYMAL APPARATUS.)

TEETH. A tooth is made up of a crown a neck and one or more roots or fangs. The greater part of the tooth is composed of dentine, or ivory, and over the crown there is a hard, brittle, white shell called enamel. The dentine surrounds a cavity containing the pulp. This consists of fine blood vessels, nerves, and connective tissue. On top of the crown are two or more elevations or cups which aid the chewing of the food. The teeth are fixed in sockets in the upper and lower jawbones, and between the root of the tooth and the wall of the socket is a substance called the cement or crusta petrosa. The gum covers the borders of the jawbones, embraces the teeth at their necks and occupies the space between the teeth.

In a grown-up person there are thirty-two teeth, eight on each side above and below. These are called the second or permanent teeth. The upper row consists of four incisors in the center, sharp and chisel-shaped; on each side of the incisors is one pointed canine; next to the canines are two premolars; then there are three molars on each side. The bottom row is placed in the same way, each upper tooth having a similar one opposite to it. The incisors and canines are for cutting purposes, the premolars and molars, with their broad ridged tops, are for grinding the food. The so-called wisdom teeth are the last molars and they do not erupt till about the twenty-first year. Occasionally they do not appear at all.

The first or milk teeth are cut gradual-

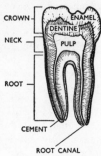

CROWN
NECK
ROOT
ENAMEL
DENTINE
PULP
CEMENT
ROOT CANAL

Structure of Tooth.

ly, the first to appear being the lower central incisors about the sixth month. Then follow the upper central and lateral incisors, and, in this order, the first molars in the twelfth month, the canines in the eighteenth, and the second molars in the twenty-fourth month. There is some degree of variation of the times of eruption even in normal children, but in rickety children, dentition is very much delayed. The second dentition begins to appear about the sixth year with the appearance of the first permanent molars and each year after this the other permanent teeth are cut; the central incisors, the lateral incisors, the first premolar, the second premolar, the canines, and the second molars.

Teething is often accompanied by unpleasant symptoms in the young child. The gums may become hot, swollen and tender and the child feverish, irritable and restless. Many other ailments of infancy are often attributed to teething yet without good reason. Teething difficulties should not require the child to be taken off the breast. Cool boiled water should be given to relieve the hot gums and fluid magnesia to relieve constipation. It is no longer considered good medical practice to lance the gums. In the intervals between eruption of the teeth, hard crusts or slices of hard apple should be given to the child. This practice helps also to develop the jaws and so tends to prevent overcrowding of the teeth with their subsequent deformity and irregularity.

If the teeth are overcrowded, the only remedy is extraction of the offending tooth or teeth. Another important aid to proper jaw development is breast feeding; the vigorous suction required is the natural and best stimulus to growth and expansion of the jawbones.

Note. The constant use of a baby's pacifier is strongly to be condemned.

Care of the Teeth. Diseased teeth and gums may be responsible for many grave diseases, rheumatism, anemia, stomach disorders, etc., therefore great effort should be made to maintain them in a healthy condition. Visits to the dentist should commence from the first year and be continued at regular intervals throughout life. Tooth and gum brushing should be practised from childhood, regularly twice a day—night and morning—and there should be a sufficiency of lime and vitamin foods in the dietary, for these are essential for the correct nutrition and growth of the teeth. Such foods are milk, wholemeal cereals, fruits, green vegetables and dairy produce generally. Caries (dental decay) and pyorrhea (gum suppuration) are always a result of faulty hygiene. Pain in a tooth, or toothache, may be due to exposure of the sensitive pulp through caries. If a cavity is obvious, to relieve the pain a little flat pad of cotton-wool soaked in oil of cloves should be applied temporarily. It is the painless type of abscess at the roots of the teeth which is most liable to cause disease in other parts of the body. These abscesses are little poison factories fouling the bloodstream, and removal of the tooth is the

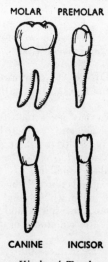

MOLAR   PREMOLAR

CANINE   INCISOR

Kinds of Teeth.

only remedy. Very often it requires an X-ray photograph to detect the offending tooth.

To Stop Bleeding After Extraction. Excessive bleeding after a tooth is extracted may be stopped by plugging the socket with a pad of cotton-wool and biting firmly on to it.

Care of Artificial Teeth. Those who wear artificial teeth should strive to keep the mouth clean and healthy. The teeth should be removed after every meal and the denture brushed with a mild antiseptic lotion. The mouth ought also to be rinsed and any natural teeth brushed. For a vulcanite plate, hydrogen peroxide makes a pleasant lotion; but for a metal plate a weak solution of chlorinated water will be necessary to keep the metal bright. Tooth powders should not be used for artificial teeth, as they tend to remove the polish. The surface is best cleaned with soap on a cloth rubbed vigorously the long way of the tooth.

TELANGIECTASIS. This is a term used to denote dilatation of the small blood vessels in the skin. It is seen most commonly on the face in a localized area and has the appearance of a birthmark. A variety resulting from exposure to the weather, or from a local injury is called a "spider naevus." If the patches of telangiectasis are not very large, they can be removed by carbonic acid snow or radium. It is inadvisable to use caustics for this purpose. (*See also* BIRTHMARKS.)

TEMPERATURE. The degree of heat or coldness of any substance or body is known as its temperature. The body temperature of man is remarkably constant in health, being about 98.6 deg. F. There is a daily variation of about 1 deg. F., the highest level being reached in the evening. After a meal or hard exercise, the temperature may be raised slightly. Regulation of the body temperature is under control of the brain. Heat is produced chiefly in the muscles and larger organs, and it is got rid of by radiation and conduction from the skin and by sweating. A balance is maintained between heat production and heat loss. If a large amount of heat is produced the skin vessels relax and dilate, more blood passes to the surface of the body and is so cooled; also, sweating takes

place and the evaporation of sweat cools the circulating blood.

Disease may upset the temperature regulating mechanism in the brain and the temperature may rise or fall much below normal. Poisons from germs are liable to affect the temperature centre and raised temperature or fever results. This fever is really a protective response on the part of the body, as a high temperature hinders the activities of the germs. In certain diseases, notably general paralysis of the insane, high temperatures are produced artificially, e.g. by malarial infection, in order to relieve the symptoms of the disease. An exceedingly high temperature—above 105 deg. F.—is called hyperpyrexia and calls for special measures to lower the temperature. A subnormal temperature below 96 deg. F. may be evidence of shock or collapse and may be equally serious. The temperature of the body is measured with the clinical thermometer.

TEMPORAL BONE. This bone takes part in the formation of the temple. The internal ear is placed deeply in it, protected by the mastoid air cells. It is irregularly shaped and is made up of several parts. There is a thin plate-like portion which helps to form the side wall of the skull. Below and behind this part it becomes thickened and projects downwards to form the mastoid process. This process forms an attachment for the powerful sternomastoid muscle. Above and in front of this process is the opening of the bony part of the outer air passage, and forwards there is a thin piece of bone called the styloid process giving attachment to various muscles.

Projecting in front of the ear opening is the zygomatic process which helps to form the arch of the cheek. Beneath the back part of this process is the joint surface for the mandible or lower jaw. Another portion of the temporal bone is directed inwards and forms part of the base of the skull. It is pear-shaped and contains the internal ear. The internal carotid artery runs through a part of this bone and the internal jugular vein is in close relation to it.

TENDERNESS. When pressure on a part of the body produces a sore painful sensation the part is said to be tender.

Often tenderness is associated with inflammation. Muscle tenderness may be due to injury, but very often it is caused by a rheumatic inflammation.

TENDON. The white fibrous structure which connects a muscle to the bone is termed a tendon. Its fibers are tough and strong and do not give much. Tendons vary in their shape; they may be rounded like cords—long and slender as in the limbs, while others may be flat and sheet-like as in the case of the abdominal (belly) muscle. Where it passes over a bone, a tendon usually runs in a fibrous sheath lined with a smooth moist membrane. Small bones (sesamoid bones), may develop in a tendon where it is subjected to special stress, the kneecap being an example of this.

The tendons of the wrist and hand are sometimes subject to acute inflammation especially following a poisoned wound of the thumb or little finger. This condition is called teno-synovitis. Teno-synovitis may also arise as a result of rheumatic disease. Occasionally, the tendon of the heel (tendo Achilles) may be snapped by a sudden severe strain. The muscles tend to pull the severed ends apart and an operation is necessary to join them together again. In some deformities of the feet, it may be necessary to sever tendons, an operation called tenotomy.

TENDON JERK. This is the response by contraction of a muscle when the tendon is tapped briskly. The knee jerk is an example of this and its presence denotes that the nerve continuity to and from the spinal cord is intact.

TENESMUS. Painful, frequent straining to empty the bowel, usually ineffectual, is termed tenesmus. Sometimes a little blood or mucus is passed. It may arise when the bowel is loaded with hard masses of feces, or it may be provoked by a fissure of the anus or a growth in the rectum. Tenesmus is quite frequently caused by diarrhea, particularly the diarrhea associated with dysentery. In young children it may be produced by worms in the bowel or it may be caused by intussusception. In this latter condition the infant has fits of screaming and blood and slime are passed.

TENNIS ELBOW. This injury is most frequently caused by playing tennis, though it can easily be caused otherwise. The pain may arise suddenly during a game or it may develop slowly. It is felt on the outer side of the front of the elbow and runs down the arm, rendering it impossible to use the arm. Backhand strokes at tennis are more liable to cause this disability than forehand. There is usually a particularly tender spot below the bony prominence on the outer side of the elbow. With rest there is a temporary recovery, but when play is resumed the symptoms are apt to recur.

The cause of tennis elbow is either a small rupture of some of the fibers of the muscles which extend to the wrist and fingers, or an inflammation of a small bursa or bag which exists between these muscles and the head of the radius bone which rotates underneath.

Treatment. Immediate treatment is to apply a firm pad to the painful spot and control it with strapping. Rest is essential and it is generally necessary to discover if there is any small area (focus) of germ infection in the body (i.e. teeth or tonsils), for a permanent cure will not be obtained until such focus is eradicated. In some cases a minor operation for the removal of the bursa may be necessary. (*See also* BURSITIS.)

TENOTOMY. *See* TENDON.

TERATOMA. This is a tumor or growth which contains developmental (embryonic) remains such as teeth, hair, and muscle. It is derived from the primitive cell layers of the embryo and the cause of its development is obscure. Most often this tumor is found in the genital (sex) organs—e.g., the testicle or ovary. Such tumors are easy to remove by surgical operation.

TERRAMYCIN. This is one of the newer antibiotics, derived from a mold growing in the soil. It is particularly useful in people who are sensitive to penicillin and in certain diseases in which penicillin is ineffective. It is usually given by the mouth, in capsule form, and is used successfully in pneumonia, septicemia, whooping cough, Malta fever, and urinary tract infections. (*See also* PENICILLIN.)

TERTIAN FEVER. This is a variety of the tropical fever called malaria. (*See also* MALARIA.)

TESTICLE. The testicle is the male sex

gland and corresponds to the ovary in the female. There are two, a right and a left, each occupying a compartment in the scrotum, a purse-like bag. The testicles develop originally in the cavity of the abdomen (belly), and just before or after birth reach the scrotum. The testicle has a complicated journey to make before it finally arrives at the scrotum and it carries with it a tubelike process of the lining of the abdomen (the peritoneum) which becomes closed at its upper end and which covers the testicles in front and at the sides. This lining is called the *tunica vaginalis* and, being smooth, it diminishes any friction that might arise from movements of the testicles. Sometimes fluid collects in the bag, a condition called *hydrocele.*

Not infrequently, one or other of the testicles may fail to descend completely. They may remain in the abdomen, or just above the entrance to the scrotum (in the inguinal canal). Such a condition is described as an "undescended testicle," and, if both testicles remain in the abdomen, the individual affected is called a "cryptorchid." If the testicles are in the inguinal canal they may descend at puberty (about fourteen years), but sometimes an operation is necessary. Should the testicles remain in the abdomen, they do not develop properly and the mature sex characteristics do not become manifest. With undescended testicles there is also a danger of an accompanying hernia (rupture), and in such a case an operation is essential to cure the defect. Undescended testicles are more liable to become involved in malignant growths than is normally the case.

The testicle produces sperm cells or spermatozoa. These are the male seeds which, when they fertilize the female eggs, produce a new individual. The sperms are contained in small tubes and make their way along a number of small ducts to reach the main duct of the testicle, called the vas deferens. This leads to the seminal vesicle (reservoir), from which the sperms are discharged during sexual intercourse.

In addition to producing spermatozoa, the testicle has another equally important function. Certain cells (interstitial cells) in the gland produce a secretion which is passed directly into the bloodstream, called an "internal secretion," and it is this secretion which is responsible for the development of the mature sex characters. Absence of the secretion, which may arise after castration (removal of testicles), causes the individual to remain boyish in figure; the skin is smooth and hairless, penis small, voice high-pitched, and there is a tendency to fatness. Such a person is described as a eunuch.

Inflammation of the body of the testicle is called orchitis, and of the upper tubular portion, epididymitis. Orchitis is liable to arise as a complication of mumps, and epididymitis is a common sequel to gonorrheal infection. Treatment is rest in bed, support for the testicle by raising it on a pillow, and hot or cold applications. Sulphonamides or penicillin should be given when the cause is gonorrhea. Chronic inflammation of the testicle may follow acute attacks or arise from syphilis or tuberculosis. The gland tends to break down, becomes adherent to the scrotum, and may ultimately discharge through the skin. Treatment depends upon the cause. In some cases the testicle may have to be removed by operation. Injuries to the testicles from kicks, etc., cause a sickening pain and may lead to dangerous shock. (*See also* EPIDIDYMIS; HYDROCELE; SCROTUM; SPERMATIC CORD; VARICOCELE.)

TEST MEAL. A meal given to obtain information concerning the digestive function is described as a test meal. Generally the patient takes a light supper and, first thing in the morning, a stomach tube is swallowed and the stomach contents, if any, drawn off for examination. If food is present it is evidence of stagnation in the stomach. Then the meal is given: it usually consists of a pint of gruel. One hour afterwards the stomach contents are drawn off and their examination reveals much useful information to the physician, especially with regard to the quantity and quality of the stomach secretion. Another method is to carry out a fractional test, i.e. successive portions of the contents are withdrawn from the stomach at fifteen-minute intervals. Opaque meals, consisting of bismuth carbonate along with milk, bread, and corn-flour, are given before X-ray examination to determine the position, size, and shape of the stomach and the way in which a meal passes down the digestive tract.

TETANUS. Tetanus, which is more commonly known as lockjaw, is due to a germ which enters the body and then produces a virulent toxin which poisons all the tissues. The germ is found in soil, and as it is extremely resistant to the effects of heat and cold it may go on living for years. It is even resistant to the effects of ordinary antiseptics, so it is easy to understand why the control of this disease presents a difficult problem. The germ lives in the intestines of horses and cattle, and any manured soil is liable to be infected. For the development of tetanus it is necessary that there should be some opening in the skin through which the germ can gain entrance to the body, and the wound must come in touch with the germ through soil. During the first World War numerous cases occurred, but preventive measures were taken by injecting all cases of wounds with antitetanic serum.

Symptoms. Symptoms usually begin to appear seven or eight days after infection of the wound, but the longer the symptoms take to appear, the better the chances are of recovery. The first signs of the disease are stiffness of the throat muscles, with difficulty in swallowing. The patient has difficulty in opening the mouth, and gradually the neighboring muscles begin to contract, giving the face a peculiar expression. The spasm extends to the muscles of the back, chest, abdomen, and limbs, and the patient has frequently recurring seizures which are terrible to watch. The skin is moist or sweating, but the patient never loses consciousness and is unhappily aware of his serious condition.

In *local tetanus,* the contractions are limited to the muscles surrounding the wound, but such cases never become severe. *Tetanus neonatorum* may occur in newborn infants, the symptoms showing themselves within a week or so of birth. Infection usually takes place through the severed umbilical cord, and convulsions may be the first sign of the disease.

Treatment. The early administration of antitetanic serum should be carried out in any case of a wound which may have been contaminated by soil. Once the symptoms of tetanus appear much larger doses are given, and they should be injected into the spinal canal or into the skull cavity.

Penicillin is given by injection because it destroys the tetanus germ, though it has no effect on the toxin already produced. Various drugs are given to relieve the spasms and to allow the patient to take nourishment. Only liquid food is given and a feeding-tube may be used if necessary. The patient must be kept absolutely quiet in a darkened room as the slightest disturbance is liable to cause a spasm. When the spasms are very severe, relief may be given with inhalations of chloroform. People exposed to an unusual risk of contracting tetanus such as agricultural workers and members of the fighting forces can be protected by immunization with tetanus toxoid. (*See also* SERA.)

TETANY. This is an affection in which there arise spasms of certain muscles. It is due to overexcitability of the nervous system. The muscles most often affected are those of the arms and hands. The elbows and wrist are bent and the fingers squeezed together. Sometimes the lower limbs are similarly affected and occasionally the face. In children, rickets is the chief cause, especially if it is associated with some derangement of digestion. In adults the condition follows removal of the parathyroid glands, tiny structures situated in the thyroid gland in the neck. The actual disorder is due to some disturbance of the calcium (lime) salts in the blood.

Treatment. Tetany in the child calls for the remedying of the coexisting rickets. Sunshine, ultraviolet rays, codliver oil, and nourishing food generally are indicated. Large doses of calcium chloride also help. Occasionally, it may be necessary to prescribe small doses of a nerve sedative such as chloral hydrate. Extract of parathyroid gland with calcium is also given for this affection. (*See also* RICKETS.)

THERAPEUTICS. This word signifies the branch of medicine which deals with the treatment and cure of the sick in all aspects.

THERMOCAUTERY. This is an instrument for burning or destroying unwanted tissues, e.g. tumors, in the body. There are many varieties and those commonly used today are heated electrically. They consist of a handle through which wires carrying an electrical current are led and to which various platinum burners—

pointed, blunt, or flattened like a knife—
are attached. The cautery is useful for
removing polypi and for arresting bleeding.

THERMOMETER. This is an instrument for recording and measuring temperature. The essential part is a substance
which expands under the influence of heat,
and the substance most commonly used is
mercury. When it is desired to measure
very low temperature, a spirit (alcohol)
thermometer is used. The instrument consists of a small glass bulb, the reservoir
for the mercury, connected with a glass
tube to which is attached a graduated
scale. No air must be present in the tube,
which is sealed.

To graduate the thermometer, two fixed
points are determined, the freezing point
of water and its boiling point. The gradua-
tion between these points is arranged in
three recognized scales. In the U.S. we
use the Fahrenheit scale, the freezing point
being fixed at 32 deg. and boiling point
at 212 deg. In Europe the Centigrade scale
is used in which the freezing point is 0,
or zero, and the boiling point 100 deg.

To convert the Fahrenheit scale to Centigrade, substract 32, divide by 9 and
multiply by 5; to convert Centigrade to
Fahrenheit, divide by 5, multiply by 9 and
add 32.

The instrument used to take the temperature of the body is called the clinical
thermometer. It is generally graduated
from 95 deg. to 110 deg. in the Fahrenheit scale, each degree being divided into
fifths, corresponding to the decimal .2. In
some varieties the glass in front magnifies,
and so renders reading easier. Normal body
temperature, 98.6 deg., is generally marked
with an arrow.

Taking the Temperature. First cleanse
the instrument by placing in an antiseptic
such as carbolic lotion and then wash in
ordinary water. Shake the thermometer
vigorously to make sure that the mercury
is well below the normal mark. In an
adult the temperature is generally taken
in the mouth or armpit, and in the child
in the groin with the thigh folded upon the
abdomen. It may also be taken in the
rectum. In the mouth, the thermometer
should be placed just under the tip of the
tongue and the lips kept tightly closed.
In the armpit, it is important to ensure

that the skin surfaces are quite dry and
that no clothing is allowed to lie between
the bulb and the skin.

Leave the thermometer in position for at
least two minutes. Some thermometers are
less sensitive than others—so it is well to
make sure of getting the correct reading
by leaving the instrument in position a
sufficiently long time. After use, the
thermometer should be rinsed in antiseptic,
shaken down, and either returned to its
case or placed in a little jar, with a plug
of wool at the bottom to prevent breakage,
and containing some antiseptic lotion. (*See
also* TEMPERATURE.)

THIGH. That part of the lower limb
from the hip to the knee is described as the
thigh. The large bone of this region is
called the femur, and it is clothed with
large and powerful muscles. In front are
the quadriceps which straighten the leg at
the knee, behind are the hamstrings which
bend the knee, and on the inner side are
the adductor muscles passing from the
haunch bone to the femur and serving to
adduct or bring the thigh towards its fellow. All the muscles are enclosed in a
strong fibrous sheath from which partitions
arise and pass between the different muscles. In men, the outlines of the various
muscles are visible to the eye; but in wom-
en the greater amount of fat under the skin
obscures them.

There are two other very important
structures in the thigh, the femoral artery
and the sciatic nerve. The main artery
enters about the middle of the groin, where
it can be compressed against the bone in
an emergency, and runs down to the inner
side of the knee where it passes behind
into the space behind the knee. The sciatic
nerve, the largest in the body, runs down
the middle of the back of the thigh and
in the lower part divides into two branches.
Painful conditions of this nerve are called
sciatica; frequently this affection is of
rheumatic origin, but it may, though less
frequently, arise from some pressure within
the pelvis.

THINNESS. Excessive thinness may be
evidence of disease especially if it is of
recent development. In such cases the doctor should always be consulted, for loss
of weight may be caused by such grave
diseases as tuberculosis, diabetes, kidney

disease and cancer. Thinness in healthy persons can often be overcome by correct exercise and by attention to the diet. Anxiety is often a cause of thinness and is inconsistent with perfect health.

THIOURACIL. This is a chemical substance that combats the effects of the natural secretion of the thyroid gland, and is given in cases of toxic goiter (Graves' disease), and also before operations on the thyroid gland. (*See also* THYROID GLAND.)

THIRST. This is the expression of the need of the body for replenishment with fluid. The sensation is associated with dryness of the throat and mouth. During 24 hours the kidneys get rid of about 2½ pints of water, while the lungs and skin lose considerable quantities. Therefore, to make good the loss, fresh supplies of fluid are needed, and thirst is the signal that this is necessary. Thirst arises after vigorous muscular exercise owing to the excretion of sweat; it is very intense if a large quantity of blood is lost from any cause, or after profuse watery diarrhea, as in cholera. In fevers, thirst is generally a prominent symptom owing to increased heat production and sweating. The thirst which follows the taking of salt or sugar is an indication of the need for dilution of those substances in the digestive tract and the blood.

Inadequate water drinking is a cause of constipation. People working in great heat usually find oatmeal or barley water more efficacious as a thirst quencher than plain water. Iced drinks should always be used in moderation as the stomach may easily be upset by the extreme cold. (*See also* DIET.)

THOMSEN'S DISEASE. This condition is called after the Danish physician who first described it. Technically, it is known as myotonia congenita, and it is shown by stiffness of the muscles on voluntary movement. There is a delay in carrying out muscular actions, in some cases the muscles becoming rigid. In a few seconds this rigidity passes and the muscles can be used again quite normally. The spasms are most marked in the limbs, and emotion aggravates the affection. The cause is unknown, but it is believed to be associated with excessive excitability of the muscle fibers. The disease first shows itself in childhood and usually several members of the same family are affected. No cure is known, but quinine often gives relief, and regular exercise seems to help to some extent.

THORACIC DUCT. This is the main lymphatic channel of the body. It is a tube about 18 in. long, commencing in the upper part of the abdominal cavity and passing upwards through the diaphragm, thence through the thorax or chest to reach the root of the neck where it joins the junction of two large veins, the left internal jugular and the left subclavian veins. The lower extremity is dilated in the form of a small cistern, called the *receptaculum chyli,* which receives lymph from the lower part of the body and the intestines. It is by the thoracic duct that a great deal of the nourishment derived from the intestines eventually reaches the bloodstream.

Poisons absorbed from the intestines may also gain access to the bloodstream through this channel. The thoracic duct also gathers lymph from the left side of the chest and the left side of the neck and head. There is a much smaller tube, the right lymphatic duct, which gathers lymph from the right side of the upper part of the body.

THORAX. The bony cage forming the skeleton of the chest is called in anatomy the thorax. It is bounded in front by the sternum or breastbone, behind by the vertebral column, and at the sides by the ribs. Separating it from the abdomen is the diaphragm muscle. The operation of withdrawing fluid from the thoracic cavity is termed *thoracentesis,* while the operation of removing portions of ribs to enable the lung to collapse is termed *thoracoplasty.* (*See also* CHEST; LUNG; PLEURA.)

THREAD WORM. *See* WORM.

THROAT. This is rather a wide and general term, but should be limited in medicine to the upper part of the digestive canal, from the tonsils to the beginning of the esophagus or gullet. It is described as the pharynx, and is dealt with under that heading.

THROBBING *See* PALPITATION AND PULSATION.

THROMBOSIS. This term refers to the clotting of blood within the heart or blood

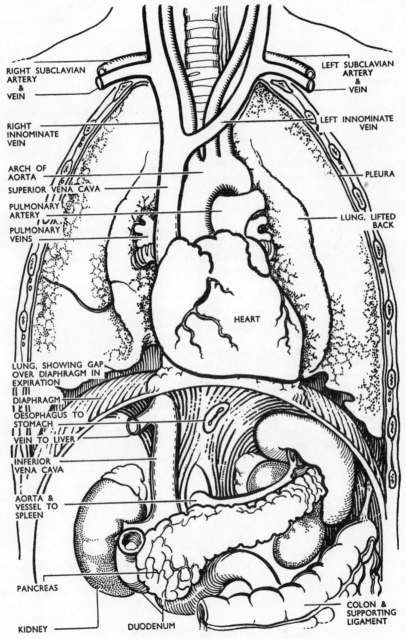

RIGHT SUBCLAVIAN ARTERY & VEIN

RIGHT INNOMINATE VEIN

ARCH OF AORTA

SUPERIOR VENA CAVA

PULMONARY ARTERY

PULMONARY VEINS

LEFT SUBCLAVIAN ARTERY & VEIN

LEFT INNOMINATE VEIN

PLEURA

LUNG, LIFTED BACK

HEART

LUNG, SHOWING GAP OVER DIAPHRAGM IN EXPIRATION

DIAPHRAGM

OESOPHAGUS TO STOMACH

VEIN TO LIVER

INFERIOR VENA CAVA

AORTA & VESSEL TO SPLEEN

PANCREAS

KIDNEY

DUODENUM

COLON & SUPPORTING LIGAMENT

The Thorax and Upper Part of the Abdomen.

vessels during life, and the clot is itself described as a thrombus. Healthy blood does not clot in healthy vessels, but if the circulation is slow or there is any roughening in the vessel walls, or if there are certain blood changes, clotting readily occurs and often extends to where the blocked vessel joins a larger one.

Symptoms. These depend upon the stopping of the blood flow. In some cases, thrombosis is beneficial, as in aneurism where there is a dilation of an artery and the walls are consequently weakened. In this condition the clot tends to strengthen the arterial wall and prevent its rupture. In general, however, the effects of thrombosis are harmful. If it occurs in the leg, pain, swelling and disablement arise. Vein thrombosis in the leg sometimes occurs after childbirth or during typhoid fever. In the brain, thrombosis leads to some degree of paralysis which tends to become more extensive, while in the heart thrombosis may cause sudden death.

Sometimes a clot may soften and there is a danger that a small piece may be washed off and carried to a distant organ to block a blood vessel. This is called embolism. Should there be any infection in the clot, the septic fragments may give rise to abscesses in various parts of the body, a grave state of affairs. In other cases, the clot may be converted into scar or fibrous tissue, obliterating completely the aperture of the blood vessel. It is in this way that a varicose vein may be cured naturally.

Treatment. This naturally depends upon the cause. The immediate remedy is rest for the affected part, and nowadays the doctor will probably use an anticoagulant drug, such as heparin. In the case of a limb, it should be well padded with cottonwool and the patient is not permitted to move the limb. Thrombosis in a varicose vein is usually treated by strapping the affected limb and encouraging the patient to remain up and about. (*See also* EMBOLISM; PYEMIA; WHITE LEG.)

THRUSH. This is an inflammatory disease of the mouth and throat occurring chiefly in delicate and poorly nourished children. It is due to an infection with a fungus, called *oidium albicans,* and it shows itself as grayish-white patches scat-

tered over the mouth. Tenderness of the mouth, digestive disturbance, diarrhea with green stools, and general irritability are the chief symptoms. Occasionally, the disease may spread to the stomach and intestines and it may infect the vagina. Cleanliness and the use of an antiseptic lotion, weak peroxide of hydrogen, along with a purge of castor oil, are the main methods of treatment.

THUMB. The thumb is the most movable of all the digits. There are only two segments as compared with three in the case of the fingers, but the metacarpal bone moves very freely on the wrist bones, while those of the fingers are much more restricted. Certain muscles in the forearm move the thumb, but there is also a small group of muscles forming the ball of the thumb, called the thenar muscles, which widens the range of muscular activities of the thumb. The utility of the thumb depends upon its free range of movements and its power to oppose the other fingers. Loss of the thumb is one of the most crippling accidents that can occur to the hand. Therefore every effort is made to save the whole or even a small portion of an injured thumb. Whitlows sometimes develop in the thumb and there is always danger of spread of infection to the wrist. Dislocation of the thumb is usually a backward one and its reduction often gives rise to considerable difficulty. The thumb is very well supplied with blood vessels and bleeds freely if cut. A firm bandage wound round the thumb from the tip upwards will generally control the bleeding. (*See also* FINGER; HAND.)

THYMECTOMY. This is the operation of removing the thymus gland, carried out in the treatment of myasthenia gravis, a disease of the muscles. (*See also* THYMUS GLAND.)

THYMOL. This is a crystalline substance with the odor of thyme and a burning taste. It is obtained from the essential oil of thyme, horsemint and other plants, and it is a powerful antiseptic; it is of specific value in the treatment of hookworm disease and it is given in large doses to the fasting patient and followed by a saline purge. No oil or alcohol must be taken at the same time, as these dissolve the thymol and cause its rapid absorption with the danger of poisoning. Thymol is used in saturated watery solutions for mouth washes, gargles and lotions. Dissolved in alcohol, it can be used as an inhalation in nasal and bronchial catarrhs.

THYMUS GLAND. This is a pear-shaped gland with the point upwards, consisting of a right and left lobe, situated in the chest immediately beneath the breastbone. It extends upwards into the neck and its base lies upon the heart. Under the microscope, the thymus is seen to consist of masses of lymphocytes (white blood cells) with groups of characteristic cells arranged concentrically called Hassall's corpuscles. Before birth there are two ducts connected with the gland, but these become closed and disappear. The gland grows until about the age of puberty (14 years) and then withers, being replaced by fat and fibrous tissue.

As with other lymphoid tissues, the thymus manufactures white blood cells; but its other functions are a matter of doubt. There appears definitely to be some connection between the thymus and the sex glands. Removal of the sex glands causes persistence of the thymus, and when the thymus is unduly enlarged (status lymphaticus) the sex development is delayed. It would appear as if the secretion of the thymus gland restricts and controls the activities of the sex glands and prevents their precocious development. It also has some effect on causing the disease called myasthenia gravis, which is treated by surgically removing the thymus gland. (*See also* STATUS LYMPHATICUS.)

THYROID CARTILAGE. This cartilage consists of two plates of gristle encasing the main part of the larynx. The meeting-point of the plates forms the prominence of the neck called the "Adam's Apple." (*See also* LARYNX.)

THYROID EXTRACT. This extract is obtained from the fresh thyroid glands of sheep which are dried and reduced to a powder. The extract is standardized to contain a definite percentage of iodine; the synthetic thyroxin is now preferred. Thyroid extract is used extensively in medical practice, particularly in the treatment of thyroid deficiency in children (cretinism) and in the same condition in adults (myxedema). Occasionally it is taken in the treatment of obesity, but in all cases it must be used with care and under a doctor's control.

THYROID GLAND. The thyroid gland belongs to the endocrine system or "ductless" glands of internal secretion. It is situated in the neck and consists of two lobes with a narrow portion (isthmus) joining them together. Each lobe is about two inches long and lies alongside the larynx and upper part of the windpipe. The gland is attached to the cricoid cartilage so that it moves up and down in the act of swallowing. Under the microscope, the thyroid gland is seen to consist of a great many little spaces lined with cube-shaped cells and containing an opaque substance (the colloid secretion of the gland). This secretion is absorbed directly into the bloodstream, the blood supply of the gland being particularly liberal for its size.

The secretion of the thyroid gland, called thyroxin, has a very important effect upon the whole body. It controls the building-up and breaking-down processes (metabolism). It speeds up these processes or slows them down according to the amount of secretion which passes into the bloodstream. Failure of the thyroid gland from birth or an early age leads to a breakdown in development, and the child is stunted in mind and body. This condition is called cretinism and it occurs in all degrees of severity. The cretin is dwarfed, with thick harsh skin, scanty hair, protuberant belly, and is intellectually dull, sometimes to the extent of idiocy. If replacement of the deficient secretion by thyroid extract is commenced sufficiently early, good results are obtained.

In adults, particularly women, a deficiency of the secretion of the gland may occur about the time of the change of life. The woman becomes heavy in mind and body, the hair falls out and the skin becomes coarse. Early treatment with thyroid extract is very beneficial. In contrast, excessive secretion of the thyroid gland causes the condition known as hyperthyroidism. The pulse is rapid, the eyes are prominent and staring, the skin warm and moist, and there is a marked tremor of the hands and fingers. Treatment is by thiouracil or carbimazole, or by radioactive iodine, or, less often, by surgery.

Goiter is the general name given to any enlargement of the thyroid gland, whether accompanied by increase of the internal secretion or not. A simple goiter of slight degree is common in young women and not of much importance. (*See also* CRETINISM; DUCTLESS GLANDS; ENDOCRINE GOITER; MYXEDEMA.)

TIBIA. This is the shinbone, and it is the larger of the two bones of the lower leg. The bone is triangular in section, ending above in two expansions which joint with the thighbone and below by forming the inner prominence of the ankle. The greater part of the tibia is immediately under the skin and can be felt by the finger.

Owing to its exposed position, the tibia is frequently subject to blows and kicks which may result in fracture of the shaft. Such a fracture is usually oblique and not infrequently compound; i.e., the skin is broken and a portion of the bone may protrude. Inflammation of the surrounding membrane of the bone, periostitis, or of the bone itself, osteomyelitis, is a fairly common disease. The tibia may also be affected in rickets, and, becoming curved, is described as a saber shin. Syphilis and tuberculosis sometimes involve the tibia. (*See also* FIBULA; LEG.)

TIC. This is a movement which is repeated time after time without any definite cause or object and which is due to a neurosis (q.v.). A tic or habit spasm, as it is often called, usually represents a movement which would be useful in its proper place, and its origin can often be traced to the continued performance of a movement which at one time was made with a definite and proper purpose. For example, a tic of blinking the eyes may result from bad sight which has been corrected by glasses or from some injury to the eye. Normally, these movements should stop when the causes which called them forth are removed, but in nervous people, especially in nervous children, the movements become a habit and keep on for a very long time.

Mimicry is a very important cause; or a tic may arise as a result of overwork or general ill health, in which case it usually disappears as the general health improves. The types of tic which may occur are very large in number. Simple tics like sniffing or blinking are the most common, but quite complicated movements of the arms and face may take place. The movements are generally quick, and consist of short spasms, which are something like the movements resulting from an electric shock.

During sleep a tic disappears. In children there is apt to be confusion between the movements of a simple tic and those of St. Vitus's dance (q.v.). In view of the great importance of recognizing the latter condition, any child who has uncontrollable movements for more than a few days should be seen by a doctor. In St. Vitus's dance, however, the same movement is never repeated twice running; in a tic it is the same movement that is repeated over and over again. The treatment of tics is difficult, especially in adults. In children, wholesome neglect of the habit, attention to the general health and mental development is sufficient to cure many cases. In adults, the habit of a tic is usually part of an obsession (q.v.) and is suitable for treatment by psychotherapy.

Tic douloureux is a spasm of the muscles of the face which must not be confused with ordinary tics, as it is due to a neuralgia of the trigeminal nerve. (*See also* NEURALGIA; TRIGEMINAL NERVE.)

TICK. This is a small parasite, belonging to the spider class, which depends upon blood-sucking for its growth and development. Ticks lurk about the ground, in the undergrowth, and, when they obtain a host, man or animal, they fix themselves with a probe furnished with teeth or hooks to the skin and engorge themselves with blood. Both male and female draw blood, but the male undergoes little change during the operation while the female swells up to resemble a reddish purplish berry.

A considerable number of infections are carried by ticks, including the relapsing fever of Equatorial Africa, the spotted fever of the Rocky Mountains, and Texas fever in cattle.

When a tick is fastened to the skin, do not try to pull it off roughly, but bathe it with weak ammonia solution or a little gasoline. Bleeding from the wound should be encouraged, as any possible infection may be washed out in this way. Afterwards, the bite should be dabbed with iodine.

TIN. This is white metal which has a very limited use in medicinal treatment. The oxide of tin is sometimes used for the relief of boils, acne, and pimples, for it has been noticed that workers with tin never suffer from such infections. Occasionally tin-poisoning may arise owing to the acids of preserved fruits dissolving off some of the metal from the can. (*See also* POISONS in FIRST AID SUPPLEMENT.)

TINCTURE. A medicinal solution of a drug in alcohol is termed a tincture. Simple tinctures contain only one drug, examples of such being tinctures of digitalis, opium, and nux vomica. Compound tinctures contain several drugs, e.g., benzoin, camphor, chloroform, and gentian.

With regard to dosage, there are four very poisonous tinctures—aconite, cantharidin, strophanthus, and iodine mitis, the doses of which are from 2–5 minims. Others have a dosage of from 5–15 minims, while strong tincture of iodine and tincture of pyrethrum are only used externally.

TINEA. This is the common name applied to a group of vegetable parasites or fungi which cause a number of skin diseases. The fungi produce spores, and while some varieties of tinea produce disease exclusively in man, others affect both animals and man. The tinea microsporon is the cause of scalp ring-worm in children. Cats and dogs are susceptible to a variety of this tinea and can communicate this to human beings.

TINNITUS. This is a term used to describe noises in the ears; not serious in itself, but annoying and difficult to get rid of. It is usually, but not always, accompanied by deafness, and in a young woman with commencing deafness is usually looked upon as one of the symptoms of otosclerosis. Tinnitus is usually treated by giving the patient a mild sedative (such as phenobarbital). (*See also* DEAFNESS; OTOSCLEROSIS.)

TISSUE. This is a collection of the microscopic cells or elements of the body to form a distinct structure, from which the various parts and organs are built up.

Some structures, such as cartilage, are formed of one tissue only with but the slightest admixture of another; other structures are simple in form, such as the blood vessels, which are formed of fibrous tissue, elastic fibers, and muscular fibers, with an inner layer of endothelial cells; while other structures are much more complex, such as the liver.

TOBACCO. The most important constituent of the tobacco leaf is nicotine, which is present to the extent of from 2 to 5 per cent. This is an oily alkaloid which is volatilized to some degree by heat and so is present in tobacco smoke. Numerous other substances are present in the smoke of tobacco, including hydrocyanic acid, carbon monoxide, pyridine, and ammonia. It is the latter two products of combustion which are responsible for the irritating effects of tobacco smoke.

The poisonous effects of tobacco are produced chiefly through the absorption of the alkaloid nicotine. In very small quantities, nicotine is harmless, but large quantities cause sickness, vomiting, sweating, and diarrhea, and profound muscular relaxation. These are the symptoms which a novice smoker often experiences after his first experiment with tobacco. Tolerance is rapidly gained to tobacco, however, and in moderation no harmful effects arise. It is a useful and pleasurable adjunct to life if used with discretion. Many people find it is stimulating to the brain, others that it has a sedative or quietening effect. The pleasure of smoking is difficult to explain, but probably the rhythmic sucking movements have a good deal to do with it. In some people, a cigarette or pipe of tobacco appears to act as the stimulus to the normal evacuation of the bowels. Smoking by young people is definitely harmful as it affects the digestion and hinders development.

Immoderate use of tobacco in any form is also detrimental to health. Irritation of the throat, loss of appetite, sickness, and diarrhea may arise. The heart becomes irritable, palpitations are experienced, and breathlessness on the slightest exertion is produced. Heavy tobacco smoking may have a serious consequence in impairment of vision. It commences with a dimness of vision and inability to read fine printing.

The color sense is often affected and unless the tobacco consumption is immediately cut down the condition may go on to blindness (tobacco amblyopia). Both eyes are affected equally in this disease.

There appears to be no doubt that long-continued, heavy cigarette smoking is at least one of the most important factors in the causation of cancer of the lung, a disease which has enormously increased in recent years, and which, in spite of the achievements of modern thoracic surgery, is usually fatal.

TOE. The human toes have lost a considerable amount of their freedom of movement in the course of evolution. The great toe is the most useful member, the other four being relatively unimportant from the functional point of view. Each toe consists of three segments, or phalanges, except the great toe, which has only two. In newborn babies the great toe shows much resemblance to a thumb in its grasping power and free movement.

Diseases and deformities of the toes are exceedingly common, mainly as a result of wearing ill-fitting footwear. The pointed shoe or boot causes the big toe to bend inwards towards the second and it may actually be over or under it. This condition is called *hallux valgus,* and to relieve the pressure on the projecting part of the great toe a bursa or serous bag forms. This is very liable to become inflamed and is known as a bunion. Radical treatment for this condition requires the removal of part of the bone by surgical operation. Stiffness of the great toe causing immobility at the chief joint is usually associated with flat-foot. Correction of the flatfoot and the use of proper footwear is necessary in treatment, but an operation may be required in severe cases.

Hammer toe may affect any of the toes, but is most often seen in the second. In this condition there is over-extension at one joint, with marked flexion at another, with the result that the first two segments of the toe become V-shaped with the point upwards. Operation is required to relieve the deformity. Deficient blood supply due to overtight footwear favors the development of chilblains in the young and gangrene in the old. The poor nutrition from this cause also leads to osteoarthritic changes in the joints. (*See also* CORNS; FOOT; HALLUX VALGUS; HAMMER TOE.)

TOLERANCE. People who take certain drugs habitually are able to withstand quantities of the drug which would be dangerous or even fatal to persons not so accustomed. Familiar examples of this are provided by the habitual use of alcohol, tobacco, and opium. In the case of narcotic drugs this tolerance is most marked, and very large doses may become necessary before any effect can be produced. Tolerance probably depends upon an adaptation of the tissues whereby the drugs are readily broken up and excreted.

TOLU. This substance is generally known as Balsam of Tolu. It is fragrant, aromatic, and is used in perfumery, for the making of pastilles, and in medicine as an expectorant, i.e. to stimulate coughing. Balsam of Tolu is used in compound tincture of Benzoin. (*See also* BALSAM.)

TONGUE. The tongue is the mobile muscular organ occupying the floor of the mouth. Its muscle fibers go in various directions and are interlaced. Covering the surface of the tongue is a moist mucous membrane. At the back of this organ there is a V-shaped series of red spots which are called the circumvallate papillae. In front of the V there are numerous little elevations termed the filiform papillae, and dotted here and there are somewhat larger and redder elevations called the fungiform papillae.

The tongue is symmetrical and has a median groove representing the position of the fibrous partition which divides the tongue into lateral halves. The back part of the tongue is bound down to the floor of the mouth. In front the tongue is free, and its undersurface has a smooth covering which is prolonged forwards to form a fold attaching the tongue to the floor of the mouth. This fold is called the frenum and, on either side of it, open the ducts of the submaxillary salivary glands. Occasionally the frenum is too short and hampers the movements of the tongue in speaking. This condition is called tongue-tie.

The tongue is richly supplied with blood, large branches of the external carotid artery, called the linguals, passing into the organ on both sides. All the muscles have a special nerve supply, the hypoglossal

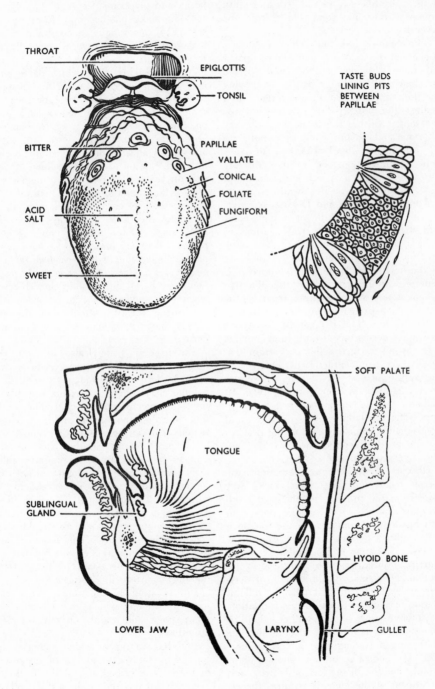

THROAT

EPIGLOTTIS

TONSIL

TASTE BUDS
LINING PITS
BETWEEN
PAPILLAE

BITTER

PAPILLAE

VALLATE

CONICAL

FOLIATE

FUNGIFORM

ACID
SALT

SWEET

SOFT PALATE

TONGUE

SUBLINGUAL
GLAND

HYOID BONE

LOWER JAW

LARYNX

GULLET

The Tongue and its Surroundings.

523

cranial nerve. The mucous membrane is supplied by fibers from the fifth and ninth cranial nerves and some fibers from the seventh cranial nerve.

The tongue has four chief functions, concerned respectively with taste, mastication, swallowing of food, and speech. In chewing, the tongue assists by moving the food to and fro in the mouth and against the hard palate. In swallowing, the tongue pushes the food mass into the pharynx and at the same time pulls up the opening of the larynx (air passage) and so allows the food to pass directly into the gullet. For speech and taste functions see under respective headings.

Tongue in Health and Disease. Normally, the tongue should be of a pink color and slightly moist all over. Variations in the appearance of the surface of the tongue give valuable information as to the state of the health. If the tongue is furred it is generally an indication that the digestive system is out of order either from constipation, dyspepsia, fever, or some constitutional disease. The fur consists of molds and other germs mixed with food remains and cast-off surface cells. In certain diseases there are characteristic changes in the appearance of the tongue. In scarlet fever a strawberry tongue is observed. In diabetes the tongue is red and beefy in appearance; in kidney disease, it is dry and cracked; in certain diseases of the nervous system, notably general paralysis, the tongue is very tremulous.

Diseases of the Tongue. Sometimes the tongue is affected with ulcers. These may arise from the pressure of a jagged tooth or may simply be evidence of poor general health. Inflammation of the tongue is called glossitis. This may be caused by excessive smoking, or by drinking hot and pungent liquids, or from some germ infection. There is a certain amount of swelling and pain and occasionally the inflammation may go on to an abscess formation. In inflammation of the tongue, there is sometimes a danger of extreme swelling of the organ leading to complete suffocation. If such a condition should arise, prompt incision of the tongue is necessary. Treatment of the glossitis requires the removal of the irritant, if any, and the use

of bland antiseptic mouth washes such as borax and glycerine.

White flaky patches may form on the surface of the tongue, a condition called leukoplakia. This disease is generally associated with syphilis and excessive smoking and drinking. The white flakes may peel off and leave a cracked and fissured surface which may become cancerous. In some cases, cancer commences as a wart on the tongue which is quite painless. Later, the wart breaks down, ulcerates, and the glands under the chin become involved, causing pain and swelling. Operation for removal of part of the tongue and of the glands, or radium treatment, are the only methods of cure and if these are to be successful they must be carried out in the early stages. *Therefore, it must be emphasized that any little ulcer or hard lump in the tongue should be regarded seriously and expert advice sought at an early stage.* On the other hand, nobody should worry when they suddenly notice, on examining the tongue, the little papillae on the surface at the back, which are quite usual and normal.

Simple tumors may also form in the tongue—warts, fatty overgrowths, and cysts. Underneath the tongue, a small fluid swelling may collect as a result of a dilatation of a mucous gland or duct. The condition is called the ranula and it is easily remedied by an operation. Occasionally, a black patch forms at the back of the tongue. It is due to a fungus, aspergillus niger, which leads to overgrowth of the filiform papillae. The patch should be painted with a solution of salicylic acid in glycerine, 5 grains to the ounce. *Injuries* to the tongue are often associated with considerable bleeding. This may be arrested by stitching the wound but not infrequently it is necessary to ligate (tie) the tongue artery in the neck.

Insects' stings of the tongue often lead to great swelling which may obstruct the air passage and require urgent surgical attention.

TONIC. Any agent which increases the tone of the body generally or of any organ or tissue is described as a tonic. It is not necessary for the tonic to be a drug; physical agents such as sunlight, fresh air, and water baths also come into the category of tonics. Tonics may be divided into different classes according to the organs they stimulate; thus, there are muscle tonics, blood, nerve, digestive, and heart tonics. Iron is a most valuable blood-forming element and may be given in a variety of forms, one of the best being ferrous sulphate tablets. Strychnine is a nerve tonic and can be suitably given as syrup of hypophosphites. Bitters, dilute acids and nux vomica are used as digestive tonics, while digitalis is the best heart tonic, for it has a specific invigorating effect upon the muscle of the heart; it increases the force of the heartbeat while slowing its rate. Arsenic is a useful general tonic having a beneficial effect upon the blood and upon the nervous system. For children, syrup of iodine of iron and compound syrup of hypophosphites are excellent tonics.

TONIC SPASM. A spasm of a muscle or group of muscles which is continuous, not intermittent, is described as tonic spasm. Such a spasm is observed during the first stage of an epileptic fit when the whole body becomes quite rigid. This stage is followed after 20 to 30 seconds by intermittent spasms called clonic spasms. More localized tonic spasms are seen in lockjaw (tetanus) and in strychnine poisoning. Occasionally, tonic spasms of a group of muscles may be of hysterical origin.

TONSIL. The tonsils consist of two oval masses of lymphoid tissue—the same tissue of which lymph glands are composed— about an inch in length and half-an-inch in thickness, placed at the back of the mouth, facing one another on opposite sides of the upper part of the throat. The tonsils are not the only lymphoid tissue structures in this part of the body; in addition, there is a smaller mass of it on the back of the tongue, called the lingual tonsil, which is sometimes enlarged especially in adults, and also another mass up behind the uvula, between the back of the nose and the mouth, called nasopharyngeal tonsil or, when enlarged, adenoids.

The chief function of this mass of tonsillar tissue is a defensive one, acting as a bulwark against infection.

It used to be imagined that enlarged tonsils did harm only because they ob-

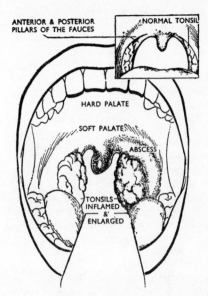

Tonsillitis.

structed the airway, and the method of treating the condition was to cut off part of the enlargement, which, indeed, often did the patient some good. It is now realized, however, that a tonsil does the real harm when it is diseased (infected by bacteria), and that while many enlarged tonsils are unhealthy, a small hidden tonsil may be more septic and may cause much more harm than an obviously enlarged but not necessarily infected tonsil.

With regard to the question of the tonsils being removed or not, there is today rather a reaction against the wholesale removal of enlarged tonsils in children. Nowadays no doctor wants to remove tonsils merely because they are enlarged; but when they are subject to repeated infection or when the glands of the neck are enlarged, and the general health suffers—in other words, when the tonsils are no longer doing their job properly and are infecting the rest of the body—then undoubtedly the tonsils ought to be removed.

Doctors today are rather disinclined to remove tonsils before the age of five, for it is up to that age that their protective function is most active, but even before that the tonsils should be removed if they are unhealthy. It is not nowadays considered so certain as it was that unhealthy tonsils cause rheumatism in children; nor will removal of the tonsils have much effect on asthma or bronchitis; but it is doubtful if the tonsils ever fully recover from an attack of scarlet fever or diphtheria, and it is probably well to remove them when a child has fully recovered from these infectious diseases.

There is no question about the removal of adenoids; the very term adenoids means that the lymphoid tissue behind the uvula is enlarged and unhealthy, and as this affects the breathing, causes deformity of the mouth (gothic-arched palate), and frequently causes inflammation of the ears and deafness, it is evident that adenoids should be removed whenever their presence is discovered. Up to the present nothing has been discovered to take the place of surgical removal of adenoids, though breathing exercises and simple nasal drops may be useful in preventing their development.

TONSILLITIS. Tonsillitis, or inflammation of the tonsils, may be either chronic or acute.

Chronic tonsillitis means the condition of enlarged and unhealthy tonsils, to which a great variety of ailments have been attributed, some justly, some unjustly; but certainly in adults they appear to have an evil influence in rheumatism, certain types of heart disease, certain types of kidney disease, persistent inflammation of the conjunctiva (white of the eye), dyspepsia, and certain types of deafness, to mention only a few that reliable authorities have catalogued. If the tonsils are not bad enough to be removed, the best treatment is to paint them regularly with Mandl's paint (which is not a proprietary preparation but is called after the long-dead physician who invented the formula).

Acute tonsillitis is sometimes divided up into different headings—catarrhal tonsillitis, lacunar tonsillitis, and parenchymatous tonsillitis, but in reality all these are merely different stages of the same disease.

A common cause of tonsillitis is infection with the germ called the streptococcus. The tonsils are the favorite entrance of the streptococcus into the body, and it causes an acute reddening of the throat, sometimes a membrane on the tonsil resembling the membrane of diphtheria (a swab should always be taken by the doctor when the membrane is present, in case it may be the latter) and a sharp rise of temperature (up to 104 deg. or 105 deg. F., sometimes).

Treatment. The patient must be kept in bed, given two aspirin tablets every four hours, and warm gargles of hydrogen peroxide or glycerine of thymol; the throat may be painted with Mandl's paint. The doctor will usually give an injection of penicillin and should always be called in, as tonsillitis may mean the beginning of scarlet fever or some other serious condition.

Quinsy, or tonsillar abscess, may develop after tonsillitis, either inside the tonsil or in the tissues behind it. When a quinsy has definitely developed a doctor should be called in to open it, otherwise the pus in it may track down more deeply and cause severe inflammation. The tonsils should be removed after an attack of quinsy, as subsequent attacks are otherwise rather common.

TOPHUS. Deposits of chalky material which form in certain parts of the body in chronic gout are termed tophi or chalk stones, though actually they are not composed of chalk but of sodium biurate. The commonest situation for a tophus is the edge of the external ear, and other common sites are the joints of the fingers and toes. In some cases, the skin over the tophus breaks down and the chalky material is exposed. (*See also* GOUT.)

TORSION. This word is used medically to signify twisting in the physical sense. Torsion of internal organs sometimes occurs, notably the intestine, a condition called volvulus. Also a tumor or growth with a stalk may twist upon itself. The term is also used to describe the stopping of bleeding during an operation, when the surgeon, by means of forceps, twists the end of a small artery which has been cut causing the inner coat to curl up and stop the flow of blood.

TORTICOLLIS. This is another name for wry neck. (*See also* FIBROSITIS; WRY NECK.)

TOURNIQUET. This is a French word used to denote any mechanical instrument for the arresting or prevention of bleeding. There are several different kinds, but in principle they consist of a pad which is placed over the main artery and an appliance for keeping this pad tightly pressed over the artery in order to stop the blood flow. This appliance may consist of a solid rubber tube, as in the elastic tourniquet, or a metal screw, as in Petit's tourniquet. The routine use of a tourniquet is not recommended, but it must be used if other methods fail. (*See also* FIRST AID SUPPLEMENT.)

TOXEMIA. Any condition of blood poisoning caused by the toxins or poisons produced by disease germs within the body is described as toxemia. It is to be distinguished from septicemia, a condition in which the germs are present and multiply in the blood. Toxemia is also used to denote the blood poisoning caused through absorption of poisons formed by the abnormal action of the body cells. Uremia, for example, is a condition of toxemia caused by failure of the kidneys to carry out their work of excretion.

TOXICOLOGY. This is a section of medical science which deals with poisons, their nature and composition, their effects upon the body and the methods of their detection. Toxicology is an important branch of legal medicine. Poisons are identified by the symptoms they produce during life, by various physical and chemical tests, and, after death by post-mortem examination.

TOXIN. This word is used to denote the poisonous substances produced by germs (bacteria) either in the body or in artificial media. Some toxins are set free from the germs and are called extracellular toxins; others are actual constituents of the germ substance being liberated when the germs break up and are called intracellular toxins. Certain extracellular toxins, notably those of diphtheria and tetanus, can be isolated and used to artificially produce antitoxins in an animal. These antitoxins are the antidotes produced by the body to neutralize the effects of the toxin. Germ toxins vary in their effects upon the body and the symptoms they produce, and each toxin stimulates the body to produce a specific antitoxin.

TRACHEA. This is the windpipe, or tube, about four inches or more in length, which conveys the air from the lower part of the throat down to the lungs. It begins just below the Adam's apple in the neck (i.e., below the larynx), and ends in the thorax by dividing into the right and left bronchi. In section the trachea is horseshoe shaped, and is composed of about a score of rings of cartilage, to keep the air passage permanently open, together with elastic membrane between them. Immediately behind the trachea is the esophagus or gullet, and close to the left side of its lower end is the aorta, which is the largest blood vessel in the body.

TRACHEOTOMY. This is an urgent operation in which the trachea or windpipe is opened from the front of the neck to allow air to get down to the lungs when the upper part of the throat is obstructed by inflammation (such as diphtheria), a foreign body, or some other cause. A tracheotomy tube made of metal is usually inserted, which permits free breathing. Sometimes tracheotomy is done as a preliminary to other operations on the throat.

TRACHOMA. This is an infective disease of the eyes, with follicles on the mucous lining of the eyelids; it is nowadays successfully treated with sulphonamides.

TRANSFUSION OF BLOOD. If a great deal of blood is lost, as when an artery is torn in an accident, or in severe cases of anemia, it may be necessary to replace the blood by transfusion. This operation consists of withdrawing blood from a person called the donor and transferring it to the bloodless person called the recipient. The blood may be passed directly to a vein of the recipient, but usually it is withdrawn into a bottle with sodium citrate to prevent clotting, and then allowed to run into the recipient's vein.

Before the operation is carried out, it is necessary first to find out if the donor's and recipient's blood are compatible. If this is not the case, there results a destruction of the red blood cells. It has been determined that all people can be divided into four classes from the point of view of blood compatibility, each class reacting in a different way to the other three. These are classified as O, A, B, and AB, determined by the presence of "agglutinogens" in the red blood corpuscles, group O containing no agglutinogens. One group, AB, can receive safely the blood of any person and it is called the universal recipient group. Another group, O, can give blood safely to any person—the universal donor group. The other two groups have blood which is compatible with members of the same group. Some red blood cells contain the so-called "rhesus" factor which occasionally gives rise to transfusion reactions, but is of greater interest as a cause of blood destruction in newborn infants.

Members of the same family do not necessarily have blood which is compatible; but, fortunately, it is comparatively simple to determine whether one person's blood can safely be given to another. In selecting a person to give blood, it is important that such a person should be free from disease and that the person should be strong and healthy enough to afford to lose the required amount of blood.

The value of blood transfusion has long been known, though not much practised until it received a marked stimulus towards the end of World War I. One serious disadvantage of transfusion with fresh blood was that a donor of the correct group had to be "on tap" when needed; in the Spanish Civil War, however, the surgeons started a "blood-bank" system of stored, preserved blood, so that large stocks of preserved blood could be laid up, for use when required. It had to be put away at once in a refrigerator and kept at a steady, low temperature, and was not of any use after about three or four weeks. It was found, too, that stored blood could cause serious reactions. The principle sources of reaction are the blood corpuscles, so in the early part of the second world war the use of blood plasma or serum was introduced, the corpuscles being removed immediately after bleeding. A further development was the use of dried plasma, which could be stored indefinitely, transported easily, and even taken from one extreme of climate to another, and when needed was reconstituted with distilled water.

During World War II blood transfusion was used more and more for the resuscitation of battle casualties by all medical units, even in the most advanced forward areas. Today, blood transfusion is an everyday affair in every hospital, and blood banks are a normal item of hospital equipment. Blood transfusion before, during, and after serious surgical operations has

been an important factor in making them safer and more successful.

TRAUMA. In medicine, a wound or injury is described as a trauma. For example, a paralysis of the arm caused by injury to the nerve would be called a traumatic paralysis, or epilepsy due to fracture of the skull, traumatic epilepsy. Some degree of shock or depression of the body vitality occurs after trauma, according to its severity. A traumatic neurosis is a condition of nervousness arising after a severe accident such as a railway smash. There need be no physical injury, but the symptoms are produced by emotional shock. A traumatic neurosis persists until any claim for compensation is suitably settled.

TREMOR. This consists of a series of rhythmical movements of a part or parts of a limb, which movements are not under the control of the will. The rhythmical effect of the movements is due to the fact that first one group of muscles contracts, and then, in quick succession, the group of muscles which moves the part of the limb in exactly the opposite direction, so that rhythm is set up, which is called a tremor. Tremor may be either fine, or coarse, according to the rate of the rhythm. Fine tremor is much more easily felt than seen, and can be best recognized in the arms by getting a person to hold out his hands in front of him and separate the fingers. Fine tremor is one of the symptoms of *exophthalmic goiter* (*see also* SYMPATHETIC NERVOUS SYSTEM), of *alcoholism,* and of poisoning by certain metals, especially mercury. A fine tremor also may be seen in states of agitation and in anxiety neurosis.

A coarse tremor is easily observed, and the most obvious condition in which it occurs is *paralysis agitans,* the disease known as the "shaking palsy." It is also a feature of the late stages of the disease "sleeping sickness" (*see also* ENCEPHALITIS LETHARGICA), when the tremor is seen at an earlier age than in the true "shaking palsy." In the very aged a coarse tremor is very common and does not necessarily mean that any disease is present. One kind of tremor which only comes on when the patient attempts to use the affected muscles is called "intention tremor." This particular tremor is seen most often in *dis-*

seminated sclerosis, and may be recognized by asking the patient to touch the tip of the nose with the pointing finger. As the finger approaches the nose, a tremor appears, and the finger shoots past the patient's nose.

TREPHINE. The operation of boring a circular opening in the skull is performed by means of a special cylindrical saw called a trephine. The trephine removes a small circle of bone from the skull and so exposes the dura mater, the tough outer membrane of the brain. The operation is carried out in cases of depressed fracture of the skull and when one of the arteries, particularly the middle meningeal, is torn and bleeding. It may also be performed to relieve pressure within the skull in cases of cerebral tumor or for the draining of abscesses.

TREPONEMA PALLIDUM. This is the organism or germ which causes syphilis. It is a long slender organism containing six to fourteen spirals and it is actively motile, moving in a corkscrew fashion. The treponema is found in the diseased tissues in the primary and secondary stages of syphilis, and it occurs in the brain in general paralysis of the insane. (*See also* SYPHILIS.)

TRICHINOSIS. This is a disease caused by eating pork infected with a tiny round worm called the trichina spiralis. The parasites invade the voluntary muscles setting up inflammation. The worms become encysted between the muscle fibers, remaining alive for years. No satisfactory cure is known. (*See also* WORM.)

TRICUSPID VALVE. This is one of the heart valves. It is situated between the right auricle and the right ventricle, and is provided with three cusps. Unlike the mitral valve, it is not frequently the seat of disease. (*See also* HEART.)

TRIGEMINAL NERVE. This is the nerve which controls the muscles of chewing, and it also enables us to feel such sensations as pain, heat and cold, and touch, on our face and in our eyes, nose, mouth, and teeth. It is the "nerve of toothache." Our sense of taste is also, to some extent, carried by the trigeminal nerve, and any damage to the nerve in a particular part of its course in the skull will cause the sense of taste to be diminished

or abolished on the front two-thirds of the same side of the tongue. The trigeminal nerve is connected with nearly every other nerve supplying the head and neck, and because it has all these connections it has situated on it, outside that part of the brain from which it arises, a mass of gray nervous tissue which is called a ganglion.

This ganglion, the Gasserian ganglion, separates out, as it were, the different parts of the nerve that are going to supply different areas of the face, and these separate parts or branches of the nerves leave the skull through separate holes.

In neuralgia of the trigeminal nerve, called *tic doulourex* (*see also* NEURALGIA and TIC), it is possible to obtain relief by injecting alcohol into whichever branch of the nerve is affected. But if the effect of the alcohol injection does not last, or the neuralgia spreads to the area supplied by another branch of the nerve, then it is possible to deal with it by either injecting alcohol into the Gasserian ganglion itself, inside the skull, or in very bad cases, by cutting the ganglion. This operation is not lightly undertaken, as it is a serious one. Fortunately it is rarely required, as an alcohol injection into the ganglion benefits all but the very worst cases of trigeminal neuralgia.

TRISMUS. This term refers to a tonic spasm of the muscles which clench the jaws. The sufferer is unable to separate the teeth and feeding becomes difficult. Trismus is a symptom of lockjaw (tetanus) and it may occur in meningitis. Occasionally, it occurs as an hysterical symptom.

TROCAR. A metal instrument for tapping collections of fluid in different parts of the body is termed a trocar. It consists of a sharp pointed perforator which fits accurately into a tube or cannula, only the sharp point projecting beyond the end of the cannula. After the trocar and cannula are plunged into the part of the body to be tapped, the trocar is withdrawn and the fluid allowed to run out into a receptacle. The trocar and cannula are used to tap pleural effusions in wet pleurisy, urine from an obstructed bladder, and fluid from a hydrocele. (*See also* SOUTHEY'S TUBE.)

TROCHANTER. The trochanters are the projections situated on the upper part of the femur or thigh bone. They serve as attachments for muscles. (*See also* FEMUR.)

TROCHLEAR NERVE. This is the fourth of the cranial nerves. It emerges from the skull through the orbit and supplies the superior oblique muscles of the eye, the function of which is to pull the eyeball downwards and outwards. (*See also* EYE.)

TROPHIC. The nervous system through the individual nerves has an important influence on the nutrition of the tissues. This is termed their trophic function. If a nerve is injured or severed, the muscles, skin, and tissues generally tend gradually to become wasted. The skin becomes smooth, thin and glossy, and readily becomes inflamed; the nails and hair are also affected. Trophic sores occur in organic diseases of the nervous system, e.g., in tabes dorsalis. Ulcers form and show little or no tendency to heal.

TRUSS. An instrument or appliance for the control of a hernia or rupture is called a truss. In principle, it consists of a firm pad to which is attached a strong steel spring which encircles the body. The pad is shaped according to the type of hernia it is designed to control, and the angle of fixture to the spring varies similarly. The spring is lined with washleather internally and prepared leather externally. For an inguinal hernia the pad is triangular and lies in a line with the spring belt. Sometimes the pad is continued down into the crotch or perineum and is attached to the back of the belt—the so-called rat-tail truss. The pad for a femoral hernia is more rounded and is fixed at a sharper angle to the belt. In the case of an umbilical hernia, the pad is circular and varies in size to suit the size of the opening.

Great care is required in the fitting of a truss, for if it is badly fitting it not only fails to perform its function but also leads to discomfort or pain. A truss is generally worn only by day and is removed when lying down in bed. It should be again fitted first thing in the morning in the recumbent posture.

In children, an all-rubber truss with an inflatable bag has advantages over the spring-pad type of truss. It can obviously be kept clean and it is not likely to lead to discomfort when worn. For the umbili-

cal hernias of children, a truss can be improvised by covering a penny with cotton wool and sewing it between two layers of plain lint. It is very seldom that a truss really cures a hernia, except in the case of the umbilical hernias of young children; they control the defect and prevent it getting worse. In a young healthy adult, an operation is to be preferred. The wearing of a truss is a great handicap to an active life. (*See also* ABDOMINAL BELT; HERNIA.)

TRYPANOSOME. This is a variety of microorganism belonging to the class of protozoa and occurring as a parasite in man and the lower animals. A trypanosome is a worm-like structure with a large nucleus centrally situated and a whip-like process or flagellum attached at the hind end. It is by means of the flagellum that the parasite moves; its multiplication may be by simple division, or in the body of the tsetse fly it undergoes a sexual reproduction. There are a number of trypanosomes, some harmless, but one is responsible for the tropical disease called sleeping sickness. This is a blood infection, and the disease is transmitted from one person to another through an intermediate host, the tsetse fly. The disease is endemic in Central Africa and South America. It is sometimes referred to as trypanosomiasis. A variety of trypanosome causes the disease called surra which affects horses, dogs, camels, and elephants. (*See also* SLEEPING SICKNESS.)

TRYPSIN. This is the protein-splitting ferment which is found in the pancreatic digestive juice which is passed into the small intestine. It requires an alkaline medium to carry out its work, and it completes the digestion of proteins which have been partially digested in the stomach by the ferment pepsin. Trypsin is a much more powerful ferment than pepsin and reduces the protein of the food to its simplest elements (amino acids), in which form they are absorbed into the bloodstream. Actually, trypsin is in an inactive form called trypsinogen when secreted, and it only becomes active in the small intestine as the result of another ferment from the intestinal juice called enterokinase. Preparations of trypsin made from the pancreas of animals are used in predigested foods. (*See also* DIGESTION; PANCREAS.)

TSETSE FLY. This fly belongs to a species known as glossina, of which there are several varieties. It is a dark-colored, narrow-bodied insect about 6 millimeters long, with brown-colored wings which have well-marked veins. The fly is found in tropical Africa and Southwest Arabia, and it inhabits thick scrub or bush near water.

The glossina is a blood-sucking insect, both male and female biting and being capable of transmitting sleeping sickness in man. The fly is the intermediate host of the trypanosome which undergoes its sexual development in the body of the fly.

TUBAL PREGNANCY. A fertilized ovum arrested in the Fallopian tube on its downward course to the womb gives rise to tubal gestation or pregnancy. As this is an abnormal place for the development of the embryo, the tube usually ruptures between the sixth and twelfth week of pregnancy—a dangerous happening, for it is associated with great shock and severe internal bleeding. An immediate operation is generally necessary.

TUBERCULIN. This is an emulsion of dead tuberculosis germs and is used in weak dilutions as a method of diagnosis of tuberculosis. A drop is injected into the skin which shows a red flare in 36 hours in subjects who have been infected with the tubercle bacillus. Many adults in this country give such a reaction, and the test is of special value in childhood as a means of detecting recent infection. It is also used to help select nurses who have already received their primary infection and are therefore suitable to work in sanatoriums. (*See also* TUBERCULOSIS.)

TUBERCULOSIS. Pulmonary tuberculosis, or **consumption,** is the term applied to tuberculosis affecting the lungs. It starts off by the formation of "tubercles," small abnormal masses of tissue due to the presence of a germ called *Koch's bacillus.* Koch was a famous German bacteriologist (1843–1910) who first described the germ which is the cause of tuberculosis. It is contagious from one person to another, from animals to man, and from man to animals. There are three main varieties of tubercle bacillus: the human, the bovine, and the avian. Infection from hu-

man sources is probably much more frequent than from any other; but quite a large amount of tuberculosis in man is caused by germs of the bovine type, which are conveyed by infected cow's milk.

Preventive Vaccination. An attenuated vaccine called by the initials of its inventors in 1920, the French scientists Calmette and Guérin (BCG), does undoubtedly give some protection, and is now being widely used to protect persons exposed to possible infection, especially child contacts, children leaving school, and hospital staff, including doctors, nurses, and domestics.

Diagnosis. It is most important that this should be early in order that the treatment may be successful. Unfortunately the onset of tuberculosis is very insidious, and the disease may be very extensively spread in the lungs without causing sufficient ill-health to make a person consider himself sufficiently ill to consult a doctor.

X-ray Examination. This is a very useful aid to diagnosis, but some degree of skill and experience is required to interpret the picture. The introduction of mass miniature radiography for selected groups of persons has resulted in revealing an average of 4 in 1,000 completely unsuspected cases of pulmonary tuberculosis. But the X-ray picture must always be regarded as subsidiary to other signs and symptoms and the diagnosis as a whole depends on the collection and weighing up of various items of evidence for and against.

Treatment. In regard to the treatment it is necessary to estimate the patient's temperament and character. It has been truly said that one cannot cure a fool of tuberculosis. The treatment is long and troublesome and may have to be carried on throughout life. Endless steadfastness, courage, self-discipline and self-denial are required, and the final result depends more on the presence or absence of these qualities than on anything else. The patient finds it hard to face the real truth and the real hardships of the road to recovery.

U.S. Surgeon General Bushnell's famous remark lies at the base of all treatment: "For tuberculosis we prescribe not medicine, but a mode of life." No certain cure for all cases of tuberculosis is known, but it is certain that in a large proportion of cases the disease is made worse by a faulty mode of life, and that if we alter the mode of life we shall be giving the correct treatment in some measure. It is very important that there should be continuous treatment, and that the patient should place himself in the hands of one doctor who is entirely responsible all the time; there are several lines of treatment that will be successful in a particular case, but often a hopeful case turns out a failure owing to lack of continuity of treatment.

Choice of Sanatorium. The conduct of the treatment and the sanatorium staff are far more important than the altitude and climatic conditions. The time spent should be not less than six months to one year.

Sanatorium Treatment. The object of this is intended to refit the consumptive for the ordinary conditions of life. Its three main objects are (1) to regain health and resistance to disease; (2) to maintain this gain; (3) to teach the individual the best way to live the remainder of his life.

The case must be suitable for sanatorium treatment and not advanced too far. The mental outlook is very important; the patient should clear up all domestic and financial worries as far as possible before the treatment is begun. No good result can be obtained in the case of a man worrying over the welfare of his family or his business, or in the case of a woman who is anxious about her children. The patient must be taught that his main object is to become as well as he can, and not to worry how soon he can return to work or to his home.

The essentials of treatment are: rest, both of mind and of body; graduated exercises; fresh air and sunlight; routine and discipline; correct feeding. All these are graduated and controlled daily by skilled medical staff. The best method of controlling the general symptoms, such as fever, shortness of breath, etc., is by rest, and the "rest" in a sanatorium means from 10 to 12 hours in bed every night, with two or three "rest" hours during the day. Complete confinement to bed is insisted on where the temperature varies too far from the normal, where there is true night sweating, or where there is a regular loss of weight. The patient is not even allowed to get out of bed for the calls of nature,

and has to use the bedpan. Bed bathing is also necessary. Visitors and outside excitements are prohibited. After a few months, and when the general symptoms have disappeared, graduated exercises are begun. These are of value in two ways: they restore the tone and efficiency of the whole muscular system; and they also restore the mental and moral tone and help to maintain that cheerful attitude of mind which is so necessary.

The exercises start with ordinary actions such as washing, eating, talking, and writing. After this, walking exercises, carefully graduated, will take many months. Much damage can be done by too much exercise, though little harm is done by taking too little. The symptoms to be watched for are undue fatigue, shortness of breath, and pain. Graduated manual labor is introduced to prevent the loss of moral tone which is so liable to occur when walking is the only form of exercise allowed. Gardening is the most convenient form of manual labor.

Fresh Air. As many hours as possible should be spent in the open air, and when indoors the windows must be widely opened, or taken out of their sashes. Direct sunlight is bad for pulmonary tuberculosis and should be avoided.

Drug Treatment. Streptomycin, a drug prepared from a soil fungus, discovered by the American, Dr. Waksman, as a result of the previous discovery of penicillin, is undoubtedly of the greatest value in the treatment of tuberculosis. It must be used with great care as it can cause severe and permanent damage to the nerve of hearing. It is best given along with para-aminosalicylic acid, or PAS, as it is popularly called, or isoniazid.

Surgical Treatment. More and more causes of pulmonary tuberculosis are being treated by surgical methods, ranging from the minor procedure when a needle is used to introduce air in order to collapse the lung, up to the removal of a lobe of the lung, or of the complete lung itself. Normally both the lungs and the inner side of the chest wall are lined by a closed bag known as the pleura. One wall of this bag is firmly attached to the lung and the other is attached to the chest wall. The sac contains only sufficient fluid to enable the walls of the lung to glide over the walls of the chest without causing friction, and the lungs are kept in contact with the chest wall by the fact that there is no air at all within the sac. The tissue of the lung is elastic, and when air is introduced into the closed sac the air pressure on both sides of the lungs is the same, so that there is nothing to prevent the elastic tissue from contracting and so pulling the lung away from the chest wall. The lung accordingly collapses. This condition is known as an *artificial pneumothorax*. Where only a little air is allowed into the pleural cavity, the degree of lung collapse is slight and the air space is quite shallow.

In most cases the air in the sac is gradually absorbed, and has to be replaced at regular intervals. Sometimes the lung is rested by paralyzing the diaphragm on one side by *evulsion of the phrenic nerve;* and in more advanced cases several ribs are partly removed to allow a thorough collapse of the lung, by the operation called *thoracoplasty*. Sometimes the lung is rested by raising the diaphragm, by means of introducing air into the peritoneal space of the abdomen, called *artificial pneumoperitoneum.*

Methods of Spread of Tuberculosis. The germs of tuberculosis are present in the phlegm which is coughed up. These germs can exist for as long as six months, though they cannot exist long in bright sunlight.

Tuberculosis of the lungs is always acquired directly or indirectly from another human being. Animal tuberculosis is sometimes responsible for disease in other tissues. Milk, however, is the most likely source of infection; not only when it comes from cows with tuberculous udders but also in cows found to be suffering from tuberculosis of any kind. In most areas the milk is usually *pasteurized,* that is to say it is heated to a temperature between 60 deg. and 70 deg. C. (boiling being 100 deg. C.) for a short time. This process kills most of the germs of tuberculosis, and again the fact that it destroys the lactic acid bacilli—the germs which make the milk go sour—tends to encourage the sale of milk which is not very fresh. The process of pasteurization also seems to

destroy properties in the milk which make it invaluable for growing children.

Milk should be able to be obtained free from the germs of tuberculosis by ensuring that the cows producing it are free from the disease, and it should not really be necessary to sterilize it later to render it free from harmful bacteria.

Tuberculosis of joints is most common in childhood and early youth, but it may occur at any age and is not uncommon in old people. It is a chronic condition and comes on insidiously, and when established there is swelling of the joint ("white swelling"), pain on movement, and the limb is often drawn up (by the pull of the muscles); at a later stage there is destruction of the joint, and deformity results. General signs of tuberculosis, such as evening rise of temperature, night sweats, and wasting are also present. When the diagnosis is made early by the doctor and time not wasted by people considering the condition "rheumatism" or "growing pains," the outlook is favorable, though treatment is always prolonged.

Treatment. The joint is usually fixed in a useful position by means of a carefully molded plaster of Paris splint or other apparatus and kept absolutely immobile for at least six months after the active disease has settled down, which may take up to two or three years. Open air and sunlight are essentials in treatment.

TUMOR. In a popular sense, a tumor refers to any abnormal swelling in the body, but pathologically it refers to an abnormal growth of cells and is sometimes also termed a neoplasm or new growth. The cell growth resembles the cells of the tissues from which it is developed, but these new cells serve no useful purpose and grow at the expense of the body.

Any tissue of the body can develop a tumor, and tumors are classified according to the type of tissue involved. Broadly, there are two main classes, the connective tissue tumors and the epithelial tumors. These, in turn, can be each divided into malignant and benign (harmless) tumors, according to whether they endanger life or not. Tumors are also named according to the name of the actual tissue affected. Thus, there are *lipomas*—fatty tumors;

fibromas—fibrous tumors; *angiomas*—blood-vessel tumors; *neuromas,* nerve tumors, and so on. Sarcomas are so called because to the eye their substance resembles a fleshy mass. Carcinoma is a cancer, and is so called because processes grow out from the parent tumour like the claws of a crab.

The actual causation of tumors is unknown and it is probable that a variety of causes are operative. Some form of irritation, chemical or bacterial, is certainly very often a precursor of cancer. Also, cancers can be produced artificially in animals by the application to the skin of irritant tars. Some tumors are probably of embryonic origin, i.e., groups of cells get misplaced during development within the womb and in later life they commence to grow in an uncontrolled manner. Teratomata probably arise in this way.

The appearance of a tumor need not be a cause for alarm, but it is always advisable to seek medical advice immediately. In a majority of cases, the person concerned will be reassured that the tumor is harmless; but should the verdict be otherwise, the chances of cure are very much greater in the early stages of a malignant tumor as compared with the later stages. Pain does not necessarily accompany a tumor, but that in itself is not evidence that the tumor is harmless. The early stages of cancer are nearly always painless. Simple tumors are only removed if they are disfiguring or are pressing on some organ. With malignant tumors early removal by surgical operation, or radium treatment, are essential as soon as they are detected.

TURPENTINE. The oil of turpentine is obtained from several species of pine found chiefly in America, Russia, and France. It is distilled from the resin and occurs as a colorless liquid with a characteristic odor and a pungent taste; it is insoluble in water but freely soluble in alcohol. If applied externally to the skin, turpentine is a counterirritant, producing redness and a feeling of warmth. It is therefore commonly used as a liniment. Internally, turpentine is sometimes used to kill intestinal worms, especially the tapeworm. It is a dangerous drug to use internally, however, as it has a powerful irritant effect upon the delicate mucous membranes. It is also absorbed and, being excreted by the kidneys, produces an intense inflammation of these organs, as shown by the presence of blood and albumin in the urine. If an overdose of turpentine is taken, an emetic (salt and water) should be given at once and, after it has acted, a dessertspoonful of Epsom salts in water. Water should then be drunk freely to relieve the irritation in the stomach.

There are two preparations of turpentine, both liniments: one, acetic turpentine liniment, is clear; the other, containing soap, is creamy.

TYMPANUM. This is the middle ear, an air-filled cavity in the temporal bone of the skull. It lies just behind the eardrum or tympanic membrane and contains a chain of three small bones, the malleus, the incus, and the stapes, which lead from the drum to the internal ear and probably have a protective function. It also contains two tiny muscles which act upon the ossicles. The tympanum communicates with the throat by a small canal called the eustachian tube, and is also connected with the air cells in the mastoid process of the temporal bone. (*See also* EAR.)

TYPHOID FEVER. This is an acute disease characterized by a special ulceration of the small intestine, with severe diarrhea, the eruption of rose-colored spots, and a typical course of temperature. It is caused by a germ, the typhoid bacillus, which is a rod-shaped organism with a number of whip-shaped processes—flagellae—enabling it to move. The bacillus is found in the blood, and in the urine and stools of typhoid patients, and it may persist in these excretions for many years after recovery. Such a person who harbors the bacilli is called a typhoid carrier and may be a menace to the community by spreading infection.

The infection is spread chiefly through the drinking of contaminated water, milk, food (particularly shellfish), uncooked vegetables, and ice cream. Flies and other insects may be the agents of infection by feeding on infected sewage and transferring the bacilli to water, or food. Typhoid fever is most common in adolescents, but it occurs at all ages. It may be found in all countries though it appears to be dying out in the U.S., and tends to be most prevalent during hot weather.

Paratyphoid fevers. These are illnesses which closely resemble the less severe forms of typhoid. They are caused by two different organisms or germs, paratyphoid A and paratyphoid B, and infection is acquired in much the same way as in true typhoid. The diagnosis depends on bacteriological examination in the laboratory.

Treatment. Chloramphenicol (or chloromycetin, as it was first called), one of the newer antibiotics, has a rapid curative effect in typhoid (and also paratyphoid) fever, and the temperature falls to normal in two or three days under its action. Convalescence, however, may still be rather prolonged, as the patient is weakened by the severe infection.

Prevention. Since water supplies have been carefully controlled and food supplies inspected by public health authorities, the occurrence of typhoid fever has greatly diminished. The possibilities of infection from oysters and mussels which have been contaminated are being diminished by special methods of purification, and the danger from this source is today far less common than formerly.

The carrier problem is hard to overcome, as such a person may remain undetected for a long time. Should such a carrier be found, it is essential that he or she should have nothing to do with the handling or preparation of food, and should be instructed on the methods of sterilizing the urine and feces. During epidemics, there may be very mild cases who are able to get about and are possible sources of infection—a type called ambulant typhoid. If the disease is prevalent in an area, protection can be obtained by inoculation with antityphoid vaccine. The vaccine is usually prepared to protect also against paratyphoid and is called typhoid-paratyphoid vaccine. This gives certain prevention for about two years and, should the disease develop, it is of a very mild kind.

TYPHOID STATE. This is the expression used to denote the profoundly exhausted condition which may arise during any severe feverish illness and which resembles the prostration of typhoid fever. The patient generally lies upon his back, with eyes open and staring. The tongue is very dry, brown and cracked, and the lips and teeth become covered with collections of mucus (sordes). The pulse is rapid, feeble, and the respiration shallow. Very often there is a muttering delirium, and the patient keeps plucking nervously at the bedclothes or makes passing movements in the air with his hands. Sometimes the bowels and bladder are emptied quite involuntarily. The patient has a peculiar tendency to slip downwards in the bed. The typhoid state calls for skilled nursing and medical attention. The time of greatest danger is the early hours of the morning, when the body vitality is naturally at its lowest ebb.

TYPHUS FEVER. This infectious disease, once very prevalent in this country, is now fortunately very rare. Its eradication is due to improvement in the standards of personal hygiene. Typhus is still prevalent in certain parts of the world. It has been variously described as spotted fever, putrid, jail, and hospital fever. Essentially, it is a disease of dirt, overcrowding, starvation and fatigue. The cause is a minute microorganism known as a rickettsia, and infection is carried from person to person by lice, ticks, and fleas.

Symptoms. The onset is revealed after eight to twelve days by shivering attacks, aching pains in the head, back and limbs, a feeling of prostration, and a rising temperature. The tongue becomes swollen and dry, the bowels are constipated, the face is flushed and somewhat dusky, and the eyes are bloodshot. The eruption or rash appears about the fourth or fifth day and shows itself as mottled mulberry-like spots, with tiny bleeding spots in some of them. It spreads over the trunk, back and limbs, the face not usually being affected.

A peculiar smell is associated with the typhus patient, being described as resembling the odor of mice. As the disease advances the patient becomes more and more prostrate; he shows a characteristic vacant and apathetic look. There is a muttering delirium by day and night, and coma or unconsciousness may supervene at any time. The fever remains high until about the end of the second week, when in favorable cases, it abates by crisis, at which time there is general improvement in the condition of the patient. The mind clears, refreshing sleep is obtained, and there is a return of the appetite. Convalescence is very slow and marked weakness and debility persist for some months.

During the fever, heart failure, bronchitis, bronchopneumonia, meningitis, and excessively high temperature (hyperpyrexia) may arise as complications and may produce a fatal result. Bedsores may also develop, and attacks of melancholia and mania sometimes complicate the convalescent period.

The diagnosis of typhus fever is not difficult during an epidemic, but solitary cases present some trouble. It may be confused with typhoid fever, but laboratory tests should be able to settle any confusion on this point. There is a test for typhus fever —similar to the Widal test for typhoid; it is called the Weil-Felix reaction.

Treatment. Strict isolation is essential in cases of typhus fever. Good nursing is vital. The skin should be sponged two or three times daily with some cool antiseptic lotion. In the acute stage the diet must be restricted to nourishing fluids. Stimulants in the form of whisky or brandy may be necessary at any time—especially at the crisis. Sleeplessness may require the use of hypnotic drugs. Specific treatment is with aureomycin, one of the antibiotics, which rapidly controls the disease.

ULCER. An ulcer may be described as an open sore resulting from inflammation on the surface of the skin, or mucous membrane. Death occurs in the tissues of the infected area, and because of this loss the ulcer is usually depressed below the surface of the healthy tissue. Any irritation to the skin may produce ulceration, but the commonest cause is infection. Other factors which often encourage the development of ulcers are poorness of the blood, general bad health, or poor circulation which leads to varicose conditions of the veins. Constant pressure or friction is liable to cause ulceration of the skin, for example, bedsores. Any malignant growth, cancer or sarcoma, is liable to break down and ulcerate, especially growths, known as rodent ulcers, which occur on the face.

Varieties. Ordinary simple inflammatory ulcers are usually rounded, depressed areas consisting of a "floor" or surface covered with greyish-yellow material, from which there is a discharge. The surrounding parts are red and swollen, and there is a blue line which marks the edge of the healthy tissue. When the destructive process has ceased, the ulcer becomes cleaner and the floor covered with red granulation tissue. The parts surrounding the ulcer then become less angry-looking and the discharge more watery in appearance.

During healing, the new tissue contracts, giving a puckered appearance to the scar and the edges show the blue line of advancing healthy skin. Ulcers may be described as *local* when they occur at one spot only, and *constitutional* when there are several of them on different parts of the body. Constitutional ulcers are generally the result of some disease such as syphilis, tuberculosis, anthrax, Oriental sore, and yaws, and they are known as *infective ulcers*. Local ulcers include many varieties according to their cause and appearance. *Indolent ulcers* are chronic, slowly healing ulcers, which occur usually on the legs of obese, middle-aged women with varicose veins. *Varicose ulcers* are met with on the legs of patients who suffer with bad varicose veins, and there is danger of the vein rupturing and severe bleeding occurring. Such ulcers are often indolent, and occur chiefly around the ankle. *Internal ulcers* tend specially to develop in the mouth, stomach and intestines. *Gastric* ulcer is fully described under GASTRIC or STOMACH ULCER and ulcer of the upper part of the intestine will be found under DUODENAL ULCER.

Treatment. For ordinary inflammatory ulcers the treatment consists of rendering the part clean with moist, warm, antiseptic applications, such as acriflavine or perchloride of mercury solution, and the dressing covered with oiled silk. Applications containing phenol should not be used. As soon as the ulcer is rendered clean, these antiseptics must be stopped, as they interfere with the healing processes. The importance of complete rest cannot be too strongly emphasized and the patient should be given good nourishing food and tonics. Exuberant growth of granulation should be treated with blue stone (copper sulphate), silver salts, or other substances which have a reducing effect upon the proud flesh. Once an ulcer has reached the healing stage, all that is necessary is to keep the surface clean and free from irritation and at rest as much as possible. The ulcer may be kept covered with a piece of lint spread over with boric ointment, or an elastic plaster bandage may be applied over zinc gelatin dressing on the leg. The usual interval allowed to elapse between dressings is three days, but if there is any discharge or if the ulcer is not clean, the dressing must be changed oftener. The lint must be thoroughly soaked before removal, and never pulled away roughly. The healing of a large ulcer, after it has been rendered clean, may often be hastened by grafting its surface with skin from another part of the body. In varicose ulcers of the leg, rest, with the foot elevated, is of the utmost importance. At night the foot of the bed should be put on blocks. (*See also* DUODENAL ULCER; GASTRIC ULCER; GRANULATION TISSUE; PROUD FLESH; PUPUS.)

ULNA. The inner of the two bones which form the skeleton of the forearm is known as the ulna, and when the palm of the hand is turned upwards it can be traced with the finger from the point of the elbow down to the wrist. At the lower end of the ulna is a small rounded knob which stands out prominently, especially in thin people. (*See also* BONES; FRACTURE; ARM; ELBOW.)

ULNAR. The *ulnar artery* is one of the branches of the brachial artery. It commences at the elbow, passes down the forearm and eventually joins the arteries which supply the palm and fingers. The *ulnar nerve* lies very close to the ulnar artery and the two structures travel together down the forearm into the palm. This nerve supplies sensation to the palm

and back of the hand and to the little finger and ring finger. (*See also* ARM; ELBOW; FINGERS.)

ULTRAVIOLET RAYS. The invisible rays of light given off at the higher (violet) end of the spectrum are described as ultraviolet rays. They have a powerful action upon all forms of life, and nowadays are widely used in the treatment of many diseases. (*See also* LIGHT TREATMENT; SUN-BATHING.)

UMBILICUS. More commonly referred to as the navel, the umbilicus is the little depressed button-like scar lying somewhat below the middle line of the abdomen. It represents the separation of the umbilical cord, which is the means of communication between the mother and the developing child while it is still in the womb. (*See also* CORD; HERNIA; RUPTURE.)

UNCONSCIOUSNESS. This is a state of insensibility in which the patient does not respond to external stimuli. It varies greatly in depth and duration and is due to a variety of causes, all of which affect directly or indirectly the brain.

The commonest cause is fainting. In elderly people and those with high blood pressure, apoplexy may be responsible. Conditions such as diabetes and Bright's disease, and poisoning due to overdosage of phenobarbitone or alcohol may all produce unconsciousness.

In simple fainting attacks, the patient should be allowed plenty of fresh air and the garments should be loosened around the neck. An inhalation of sal volatile will rapidly restore consciousness. When unconsciousness persists in spite of these measures, a doctor should be consulted without delay. (*See also* APOPLEXY; COMA; EPILEPSY; FAINTING; FIRST AID SUPPLEMENT; FIT; HYSTERIA; SHOCK.)

UNDULANT FEVER. This disease is more commonly known as Brucellosis or Malta fever, but it also occurs in this country. It is due to infection of milk by a germ, Brucella abortus. It can be prevented by thorough pasteurization of the milk. Aureomycin, one of the new antibiotics, is very effective in the treatment of this disease, and is usually given along with Vitamin B complex. Chloramphenicol, another antibiotic, is also used successfully in its treatment.

UNGUENTUM. This is Latin name for ointment. (*See also* OINTMENT.)

UREMIA. This is a serious condition due to impaired renal function. Poisonous materials, normally excreted in the urine, are retained in the blood. It is commonly due to advanced Bright's disease (nephritis), but may follow obstruction to the urinary outflow, as in stone of the kidney, or enlargement of the prostate.

Symptoms. In cases that develop in a few hours or days the term *acute* is given; while the *chronic* type includes cases in which the symptoms are less severe and may last over weeks, months, or even years. The chief symptoms of uremia are nausea, vomiting, and diarrhea; headache, shortness of breath, muscular twitchings, convulsions, and unconsciousness. There is no sharp dividing line between the acute and the chronic types, and chronic uremia is liable to develop into the most severe or acute form. Headache is the most constant and earliest symptom and it may be very severe in character. Convulsions may occur without any warning, and other common nervous symptoms include tingling and numbness of the fingers, muscular twitching and cramps in the legs. Drowsiness may be present, but on the other hand persistent sleeplessness is not uncommon. The breathing assumes a peculiar asthma-like character and the patient may gasp for breath. In some cases delusional insanity occurs.

Treatment. The first step is to remove the cause, where this known (e.g., operation for removal of stone in kidney). The patient should be given plenty of fluids to drink, and his diet should contain very little protein. Hot packs to the kidneys may help.

UREA. Urea is a compound which is always present in the urine and sweat; but in disease, especially disease of the kidney, its concentration in the blood may be greatly increased. One of the uses of this compound is to stimulate the functions of the kidney, and it is sometimes given for this purpose in cases of dropsy. The hypnotic drugs known as veronal, dial, medinal, and luminal are very closely allied to urea. (*See also* HYPNOTICS.)

URETER. The ureters are two in number, and they are the tubes which convey the urine from the kidneys to the urinary bladder. Each ureter measures from ten to twelve inches in length and is lined by a delicate mucous membrane. Obstruction of the ureter may be a serious condition; it is usually caused by a stone, the passage of which along the ureter gives rise to severe pain, known as renal colic. (*See also* BLADDER; URINE.)

URETHRA. In the male, the urethra is the tube inside the penis which extends from the neck of the bladder to the exterior. It measures from seven to eight inches in length and is the passage for both urine and seminal fluid. The female urethra is a narrow canal about one and a half inches long and lies embedded in the wall of the vagina. Inflammation of the urethra is known as urethritis, and it is nearly always due to gonorrhea. (*See also* GLEET; GONORRHEA; KIDNEY.)

URIC ACID. Uric acid is present in the urine and blood and it is formed by the breakdown of proteins in the tissues. Its presence is greatly increased in disease, but whether this increase is a cause or a result of a particular disease has not yet been proved. People who suffer from rheumatism and gout very often have uric acid crystals deposited in the urine, and these may give rise to severe colic or the passage of blood. But "uric acid" is not nowadays blamed for as many ailments as used formerly to be the case. (*See also* GOUT.)

URINAL. A vessel for receiving urine is described as a urinal.

URINARY SYSTEM. This consists of the two kidneys, the two ureters, the bladder and the urethra. These various parts are described under their own headings.

URINE. This is the water solution excreted by the kidneys by way of the ureters to the bladder, which is emptied periodically through the urethra. It consists of waste substances which result from the activity of the body, and is normally of a pale yellow color with a distinctly aromatic smell and a slightly acid reaction. It has a specific gravity by day of 1018, and by night of 1026—water has a specific gravity of 1000; but the specific gravity of one specimen of urine is of no value as an index to health, and a 12- or 24-hour specimen is necessary to judge this. The amount of urine excreted by a normal adult in 24 hours is 50 ounces, about 38 ounces by day and 12 ounces by night.

The color of urine may vary in different diseases and also after taking various drugs. A deposit may be due to phosphates or urates (which are of little or no importance), or may be due to pus or blood (which are important as indicating disease in some part of the urinary system). Black urine may be due to taking carbolic acid; green urine to bile or to taking methylene blue—blue urine may also be due to the latter drug; orange urine to taking santonin or rhubarb; pink urine to the presence of urates; and red urine to the presence of blood. Oversecretion of urine may be due to such diseases as diabetes or chronic Bright's disease (of the kidneys), but it may also be due to such comparatively trivial causes as nervousness or drinking too much coffee or beer.

Undersecretion of urine may be due to inflammation of the kidney, various fevers, or it may be due only to sweating or violent exercise. Albumen in the urine often occurs in nephritis, and sugar may denote diabetes.

URINE, RETENTION OF. *Retention* of the urine is the term applied to the involuntary holding back of the urine in the bladder, although the urine is secreted by the kidneys; *suppression* of urine is an even more serious condition, as it is due to the failure of the kidneys to produce urine. Retention of urine, is usually due to obstruction from a stricture, or a stone, or enlargement of the prostate gland at the neck of the bladder (common in old men). Sometimes a warm bath will relieve the condition, but it is usually relieved by the passage of a sterilized catheter. This may have to be repeated frequently. Should this fail, operation is indicated. (*See also* CATHETER.)

URTICARIA. This is popularly known as hives and it is characterized by weals on the skin. The eyelids or lips may swell and become very tense and painful. The hives may be preceded by digestive disturbances, and in some cases there seems to be a definite connection between an outbreak of the rash and the taking of certain foods such as fish, strawberries, and various other substances. Urticaria is considered to be an allergic phenomenon, but antihistamines are not very helpful. When the hives occur the skin may feel intensely irritable, and rubbing tends to bring out the weals. Baths containing bicarbonate of soda will relieve the itching. There is a form of the disease known as *giant urticaria*, or *angioneurotic edema*, in which sudden swellings may occur in the eyes, lips, mouth and throat. The eyes may be completely closed, and swellings may develop in the tongue or larynx causing very distressing symptoms. An injection of adrenalin should be given; but in swelling of the larynx intubation of the larynx may have to be carried out in order to save the patient's life. The condition known as *lichen urticatus* is a disease similar to urticaria, the legs and trunk being the chief sites of the eruption. Children, particularly, are affected with this condition and the rash sometimes resembles the blisters of chickenpox. The diet must be carefully gone into and the regularity of the bowels maintained. The affected parts should be sponged with bicarbonate of soda dissolved in warm water. (*See also* ALLERGY; ANAPHYLAXIS; LICHEN.)

UTERUS. This is the womb, or hollow maternal organ in which the fetus grows. (*See also* WOMB.)

UVULA. This is the small muscular mass that hangs down from the middle of the soft palate between the pillars of the fauces.

VACCINATION. Vaccination is simply the introduction into the human body of the virus of cowpox, a modified form of smallpox, with the object of producing a mild attack of the disease and stimulating the natural resist-

ance of the body to gain an immunity to smallpox. The material now used for vaccination is extracted from the skin pustules of calves which have had cowpox. Glycerine is added to the fluid obtained and the material called "glycerinated calf lymph." It is stored in fine glass tubes, and in the actual operation, performed when the child is about four months old, the skin of the arm or leg is first cleaned and two or three drops of lymph placed on the skin about one inch apart. The skin at these points is then gently scarified, not sufficiently deeply to draw blood, and the lymph then allowed to dry on the arm. In girls vaccination is frequently done on the leg or buttock to prevent disfigurement of the arm.

In about three days a small red pimple or papule appears which becomes a blister by the sixth day, and, by the ninth or tenth day pus forms. Then the pustule dries up and a scab forms which falls off by about the fourteenth to twenty-first day, leaving a depressed scar. As a rule, in healthy persons there is comparatively little constitutional disturbance, but occasionally there may be a certain amount of feverishness. The protection afforded by vaccination is not absolutely permanent in all cases, so that it is necessary to be revaccinated after the tenth year and again at the twenty-first year. Should smallpox be epidemic in a district it is generally advisable to be vaccinated, unless this operation has been carried out a short time previously. If a first vaccination is unsuccessful, another attempt should be made, as the lymph may have become inactive, but it is necessary to wait about four weeks after the first attempt. (*See also* SMALLPOX.)

VACCINE. This term is used to describe preparations of the bodies of bacteria which are administered by injection under the skin with a view to preventing or curing certain diseases. In most cases, dead germs are used and the vaccine is so prepared as to contain so many germs to a cubic centimeter, so that accurate doses can be given. If the germs from which the vaccine is to be prepared are obtained from the patient's own body, the vaccine is termed *autogenous*. Most often *stock* vaccines are used, i.e., vaccines are made up from germs of various diseases, and are administered according to the disease in question. (*See also* IMMUNITY.)

VAGINA. This is the passage between the womb and the vulva or external genital organs in the female. It lies between the urinary bladder in front and the rectum behind, the urethra being embedded in the lower half of the front wall. The lower opening of the vagina is partially closed by the hymen in the virgin. Inflammation, or vaginitis, may be caused by gonococcal infection or by the presence of a foreign body such as a pessary or tampon. It may occur as a complication of measles, scarlet or other infectious fevers. There is generally a certain amount of discharge, and the passage may become painful and tender, according to the severity of the inflammation. Leucorrhea, or "whites," is the term applied to a discharge from the vagina.

In women who have borne children the walls of the vagina may prolapse, leading to the production of a *cystocele* or *rectocele,* i.e. part of the bladder or rectum protrudes into the vagina. An operation is necessary to remedy this defect, but this is only advisable if no further children are expected. In young women, where operation is contra-indicated, the condition may be held in check temporarily by the use of a pessary. As a result of a difficult labor an opening or fistula may arise between the bladder and vagina so that incontinence of urine results. Less often a fistula may arise from the same cause between the rectum and the vagina. An operation is the only remedy. (*See also* DOUCHE; LEUCORRHEA; REPRODUCTIVE SYSTEM.)

VAGINISMUS. This is a condition of hypersensitiveness of the vulva and vagina which leads to painful spasms of the muscles at the entrance of the genital canal whenever an attempt at sexual intercourse is made. It may be caused by excessive smallness of the opening, rigidity of the hymen, or some painful inflammatory disorder of the parts, but is often merely a reflex spasm in a nervous, highly strung woman. The treatment naturally depends upon the cause; sexual intercourse should be avoided until the condition clears up.

VAGUS. The pneumogastric nerve is known as the vagus and is a very important nerve sending branches to several vital organs. (*See also* NERVOUS SYSTEM.)

VALERIAN. From the root of the valerian plant—a native of Europe and North America—is obtained a volatile oil which has a strong and disagreeable smell

and a bitter unpleasant taste. Owing to
its evil odor and taste it has had a reputation for benefiting hysterical conditions
and it is often prescribed along with bromides. The effect of valerian is purely
psychological.

VALVE. In the heart, veins, and lymphatics of the human body there are flaps
of tissue which permit of the blood or
lymph flowing in one direction only. Such
flaps are termed valves, and they are an
essential part of the mechanism of the
heart and veins.

VARICELLA. This is another name for
the infectious disease called chickenpox.

VARICOCELE. This is a dilated and
twisted condition of the veins of the spermatic cord. These veins drain the testicle
and its coverings, and the condition shows
itself as a slight swelling in the scrotum
which disappears when the patient lies
down. It feels like a bag of worms, and
the condition occurs most often on the left
side. Varicocele occurs in young adults and
its production is favored by constipation.
Very often no symptoms are produced,
but sometimes there is experienced a feeling of weight and discomfort—the latter
occasionally amounting to a neuralgic pain.
The discomfort is generally worse during
vigorous exercise and during hot weather.

In mild cases, the best treatment for
a varicocele is to ignore it; in more severe
cases a suspensory bandage may be worn.
The affection can often be relieved by
cold baths, which have a bracing effect
generally, and by attention to the bowels.
If the condition is causing anxiety, an
operation can be performed to remove
a portion of the venous network, or it may
be obliterated by injection. (*See also* SPER-
MATIC CORD; TESTICLE.)

VARICOSE VEIN. A vein is called
varicose when it is dilated, twisted and
knotty in appearance. Actually, the twisting is due to the elongation of the vein.
Many veins in different parts of the body
can be so affected, but the commonest
situation is the leg. Most often it is the
saphenous vein which passes up the inner
side of the leg and thigh which becomes
varicose.

The fundamental cause of varicose veins
of the leg is a hereditary weakness of the
walls of the veins and of the valves. These

valves are unable to withstand any extra
call upon the blood circulation, so that
they become incompetent and do not help
to support the long column of blood. The
result is that there is a certain amount of
sluggishness of the venous return of blood
—and sometimes a back flow so that the
veins become dilated, lengthened and finally twisted. There are certain contributory
factors which tend to produce varicose
veins. Anything constricting the limb, such
as tight garters, leads to this affection, and
the strain of standing for prolonged periods is a common precipitating cause. This
explains the frequency of the condition in
store clerks and policemen. Athletes are
liable to develop varicose veins. In women,
the pregnant womb, by pressing on the
great veins in the pelvis, may lead to
varicose veins and similarly any abdominal
tumor or even an overloaded bowel, as in
constipation, may have the same adverse
effect.

The earliest symptom is a feeling of
weight and fullness in the limb after standing or after a long walk. On examination,
the veins will be seen to be prominent and,
as the condition develops, the veins bulge
out and are seen to be twisted and knotted
under the skin. The feeling of weight increases and there is a marked weariness
of the limbs after even a short period of
standing. There is nearly always a certain
amount of swelling of the ankles, for the
obstruction of the venous flow causes a
local dropsy. This leads to impairment of
the nutrition of the skin and blood pigment is deposited which is irritating. Any
friction on the part is then apt to lead to
dermatitis which may ultimately cause a
breakdown of the tissues, or, in other
words, a varicose ulcer.

There are two other possible complications. The thin skin over the dilated veins
may rupture and so lead to bleeding. It
may happen also that clotting or thrombosis takes place, especially after an injury
or during some infectious illness. In such
a case, the clot may become changed into
fibrous tissue, obliterating the vein and
thus curing the condition, or fragments of
the clot may become detached and block
a vessel in the lungs or some other organ.

A certain amount can be done to prevent this relatively crippling affection. A

garter belt should always be worn instead of garters. Store clerks and other workers who have to stand about a great deal should be provided with seats for occasional rests. Constipation can readily be prevented by appropriate dieting. During pregnancy, the weight on the veins can be relieved by periodic rests and by gentle massage of the limbs.

Treatment. Once the condition is established, it is difficult to cure except by the modern method of injecting chemical substances which lead to obliteration of the veins, or by operation. In some cases, the varicose veins can be controlled by the wearing of an elastic bandage. This should be put on first thing in the morning *in bed,* and should not be taken off again until the person is again in bed at night. Massage or gentle rubbing in an upward direction is also beneficial, but it must be carefully carried out so as to avoid injury to the veins. Should redness and pigmentation of the skin in the lower part of the leg develop, the part affected should be freely dusted with a zinc oxide and fine boric powder. For the treatment of eczema and ulceration *see* under respective headings.

The most recent treatment for varicose veins is by the local injection into the veins of a solution of ethamolin or sodium morrhuate, which produce a firm clot within the veins. This clot ultimately becomes hard and fibrous and so obliterates the venous channel. This treatment may take some time, but it does not necessitate the patient remaining in bed and it prevents the need of a more extensive surgical operation. Some people might imagine that the formation of a clot in the vein is dangerous, but this is not so, as there should be no sepsis. Thousands of cases have been treated in this way without fatality. (*See also* VEIN.)

VARIOLA. This is the technical name for smallpox.

VARIX. This term is used to denote a dilated, twisted, or varicose condition of a vein. If a vein communicates directly with an artery, as a result of a puncture wound, the expression aneurismal varix is applied; while a varicose aneurism means the communication of a vein with an aneurism. (*See also* ANEURISM.)

VASA VASORUM. These are the tiny microscopic blood vessels which supply the walls of the arteries and veins. Like all other tissues, the large blood vessels need constant nutriment.

VAS DEFERENS. This is the main duct of the testicle along which its secretion is conveyed to its temporary storehouse in the seminal vesicles.

VASELINE. A variety of soft yellow paraffin, or petroleum jelly is known by the trade name of Vaseline. It serves as a protective covering to the skin and is used as a basis for many ointments. Unlike fats of animal or vegetable origin, it does not go rancid.

VASOMOTOR NERVES. The nerves which supply the muscle-coat of the blood vessels are termed vasomotor. They are derived from the sympathetic nervous system. Certain diseases are dependent upon disorder of these nerves, notably Raynaud's disease, angioneurotic edema and some forms of asthma. (*See also* SYMPATHETIC NERVOUS SYSTEM.)

VEGETABLE FOODS. See DIET; FOOD; VITAMINS.)

VEGETARIANISM. This is the dietetic system in which, strictly speaking, only vegetable foods are eaten. It is more generally used to denote the abstinence from all animal foods excepting milk, eggs, and cheese. It is doubtful whether a purely vegetarian diet is completely satisfactory from the nutritional point of view, but when dairy produce is included a perfect diet which satisfies all the needs of the body can be obtained. (*See also* DIET; FOOD.)

VEGETATION. In medicine, this term is used to denote small lumps or growths which arise as a result of some inflammatory process on the heart valves. Rheumatic fever is the commonest cause. (*See also* EMBOLISM.)

VEIN. The tubes which carry the blood to the heart are called veins. They are similar in structure to the arteries, and possess three coats—an inner elastic lining, a middle muscular coat, and an outer covering of fibrous connective tissue. In contrast with an artery, the middle muscle-coat of a vein is much less developed, so that the vein collapses when empty while the artery retains its tubular form. The veins are provided with valves which permit the blood to flow in one direction only. A vein commences as a tiny tube which is connected with the microscopic blood vessels called the capillaries. These small veins or venules unite to form larger veins until the main venous trunks are formed. These are two in number, the superior and the inferior vena cava, and they open into the right auricle of the heart. The superior vena cava is formed by the internal jugular and subclavian veins which unite to form the innominate veins, and the inferior vena cava is formed by the two iliac veins which drain the lower limbs and pelvis. In its course through the abdomen and chest, the inferior vena cava receives numerous tributaries.

The portal vein is important in that it drains the blood, rich in nutriment derived from the stomach and intestines, and carries this blood to the liver where it ends by breaking up into small capillary vessels.

The flow of blood in the veins is dependent upon a number of factors: there is the force from the heart carried through the arteries and capillaries; most important of all there is the action of the skeletal muscles which tend to drive the blood towards the heart, and there is also the suction effect of breathing.

The blood in the veins is dark purplish in color, for much of its oxygen has been lost to the tissues. There is one exception to this in the case of the pulmonary veins which take the pure oxygenated blood from the lungs to the heart. The veins generally follow the course of the arteries

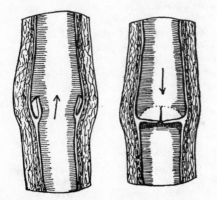

Vein showing closure of valve.

and are named after the arteries they accompany throughout the body.

Diseases and injuries of veins. An injury to a vein is usually a much less serious affair than an injury to an artery, as the blood flows slowly and the flow can easily be controlled by pressure. Bleeding from a large vein, however, such as a ruptured varicose vein in the leg, may be dangerous, as may be a wound involving one of the large veins in the neck or armpit. In the latter case, there is the added risk of air being sucked into the vein, causing an air-embolus which may lead to death. Veins which have become dilated, twisted, and knotty are termed *varicose*. (See VARICOSE VEINS.) Clotting of blood in a vein is termed *thrombosis;* it causes stoppage of the flow of blood; the vein swells and the function of the part involved is handicapped. This condition may arise during the course of prolonged illnesses, as in typhoid fever.

Inflammation of a vein is called *phlebitis.* It may be caused by germs circulating in the blood—or by an infected wound in the vicinity of a vein. This is a dangerous condition, as clotting is apt to occur, and should portions of clot become detached, abscesses may be formed in different parts of the body (pyemia). Injury may produce a simple phlebitis, which may also follow thrombosis in a vein.

Symptoms. The onset of phlebitis is marked by pain and tenderness along the line of the vein, which becomes hard and cord-like to the touch. The skin over the vein is reddened and may be swollen. If a large vein of the leg is involved, the limb becomes swollen and hard, and there is generally some degree of fever.

Treatment. Phlebitis of superficial veins of the leg calls for the application of a firm crêpe bandage. The patient should remain up and about.

When phlebitis involves the deeper veins, however, thrombosis often occurs, and such cases must be confined to bed and given a course of an anticoagulant drug—either heparin or dicoumarol. (*See also* CIRCULATION OF BLOOD; THROMBOSIS; WHITE LEG.)

VENA CAVA. The two great veins which collect the blood from the whole of the body and pass it into the right auricle of the heart are called the superior and the inferior vena cava. (*See also* VEIN.)

VENEREAL DISEASE. A disease acquired through sexual intercourse is termed a venereal disease. Into this category come *syphilis, gonorrhea* and *soft chancre* or sore. All these diseases are dependent upon microorganisms or germs, and they may in rare cases be acquired without any sexual contact, e.g., by contact with infected towels in the case of gonorrhea or drinking vessels in the case of syphilis. Gonorrhea responds well to penicillin, and this drug, along with bismuth and arsenicals, is used in the treatment of syphilis. (*See also* GONORRHEA; SOFT CHANCRE; SYPHILIS.)

VENESECTION. The operation of opening the vein to allow the escape of blood for the treatment of disease is termed venesection or blood-letting. Formerly, it was a very popular method of treatment, but nowadays its use is more restricted. (*See also* BLEEDING.)

VENOM. This term is applied to the poisons secreted by reptiles and insects. (*See also* BITES AND STINGS.)

VENTILATION. Ventilation is the continuous change of air in a room, without production of a draft.

Why air should be kept moving. We should not breathe second-hand air. Such an atmosphere makes us sleepy and dull; it does not stimulate our nerves or our brains, and we are very likely to catch a cold in a stuffy place. The air we have been breathing contains a high percentage of carbon dioxide and water vapor and is laden with bacteria.

No need for drafts. A draft is a little current of air that blows on one spot—the neck, perhaps, so that a stiff neck results—or on the floor, making the feet cold. Hot air rises—this is why we open our windows at the top to let it out, while the fresh air comes in by way of the lower part of the window. What we want to do is to let the bad air out and let the good in, without creating a draft.

The livingroom. We can let in the fresh air by opening the window—and there will be no draft if a strip of wood the same width as the window, and about three inches deep, is put at the bottom of the window. Now, with the lower sash pushed

up those three inches, the good outside air will come in; to get more of it, the window may also be opened at the top. There will now be a regular stream of bad air going out and good air coming in, by which means the air of the room is constantly and gently changed. That is the secret of ventilation.

The bedroom. Good ventilation is of even more importance here. No one should ever sleep in a room with a tightly shut window. A curtain is sufficient to prevent drafts.

The sickroom. In a small house it is sometimes difficult to keep the patient out of drafts, but there is usually space enough for the bed to be between neither door nor window nor two windows. When the window is open the door should be closed. Ventilating by way of the door is not a good plan, for the air of the house is not likely to be so pure as that outside. It is best to open the window at the top and use a board such as that previously described below the lower sash. If outside air is allowed to come in at the bottom of the window, it will chill the air below the patient's bed.

VENTRICLE. The literal meaning of this word is "little stomach," and it is used to describe two of the muscular chambers of the heart, the spaces in the brain filled with cerebrospinal fluid, and to certain spaces in the larynx or voice box.

VERMIFUGE. This is the term applied to any agent which expels intestinal parasites or worms from the body. (*See also* WORM.)

VERONAL. This is a drug which has a sedative or calming effect upon the nervous system and helps to induce sleep. Its chemical name is barbital and it occurs as a white crystalline powder; it is commonly given dissolved in warm milk, and the dose is approximately five grains. As its action is sometimes uncertain, and even small doses may have unexpectedly severe effects, it should be taken only under medical advice. Today it is rather out of date, or out of fashion, and its place has been taken by the derivatives called barbiturates. Veronal is of little value if the sleeplessness is caused through physical pain. In susceptible persons it may produce a skin eruption, and in large doses it has a very depressing effect upon the nervous system and upon the heart. In veronal poisoning there is unconsciousness with shallow breathing and coldness of the body.

In the case of an overdose of veronal the patient should be given an emetic of mustard and water, if conscious, and a cup of hot strong coffee. If unconscious, expert treatment will be required, which is best carried out in hospital. (*See also* HYPNOTIC.)

VERSION. This is the term used to describe the operation of turning the child within the womb to enable it to be born in the normal manner. (*See also* CHILD-BIRTH; LABOR.)

VERTEBRA. The backbone is made up of a number of segments, each super-imposed upon the other, and the individual bones are called vertebrae. There are thirty-three vertebrae, varying in size and shape, but they are all constructed on a similar plan.

There is a rounded or oval body from which two portions are directed backwards to form an arch which ends in a spine-like process. The body is composed of spongy bone, and between the bodies of the vertebrae are disks of fibrocartilage, thus making a solid yet flexible column. Projecting from either side of the arch is a bony outgrowth called the transverse process, and in the neck region this is perforated for the transmission of the vertebral artery. On the arch there are also articular processes by which the arch of one vertebra joints with that of another. The superimposed arches with their ligaments form the spinal canal, in which is placed the delicate spinal cord. There are seven cervical, twelve dorsal, five lumbar, five sacral, and four coccygeal vertebrae. The neck vertebrae are small and permit of free movement. The first cervical vertebra is called the atlas, and it joints with the occipital bone of the skull. The second cervical vertebra is called the axis. To the dorsal vertebrae are attached the ribs. The lumbar vertebrae are very strong, while the five sacral vertebrae are fused together in early life to form a solid triangular bone. The coccygeal vertebrae are very small and insignificant and are often fused together.

The vertebral column may be affected by tuberculosis as in Pott's disease, and it is sometimes the site of secondary cancer. Ankylosing spondylitis is a form of arthritis of the spinal column which converts the flexible column into a rigid, unbending mass. (*See also* POTT'S DISEASE; SPINAL CORD.)

VERTIGO. *See* DIZZINESS.

VESICAL. This is an adjective used to denote anything referring to the urinary bladder. Thus the blood vessels supplying the bladder are called the vesical arteries and veins, and a stone in the bladder is called a vesical calculus.

VESICANT. *See* BLISTER.

VESICLE. *See* BLISTER.

VILLUS. This is a small finger-like process which is found in the lining membrane of the small intestine. Villi are present in great numbers and give the interior of the intestine the appearance of velvet pile. Each villus contains blood vessels and one or more lacteals (small tubes which carry off the fat absorbed from the intestine). By means of villi the absorptive capacity of the bowel is greatly increased.

The term villi is also given to the small processes on the outer surface of the chorion, which is one of the membranes of the developing embryo in the womb. On one part the chorionic villi are greatly developed and form the placenta, by means of which nourishment is conveyed from the mother to the child.

VINCENT'S ANGINA. *See* ANGINA.

VINEGAR. This is a dilute solution of acetic acid containing varying amounts of sugar, gum and coloring material. It is a by-product in the manufacture of wine. It is commonly used in the preparation of salads, the weak acid softening the cellulose fibers of vegetables and rendering them more easily digested. The addition of an aromatic vinegar to water makes an astringent lotion which has a hardening effect upon the skin and diminishes the disfigurement caused by dilated blood vessels. (*See also* ACETIC ACID.)

VIRUS. This is the term which signifies the morbid material produced in the course of an infective disease, by which the disease can be reproduced when it is inoculated into another person. The virus may contain germs visible through the microscope, but in some cases these cannot be demonstrated, though they are presumed to exist. Certain types of virus, such as those of smallpox, rabies, and foot-and-mouth disease, are able to pass through a fine porcelain filter and they are described as filterable viruses. (*See also* BACTERIA.)

VISCERA. This is the term applied collectively to the internal organs of the body. A single organ is described as a *viscus*.

VISCEROPTOSIS. Sagging of the abdominal organs is termed visceroptosis. The condition is also known by the name Glenard's disease or abdominal ptosis. It is a fairly common complaint, being much more frequently observed in women. It rarely gives rise to symptoms, and when it does they are usually unimportant. Normally, there is a certain range of movement permitted to the stomach, intestines, and other organs, but, in visceroptosis, the movement downwards is excessive. The actual displacement is due to several causes; stretching of ligaments, feebleness in the abdominal muscles, compression of the chest and upper abdomen by wearing tight corsets. Weak abdominal muscles may be a result of underfeeding and lack of exercise, or, in women, frequent pregnancies.

VISION. Vision is a function of the brain; the eye is the instrument by which we see. When the image of an external object is formed on the retina, a nerve current passes through the optic ("eye") nerve to the brain, and stimulates the cells in the two vision centers, which lie at the back of the brain. There is not one center for each eye, but each shares in both. For example, if one center were destroyed, half of each retina would lose the faculty of sight, and we should be blind on one side.

Vision includes also the formation of judgments of seen objects. These judgments are based on experience and can be increased by practice, as in the detective, medical, and artistic professions. Visual illusions, however, are quite common, e.g., the stationary moon seen through flying clouds seems to our eyes to move.

The visual center on the left side appears to store visual memories. If, for instance, the center for "visual speech" were destroyed, we should be able to see words, but not to understand their meaning. If complete destruction took place, we should still *see* objects, but should only be able to *recognize* them by handling them.

Infants under six months cannot see clearly because they have not learnt to focus accurately, and cannot keep a moving object in view. Even after they can focus easily, and move head and eyes quickly, they are very apt to make mistakes in visual judgment, and naturally try to correct their mistakes by using their other senses. An infant "puts everything into his mouth" not because he is hungry or greedy, but because he is inquisitive. An older child handles everything he sees not because he is naughty but because he wants to find out all about it. As far as possible, children should be encouraged to examine a large variety of objects as a part of their education.

VITALLIUM. A metal alloy, used for screws and nails in bone surgery, as it is nonirritant and noncorroding.

VITAL STATISTICS. The statistics which deal with births, deaths, causes of deaths, and marriages are described as vital statistics. They are of great importance in the solution of public health problems. (*See also* BIRTHRATE; DEATHRATE.)

VITAMINS. These are substances present in various foodstuffs which are essential for the maintenance of health. If any of them are deficient in the dietary, serious disease results. There are many more vitamins than was at first realized: Vitamin A is a fatsoluble crystalline hydrocarbon and is found in animal and fish fats; lack of it causes xerophthalmia or night-blindness and diminishes powers of resistance to infection. Vitamin B is found in many plants and in yeast and wholegrain bread; it is now known to consist of at least a dozen separate chemical substances, the chief of which are called aneurine, riboflavin, and nicotinic acid. Lack of Vitamin B_1 (which is destroyed by boiling) causes constipation, mental depression, and polyneuritis—when in a marked degree, heart weakness results, with swelling of the body (edema) and neuritis, the signs of beri-beri.

Lack of Vitamin B_2 causes fatigue, palpitation, depression, diarrhea, a sore tongue and skin disorders—signs of the disease called pellagra, which is known chiefly among the poor, owing to their inadequate dietary. Lack of Vitamin B_{12} causes pernicious anemia. Vitamin C, or ascorbic acid, is found in fruits and vegetables, and its lack causes fatigue, spongy gums, bleeding under the skin and into the joints, and poor healing of cuts and wounds.

Vitamin D is the vitamin which prevents rickets; there are at least ten chemical substances with Vitamin D activity, but only two of them, D_2 and D_3 are important. D_2 is calciferol, a substance obtained by exposing the chemical ergosterol to ultraviolet irradiation; D_3 is the naturally occurring vitamin present in animal fats and fish oils, especially cod-liver and halibut-liver oil, and is also formed in the human skin by the effects of the rays of the sun. It is important not to take too much Vitamin D, as overdosage causes lethargy, and, when long continued, may cause the formation of kidney stones or thickening of the walls of the blood vessels.

Vitamin E is a fat-soluble alcohol, found in wheat germ, seeds, oats and corn; its absence causes sterility in animals, but there is no proof that it does this in human beings. Vitamin K is a yellow oil, naphthoquinone, obtained from alfalfa, spinach, and some vegetable oils; when given to a pregnant mother a week before her baby is due to be born, it prevents the severe bleeding that sometimes occurs in newborn babies. Vitamin P, citrin, exists in fruit and vegetables, especially paprika and lemon rind; its lack causes bleeding from the smallest blood vessels (purpura). Combined deficiency of Vitamins C and P is the cause of scurvy.

A very striking feature of the vitamins is the exceedingly small amount of them that is necessary compared with the total daily ration of food. It has been calculated that a tablespoonful of one of the chemically-produced vitamins that helps to prevent the appearance of rickets would be enough to give a million children an adequate daily dose. (*See also* DEFICIENCY DISEASES; PERNICIOUS ANEMIA.)

VITRIOL. Oil of vitriol is another name for sulphuric acid. Blue vitriol is the common name for copper sulphate.

VIVISECTION. Any scientific experiments conducted on living animals are popularly described as vivisection, even though such experiments involve no actual cutting. Most states and many cities have their own laws pertaining to vivisection. If information is desired regarding those applicable to your community, it is suggested that you contact the local branch of the Society for the Prevention of Cruelty to Animals or else write to the Humane Society of New York, 313 East 58 Street, New York City.

VOCAL CORDS. These are two cords consisting of tense elastic bands which stretch from back to front of the larynx. Each is controlled by small muscles supplied by nerves under the control of the will. It is through the vibration of these cords that speech is chiefly produced. During swallowing, the vocal cords approximate and so prevent food from passing into the larynx on its way to the gullet. Above the "true" vocal cords are the false vocal cords, which are simply folds of tissue which take no part in phonation. (*See also* LARYNX.)

VOICE. *See* SPEECH.

VOLVULUS. The twisting of a length of bowel upon itself so as to obstruct the passage of the bowel contents is called volvulus. The portion most usually affected is the sigmoid colon. (*See also* INTESTINE; OBSTRUCTION.)

VOMITING. The forcible expulsion of the stomach contents through the mouth is called vomiting. This act is generally preceded and accompanied by a feeling of sickness or nausea and by a free flow of saliva. The mechanism of vomiting is fairly complex: first a deep breath is taken and the opening to the larynx is closed; then the abdominal muscles contract quickly and force the stomach against the diaphragm; at the same time the upper opening of the stomach relaxes and the stomach contents are forced upwards. Actually, the contractions of the muscular walls of the stomach are insignificant in the production of vomiting.

The causes of vomiting are exceedingly numerous and many are not related to the digestive organs. The commonest cause, however, is irritation of the stomach from eating unsuitable food, drinking excessive amounts of alcohol, or swallowing irritant chemical poisons. Vomiting is a symptom of gastric catarrh, acute or chronic, and of other organic diseases of the stomach such as ulcer, cancer, and dilatation. In dilatation of the stomach there is vomiting of large quantities of fluid at considerable intervals of time. After very severe vomiting from any cause, the vomit may be streaked with blood, and this is merely due to the effects of straining upon the membranes of the stomach. In ulcer or cancer of the stomach the vomit may be frankly bloodstained or it may look like "coffeegrounds." This appearance is due to chemical alteration of blood by the action of gastric juice.

Vomiting may arise from reflex causes, i.e. from irritation in some distant organ. Thus it may arise from tickling of the throat, from coughing, in colic, appendicitis, worms, gall-stones, gall-bladder inflammation, liver and pancreatic disorders, and strangulated hernias. It may also occur in nervous and mental disorders, in hysteria, migraine, tabes dorsalis, brain tumor and abscesses, concussion, and compression of the brain and meningitis. Any disagreeable smells or unpleasant sights may evoke vomiting in sensitive persons. The motion of a boat at sea is a common cause of vomiting.

In children, periodic attacks of vomiting may arise—cyclical vomiting, which is associated with a diminution of the alkalinity of the blood (acidosis). In the early months of pregnancy, sickness, sometimes amounting to actual vomiting, is a common symptom. Finally, vomiting can be caused by direct irritation of the vomiting center in the brain through the action of an emetic drug such as apomorphine or from the circulation in the blood of the poisons of certain infectious fevers.

Treatment. It should be remembered that vomiting is in itself merely a symptom, and it is the fundamental cause which requires treatment. If it is due to irritant foods or drinks, the vomiting will rid the stomach of the cause of the trouble, and in such cases the vomiting is to be encouraged. Plenty of warm water should be drunk as this helps to wash out the stomach and also relieves the distress and discomfort of the vomiting. In gastritis or gastric catarrh, regulation of the diet is all important. For some days the diet should be limited to fluids, milk, egg and albumen water and, when all vomiting has ceased, semisolid foods can then be taken.

Distressing vomiting from any cause may be relieved by sipping hot water or iced soda water. In children who suffer from cyclical vomiting, large doses of alkali (sodium bicarbonate) and of glucose will cut short the attacks. Alcoholic cases will benefit by a saline purge every morning. A great many drugs are used in the treatment of vomiting—tincture of opium, chloretone, dilute hydrocyanic acid, and others; but an effective remedy is to use a drop of tincture of iodine in a tablespoonful of tepid water and repeat the dose four or five times at fifteen-minute intervals. (*See also* DYSPEPSIA; EMETIC; GASTRITIS; SEA SICKNESS.)

VULVA. This is the name given to the external genital organs of the female. It consists of two pairs of lips or double folds of skin which surround and conceal the vaginal opening. These lips are called the labia majora and the labia minora. The front ends of the labia minora surround the clitoris, which is a sensitive erectile structure developmentally the same as the penis in the male sex.

Inflammation of the vulva, or vulvitis, may arise from lack of cleanliness or from the irritation of threadworms (especially in the case of children). The symptoms include a feeling of itching and burning with intense discomfort and the presence of a purulent discharge. The vulva become red and swollen. Treatment necessitates rest in bed with frequent bathing and douching and the use of a mild antiseptic ointment. Gonorrheal vulvitis is a more serious condition which always requires special treatment under the direction of a doctor. (*See also* REPRODUCTIVE SYSTEM; SEX HYGIENE.)

WARTS. Warts are small harmless tumors of the skin. They may appear on any part, and are thought to be due to an infectious virus. They are certainly contagious. There are four varieties: (1) the common raised wart found on the hands; (2) the flat wart found on the hands and face, and most commonly in children; (3) the corn-like warts found on the soles, rarely on the palms, at sites of pressure; (4) "cauliflower" or venereal warts, found chiefly about the genitals and anus. Warts may also occur on a skin affected with seborrhea, and on a senile skin. These may become cancerous.

Treatment. The simplest method is to freeze the warts with ethyl chloride and snip them off with scissors; or they may be destroyed by freezing with carbon dioxide snow. Caustic, such as salicylic or acetic acids, are efficient but slow, and the pain naturally lasts over a longer period. Venereal warts owe their size to the heat and moisture of the parts, and when treated with a simple drying powder containing 5 per cent salicylic acid, readily shrivel up. Seborrheic and senile warts are treated by curetting and cauterizing.

The effect of X-rays on warts is, in careful hands, remarkable, large crops often disappearing in a very short time. On the other hand, in some cases this treatment may fail entirely.

Internally, arsenic in small doses, Epsom salts, or green iodide of mercury will sometimes produce a cure; and the injection of salvarsan (an arsenical preparation) is also successful in some cases.

WASP STING. *See* BITES AND STINGS.

WASSERMANN REACTION. This is a test introduced by Wassermann in 1906 for the detection of syphilitic infection. It is a very complicated reaction and requires to be carried out by a skilled pathologist. The test can be applied to the blood or to the cerebrospinal fluid. It is exceedingly valuable as an aid to diagnosis and also as a means of controlling treatment. The Wassermann reaction is also given by certain tropical diseases, yaws, trypanosomiasis, and occasionally leprosy, but with these exceptions a positive test is conclusive evidence of syphilitic disease. (*See also* SYPHILIS.)

WASTING. *See* ATROPHY; EMACIATION.

WASTING PALSY. *See* PROGRESSIVE MUSCULAR ATROPHY.

WATER. Chemically, water is a combination of hydrogen and oxygen. Water is an essential requirement of the living organism. Two thirds of the weight of the human body consists of water, a proportion which must be kept constant. Since the body is continually losing water at the rate of four or five pints a day, the loss

must be made good by at least as much taken in the form of fluid or water-containing food.

The channels by which water escapes from the body are the skin, kidneys, lungs and bowels, and, as water is essential to enable these organs to carry out their work as waste eliminators, the need for drinking ample amounts of water is obvious if good health is to be maintained.

Hard and Soft Waters. Hardness is classified as temporary or permanent. Temporary hardness is removed by boiling; permanent hardness is not. These qualities depend on the salts present. If they are in the form of bicarbonates, boiling causes their precipitation as carbonates. It is these salts which constitute the fur in kettles and boilers. Permanent hardness is caused by salts of lime, magnesium, iron, and alum. Hard water is wasteful from the domestic point of view as it leads to destruction of soap and to the furring of pipes and cisterns.

Soft waters contain mineral salts in very small proportions. There is some danger with very soft waters, especially those derived from peaty soils, because of their solvent action on the lead used in the construction of pipes and cisterns. This has been known to cause lead poisoning.

A hard water may be softened by boiling, but on a large scale slaked lime in quantities dependent upon the degree of hardness is used. To correct permanent hardness soda must be added. Special domestic water-softeners are now on the market and lead to considerable saving in soap and in the preservation of pipes, etc.

Water and Disease. Water is a ready medium for the spread of certain types of disease. Ordinary organic pollution may cause diarrhea, but the greatest danger lies in water which has been contaminated with disease germs. Sewage pollution of water may cause its infection with the germs of typhoid, paratyphoid, cholera, and dysentery, while certain worms and their eggs may exist in water and cause infection in human beings. The most efficient method of removing germ impurities from water is by boiling, but this is inapplicable on a large scale. Therefore, it becomes necessary to adopt some method of filtration.

The usual type of filter is one containing a 2 foot layer of sharp sand supported upon a bed of gravel and stones which increase in size till the bottom of the filter, where the outlet pipe is situated, is reached. As a preliminary to filtration, water is stored in special reservoirs for about 30 days as this greatly reduces the number of germs present.

Mechanical filters are often used for domestic purposes, some of these combining a means of chemical purification. The best domestic filters are those made of mixtures of porcelain and clay and molded into candles, the water being forced through them by pressure. They must be kept clean by regular washing and boiling.

Chemical substances can completely purify water and are widely used. The great objection to this method is that large quantities of germicide must be added thus imparting an objectionable flavor to drinking water. One of the commonest agents for this purpose is chlorinated lime or bleaching powder. This sets free chlorine which is destructive to germ life. A stock solution of this re-agent may be made by adding half a teaspoonful of the powder to a pint of cold water; a teaspoonful of this solution is added to ten gallons of water and in half-an-hour the water can be reckoned safe for drinking. The unpleasant taste of the chloride can be got rid of by adding sodium hyposulphate. Both preparations can now be had in tablet form for treating water of doubtful purity.

Potassium permanganate is often used for chemical purification. It oxidizes organic vegetable matter and kills germs. Sufficient permanganate is added to turn the water a very pale pink and the water is allowed to stand for half an hour. Acid sodium sulphate, used in a strength of 15 grains to the quart and allowed to act for 15 minutes, is also an effective purifier and tablets of this chemical are available for this purpose. Electrically produced ozone has been utilized for water sterilization, but this is an expensive method though the results are good. Ultraviolet rays have been used for the same purpose.

It is impossible to judge from the appearance, clearness, and taste of a water whether it is fit for consumption. A water that is clear and sparkling may be highly dangerous. Therefore the source of the water should always be considered and precautions adopted accordingly.

WATER-BED. A large rubber bag, formed like a mattress, and filled with water, is called a water-bed. It is valuable in the nursing of chronic bed patients who are liable to develop bed-sores. (*See also* NURSING.)

WATER-BRASH. This is the regurgitation into the mouth of a hot, bitter fluid from the stomach. Very often it is accompanied by heartburn. Water-brash is a symptom of acid dyspepsia. (*See also* HEARTBURN.)

WATER-HAMMER PULSE. In severe disease of the aortic valve of the heart, in which there is regurgitation of blood, the pulse has a characteristic up and down movement. There is a strong impulse at the pulse which falls away very rapidly. This thumping pulse is called the water-hammer or Corrigan's pulse. (*See also* HEART.)

WATER ON THE BRAIN. *See* HYDRO-CEPHALUS.

WEANING. *See* INFANT FEEDING.

WAX. (Cerumen). *See* EAR.

WEIGHT. This is a useful indication of the general health of an individual, as there is some correlation between weight and height and weight and age. (*See* tables under heading of OBESITY.) Naturally, weight varies with habits of diet and exercise, but thinness and stoutness are to a large extent constitutional. Some people are born to be thin and others to be fat. Progressive loss of weight—not definitely of dietetic origin, as from fasting—is evidence of constitutional disease, and is a symptom always to be regarded seriously. Diabetes, tuberculosis, and cancer are important among the diseases which produce rapid and progressive loss of weight. (*See also* GROWTH.)

WEIGHTS AND MEASURES. *See* APOTHECARIES' WEIGHTS AND MEASURES.

WEIL'S DISEASE. This is a febrile disorder associated with jaundice and bleeding and occurring in epidemic form. The disease is caused by a spirochete, a spiral germ, which is conveyed to man by the bites of insects or by water contaminated by rat's urine. It may also be acquired by bathing in infected waters.

The onset of the disease is sudden and marked by headaches and shivering. About the fourth day jaundice sets in, and increases in severity till about the tenth day. Bleeding occurs from different parts of the body, from the nose, stomach, bowel, and lungs. The liver becomes enlarged and tender. Within a fortnight the temperature subsides and recovery gradually takes place. During the course of the disease, the spirochetes are found in the blood and urine.

Treatment. The patient must be nursed in bed and kept on a fluid diet. The bowels are kept open. Pencillin and aureomycin are effective against this disease.

WEN. This is the popular term for a sebaceous cyst. It forms in the skin, most often of the scalp, face, or back, and results from the blocking of a duct of a sebaceous gland. Normally, the oily secretion of these glands is poured out on the skin, but should the duct of the gland be obstructed the secretion accumulates and a soft swelling forms which gradually enlarges to considerable dimensions if untreated. The skin over the wen in time becomes thin and red and may become inflamed. Suppuration may then arise, and the wen ruptures with discharge of offensive pus. Apart from this complication, wens are disfiguring, and they should be removed when of quite moderate size. The operation is very simple and is carried out under a local anesthetic. It consists of opening the cyst, evacuating its contents, and then removing the whole of the cyst wall.

WHEY. This is the watery fluid which remains when the clot formed in milk by the action of the ferment, rennet, is removed. It contains sugar, proteins, salts, and fats in small quantities, and also Vitamins A and B. Though of comparatively slight nutritive value, it is sometimes used in conjunction with fruit and vegetables to form a dietetic regime called the whey cure. It is recommended in some forms of dyspepsia, especially if due to overeating. Whey is also a useful drink in certain fevers and in kidney disease, especially if whole milk cannot be tolerated. Wine whey is a pleasant drink for convalescents.

It is made by adding half a glass of sherry to a teacupful of milk in a saucepan and heating till clotting has occurred. The milk is then strained and the whey sweetened with sugar if desired.

WHIPWORM. *See* WORM.

WHITE LEG or Phlebitis. This is the popular expression used to describe a swelling of the leg which sometimes complicates the puerperium, i.e., the first 2 or 3 weeks after childbirth. The condition is due to inflammation of the deep veins of the leg, thus obstructing the return of blood. The infection probably enters through injury of the tissues at the neck of the womb. The left leg is most often involved.

The swelling is first noticed in the thigh and gradually extends to the whole leg. It is dead white in color, and the swelling is hard and unyielding. There is usually a certain amount of fever which persists for a few days. Treatment consists in absolute rest in bed. Extension of the clot in the vein is prevented by giving drugs which diminish the clotting power of the blood. The most commonly used drugs for this purpose are heparin and dicoumarol. Within a few weeks, the condition subsides and recovery is complete, although in a few cases the swelling of the leg may reappear on exertion. An elastic stocking or a crêpe bandage is useful in such cases. Swelling of the lower limbs may also arise from clotting of the blood in deep veins during the course of infective fevers such as typhoid or pneumonia. (*See also* LYMPHATIC SYSTEM; PHLEBITIS; THROMBOSIS.)

WHITES. The name "whites" is popularly used for a thick white or yellow vaginal discharge. It is described under its medical name of LEUCORRHEA.

WHITLOW. This is a painful septic inflammation occurring in one of the fingers or thumb. It is most often caused by the prick of a dirty pin. The inflammation may only extend under the skin when it is described as subcuticular; or it may involve the tissue under the skin, the subcutaneous variety; or the sheath of a tendon may be affected, the thecal type; or the infection may be subperiosteal when it attacks the periosteum or covering of the bone. A deep whitlow, involving a

PATH OF
INFECTION

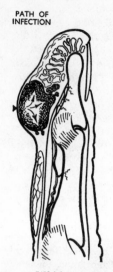

Whitlow.

tendon or bone, may arise from a superficial infection spreading deeply or from the initial injury far into the tissues.

A superficial whitlow commences as a red tender spot which becomes a blister filled with pus. If the inflammation spreads more deeply, pain and tenderness become very marked, and there is also throbbing. The whole finger commences to swell, the glands in the elbow and armpit become tender, and the pain gets progressively worse and may be so severe as to prevent sleep. There is often a certain amount of fever and constitutional disturbance, according to the degree of the inflammation.

The thecal form is most dangerous. Suppuration in a tendon sheath may extend into the palm, and this is almost certain to cause subsequent disability in the use of the hand. If the tendon of the thumb or little finger is involved, the inflammation may spread to the wrist and forearm and abscess formation may take place. In the most severe cases there may be sloughing of the tendons and the bone may be affected, causing its destruction. In such a case, it may become necessary to sacrifice the finger by amputation to prevent further spread of the suppuration, and there is always a danger of a serious blood infection or septicemia.

It is therefore clear that a whitlow is a potentially dangerous condition and should always be regarded seriously. If the whitlow does not immediately respond to home methods of treatment, there should be no delay in seeking expert treatment from the doctor. It is nearly always in cases where the sufferer has continued to attempt self-treatment that the grave complications mentioned arise.

With a superficial whitlow, the best immediate treatment is to open the blister with a sterile needle or pair of scissors, allow the contents to escape, remove any loose skin, and then apply a boracic fomentation and continue fomenting until all pain and redness disappear. Deeper types of whitlow require free incision deeply into the skin in order to allow any pus to drain away. This should be performed by the doctor. Subsequently hot boric acid fomentations are applied at frequent intervals until the condition clears up. Meanwhile the arm should be supported by a sling with the hand well raised. It is often possible to arrest the progress of a whitlow in its early stages by injections of penicillin. (*See also* ABSCESS.)

WHOOPING COUGH. This is an acute infectious fever characterized by peculiar spasmodic outbursts of coughing; whooping cough is also known by the technical term pertussis. Immunization should be carried out preferably before the age of six months, as the disease is serious in infancy. It is caused by a germ called the bacillus of Bordet and Gengou which it is found in the sputum and nose discharges of sufferers. Infection is conveyed by droplets laden with germs, but the risks of infection diminish after early stages of the fever are past, and during the spasmodic coughing stage, the danger is slight. One attack of the disease confers complete immunity for the rest of life.

The incubation period is from one to two weeks and the fever is conveniently divided into three stages. Firstly, lasting from 7 to 10 days, there are symptoms suggesting a severe cold in the head with a certain amount of feverishness. There is some degree of bronchitis with a hard cough, and then in the second stage there develops the typical spasmodic cough. This consists of a series of short expiratory coughs, the sufferer becoming blue in the face at times. Then follows a long crowing inspiration, producing the characteristic "whoop." A number of attacks usually follow on each other and, as a rule, relief does not arise until either vomiting occurs, or a considerable quantity of sticky mucus secretion is brought up. The paroxysms come on most often at night before sleeping, and sometimes after meals. They are liable to be induced by a fright or by hearing someone else cough.

During the attacks the eyes bulge and may become bloodshot and bleeding may occur into the conjunctiva. The child holds on to the bed or an adult and is in great fear. Bleeding from the nose not infrequently arises, and very occasionally bleeding into the brain may result. Convulsions may also occur in very young children. Interference with the child's sleep and his inability to take proper nourishment may produce considerable exhaustion and wasting.

In the third stage, the whooping cough gets gradually less and within three or four weeks the child should be practically well. In some debilitated children an occasional whoop may persist for some months. The complication most to be feared in whooping cough is catarrhal pneumonia, and for the prevention of this everything depends upon careful nursing and treatment of the child. Persistent bronchitis and emphysema may also be sequels to severe attacks. There is also a danger that the weakened resources of the child may render it a prey to tuberculosis. As whooping cough is very infectious in the early stages, complete isolation of the child is essential in the interests of other children. Six weeks is generally reckoned an adequate time; and children who have been in contact with a known case of the disease should be isolated for three weeks as a precautionary measure. During an epidemic of whooping cough, a child who develops an acute cold in the head with bronchitis should be carefully watched and preferably isolated until the real nature of the illness is manifest.

Treatment. In the case of strong children there may be no need to put them to bed, especially in the summer. They should have as much fresh air as possible and should be kept warm and given nutritious food. With more delicate children—and in winter—they should be kept in bed exclusively in one room until the temperature has subsided and the symptoms have considerably abated. If there is much vomiting, the diet should be restricted to bland foods such as milk, beaten eggs, and custard.

The antibiotic terramycin, given as a syrup, has been found to reduce the severity of whooping cough. During a paroxysm, someone should always be present to comfort and reassure the child, as the mental strain to a young child so induced is very great. Care should be taken to disinfect and destroy any sputum from the child, especially in the early stages. There is evidence to show that children can be protected from the disease, or at least have its course modified if they contract it, by injection of a vaccine of dead germs. Immunization is best carried out before the first birthday by means of three separate injections at four- to six-weekly intervals. (*See also* Bronchopneumonia; Disinfection; Infectious Disease.)

WIND. *See* Flatulence.

WINDPIPE. The windpipe is described under its medical name of Trachea.

WINTER COUGH. A winter cough is usually Bronchitis and is described under that name.

WITCH HAZEL. The hamamelis virginiana, or witch hazel, is a shrub which grows in North America, and from its bark and leaves are obtained tannic acid and a volatile oil. The tincture of hamamelis is made from the bark and the liquid extract from the leaves. Owing to its astringent properties, the extract is commonly used in the treatment of bruises and sprains. In ointment form, witch hazel is a popular remedy for piles.

WOMB. The uterus, or womb, is a pear-shaped organ freely movable in the pelvis and situated between the bladder and the rectum. It measures $3\frac{1}{2}$ inches long, 2 inches wide, by 1 inch thick; its narrow end or neck projects into the vagina, while its upper expanded end, or fundus, has the Fallopian tubes springing from its sides. These pass outwards to be loosely attached to the ovaries from which they convey microscopic ova (eggs) to the womb.

The womb consists of an outer or serous coat, a middle or muscular coat, and an inner or mucous coat. The mucous membrane is of peculiar structure and is constantly undergoing changes. During the childbearing period it periodically becomes engorged with blood, culminating in menstruation. The membrane is reconstructed every month unless pregnancy takes place, when it undergoes another complete change. After birth, it slowly returns to its normal condition and remains quiescent until lactation has ceased.

Owing to its mobility, the position of the womb is constantly being affected by neighboring organs, especially the bladder, the varying size of which necessitates accommodating movements of the womb. In close association with the Fallopian tubes are two muscular cords, the round ligaments, which extend upwards and pass to the external genital organs (labia majora) and help to support the womb. There are six other supporting ligaments which are composed of folds of peritoneum. Inside the uterus there is a triangular cavity into which the Fallopian tubes open above, and which is prolonged downwards into the cavity of the neck of the womb as the cervical canal. This opens into the vagina, the opening being termed the external os (to distinguish it from the internal os which is the place where the cervical canal joins the cavity of the body of the womb).

Displacement of the Womb. Normally the womb is bent forward upon itself at the junction of the neck with the body, this position being described as *anteflexion*. It is also bent forward in the pelvic cavity and this is termed *anteversion*. When it is bent backwards this is called *retroflexion,* and when it is tilted right back on itself this is called *retroversion*. One of the commonest forms of womb trouble is one or other of the displacements to which the organ is subject. It may be displaced in various directions by pressure exerted by tumors or swellings in the abdomen, or by adhesions to other organs which drag upon it, or by its own weight, especially if there is weakness of the supporting ligaments and muscular floor of the pelvis.

Prolapse. This, also known as "falling of the womb," is a downwards displacement. It is most common in elderly women whose muscles have lost tone or who have become thinner, and so have lost the support of the internal pads of fat which help to maintain the womb in position. It usually arises after a confinement in which the birth passages have been injured and torn. Frequent straining as a result of chronic constipation or a chronic cough also gives rise to downward displacement, especially if there is any weakness of the ligaments and the plevic floor.

The first symptom is generally a feeling of inward heaviness, with backache. There is also frequent desire to pass water and to empty the bowels, while menstruation is often excessive and more prolonged than usual. At this stage the patient should consult a doctor, for much can be done by exercises, general tonic treatment, fresh air, correct dieting, and the relief of constipation to prevent further trouble and avoid the need for an operation. Once a displacement is definitely established, a pessary or womb support will be required or an operation resorted to. In an otherwise healthy woman the latter is preferable, as a pessary is only palliative, and unless correctly fitted is of no value. In very severe cases, the womb may appear outside the body and then it is apt to become ulcerated and bleed. Part of the bladder and bowel may also protrude (cystocele and vectocele) and cause discomfort. In such cases an operation is desirable.

Tumors of the Womb. In the womb the commonest simple tumor is the fibroid or fibromyoma. It is a solid tumor composed of a mixture of fibrous, muscular, and sometimes glandular tissue. The growth may occur at any time of life, but it is rare before the age of thirty, and is most frequent about the change of life. It occurs most commonly in childless or unmarried women. In size, a fibroid varies from that of a small marble to that of a child's head, and it may be situated under the peritoneum lining the womb, in the wall of the womb, or may bulge into the cavity of the womb.

If situated on the inner surface, bleeding is a common symptom and may be severe. Such a fibroid is apt to become stalked or pedunculated. It gives rise to pain at the menstrual period, and .there is often leucorrhea. A small fibroid in the wall of the womb may give rise to no symptoms, but as it tends to increase in size it may cause effects through pressure. Fibroid tumors in the womb are often multiple and may grow to an enormous size—shown by considerable abdominal swelling. Such a swelling is often mistaken for pregnancy until a medical examination is undergone.

Fibroid tumors may occasionally disappear spontaneously, after a pregnancy or at the menopause, but generally it is advisable to have them removed by surgical operation, as there is always a danger of their undergoing a malignant degeneration. The presence of symptoms from pressure, or the occurrence of bleeding are definite indications for operation and there should be no delay. In some cases, X-ray or radium may be used to control the growth, but this treatment is apt to hasten the onset of the change of life. In a comparatively young woman, a fibroid should always be removed, as, should pregnancy occur, there may be danger to the mother and child. (*See also* FIBROID.)

Malignant growth or cancer of the womb is of fairly frequent occurrence, and generally arises in women who have borne children. It is most commonly situated at the cervix or neck of the womb, and it is apt to spread locally and also to set up secondary growths in other parts of the body. The early symptoms are important. Bleeding at irregular intervals, at the time of or after the menopause, and an unpleasant discharge are the first signs. Pain is a late symptom. In such cases, a doctor should immediately be consulated, for in the early stages much can be done to cure the condition. Cancer treated early is curable, but when not detected till well advanced it is one of the deadliest of all diseases. Surgical operation and radium treatment give the best chances of cure. The sarcoma, another malignant growth, may also occur in the womb, though less frequently. The outlook in such a case is unfavorable. Yet another malignant tumor, fortunately comparatively rare, is the chorion epithelioma. It is an overgrowth of the villi, finger-like projections of the chorion, which is one of the membranes surrounding the embryo within the womb.

Inflammation. Inflammation of the womb mucous membrane is termed endometritis; of the muscle—metritis; and of the tissues surrounding the womb—perimetritis. It is treated usually by hot douches; but an operation (curettage) may sometimes be necessary. (*See also* REPRODUCTIVE SYSTEM; MENSTRUATION; PESSARY; VISCEROPTOSIS.)

WOOLSORTER'S DISEASE. *See* ANTHRAX.

WORM. Various types of worm are parasitic in the human body and are productive of disease. There are two main groups, the flatworms which consist of the tapeworms and flukes, and the roundworms. These parasites gain entrance to the body through eating infected food, drinking infected water, or directly through the skin.

The roundworms most often infecting man are the thread or pinworm, the ascaris lumbricoides or intestinal roundworm, and the whipworm or tricocephalus dispar. There is one other variety, the ankylostoma, but this worm is not uncommon in this country. The *ascaris lumbricoides* resembles the ordinary earthworm; it has a pinkish color, tapers at each end, and the mouth is surrounded by three projections armed with fine teeth. In length it varies from 4 to 12 inches. It is probable that the mouse or rat is the intermediate host by swallowing the eggs. These develop into larvae and are deposited on human food, and the infection so conveyed to man. The worms live in the small intestine and may make their way into the bile ducts, stomach, gullet and thence to the air passages. They are expelled by the bowel or they may be vomited. As a rule only two or three worms are present, but occasionally there are large numbers.

If only a few are present, there may be no symptoms and the condition is only discovered when a worm is detected in the movement. On the other hand, there may be a capricious appetite, with sickness and vomiting, and sometimes blood in the movements. If a worm enters the bile duct, jaundice may be caused, and if a large number of worms are present, they may lead to obstruction of the bowel. The best treatment is the correct administration of the drug santonin or oil of chenopodium. A light diet precedes the use of the former drug, which is given in doses from 1 to 5 grains along with 2 grains of calomel at bedtime. In the morning a saline purge is taken. Santonin must be administered with care as it sometimes upsets the patient, producing yellow vision among other unpleasant symptoms, and two nights should elapse before the dose is repeated.

The **threadworm** or *oxyuris vermicularis* is an exceedingly common infection in children. This worm is about ½ to 3-inch in length, the female being 2 to 3 times larger than the male. The worm gets into the body by the swallowing of the eggs which hatch out in the intestine where the worms mature. Their habitat is the large intestine from the caecum to the anus, and the impregnated female wriggles out of the anus at night to lay her eggs on the neighboring skin.

In females they may enter the vagina, causing irritation and discharge. Children are apt to scratch these parts and convey the eggs to the mouth and so infect themselves. Children so infected are peevish, irritable, complain of colicky pain and exhibit reflex symptoms such as grinding of the teeth at night, night terrors, and occasionally convulsions. The appetite may be capricious. The condition is easily detected by finding the worms in the movements. They resemble small wriggling pieces of white thread.

To rid the bowel of the worms, frequent enemas of infusions of quassia are necessary. The young child should be given an injection into the bowel of about 6 ounces and older children up to ¾-pint. Internally, gentian violet in capsules is effective, but this should be administered only under medical supervision.

On rising in the morning the child's anus should be washed after the bowels move, and a weak mercurial ointment applied fairly liberally to the part. Regular action of the bowels is essential, and if the child scratches at night a close pair of underpants should be worn. Every precaution should be taken to prevent the child from reinfecting itself.

The **whipworm** or *tricocephalus dispar* is a very common parasite in man. It is especially prevalent in warm countries and infects man and monkeys. The whipworm measures about 2 inches in length, the female being slightly larger. It owes its name to the fact that it has a head and a slender neck with a thick body, thus resembling a minute whip. Its home is the caecum, the first part of the larger bowel, but it wanders about the large intestine and may reside in the appendix. It attaches itself to the mucous membrane by its head, the rest of the worm being free. The symptoms are very variable; often there are none at all. Its presence may only be known by the discovery of its eggs in the movements. The whipworm is very difficult to expel, but oil of chenopodium is the best remedy. Infection usually arises from drinking contaminated water, so that any questionable water should always be boiled.

The **ankylostoma** is a small round worm armed with hooks, and the disease it produces is sometimes called hookworm disease or tunnel disease, for it was prevalent among workers during the construction of certain tunnels. It occurs to people who walk barefoot, especially in southern U.S. The worm finds entry in the larval state, and an eruption appears on the hands and arms—the so-called "ground itch." The most important symptoms are a profound anemia, with diarrhea and great debility. Treatment is by administration of thymol or carbon tetrachloride taken on an empty stomach and followed by a purge. The anemia also requires special treatment.

There are three varieties of **tapeworm,** known technically as the taenia solium, taenia saginata, and bothriocephalus latus. Common to all are a head and neck called the scolex, and a segmented body. The terminal segments contain the testes and uterus, and the latter is full of eggs which are evacuated. The total length of the tapeworm is anything up to 30 feet. It depends for its nourishment upon digested foods which are absorbed into its tissues from its host. Periodically, some of the segments pass out of the bowel, the eggs are set free, and for their further development they require to be swallowed by an animal.

The **taenia solum** or pork tapeworm is a flat ribbon-shaped worm, 8 to 15 feet in length, with a head the size of a pin-head with two rows of hooklets and four sucking discs. Each segment possesses the reproductive organs of both sexes. It is the pig which swallows the fertilized eggs, usually by eating contaminated vegetables. In the pig's stomach the shell of the egg is dissolved by the gastric juice and the embryo, armed with six hooks, bores its way into the stomach blood-veins and so makes its way to the liver, muscles, or other organs. Here, it develops a small sac about the size of a pea, in which the hooklets are discarded and a head develops similar to that of the adult worm. The worm at this stage is described as a cysticercus. If the cysts are in the pig's flesh, the pork is said to be "measly," and consumption of such pork if inadequately cooked causes infection in man.

The **taenia saginata** has a larger head than the former, and it has four sucking discs but no hooklets. The intermediate host is the ox.

The **bothriocephalus latus** is 20 to 30 feet long and has a long head with a sucking grove on either side. The larval form is found in fresh water fish—pike, salmon, perch and trout.

In all forms of tapeworm, when infected meat is eaten, the cyst is dissolved in the stomach, the head is set free and fixes itself to the mucous membrane of the intestine and develops segments. The symptoms are variable and the infection may only be discovered by finding segments of worms in the expelled motions. Colic may occur. Occasionally, there is headache, depression, and irritability, these nervous symptoms being attributed to poisons liberated by the worm. Tapeworms may live for years in the human body, and there may be several present at the same time.

Treatment. The most usual remedy is oil of male fern. This is administered with some carminative such as peppermint or cinnamon first thing in the morning before breakfast and after a fast which has commenced at 6 p.m. the night before. Two hours afterwards a saline purge is taken, and the movements are passed into warm water. It is essential that the head be sought for; unless it be passed, the segments will grow again. Should the head not be passed, it will be three months before more segments are passed, and it is therefore advisable to wait until that time before recommencing treatment. *It is important* that castor-oil should never be

taken at the same time as the male fern, as it dissolves a harmful substance in the latter. Other remedies used to kill tapeworm are oil of turpentine and decoction of pomegranate bark.

There is a variety of tapeworm, **taenia echinococcus,** which exists in its adult stage in the dog or cat, but may be present in its immature larval form in man. It gives rise to what is called hydatid disease. The infections is rare in this country, but occurs in parts of the world where dogs and men live in very close contact. Hydatid cysts form in various organs of the body, lung, kidney, brain, and notably the liver. Symptoms are produced through pressure. The disease is very difficult to cure, a surgical operation usually being necessary.

The only flukeworm which is common in man is the bilharzia haemotobia, and it causes the disease bilharziasis. It is common in Egypt, India, and Africa. Fresh water snails are the intermediate hosts, and infection results from the parasite entering the body through the skin or mucous membrane when bathing. The adult worms are found in the veins of the kidney and the ova, pierce the urinary mucous membrane and cause bleeding. Male fern is used in treatment, but it is impossible to destroy the adult worms in the veins. (*See also* BILHARZIASIS; HYDATID DISEASE; MALE FERN; SANTONIN; TILARIASIS).

WOUND. Broadly speaking, a wound means any injury to the tissues of the body; but, in practice, it is generally confined to a breach of one of the surface tissues, an open injury involving a breaking of the skin. Open wounds are conveniently classified as incised, lacerated, punctured, and gunshot. They also may be clean or infected.

An incised wound implies that the edges are not ragged and bruised. The wound gapes and arteries and nerves may be severed if the injury is a deep one. Such wounds are caused by sharp-cutting instruments, but may also arise if a hard blow catches the skin over a ridge of bone as in the case of the eyebrow. In these circumstances, there may be bruising of the tissue; the wound is then described as contused.

Treatment. For a small incised wound this is simple. A little bleeding is beneficial, for it washes away dirt or germs. The wound should be touched with some cotton-wool or gauze soaked in tincture of iodine and a small piece of sterile white lint then applied and kept in position with a bandage. If bleeding is very free, the bandage should be tightly wound round the part for half an hour or so and then released and fixed more loosely. If the edges of the wound gape, a strip of adhesive plaster may be used to bring them together. Extensive incised wounds must be stitched, and this is also advisable in the case of face wounds in order to minimize any subsequent disfigurement. If nerves or tendons are severed, it may be necessary to extend the wound in order to unite these structures. In incised wounds of the wrist, the possibility of cut nerves and tendons must be borne in mind.

In **lacerated wounds** the tissues are torn, and the edges of the wound are irregular and bruised. This is the type of wound liable to be caused by machinery, and it is more dangerous than an incised wound as it more readily goes septic. Also, the resultant scar is apt to be unsightly. Bleeding may not be severe, as the coats of the arteries, being torn, tend to curl up and block the vessel. Should extensive bleeding arise, however, this must be attended to first. In the case of a limb, it should be elevated and pressure applied with a sterile dressing over the bleeding point. The dressing should be held in place by a tight bandage, but if this fails to arrest bleeding an improvised tourniquet should be applied to the limb. If possible, stitching of the separated tissues will help to diminish unsightly scarring.

Punctured wounds are dangerous, as it is often impossible to tell the extent of the concealed injury, and also because infection may be conveyed deeply into the tissues. Such wounds are caused by stabbing instruments, needles, etc., or by thorns or splinters of wood. There is always the risk that an organ such as the lung or even the heart may be damaged, or the stomach or intestine perforated. In treatment, bleeding must be arrested and the wound covered. Then, the patient should be carefully watched, and if there is any doubt as to the depth of the wound, a doctor should be immediately summoned.

A gunshot wound is one which is produced directly or indirectly by explosives. It may thus be a bullet, a fragment of a shell, or masonry dislodged by an explosion. Such wounds are very varied. In the case of a bullet wound, there may only be a small hole at the point of entrance but considerable damage to deeper tissues and, if it penetrates right through, the point of exit may be large and lacerated. If the bullet is projected from a near range there may be some scorching or burning of the skin. The dangers of gunshot wounds lie in the possible injury to vital structures and organs, such as arteries, nerves, lungs, heart, or intestines, and in the likelihood of septic infection. The projectile very often traverses clothes, and germs are introduced into the wound from this source. In the treatment of such wounds, it is generally advisable to remove the layer of tissue which surrounds the damaged area, in this way removing a possibly infected zone.

Wounds from which all germs have been excluded heal by what is called "first intention." The edges of the wound become glued together by blood serum and the cells of the adjoining tissues multiply and ultimately the wound is replaced by fibrous or scar tissue. If germs are present, however, the wound may suppurate and the process of healing is greatly delayed. Ultimately the germ infection is overcome and the tissues then heal by what is called "second intention." Poisoned wounds may be caused by bites from insects, such as wasps or mosquitoes, snakes or rabid animals. In such cases, the wound should be thoroughly cleaned with iodine or other antiseptic. In snake bite, crystals of permanganate of potash should be rubbed in and the limb encircled with a tourniquet for about 20 minutes. In the case of a dogbite, if there is any suspicion that the animal is rabid, the wound should be cauterized with pure carbolic.

If there is any likelihood of *any* wound being contaminated with soil, especially manured soil, the patient should receive immediately an injection of *antitetanic serum* in order to prevent the possible development of tetanus or lockjaw. (*See also* ANTISEPTIC; BANDAGE; BITE; BLEEDING; FIRST AID SUPPLEMENT; IODINE;

LOCKJAW; SHOCK; SEPTICEMIA; TOUR-
NIQUET.)

WRIST. The region between the hand
and the forearm is popularly described as
the wrist. The bony framework of this
region is made up of the lower ends of
the radius and ulna, the eight carpal or
wrist bones, and the adjacent parts of the
metacarpal bones. The eight small bones
are arranged in two rows of four, the upper four joining with the radius to form
the radiocarpal joint, or the wrist joint
proper. There is a considerable range of
movement at the wrist, flexion (forward
bending), extension (backward bending),
adduction (bending to little finger side)
and abduction (bending to thumb side).
Forward and backward movements are
also combined with side movements so that
the wrist is exceedingly flexible. Consequently, dislocation is an infrequent injury, though sprains are comparatively
common, especially among athletes.

The wrist region is devoid of muscles,
but there are numerous tendons by which
the hand and fingers are moved and these
strengthen the part considerably.

Fracture of the lower end of the radius,
Colles' fracture, often results from a fall
on the outstretched hand. A characteristic
spoon-shaped deformity results. Reduction
is, as a rule, easy if carried out immediately after the accident. It is important that
a good result be obtained, otherwise the
efficiency of the wrist joint may be seriously impaired. Fracture of one of the
small wrist bones is difficult to detect, as
there is little or no displacement, and an
X-ray examination is necessary. Here
again, the main risk is that the tendons
may be interfered with and a crippling
fixation of the joint will result. Therefore,
as soon as it is thought that the fracture is
firmly reunited, active movements should
be carried out at the joint to prevent
adhesions.

Rheumatism, tuberculosis and gonorrheal arthritis may involve the wrist. In
all these diseases there is swelling, pain,
and restriction of movement. Rest for the
part is necessary, a splint which cocks up
the hand being advisable to prevent the
powerful flexor muscles drawing down the
hand and causing permanent disability.

In the condition of **wrist-drop,** the hand
is flexed and cannot be raised owing to
weakness or paralysis of the extensor muscles. This arises if the musculo-spiral nerve
is injured from a penetrating wound or if
it is inflamed from alcoholic, lead, or
arsenical poisoning. In treatment, the hand,
including the thumb, should be raised upon
a splint, for in this way the extensor
muscles are rested and the flexor muscles
are prevented from drawing the wrist
down. To keep the muscles healthy, massage should be practiced at regular intervals. Where the nerve is inflamed, the
source of the poisoning must be removed,
otherwise the condition will become permanent. (*See also* FOREARM; GANGLION;
RADIUS; SCAPHOID SPRAIN.)

WRITER'S CRAMP. Also known as
scrivener's palsy, this affection is of psychological rather than of physical origin
and comes into the category of the occupational neuroses. Of similar nature are
telegraphists', pianists', and typists' cramp.
The condition shows itself by an inability
properly to carry out the muscular movements entailed in writing, typing, and so
forth. There are cramps or spasms, with
tremors, and frequently pain in the affected
groups of muscles. In time, the muscles
may become wasted and the skin of the
fingers glossy and thin.

Mental conflict is probably the root
cause, the muscle cramps being evidence
of the psychological tension and constitut-
ing a means of escape from difficulties
associated with work. The treatment therefore must be mainly directed to this cause.
A complete rest from all work is desirable,
and if possible a change of environment.
Tonic treatment and massage are beneficial, but every effort must be made to
investigate the sufferer's mind and discover
the nature of the mental conflict. If this
remains unsolved, any improvement is
likely only to be temporary and a relapse
occurs as soon as the person returns to
work. It is a difficult condition to cure
and not infrequently a change of occupation is considered the best solution. (*See
also* NEUROSIS.)

WRY-NECK. In this condition the neck
is bent to one side or the other. It is also
termed torticollis and it occurs in two

forms, either fixed or spasmodic. In the first variety, there is a shortening of the sternomastoid muscle, the muscle which turns the chin to the other side and bends the head sideways. It is generally inherited, though occasionally it may arise from injury at birth or later in life. Torticollis is not usually obvious in a baby, owing to the shortness of the neck, but later it becomes quite evident. If manipulation of the neck is carried out in early life, or an apparatus is worn, the deformity may be cured, but if the condition is definitely established, an operation to divide the shortened muscle becomes necessary.

XANTHELASMA. This is the term applied to the yellowish deposits which sometimes form on the eyelids as a result of degeneration in the muscle fibers. It is a comparatively harmless condition.

XANTHOMA. Occasionally, during the course of diabetes mellitus, yellowish swellings appear in the skin. They are surrounded by a red congested area and are termed xanthoma. The underlying cause is unknown, but it is related to some disturbance of the chemistry of the body. Apart from the disfigurement, they do not cause any symptoms. Another variety of xanthoma is described, a rare condition, in which yellow tumors develop extensively in the body. No cause is known.

XANTHOPSIA. This is the technical name for yellow vision. To a person suffering from this affection, everything appears to be tinted yellow. It occurs sometimes after the administration of the drug santonin, which is given to persons infected with roundworm. It is a transient condition and disappears very soon after the drug has been withdrawn.

XEROPHTHALMIA. This is an inflammation of the cornea and eyelids, observed sometimes in children, and due to deficiency of Vitamin A. Permanent blindness may result if Vitamin A is not added to the diet. Vitamin A is found chiefly in codliver and halibut oil, animal fats, milk and butter. (*See* VITAMINS; DEFICIENCY DISEASES.)

X-RAYS. Known also as Röntgen rays, after their inventor, X-rays are a form of radiant energy. A vast number of radiations are given off by the sun which travel through space in waves of different length and vibration. There are the obvious luminous rays, but there are many more invisible rays, the ultraviolet rays, X-rays, and certain rays of radium.

X-rays are produced by passing an electric current through a glass tube from which a certain amount of air has been withdrawn. From the cathode or negative pole a discharge of electrons is made to focus upon a tungsten plate called the anticathode. From the impact of these rays, X-rays and heat are produced and the X-rays are directed through the tube at a certain desired angle.

The character of the X-rays varies with the degree of evacuation of the tube and the voltage of the electricity passed through it. If the amount of gas in the tube is large and the voltage relatively low, "soft" rays are produced; these have but little power of penetration of the tissues, and are largely absorbed by the superficial tissues. In contrast, the greater the degree of evacuation and the higher the voltage, the "harder" do the X-rays become. Various devices are therefore used to vary the softness or hardness of the X-rays by altering the amount of gas contained in the tube.

An essential part of an X-ray plant is the transforming unit, because the electrical supply from the main must be converted into high-tension current. The average electrical supply varies from 200 to 500 volts, but the tensions required for X-ray work vary from 50,000 volts for diagnostic work to 1,000,000 for modern treatment purposes.

X-rays are used for investigating and also for the treatment of disease. These rays possess the power of penetrating the body tissues according to their density, so that where only partial penetration takes place shadows are cast, the depth depending on the extent to which the transit of the rays has been blocked. An impression of these shadows can readily be obtained on a screen rendered fluorescent, or on a photographic plate or film. Screening, as the operation is called whereby an impression is thrown on a fluorescent screen, is generally used for the immediate examination of a patient. It is possible then to observe the action of the heart, lungs and abdominal organs. A photographic record on a film is made as a permanent record for detailed study.

Today, the X-ray examination adds greatly to the accuracy of diagnosis. There is the obvious value of X-rays in detecting fractures, dislocations, and in locating needles, bullets, and other metallic objects in the tissues; but the X-rays are equally valuable in investigating the deeper organs. The condition of the heart, great vessels, and lungs can be determined by X-ray examination of the chest; the alimentary canal can be photographed by giving the patient a meal containing barium, which is opaque to X-rays. It is even possible to bring such organs as the brain, kidneys, and, gall bladder within the scope of accurate X-ray diagnosis by the injection into these organs of opaque substances.

A recent and very important development of X-ray diagnosis is in the detection of dental disease. It is impossible to tell the condition of the roots of teeth other than by the use of X-rays. It has been shown that abscesses may exist without any pain or other symptom, yet be responsible for ill-health. X-ray films give well-defined pictures of the teeth and reveal clearly any infection at the roots.

X-rays as Curative Agent. Radiotherapy, or treatment of disease by means of X-rays, has made rapid strides in recent years. In the treatment of cancer the value of X-rays is considerable. In some cases, the growth may be completely destroyed, and in others it is so reduced that it is easily removed by operation. In inoperable cancers, X-ray treatment enables the sufferer to live for a longer period and in greater comfort than would otherwise be the case. The term "deep therapy" is applied to X-radiation designed to reach organs affected with malignant disease deeply situated within the body and inaccessible to the surgeon. In the treatment of skin diseases, X-rays are of established value. In ringworm of the scalp, the hair can be caused to fall out so that it may grow again in a healthy state. Chronic eczema and pruritus, or itching, can also be benefited. The X-rays in small doses benefit the skin, but in large doses will produce redness which may go on to actual destruction of the tissue—a so-called X-ray burn. These burns are extremely resistant to treatment and may be followed by cancerous growths, so that great care must be exercised in the dosage of X-rays during all forms of treatment. X-rays are also used in the treatment of certain blood diseases and diseases of the blood-forming organs.

The dangers from the use of X-rays may be grouped as immediate and remote. During an actual exposure, the possibility of making a contact with a high-tension lead carrying a very high voltage has to be guarded against. An accident of this kind may easily be fatal, but fortunately most modern forms of apparatus are reasonably protected against such a contingency, though there is need for constant carefulness.

The remote effects are those which may arise from the absorption of the X-rays by the tissues. They do not manifest themselves till long after the exposure. Too large an exposure may lead to burns, warts, and cancerous growths; while frequent exposures, even in small doses, may cause a dermatitis which may ultimately become the seat of malignant disease. Also, telaangiectasis, a condition in which the blood vessels of the skin become dilated and prominent, may develop. Constitutional disorders, anemia, and sterility not infrequently arise in operators who are constantly exposed to X-rays. It may be said, however, that with modern methods of application and protection, the risk and dangers associated with X-ray work are fast diminishing, while the scope of this agency in the treatment and diagnosis of disease is constantly increasing to the great benefit of humanity.

YAWS. This is a tropical disease variously known as frambesia, purru, parangia, and coko, and it is seldom met with in the U.S. Yaws is a very contagious disease and is caused by a micro-organism called the treponema pertenue, which is somewhat similar to the organism which causes syphilis, the treponema pallidum. The disease is spread by direct contact with infected persons or their belongings, and insanitary and unhygienic conditions increase its incidence. Infection can only take place through an abrasion or wound of the skin.

There is an incubation period of from 12 to 20 days, during which there may be irregular fever, headache, joint pains, and digestive disturbance. These symptoms disappear with the appearance of the sore at the site of the original infection, the commonest sites being the thigh, leg, arm, and breast. The eruption commences as a small nodule, which increases in size and finally breaks down, exposing an ulcer which readily bleeds. This sore may heal or else may develop into a large fungating mass. The second stage follows in about two months, when there is an eruption of sores similar to the original sore all over the body. Crops of such sores appear from time to time over a varying period, but the condition may completely terminate at this stage or may pass on to the third stage, when deep-seated ulcers form, and painful swellings in the bones develop.

The diagnosis of yaws is easily made by a microscopic examination of the discharge from the sores, which contain the parasites of the disease. Treatment is by injection of penicillin in large doses; arsenic and bismuth have also been used with good results.

YEAST. Yeasts belong to the group of vegetable growths known as fungi and are found widely distributed in nature. They are chiefly found in connection with such fruits as the grape. Certain rare diseases are caused by special varieties of yeast, but ordinary yeast is used in bread making. Its value depends upon the fact that it causes fermentation: the starch of the flour is partly converted into sugar, and in turn converted into alcohol and the carbonic acid gas which aerates the dough and so fills the bread with cavities. Yeast is an important source of Vitamin B. (*See* VITAMINS.)

YELLOW FEVER. This is an acute specific tropical fever, now confined mainly to West Africa and South America, and characterized by jaundice, bleedings, gastrointestinal disturbance, and sometimes suppression of urine. The disease affects white people much more than colored people; it is most prevalent in swampy, lowlying country and in unsanitary, overcrowded towns.

Yellow fever is caused by a microorganism which is carried by a special variety of mosquito called the stegomyia fasciata. If this insect bites a patient suffering from yellow fever during the first three days of the illness, it will probably become infected with the parasite and, after an interval of twelve days, will inoculate the disease into the next person it may chance to bite.

The stage of incubation is from three to five days, and the onset of the disease is sudden, with severe headache, shivering fits, pains in the muscles and joints, sickness, and vomiting. The temperature shoots up: the face becomes flushed, the eyes bloodshot, and within two or three days marked jaundice appears and albumen is present in the urine. About the fourth day the fever remits, the symptoms become less marked, and in favorable cases, the patient recovers. In other cases, however, there is a further rise in temperature, the jaundice returns, there is severe vomiting, sometimes of blood, so-called "black vomit," and there may arise suppression of urine, convulsions and coma. A peculiar feature is that though the temperature rises, the pulse rate falls and may not exceed 70 to the minute with a temperature of 103 deg. F. Death may take place, usually about the sixth or seventh day, from heart-failure or uremia. Recovery, when it does take place, is often delayed by protracted diarrhea or nephritis. One attack confers immunity. The death rate is from 10 to 75 per cent, varying in different epidemics; it is often nearer the higher figure.

In treatment, a special serum invented by Noguchi, if injected during the first day or two of the disease, is likely to be beneficial and lead to recovery, but after the third day this serum is comparatively ineffective. Otherwise, the usual methods for the management of fever are adopted. The occurrence of yellow fever has been greatly diminished by the destruction of mosquitoes and by preventing their breeding, and by draining swamps. Persons suffering from the disease should be carefully screened to prevent being bitten by mosquitoes and so spreading the infection. A vaccine is now available in preventing this deadly disease. (*See also* Mosquito.)

ZINC. Zinc is a bluish-white metal which is used in medicine in various forms, most commonly as an external application.

Zinc sulphate occurs as thin colorless crystals, resembling those of Epsom salts. In solution, it has a sharp taste and is astringent and mildly antiseptic. It is commonly used as a lotion for the eyes in conjunctivitis, in a strength of 1 grain to the ounce. For stimulating sluggishly healing tissues, as in a varicose ulcer, zinc sulphate is dispensed as red lotion, being combined with tincture of lavender. Zinc oxide and zinc carbonate (prepared calamine) are valuable in the treatment of eczema, pruritus, and irritated states of the skin. They are insoluble in water, and if used as a lotion for the skin the bottle must always be thoroughly shaken up before application.

Zinc ointment consists of zinc oxide and benzoated lard. It has a mildly astringent and antiseptic action, and it is soothing to the skin in slight irritating conditions. Zinc oxide is also contained in Lassar's paste. Along with starch and boracic powder, zinc oxide makes a useful dusting power and is used where the skin is red and chafed. Many adhesive plasters contain zinc oxide. Zinc chloride is a powerful caustic. In weak solution it is antiseptic and is used to stimulate healing in wounds, and also as a lotion for the eyes in conjunctivitis.

ZOSTER. Herpes Zoster is the medical name for a form of shingles, and the condition is described under the heading Shingles.

ZYGOMA. This is the name applied to a bridge of bone which joins the temporal bone with the malar bone. (*See also* Bone; Temporal Bone.)

APPENDIX I

FIRST AID IN EMERGENCIES

The aim of First Aid is to relieve suffering and to prevent the development of further injury pending the arrival of medical aid.

It covers all emergency measures, from the application of iodine or other disinfectant to a wound, to artificial respiration to persons overcome by suffocation and drowning. Various kinds of poisoning also call for suitable first aid measures.

In a city, a doctor can be quickly summoned, but if the accident occurs in outlying parts there may be considerable delay. In such cases, prompt action on the right lines will do much to promote the patient's mental, as well as physical, well-being, and may even save his life.

How to act in various emergencies is described in detail in the following pages, but these general rules apply to all cases of rendering First Aid to the injured.

1. Keep cool yourself, and avoid all appearance of panic.
2. Send someone for a doctor.
3. If there is serious bleeding, tackle this first.
4. Guard against shock by keeping the patient warm.
5. Determine the nature of the accident, and decide upon what treatment should be given.
6. Decide whether the initial treatment should be for injury or for shock.
7. See that the patient is in a position which permtis him to breathe. If in a city, do your best to keep him free from the attentions of well-meaning spectators who crowd around and prevent the proper circulation of air. If breathing has ceased take prompt measures to restore it.
8. Do not heedlessly alter the position assumed by the vital functions.

First Aid Box. In every camp or workshop a First Aid box must be kept. This should be painted white and carry a distinctive red cross. It should be in the charge of one individual who has a knowledge of First Aid, and who will be responsible for the box being replenished after use.

Where fifty or more persons are employed, the box should contain the following articles:

1. Red Cross First Aid manual.
2. Two dozen small, 1 dozen medium, 1 dozen large, sterilized dressings.
3. One tin or jar of petroleum jelly or cold cream.
4. Two dozen half-ounce packets of absorbent cotton.
5. Six ounces of 2 per cent alcoholic solution of iodine in a stoppered bottle.
6. A bottle of sal volatile with directions for use on the label.
7. One packet of bicarbonate of soda and one of boric acid crystals.
8. Splints and absorbent cotton or other padding.
9. Adhesive plaster, one 2-inch reel.
10. A tourniquet.
11. One dozen roller bandages, 1 dozen triangular bandages.
12. Safety pins.

ABDOMINAL INJURIES. Most of the accidents to the soft parts of the body, especially the abdomen, are very serious and unfortunately common in these days of industrial and road accidents. When a person has been run over or crushed, the skin and flesh of the abdomen are likely to give way, and the direction in which they have been torn or have given way is of importance when considering what to do for the best until the doctor arrives. Three things may happen: the belly may be burst open and various organs, such as the bowels, may protrude through the opening. If this happens, keep the person lying down flat on the back. Uncover the injury by removing or cutting away the clothing. Take a towel, napkin, or other large piece of cloth, whatever may be clean and handy. Wring it out in warm water and lay it over the wound, covering it and the area around thoroughly. Cover with a clean bandage and keep the patient warm. Do not give any food or drink.

If no organs are protruding, proceed as follows: If the skin is broken in an up-and-down direction, keep the person lying flat on the back with the legs stretched out. If, however, the injury is from left to right, still keep the patient on his back, but in this case draw up the knees and put a pillow under them and under the head and shoulders. Dress the wound and bandage firmly. Keep the injured person as warm as possible, give no food or drink. Of course, in all abdominal injuries a doctor should be sent for at once.

Sometimes an internal organ, usually a loop of the bowel, pushes through a weak place in the wall of the abdomen under the skin. This is called a rupture or hernia. When it gets fixed or "strangulated" it causes swelling, pain, and severe sickness. When this occurs, treat it as you would an accident. Send for the doctor. Lay the patient on his back with knees drawn up and head and shoulders supported by a pillow. Apply ice or cold water compresses to the swelling.

ARTIFICIAL RESPIRATION.

The importance of artificial respiration is the urgent necessity of getting the blood oxygenated for it has been found that if the brain is deprived of blood for only four minutes the tissues cannot revive and death ensues.

Nowadays the method of choice in emergency resuscitation is considered to be mouth-to-mouth or mouth-to-nose, which can be used in situations where it is difficult or impossible to employ the older well-tried methods. The vital need is to get air into the lungs and oxygenate the blood, even if it has to be blown past an obstruction in the patient's throat or windpipe. The patient lies on his back (sometimes even in shallow water); the first-aider holds the patient's head in both hands, one pressing the head backwards and the other pressing the lower jaw up-

wards and forwards, opens his own mouth wide, takes a deep breath and, sealing his lips round the patient's mouth, blows into the lungs, watching the chest rise, ten times per minute; the patient's nostrils must be closed, by pinching them if necessary. In an infant or young child, the first-aider seals both mouth and nose with his own mouth. If, because of spasm or other cause, the patient's mouth cannot be opened, the mouth-to-nose method is used, taking care not to obstruct his nostrils and keeping his mouth closed.

When the patient begins to breathe naturally, adjust the rhythm of your movements to his respiration.

Be ready to recommence the treatment at once if his breathing should again fail. (*See also* ARTIFICIAL RESPIRATION for other methods.)

BANDAGING. (*See* BANDAGES AND BANDAGING.)

BITES AND STINGS. Snakes, dogs and rabid animals.

In the case of bites by snakes, poison has been injected by the snake into the wound, causing immediate danger to life unless the poison can be stopped before it gets into the general circulation.

There is not much danger of hydrophobia in this country, but where it is suspected that the animal which caused the wound, whether dog, wolf, cat, etc., was suffering from *rabies,* the condition must be treated as if it were a venomous snake bite, and in addition arrangements must be made for the bitten person to receive the Pasteur inoculation treatment at the earliest possible moment. The local medical officer of health can give information on this subject.

Treatment. Bind a tight bandage or tourniquet of some sort with the utmost speed between the injury and the heart so as to stop the circulation. Wash out the wound by holding it under a tap, or suck it hard and spit out the blood. Keep the part low. This encourages bleeding, and thus helps to wash out the poison. Pour some tincture of iodine or rub some crystals of potassium permanganate into the wound. The tourniquet *must not* be left on for more than 20 minutes, so it is of the utmost importance to get the patient to a doctor without delay.

Insect Stings. Bees, wasps, and other insects can cause serious injury by their bites, especially if the sting is on the face or, as sometimes happens, on the tongue or in the mouth. A bee leaves its sting in the wound, so find it and pull it out. Bathe the part freely with methylated spirit, iodine, or weak ammonia. Baking soda or washing soda may be rubbed in to counteract the poison from the sting. (*See also* Bites and Stings.)

BLADDER, INJURY TO. A crush which fractures the pelvis, or haunchbone, may injure the bladder.

The symptoms are inability to pass urine, or if some is passed it is tinged with blood.

Treatment. (*a*) Send for a doctor quickly, or take the patient to hospital on a stretcher. (*b*) Keep the patient recumbent, quiet and warm, and instruct him to make no attempt to pass urine.

The passing of blood-tinged urine following an accident to the abdomen is always serious.

BLEEDING, or HEMORRHAGE. *Blood vessels.* A detailed knowledge of the blood system is unnecessary, but a general idea of the principal vessels is easily acquired and a great help in First Aid work.

The blood leaves the heart by the *aorta*, a large vessel which, forming an arch behind the breast bone, passes down the left side of the spine. Just below the level of the navel it divides into two branches —the *iliacs*—which supply the pelvic organs and lower limbs.

The aorta gives off various branches. From the arch springs the main supply to the head, the *carotid* arteries on each side of the neck. These vessels run up from the collarbone, and can be felt pulsating at either side of the throat. From the carotid flows the *facial* artery, which supplies the greater part of the face. This vessel passes across the lower jaw in a slight hollow about an inch in front of the angle of the jaw. The *temporal* artery, which supplies the forehead and front of the scalp, passes in front of the upper part of the ear, and the *occipital,* which supplies the back of the scalp, passes about 2½ inches behind the ear.

The *subclavian* is a shorter artery which runs from behind the inner end of the collarbone to the armpit; it then becomes the *brachial* artery and runs down the inner side of the arm to the elbow. There it divides into two—the *radial* and *ulnar* arteries—which run down the front of the forearm on the outer and inner sides respectively. These arteries meet again in the *palmar arches* in the palm of the hand.

The two main arteries in which the aorta ends—the *iliacs*—pass into the thighs just to the inner side of the center point of the

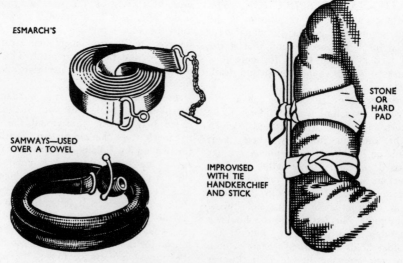

ESMARCH'S

SAMWAYS—USED OVER A TOWEL

IMPROVISED WITH TIE HANDKERCHIEF AND STICK

STONE OR HARD PAD

Types of Tourniquet.

groins. They are now called the *femoral* arteries, and pass down the inner side of the thigh for about two-thirds of its length. They then run behind the thigh bone to the back of the knee joint. Dividing into two, one part passes down the front and the other down the back of the leg to unite again in an arch in the sole of the foot.

Treatment of Hemorrhage. Hemorrhage is of three kinds.

1. **From an Artery (Arterial).** This condition is dangerous and calls for prompt treatment. It is readily distinguished from the other forms as the blood is scarlet, and, if the wounded artery is near the surface, spurts in jets corresponding to the heart beats.

Get the patient into a suitable position, preferably lying flat, and except when dealing with a fractured limb, elevate the bleeding part so as to reduce the flow of blood to it. If there is no fractured bone nor foreign body in the wound, apply direct pressure with the fingers or thumb over the wound. If a fracture or the presence of a foreign body be suspected, or if the wound is large, apply indirect pressure by pressing on the appropriate pressure point next to the wound on the heart side. Maintain the pressure by means of a *pad and bandage,* or a *tourniquet.*

A *pad* may be improvised from a folded handkerchief, a knot in the center of the bandage, with or without a stone enclosed, and should be accurately placed on the pressure point and firmly bound in position.

A *tourniquet* consists of a band of some sort, which is provided with a means of being tightened. It is passed round the bleeding limb above the injury with the object of squeezing the artery and preventing the further escape of blood. It should not be applied directly to the skin, but only outside the clothing or over a folded cloth.

A tourniquet may be improvised as follows: Place a pad accurately on the pressure point and encircle the limb with a narrow bandage, necktie, strap or a piece of cord. Opposite the pad tie a half knot and then a reef knot. Between the knots insert a short, strong piece of wood, such as a pencil. Twist to tighten the band and

so bring pressure to bear on the pad. Fix the stick in position with another bandage or in the folds of the tourniquet. The best sites for a tourniquet are the middle of the upper arm or thigh. They are not so efficient below the knee or elbow.

A piece of rubber tubing is the best kind of tourniquet. In this case no twisting is necessary, the rubber being passed two or three times round the limb and pulled tight each time.

Precautions to be observed when using a tourniquet. A tourniquet *must* be slackened off after it has been in position for 15 minutes. If the bleeding recurs, tighten up again and loosen every 15 minutes. Neglect to do this may have deplorable results. If the blood supply to the limb is cut off for too long, the limb will die. Prolonged pressure on a nerve may easily cause paralysis.

2. **From a Vein (Venous).** In this case the blood is dark red, flows evenly from the wound and does not spurt. It is always easier to stop and less dangerous than arterial bleeding. Press with the fingers or thumb, unless there is a fractured bone or foreign body in the wound. Loosen any tight clothing between the wound and the heart, e.g. collar, corsets, or garters. Place a pad over the wound and bandage firmly (lightly if there is a fracture or foreign body).

3. **Capillary Hemorrhage.** In this case the blood is medium red, and generally oozes evenly from all parts of the wound. Apply a dressing and bandage firmly.

The above are the general principles of treating hemorrhage, but it must be understood that the wound itself requires treatment as well as the hemorrhage.

Before the wound is treated, however, the hemorrhage must be stopped, and in doing this the First Aid worker should take all reasonable care that the wound does not become infected or septic. He must, therefore, endeavor to exclude germs by protecting the wound, and he must avoid doing anything which might introduce germs into the wound.

Hemorrhage from various parts of the body. The Scalp. Scalp wounds usually bleed freely, and often look more serious than they are. If there is no fracture of the skull, bleeding is generally stopped by

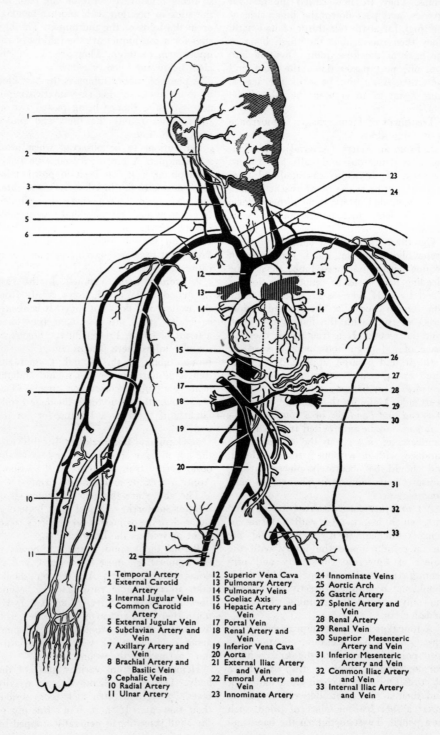

1 Temporal Artery	12 Superior Vena Cava	24 Innominate Veins
2 External Carotid Artery	13 Pulmonary Artery	25 Aortic Arch
3 Internal Jugular Vein	14 Pulmonary Veins	26 Gastric Artery
4 Common Carotid Artery	15 Coeliac Axis	27 Splenic Artery and Vein
5 External Jugular Vein	16 Hepatic Artery and Vein	28 Renal Artery
6 Subclavian Artery and Vein	17 Portal Vein	29 Renal Vein
7 Axillary Artery and Vein	18 Renal Artery and Vein	30 Superior Mesenteric Artery and Vein
8 Brachial Artery and Basilic Vein	19 Inferior Vena Cava	31 Inferior Mesenteric Artery and Vein
9 Cephalic Vein	20 Aorta	32 Common Iliac Artery and Vein
10 Radial Artery	21 External Iliac Artery and Vein	33 Internal Iliac Artery and Vein
11 Ulnar Artery	22 Femoral Artery and Vein	
	23 Innominate Artery	

tying a narrow bandage firmly round the head with the knot or a pad over the bleeding point. If this fails, firm finger pressure applied direct to the bleeding point over a clean dressing will arrest it.

If the patient is unconscious, use a ring pad. To make this, take a narrow bandage and wind one end several times round the fingers of the left hand to form a ring. When within two feet of the other end, stop and pass the free end through the ring again and again until it is used up. Place the ring pad over the wound and bandage firmly in position.

The Nose. Make the patient sit in a chair before an open window. On no account let him bend over a basin. Loosen any tight clothing about the throat or chest and make him breathe through his mouth. This is usually enough to stop bleeding, but the nostrils may also be pinched firmly and a cold compress applied over the nose.

A Tooth Socket. Wash out the mouth repeatedly with cold water. If the bleeding continues, plug the socket with absorbent cotton, place a small pad over the gum and tell the patient to bite on it. Hydrogen peroxide is very useful for stopping bleeding in the mouth.

The Ear. Bleeding from within the ear after an accident generally indicates a fractured skull. Do not plug the ear. Apply lightly a dry absorbent dressing and send for medical aid.

The Armpit. (Arterial bleeding). If direct pressure fails, compress the subclavian artery (*see* illustration on page 567). Face the patient and place the hand close in on the shoulder so that the thumb lies in the hollow above and behind the collarbone and the fingers round the back of the neck. Press the thumb downwards and backwards on to the first rib. This is more readily done if the injured side is kept well forward and the patient's head turned away.

The Upper Arm. *Arterial Bleeding.* If direct pressure on the wound has failed, compress the artery in the armpit. To do this, roll up in a piece of cloth some small hard object, such as a golf ball or stone, to form a firm pad about the size of an orange. Push this well up into the armpit and fix it in position with a narrow band-

age. Place the center of the bandage over the pad and carry up the ends one in front of, and the other behind, the shoulder. Cross the ends on top of the shoulder and pass them round the body to meet under the armpit on the uninjured side. Tie tightly. Bend the forearm across the front of the body and bandage the injured limb firmly to the side.

The Forearm. *Arterial Bleeding.* Apply a tourniquet to the brachial artery pressure point (*see* illustration on page 567); or place a pad in the elbow joint, bend the forearm right back and bandage it to the upper arm. This compresses the artery.

The Palm of the Hand. The two arteries of the forearm—the radial and the ulnar—join in a complex system of blood vessels in the palm of the hand. An injury to this part may bleed profusely from both ends of the cut vessels.

If no foreign body, such as broken glass, is present, quickly improvise a firm pad and place it in the injured palm. Make the patient grasp it and then bind the fingers tightly with a narrow bandage.

As an additional measure, or if a fracture or foreign body is present, compress the wrist arteries as follows:

Procure two small objects such as corks or pieces of pencil, lay them on the wrist pulses and bind firmly. The radial pulse is easily found just below the root of the thumb. The other artery—ulnar—is in a corresponding position on the little finger side of the wrist.

Should the bleeding still persist, compress the brachial artery as described under "Forearm."

The Fingers. Serious bleeding from a severed finger may be stopped by binding the stump firmly.

The Thigh. Stop arterial bleeding from the thigh by pressing on the femoral artery where it crosses the midpoint of the grain. Lay the patient on his back and raise the leg. Kneel facing him and pass the fingers of one hand inside and those of the other hand outside the top of the thigh. The two thumbs will fall together over the groin and may be jointly used to exert pressure. Meanwhile an assistant can prepare a tourniquet. The femoral artery passes from the groin down the inner side of the thigh to the back of the knee. Place the tourniquet high up on the thigh and use a firm pad the size of an average apple. Hemorrhage from the femoral artery is very serious, and prompt action is imperative if the patient's life is to be saved.

The Foot and Leg. Press with the fingers on the wound, and then fix a pad and bandage tightly.

If the bleeding is severe and the above treatment fails, compress the artery by pad and flexion. Lay the patient on his back and place a firm pad the size of a tennis ball behind the knee. Raise and bend the knee until the calf touches the back of the thigh. Fix the limb in this position with a narrow bandage, handkerchief or necktie.

Varicose Veins. Lay the patient flat and raise the limb. Apply a pad and bandage over the bleeding point.

Bleeding from the Lungs. Spitting blood (hemoptysis). Blood which is coughed up is bright red and frothy. It is the result of disease or injury of the lungs. Send for a doctor at once.

Bleeding from the Stomach. Vomiting blood (hematemesis) may be due to disease or injury of the stomach.

The blood is very dark and, being mixed with particles of food, often resembles coffee grounds.

Get the patient to bed and keep him as quiet as possible until the doctor comes. Give no food or drink.

Internal Hemorrhage. A bullet wound or stab, a run-over or similar crushing accident may damage internal organs and cause concealed hemorrhage. The symptoms are:

(*a*) Giddiness and rapid loss of strength.

(*b*) Pallor and thirst, with a rapid and feeble pulse.

(*c*) Restlessness and "air-hunger."

Treatment. Send at once for medical aid. Lay the patient down flat and loosen any tight clothing. Provide free circulation of air, but keep the patient warm with rugs, etc. Ice may be sucked but *no* food or fluid may be given by mouth. If there are signs of shock raise the feet and bandage the limbs from fingers to armpits and from toes to groins.

BRUISES. A bruise is damage to the small blood vessels beneath the skin without breaking of the skin.

Bruises rarely require treatment. If pain and swelling are troublesome, apply a piece of lint or a clean, folded handkerchief which has been soaked in equal parts of methylated spirits and water, and bandage firmly.

BURNS AND SCALDS. A Burn may be caused by dry heat, such as fire or hot metal; by lightning or an electric current; corrosive acid, such as nitric acid or vitriol; a corrosive alkali, such as caustic soda, caustic potash, or quicklime.

A Scald is caused by moist heat, such as boiling water, steam, hot oil or tar. The extent of the damage varies from mere reddening of the surface of the skin to charring of deep tissues. The degree of the damage depends upon the intensity of the heat and the length of exposure.

The dangers are *shock* and *infection.*

Treatment of Scalds and Burns caused by Dry Heat, Electricity, or Friction. Cautiously remove the clothing and, if it sticks to the skin, cut round it with scissors. Put the injured part immediately into a bath of water at body heat (98.4 deg. Fahr.) while the dressings are being made ready. Apply strips of lint, gauze, or linen soaked in a solution of one dessertspoonful of baking powder (sodium bicarbonate) in a pint of warm water. Keep the dressing moist. If the burn is slight, take the patient to the doctor. If it is severe, treat for shock and send for the doctor or the ambulance.

The application of an oily dressing relieves the pain at the time, but as it complicates the subsequent treatment a watery lotion is to be preferred. The best modern treatment of burns is by the application of tulle gras impregnated with penicillin. Penicillin may also be given by injection.

If a person's clothes catch fire, anyone coming to the rescue should first *make the sufferer lie flat on the ground* with the burning side uppermost, then *seize a blanket, rug, coat or tablecloth* and smother the flames. The person whose clothes are afire must lie flat, because flame rises and will quickly reach the head and neck if he or she remains standing or kneeling. Similarly he or she must not lie with the flames underneath, or they will pass round and burn the body. As soon as the flames are extinguished, reassure the patient, treat for shock by giving coffee, etc., and attend to the burns. Anyone whose clothing is afire should not rush to the window, or into the open air.

If a face is burned, cut out a mask of lint or linen with holes for eyes, nose and mouth. This should be soaked in bicarbonate of soda dissolved in warm water and applied, and the lips, eyelids and nostrils smeared with a little petroleum jelly or cold cream and a drop of castor oil put into each eye.

Burns Caused by Acids. If it can be obtained *quickly,* bathe the part in an alkaline solution, such as ammonia, or fluid magnesia, or a dessertspoonful of baking powder or washing soda may be used in a pint of warm water. Otherwise, flood the part with warm water, and treat as a burn.

Electric Burns. These resemble burns caused by fire, but are often deeper and more severe. If possible switch off the current. If this cannot be done, try to drag the sufferer out of contact with the current, by means of a nonconductor, such as a loop of rope or the crook of a walkingstick. Protect the hands by using gloves, a rubber tobacco pouch, dry raincoat, or other dry garments. If the rescuer fails to adopt these precautions, he risks receiving a dangerous shock himself. Remember that moisture is a conductor of electricity, and do not make use of any damp or wet article. As soon as the patient is out of contact with the current, treat for shock and burns.

Burns Caused by Alkalis (caustic soda, potash, quicklime, etc.). If it can be quickly obtained, bathe the part in a weak acid solution, such as vinegar or lemon juice diluted with an equal quantity of water. Otherwise, flood the part with warm water, first having taken care to dust off any quicklime remaining on the burnt part.

Burns of the Eye. Burns of the eye may occur from hot metal, acids, or other destructive chemical fluids. A slight burn, severe enough to injure but not destroy the nerves of the cornea (the transparent membrane through which we see), causes great pain. This is best treated by albucid drops (a preparation of a water-soluble sulphonamide).

The more serious burns are those caused by lime, strong acids such as sulphuric (vitriol), and a splash of molten metal, usually lead. As time is everything in a good many of these cases, even a matter of seconds making a difference, it is necessary to know the first aid treatment, though naturally the injured person should be taken to a doctor as soon as possible. In cases of lime burning, as much lime as possible should be quickly but *very gently,* without actually touching the eye, brushed away, and the eye bathed thoroughly with weak sugar and water, or vinegar and water, used warm. Two teaspoonfuls of each to the pint is sufficient. Plenty of this should be used to wash away the lime as rapidly and thoroughly as possible. It must be reiterated that the eye itself must not be touched, or the damge may be made worse. A little olive or castor oil should then be dropped into the eye, a soft clean pad put on, and the eye bandaged gently.

In cases of acid burning, a solution of sodium bicarbonate, 1 teaspoonful to the pint of warm water, may be used as a wash, the rest of the treatment proceeding as before. In lead burning, if the lead can be seen *loose* in the eye (usually in the pocket formed by the lower eyelid), it may be gently removed, but if there is destruction of the tissue, as frequently happens, oil should be used, and the pad and bandage as before, the bandage being just sufficiently firm to keep the eyeball steady until the eye can be medically examined.

Treatment of Scalds. The damage being similar to that of a burn, treatment is along the same lines.

Treat and dress as for a burn.

Scalded Throat. The danger here is from the swelling that may occur at the top of the windpipe. This may lead to suffocation through interfering with the breathing. Treat as follows:

Lay the patient down, or better, get him to bed. Give ice to suck, or, failing ice, sips of cold water. Send for medical aid.

CARRYING A HELPLESS PERSON. *When single handed* and strong enough, lift the patient by passing one arm beneath his knees and the other round his back. This is known as the "Cradle."

If the patient is too heavy for the cradle or only partially incapacitated, stand close by his side, put one arm round his waist and grasp his far hip. Then draw his nearside arm round your neck and over your shoulder, where you hold his hand with your free hand. This is known as the "Human Crutch."

Fireman's Lift. A very useful method of carrying an unconscious patient, which also leaves one hand free to use in descending a ladder, and is therefore called the "Fireman's Lift," is as follows: The helpless person is turned on his face on the ground and the bearer puts his hands under his arms and drags him to a kneeling position, then to a standing position. To get the patient to a standing position, the bearer should stoop, place the patient's right arm round his own neck while he thrusts his own right arm round the right thigh of the patient, placing his right shoulder against the middle of the patient's body to steady himself. He should then rise slowly to the erect position, grasping the patient's right hand with the right hand. This leaves the patient steadily poised on the right shoulder, while the left hand of the bearer is free. Instead of grasping the patient by the right thigh only, it may be more convenient to pass the arm round both the legs just above the knees. Alternatively, the patient may be carried "pick-a-back" where it is possible to get him into this position.

When two bearers are available.

The Two-Handed Seat. This is used if the patient is totally incapacitated. The two bearers stand facing each other, one on each side of the patient. They stoop down and each passes his rear forearm under the patient's back below the shoulders and grasps his clothing. After slightly raising his back, they pass their other forearms beneath the middle of the patient's thighs and grasp hands. They rise and step off together, the left bearer with the left foot the right bearer with the right.

In a narrow passage where the two-handed seat cannot be used, the fore-and-aft method may be employed. In this case one helper stands behind the patient, bends down, and passing his forearms under the patient's armpits, clasps his hands. The other helper stands with his back to the patient between the latter's legs. He bends down and passes his forearms under the patient's knees. Both rise together and carry patient away. For lifting and carrying a patient in a recumbent position, use the "Human Stretcher." The two bearers stand facing each other, one on each side of the patient. They bend down and clasp their left hands beneath the patient's hips as in a handshake. Then the bearer on the left supports the head and shoulders with his right hand and forearm while his companion similarly supports the legs. They rise and move off in short sidesteps, the patient's feet foremost.

The Three-Handed Seat. This is employed when a patient can use one or both of his arms but needs support for one of his legs, e.g., in the case of a sprain.

The two bearers go behind the patient and face each other. To support the right leg, the bearer on the patient's left holds his own right wrist with his left hand. The other bearer holds the first bearer's left wrist with his left hand, leaving his right hand free to support the patient's right leg. (If it is necessary to support the patient's *left* leg, substitute "left" for "right" and "right" for "left" throughout the foregoing instructions.) The bearers then stoop, the patient passes an arm round one or both of their necks and sits upon their hands. The bearer with a free arm supports the injured lower limb. They rise together and move off, the left bearer with the left, foot, the right bearer with the right.

Stretchers may be improvised thus:

1. Take two or three coats and turn the sleeves inside out. Pass two strong poles through the sleeves and button up the coats. Separate the poles by binding cross pieces of wood at either end. Instead of coats, sacks may be pressed into service, in which case holes must be made in the bottom corners.

2. Spread out on the ground a rug, tarpaulin, or blanket and roll up two strong poles in the sides. The bearers stand on either side and grasp the covered poles in the center and near the end.

3. A ladder, door, or broad plank may be utilized. Place some hay, straw, or clothing thereon and cover this with a

piece of sacking, a blanket, or a rug, by means of which the injured person may be carefully lifted off.

N.B. Be sure to test the safety of any such improvised stretchers.

DISLOCATION. When one or more of the bones at a joint are displaced, they are said to be dislocated, or out of joint.

The First Aid worker should not attempt to put the bones back.

The joints most commonly dislocated are the shoulder (adults), elbow (children), fingers, thumb, and lower jaw.

Signs and Symptoms are: 1. Severe *pain,* often of a sickening character, at or near the joint.

2. *Loss of movement* of the limb and fixity of the joint.

3. By comparison with the corresponding uninjured joint there is *deformity*; a hollow where the displaced bone should be, and a prominence where it is.

4. The limb usually assumes an abnormal attitude.

5. *Swelling* occurs, owing to damage to small blood vessels.

Dislocated Shoulder. Treatment. Support the limb in the position most comfortable to the patient, and least susceptible to jolting or jarring during transport to the doctor. Loosen the clothing round the seat of injury.

If the patient is unable to go to a doctor, send for one.

Give no food, as an anesthetic may be needed later.

Dislocated Elbow. This injury seldom happens to persons over twenty-five. Support the arm in a large sling and take the patient to a doctor.

Dislocation of Hip or Knee. This is a very serious injury, fortunately also very rare. The First Aid treatment is to use a long splint fixed outside the leg, or the two legs may be bandaged together. The patient should be carefully lifted and taken at once to a doctor or hospital.

Dislocated Jaw. A yawn or a blow may put the lower jaw "out of joint." Remove false teeth if any, and go to or send for a doctor.

Compound Dislocation. A dislocation is said to be compound when the bones protrudes through the skin.

Place a clean dressing over the damaged tissues and cover with a layer of cotton-wool.

Support the limb in the position the patient finds most comfortable and transport carefully to hospital or doctor.

DRESSINGS. A dressing should be absorbent and sterile (germ-free). Suitable materials are gauze, lint, cotton, linen, or muslin. They may be sterilized by boiling in water for twenty minutes, baking in an oven, or by soaking in an antiseptic solution, such as 1 in 40 carbolic acid (one tablespoonful of pure carbolic acid in a quart of water after taking out one tablespoonful of the water) or a weak solution of lysol.

Dressings may be improvised from a *clean* handkerchief, towel, or bandage.

Infected, or septic, wounds require wet dressings. Squeeze the dressing as dry as possible before application.

To make a *hot fomentation,* place a piece of lint, flannel, or toweling larger than the affected area in the folds of a small face towel. Still holding the ends of the towel, submerge the dressing in boiling water. Lift and wring out thoroughly and quickly. Apply the dressing as hot as can be borne and cover with jaconet, cotton-wool, and a bandage.

Cold Compress. Soak a piece of towel, lint, flannel, or cotton-wool in the coldest water obtainable. Wring it so that it does not drip, but do not squeeze it dry. Place it on the part and add a little water from a sponge every half-hour. Do not cover up a cold compress, as it is required to evaporate. If a tablespoonful of methylated spirit is added to each pint of water, the evaporation is greater.

FOREIGN BODIES. A foreign body is anything embedded in the human body which does not normally belong there, e.g., a broken needle in the hand, or a cinder in the eye.

In the Ear. If an insect enters the ear, make the patient lie down with the affected ear uppermost, and pour warm olive, castor, or sweet oil into the ear passage. The insect will float to the surface and can be removed. For any other sort of foreign body in the ear, seek the advice of a doctor. Never probe into, or syringe, the ear.

In the Eye. First prevent the patient from rubbing the eye. Then pull down the lower eyelid. If the foreign body can be seen, remove it with the corner of a clean handkerchief moistened in clean water. If the foreign body is underneath the upper lid, pull this outwards and downwards; push up the lower lid inside it and let go. The lashes of the lower lid in this way may wipe away the body. Let the patient blow his nose violently. This may dislodge the particle into a more accessible spot where it can be removed.

If an iron filing or similar object is embedded in the eye and cannot be easily removed, drop olive or castor oil under the lower lid to relieve the irritation, apply a soft pad, and take the patient to a doctor.

For *quicklime* in the eye, first brush away as much as possible. Then bathe the eye in warm water containing vinegar, one teaspoonful to the pint. If these are not handy, wash freely in warm water and apply oil.

For vitriol or other strong acid in the eye, bathe the eye in a solution of baking powder (bicarbonate of soda)—1 desertspoonful in a pint of warm water. Prevent rubbing and apply castor oil to the affected eye.

Under the Skin. *Needle.* If a needle breaks off, leaving part of itself embedded under the skin, take the patient *and the broken piece of needle* to a doctor.

If the needle is embedded near the elbow, wrist, or finger joint, paint the place with tincture of iodine, apply a dressing and support the part in a sling. If the needle is near a joint of the leg, dress the place as above, but do not let the patient walk until a doctor has seen the case.

Thorn or Splinter. If visible, a thorn or splinter can generally be extracted by means of a clean sharp needle. Enlarge the opening in the skin, and a little manipulation will enable the foreign body to be withdrawn.

If the thorn is not visible, bandage the part tightly and hold it above the head for 5 to 10 minutes to render it bloodless. Then shave away the hard skin round the puncture with a sharp knife or razor until the end of the splinter or thorn is visible and can be withdrawn. If this is impossible, consult a doctor.

Fish-hook. On account of its barb, do not attempt to draw the hook back. Try to work the point on and out through the skin in a second place. Then snip off the barb with a pair of pliers or stout scissors and withdraw the hook the way it entered. Or cut off the dressing so that only metal remains and push the hook on and out.

In either case apply tincture of iodine before and after. If the hook is deeply embedded, go to a doctor without delay.

FRACTURES. A fracture is the technical term for a broken, cracked, or splintered bone, and is the result of violence of some sort.

When a fracture occurs at the spot where violence was applied, the fracture is said to have been caused by *Direct Violence*; e.g., a car wheel going over the leg and breaking a bone, or a blow on the head which fractures the skull.

When a bone breaks at some distance from the site of the injury, the fracture is said to due to *Indirect Violence*; e.g., a fall on to the outstretched hand may break the collarbone.

Occasionally a sudden violent contraction of a muscle fractures the knee-cap or tears off a bony point. Such fractures are said to have been caused by *Muscular Action*.

There are various kinds of fracture.

1. Simple. In this case the bone is broken, but not the skin. There is a minimum of injury to the surrounding tissue.

2. Open or Compound. In a compound fracture the skin and surrounding tissues are torn, and there is communication between the outside air and the broken ends of bone. Sometimes these ends protrude; at other times the wound leads down to the fracture site, as when a bone is broken by a bullet.

3. Complicated. A fracture is termed complicated when, in addition to the fracture, there is injury to an important blood vessel, nerve, or internal organ; e.g., a fractured rib may pierce the lung, or, in a broken upper arm, the fractured end of the bone may cut a main nerve and paralyze the muscles of the lower arm and hand.

Note. A fracture originally simple may become compound or complicated if patient or attendant move the part carelessly and the ends of the bone get separated.

Fractures are also classified according to type of injury to the bone.

When the bone is broken into several pieces, the fracture is termed "comminuted." Such fractures need especial care in handling.

Owing to the softer state of the bony tissues in children, a bone may bend and crack without breaking completely. This type of partial fracture is termed "green-stick."

When the ends of a broken bone are driven into each other, the fracture is termed "impacted."

General Signs and Symptoms of Fractures. In many cases a fracture is self-evident, but it is not always so. Therefore inquire of the patient or onlookers the nature of the accident. Note any tears or mud marks on the clothing and ask if the snap of a bone was heard or felt.

Some, but not necessarily all, of the following symptoms occur in every fracture.

1. *Pain and tenderness at the site* of the fracture.

2. *Loss of power* in the limb. (*N.B.* Though impaired function strongly suggests fracture, continued power to use the limb does not exclude fracture entirely.)

3. *Swelling* of the tissues round the seat of the injury.

4. *Deformity.* The limb is misshapen, and below the suspected fracture it assumes an unnatural position. Owing to the broken ends overlapping each other, shortening of the limb may occur.

5. *Discoloration.* Bleeding within the limb may cause discoloration soon after the injury.

Only a doctor should ascertain:

6. If there is unnatural mobility of the limb.

7. If a bony grating (crepitus due to the broken ends moving upon one another) can be felt or heard.

These last two symptoms will be absent in greenstick and impacted fractures.

As the object of First Aid treatment is to prevent any aggravation of the damage already done, in all doubtful cases proceed as though the existence of a fracture had been established.

General Rules for First Aid Treatment of Fractures. All cases of fracture must be attended to by a doctor as soon as possible.

Meanwhile, the following First Aid treatment should be given:

1. No matter how crowded the street or how near at hand a more convenient or comfortable place, treat the fracture *on the spot.*

2. When there is bleeding (hemorrhage), attend to this first. (*See also* BLEEDING.)

3. Steady the injured limb.

4. Treat for shock.

5. Look about for articles from which to improvise splints, bandages, etc.

6. NEVER TRY TO ALTER THE POSITION OF A FRACTURED LIMB.

7. *Expose the injury* by cutting open the clothes, and, if the fracture is compound, remove them. Otherwise leave them to act as additional padding for the splints.

8. *Apply splints and bandages.* Splints are used to keep the limb at rest. This prevents further damage to the soft tissues and relieves pain. Splints must be firm enough to support the limb and long enough to pass beyond the joints immediately above and below the fracture. They must be padded to fit, as far as possible, the contour of the injured limb, and should be applied over the clothing. They may be improvised from walkingsticks, umbrellas, police truncheons, broomsticks, tightly rolled newspapers or maps etc.

If no suitable article is nearby, a fractured arm may be tied to the body without splinting. In all cases a broken leg should be bound to its fellow in addition to being splinted.

Bandages must be firmly applied, yet not so tightly as to impede the circulation. As far as possible they should be passed under the body or limb in the natural hollows, such as the small of the back or behind the knee. Do not lift a fractured limb in order to bandage it. Push the bandage under the limb with a piece of stick or cardboard.

9. Never attempt to remove a case of fractured leg, spine, pelvis, or skull except on a stretcher.

10. As an anesthetic is likely to be given for the setting of the fracture, it is advisable not to give the patient food.

Special Fractures. *The Skull.* A fracture of the dome is usually caused by direct violence, such as a blow on the head or a fall from a height.

A fracture of the base is usually the

result of indirect violence, such as a fall on the feet or a heavy blow on the jaw.

In both cases the patient is generally unconscious.

Signs of a fractured dome are injury to the scalp, swelling, and sometimes depression of the bone.

Signs of a fractured base are bleeding from the ear, mouth, or nose and no visible scalp injury.

The danger lies in injury to the brain, and medical aid must be sought at once. Therefore as soon and as carefully as possible transport the injured person home or to a hospital. While awaiting the doctor, keep the patient quiet and warm and apply cold to the head.

The Jaw. A fracture is generally caused by direct violence, e.g., a blow or a fall. Either or both sides of the jaw may be involved. There is pain and swelling, inability to move the jaw freely, and bleeding from the gums. The line of the teeth may be altered and the patient speaks with difficulty.

Gently press up the lower jaw against the upper; if no "four-tailed" bandage (*see also* ROLLER BANDAGES) is available, use a narrow-fold bandage or two handkerchiefs. To apply the former, place the center under the chin and carry one end up over the top of the head and down as far as the angle of the jaw. Cross the ends and pass the longer, one across the front of the chin and round the back of the neck. Tie at the side of the neck.

The Spine. A fracture of the spine may result from direct or indirect violence. A wheel passing over the back exemplifies direct violence; a broken neck resulting from a fall on the head is an example of indirect violence.

Dislocation of some of the segments (vertebrae) often accompanies a fracture of the spine. In both cases the danger lies in injury to the spinal cord or some of the nerves issuing therefrom. Such injury is likely to cause paralysis of the lower part of the body.

Treatment. If the patient is conscious, warn him not to move. Cover him up and bandage together thighs, knees, legs, ankles, and feet.

If the injury is to the *back,* roll the patient gently on to his *face* and place blankets (or other pad) under the upper part of his chest and under his groin. If the injury is in the *neck,* roll him gently on to his *back,* and place a good pad under the shoulders to allow the head to fall well back. Send for an ambulance immediately.

Method of removal. Improvise a rigid stretcher from a ladder and board, some planks, a door, gate, or shutter, and place it close to the patient's head. If a rug or blanket is available, spread it on the ground. A helper kneels by each of the patient's shoulders, works the edge of the rug under the shoulders and gradually pulls it down beneath the hips and legs. (*Do not lift up the body* to pass the rug or blanket beneath.) Poles are now rolled up in the sides of the blanket or rug, and two helpers on each side carefully lift the patient on to the stretcher.

Failing any rug, blanket, or similar article, open out the patient's coat and roll up each side firmly against the body. Five helpers are now needed. One supports the head and neck. One on each side grasps the rolled coat and another on each side takes a firm hold of the clothing about the thighs and legs. They lift together, slowly and carefully, keeping the body level.

When the stretcher reaches the place of shelter, the patient may be given water, tea, etc., (no alcohol), while awaiting medical aid.

The Ribs. Direct or indirect violence may fracture a rib or ribs. If the cause is direct violence, such as a heavy blow, the fractured ends are usually driven inwards and may damage the lungs, liver, spleen, or other organ. If the violence is indirect, the ends of bone are likely to press outwards and under these conditions internal complications are improbable.

The principal symptom of a fractured rib is a sharp, stabbing pain on coughing or taking a deep breath. Coughing up or spitting blood, pallor of face and lips, failing pulse, and "air hunger" suggest internal injury and hemorrhage.

Treatment. If there are no indications of internal injury, pass two broad-fold bandages round the chest with their centers over the painful area. The second should overlap the first by half its width. Secure them on the uninjured side tightly enough to support the ribs and restrict the breathing to some extent.

If there are signs of injury to an internal organ, do not apply bandages round the chest. Lay the patient flat and support his body so that it inclines towards the injured side. This limits the breathing movements of that side of the chest. Loosen the clothing and send for a doctor.

The Pelvis. Severe crushing violence, such as the passing of a wheel over the body or a heavy fall, may fracture the pelvis or haunch bone.

The symptoms are inability to stand, great pain and difficulty in moving the lower limbs though they themselves are uninjured, and pain on pressing the hips inwards.

Treatment. Settle the patient in the position giving greatest ease, preferably flat on the back. Bend up or straighten out the legs as the patient desires. Push a broad-fold bandage in under the small of the back and work it down under the hips. Tie it tightly enough to support and keep at rest the injured parts. Place a pad between ankles and knees and bandage the legs together.

There is always considerable shock when the pelvis is fractured, so keep the patient warm and remove him on a stretcher as soon as possible.

The danger lies in possible injury to one of the important internal organs.

The Collarbone (Clavicle). This is a common fracture and usually due to indirect violence, such as a fall on to the shoulder or outstretched hand.

The fracture can generally be felt by passing the fingers lightly along the collarbone. The fractured ends often overlap by about ½ an inch, the inner fragment being, as a rule, above the outer.

The arm on the injured side is partially helpless, and the patient usually supports it at the elbow with his other hand. The head leans over to the injured side.

Treatment. Remove the coat, uninjured arm first, and other garments as necessary. Unfasten a man's suspenders. Then:

1. Place in the armpit a firm, flat pad.

2. Gently draw back the shoulder, keeping the forearm well up and resting across the chest.

3. Apply a St. John's Sling. (*See also* BANDAGES, USES OF TRIANGULAR.)

4. Pass a broad-fold bandage round the elbow and trunk. Draw in and tie the injured limb securely to the side.

5. Make sure that the pulse is present at the wrist. If not, loosen the bandage round the body.

6. Tighten the sling.

Alternative Method. For a fracture of one or both collarbones.

1. Place a pad in both armpits.

2. Make two rings by tying the ends of two handkerchiefs, or narrow-fold bandages if available. Pass one up over each arm so that they rest one on each shoulder.

3. Go behind the patient and pass a third bandage or handkerchief through each loop. Draw fairly tight so as to "brace back" the shoulders. Tie in the middle of the back.

4. If only one collar-bone is broken, support the arm on the injured side in a narrow arm sling. (*See also* BANDAGES.) If both are broken, fold the hands across the chest, pass a bandage round arms and trunk, and tie in front.

The Shoulder blade (Scapula). Fracture of this bone is a rare accident, but may result from a crush injury.

It is not easy to detect, but if a severe blow has been received over the shoulder blade and there is sharp pain and perhaps a grating sensation (crepitus) on moving the arm, treat as a fracture.

Support the arm on the injured side in a large arm sling.

The Upper Arm (Humerus). Fractures of the upper arm may occur close to the shoulder, close to elbow, or in the middle of the shaft of the bone.

The latter kind are readily diagnosed, but those occurring close to the joints are not easily distinguished from dislocations.

The chief differences are:

(*a*) Fracture near the shoulder joint.

The arm moves freely and the elbow is close to the body. In dislocation of the shoulder the arm moves with difficulty and the elbow hangs away from the body.

(*b*) Fracture near the elbow.

The end of the upper fragment of bone is sharp and rough to the touch in a fracture. In dislocation of the elbow the projecting ends feels round and smooth.

If in doubt treat as a fracture.

Treatment. (*a*) *Fracture near the shoulder joint.* (i) Bind the injured arm to the side by passing a broad-fold bandage round the upper half of the limb and tying it on the opposite side under the armpit. If the bandage is long enough, it is better to cross the ends under the armpit and tie on top of the sound shoulder.

(ii) Support the forearm in a small arm sling, which will allow the elbow free.

(*b*) *Fracture near the middle of the shaft.*

(i) Seat the patient.

(ii) Bend the forearm at a right angle to the arm and get the patient (or another helper) to hold it so.

(iii) From such articles as pieces of wood, cardboard, or folded newspapers, improvise four splints long enough to reach from the elbow to the shoulder. Pad them.

(iv) Apply these splints to the front, back, and two sides of the injured limb, taking care that no splint presses into the armpit or bent forearm. Tie them in position with two narrow-fold bandages, one above and one below the fracture, keeping the knots on the outer side.

(v) Support the wrist and hand in a small armsling.

(vi) Test the pulse at the wrist. If it cannot be readily felt, slacken the bandages round the splint.

If only two splints can be devised, fix one in front and one behind the arm. If no splints of any kind are obtainable, bind the injured arm to the side with two broad-fold bandages.

(*c*) *Fracture near the elbow joint.* Much swelling often attends such fractures, and it is difficult to determine the nature and extent of the injury. Therefore:

(1) If the accident happens *indoors,* lay out the limb on a pillow in the most comfortable position and send for a doctor.

(2) If the accident happens *out-of-doors,* the limb should be splinted before removing the patient.

(i) Take two flat, thin pieces of wood, one long enough to reach from the armpit to the elbow, the other from beyond the elbow to the fingertips. Cross the splints near one end, tie them together to form a right angle and pad them.

(ii) Bend up the forearm and apply the splint to the side which shows least injury.

(iii) Secure by four narrow-fold bandages; two round the upper arm, one round the forearm and one round the wrist.

(iv) Support the whole arm in a large arm sling.

(v) On reaching home remove the splint and treat as if the injury had occurred indoors.

If no splint is available, take two complete unfolded newspapers. Fold them over lengthways to make two long pads about 6 inches wide by 2 feet long. Bend them at right angles in the middle and place one behind the arm and below the forearm, the other down the front of the arm and along the upper surface of the forearm. Tie them in position and place the arm in a large sling.

The Forearm. The forearm contains two bones—the radius and the ulna; either or both may be broken. Such fractures are caused by direct or indirect violence, such as a blow or a fall on the hand or forearm.

When both bones are broken, the general signs and symptoms of fracture are present. When one bone only is broken, there is pain, partial loss of power, and swelling.

Treatment. Two splints are needed, one somewhat longer than the other. To prevent the bones being pressed together, the splints should be slightly wider than the broadest part of the forearm.

(*a*) Bend the elbow to a right angle and lay forearm across the body, thumb uppermost.

(*b*) Pad the splints and apply the longer to the palm of the hand and inner surface of the forearm, so that it reaches from beyond the elbow to beyond the fingertips. Place the shorter splint on the outer surface, extending from beyond the elbow to the knuckles.

(*c*) Secure the splints with two narrow-fold bandages, one above the fracture and the other tied as a figure of 8 round the wrist and hand.

(*d*) Look at the fingernails and see if the color returns to them after being pinched. If it does not, slacken off the bandages.

(*e*) Support the splinted arm in a large sling.

Special Fractures of the Forearm.

1. *Fracture of the Elbow Tip* (olecranon process).

The prominence at the back of the elbow is called the "olecranon process." It is the upper end of the ulna and sometimes fractures. There is pain, swelling, and discoloration at the back of the elbow. A gap may be felt below the tip of the elbow between the fragments. The arm cannot be straightened.

Treatment. Procure a straight piece of wood, a short umbrella, some cardboard, or a folded newspaper, long enough to reach from the middle of the upper arm to the wrist. Place this along the front of the limb and secure with two narrow-fold bandages. Fix the arm to the body with another bandage.

(2) *Fracture of the Lower End of the Radius* (Colles's fracture).

This injury is caused by falls on to the outstretched hand.

There is swelling and pain, with marked deformity at the wrist and a characteristic inverted-spoon-like prominence on the back of the wrist.

Treatment. If the patient can be taken quickly to a doctor or hospital, apply a cold compress to the wrist and put the arm in a large sling. Otherwise, splint as for a fracture of the shaft and get the patient to bed. Remove the splint and rest the injured part on a pillow until a doctor arrives.

N.B. In this fracture the broken ends are often driven into each other (impacted.) The symptoms then are deceptive and suggest a sprain rather than a fracture. When in doubt treat for fracture.

Fracture of the Hand. (Crushed Hand.)
Place the palm of the hand upon a carefully padded splint reaching from the middle of the forearm to beyond the finger tips. Secure the splint with a narrow figure of 8 bandage round hand, wrist and forearm.

The Thighbone (Femur). This bone is one of the strongest in the body and, especially in its upper third, is well protected by soft surrounding tissues.

Fractures of it are divided into two main classes: (i) Fractures of the shaft, and (ii) Fractures of the upper end or neck.

Fractures of the shaft are usually due to direct violence, such as a fall from a height or a run-over accident. But the neck of the femur, especially in elderly people, is often broken by a slight fall or stumble. Such a fracture resembles a dislocation, but may be recognized by:

(*a*) Mobility of the limb.

(*b*) The position of the foot, which lies on its outward side.

(*c*) Inability to raise the foot when lying on the ground.

With a dislocated hip there is:

(*a*) Rigidity of the limb.

(*b*) The head of the bone can be felt, usually at the back of the buttock.

(*c*) The foot is turned inwards.

In both cases there is shortening of the leg.

Treatment. This depends upon the nature of the injury and the apparatus available.

Keep the patient warm and telephone for an ambulance to bring a Thomas splint. This is a special appliance named after its inventor, H. O. Thomas, a pioneer of bone and joint surgery, and brought to world-wide fame by his nephew, Sir Robert Jones. It was used extensively during both world wars and saved countless lives and much suffering. It is, however, not a suitable appliance for "casual" first aid, but needs for its application a trained first aid unit.

Except where there is very extensive wounding of the upper thigh or buttock, against which the splint would press, the Thomas splint can be used for all fractures of the upper third of the lower leg, the knee and the thigh.

If no hospital or ambulance is within call, proceed as follows:

1. *For a fracture of the lower two-thirds of the shaft.* Procure a straight piece of wood, such as a broom, long enough to reach from the patient's armpit to beyond the sole of the foot. Lay the patient on his back and do not move the fractured limb. If there is marked deformity at the fracture or shortening of the leg of two inches or so, it is sometimes advised to take hold of the foot and draw it gently down till it corresponds with the sound limb. It is, however, wiser in most cases not to move the limb at all; in any case stop if it causes severe pain.

Arrange some padding and lay the splint along the outer side of the body and leg from the armpit to beyond the heel. If a second, shorter splint is available, place it on the inner side of the leg from the fork to the heel. Failing this, after splinting the injured leg, tie the sound one to it.

Seven bandages are needed. The first holds the foot to the splint and both feet together. Slip it under both ankles and take a turn round the splint. Cross the ends over the instep and pass them figure of 8 fashion round feet and ankles. Tie off under the soles of the feet.

The *second* holds the splint to the chest. Slip the bandage beneath the small of the back and slide it upwards to the level of the armpits. Take a turn round the splint, pull firmly and tie the ends over the splint.

The *third* holds the splint to the hips. Slip the bandage under the small of the back and slide it downwards to the broadest part of the hips. Take a turn round the splint and tie tightly over the outer side of the splint.

The *fourth* and *fifth* hold the thigh to the splint above and below the fracture. They are pushed under the limb and worked into position.

The *sixth* goes round both knees and both splints, holding them firmly.

The *seventh* encircles the leg midway between knee and ankle.

If no splint at all is available, bind the two legs together with handkerchiefs, ties, belts, etc. Place one at the top of the thighs, another just above the knees, a third below the knees, and a fourth binding feet and ankles.

2. If the fracture occurs in the *upper third of the bone,* though the above treatment is permissible, it is better to apply short splints and to support the leg in a flexed position.

Four stiff splints are required, and after application the legs are bandaged together and the patient placed flat.

The Kneecap (Patella). A fracture of the kneecap may be caused by direct violence, but is more frequently due to muscular action. For example, if the foot slips, the front muscles of the thigh contract with such violence that in the attempt to recover balance the knee-cap sometimes snaps across.

The symptoms are pain, swelling, loss of power and a gap which can be felt between the upper and lower fragments of bone.

Treatment. (i) Put the patient on his back and support the head and shoulders.

(ii) Straighten the leg and support the heel about 12 inches from the ground on an upturned bucket, bricks, etc.

(iii) Apply a splint along the back of the limb from the edge of the buttock to the heel.

(iv) Apply three bandages. (*a*) Place the center of a narrow-fold bandage against the sole of the foot. Cross the ends over the instep and pass them round behind the ankle and splint. Cross and bring them forward again and tie off in front of the ankle or beneath the sole. (*b*) Pass a broad-fold bandage round the middle of the thigh to secure the upper end of the splint. (*c*) Place the center of a narrow-fold bandage on the front of the thigh just above the knee. Cross the ends beneath the knee and bring them up to the front again below the knee. Pull tight and tie.

The Lower Leg. The leg from knee to ankle comprises two bones, the tibia and the fibula. Either or both of these bones may fracture. If both break, the nature of

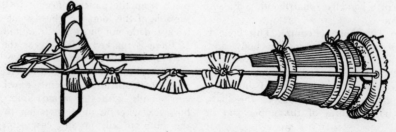

A Thomas splint in position.

the injury is self-evident. But when only one fractures, the unbroken bone may act as a splint and mask the damage.

In such a case there may be no deformity or shortening of the limb, the only symptoms being pain, swelling, and discoloration. Such a fracture occurring low down near the ankle is distinguished with difficulty from a sprain or dislocation. If in any doubt as to the nature of the injury, treat as a fracture.

Treatment *of a simple fracture:*

1. Steady the leg by holding the ankle and foot.

2. Apply splints to the outer and inner sides of the leg, extending from above the knee to beyond the foot. (If only one splint can be devised, place it on the outer side. If there is nothing at all which can be utilized, tie the knees, legs, and feet firmly together.)

3. Five bandages are needed. The *first* holds the splint to the foot. The *second* holds the top of the splint to the thigh. The *third* and *fourth* bandages encircle limb and splint, one above and one below the fracture. The *fifth* passes round both knees and the splint. If a sixth bandage is available, tie it round both ankles and the splint.

Do not put a splint down the front of the leg, nor tie a bandage over the seat of the injury.

Treatment *of a Compound Fracture of the Shaft of the Shinbone.* Owing to its position just under the skin, a fracture of the tibia is often compound, or may easily become so through careless handling of the leg.

It is a common injury in road accidents.

Symptoms and Signs. There are pain, inability to move the foot, blood on the trouser or stocking, deformity, and the foot turns outwards. When the clothing is removed, a wound is seen in the front of the leg from which blood oozes and from which a piece of bone may protrude.

1. Send immediately for an ambulance or a doctor.

2. Cut away the clothing and expose the wound.

3. Unless you have a first aid dressing a *clean* handkerchief, or a *clean* piece of paper to apply, leave the wound uncovered.

4. Do not attempt to manipulate the limb in any way.

5. Apply such splints and padding as are available. If thin sticks are used, apply several on both sides of and under the leg. Tie the legs together and remove the patient to hospital as quickly as possible.

The Foot. (Crushed Foot). This injury is caused by a fall from a height or the dropping of a heavy weight on to the foot. The symptoms are pain, swelling, and loss of power.

Treatment. 1. Remove the shoe and stocking. To do this, steady the foot, undo the laces and, if necessary, cut up the center of the toe-cap.

2. Pad and apply to the sole a flat piece of board somewhat longer than the foot itself.

3. Place the center of a narrow-fold bandage over the instep. Carry down the ends and cross them over the splint. Bring them up and back to cross behind the heel. Then take them forward round the ankle, cross again over the instep, and tie off under the sole of the foot.

4. Support the foot on a cushion or rolled-up coat.

FROSTBITE. Exposure to extreme cold may destroy any parts of the body which are not adequately protected. The edge of the ears, the nose, fingers, and toes are most likely to suffer.

The symptoms of frostbite are numbness, a waxy appearance, and coldness to the touch.

Treatment. The affected part should not be warmed in front of a fire, nor should the injured tissues be exposed to further damage by injudicious rubbing. The patient should be brought into a warm room, and his trunk should be warmed by hot-water bottles and hot drinks to restore the circulation in the extremities. The affected part should be covered with a clean dry dressing and bandaged lightly over a pad of cotton-wool.

INSENSIBILITY — UNCONSCIOUS-NESS—FITS. Loss of consciousness, other than natural sleep, may be partial—"stupor"—or complete—"coma."

The patient can be aroused with some difficulty from stupor, but not at all from coma. In stupor the pupils of the eyes react to light—i.e., they contract in a bright light and dilate in shadow, and the patient objects to the eyeball being touched—but not in coma.

The object of First Aid treatment in cases of unconsciousness is to ensure the action of the heart and lungs and to treat the cause of the condition.

General Rules for Treating Unconsciousness. 1. Put the patient on his back, the head turned to one side. If the face is flushed, prop up the head and shoulders. If the face is pallid, raise the feet and legs.

2. Loosen the clothing about the neck, chest, and waist; send for a doctor.

3. Ensure plenty of fresh air.

4. Treat hemorrhage when present, but ignore minor injuries till consciousness returns.

5. Support fractures, but do not splint or bandage extensively.

6. Cover the patient with coats, rugs, or blankets to promote warmth, and remove him to any near-by shelter.

7. Give no food or fluids whatever by mouth so long as the patient is insensible. When he recovers consciousness, give sips of water. If the pulse is feeble, and provided there is no hemorrhage apparent or suspected, give strong tea or coffee.

While carrying out these general rules, examine the patient to discover (*a*) if he is still alive, and (*b*) the cause of the unconsciousness.

Examination of an unconscious person. 1. Ascertain whether the onset was sudden or gradual, and whether it is stupor or coma.

2. Find out if the heart is beating by feeling the pulse at the wrist, temple, or throat. Or place the hand over the heart. If pulse or heartbeats can be felt, the patient is alive.

3. Watch the chest to see if the patient breathes. Note whether the breathing is quick or slow, deep or shallow, silent or noisy. Note, too, if the breath has any odor. A smell of alcohol does not necessarily mean that alcohol caused the insensibility. A stimulant may have been given or taken because the patient felt ill. If intoxication is the real cause, then the condition is serious and needs skilled medical attention.

4. Examine the head for signs of injury, the ears and nose for hemorrhage, and the mouth for blood, froth, or corrosive burns.

5. Examine the eyes. The pupils are small in *opium* poisoning and are of unequal size in brain injuries and apoplexy. They are large in (i) death, (ii) suffocation, (iii) belladonna, alcoholic, and other poisoning, and (iv) shock and excitement.

6. Examine the limbs and trunk for wounds and indications of fractures or dislocations. Compare the two sides of the body. After hemorrhage into the brain, one side may be limp and the other stiff.

7. Place the back of the hand against the patient's bared chest and note whether the skin is hot, cold, or normal.

Early Signs of Death. These are: (i) Complete cessation of breathing and heart action; (ii) the body cools; (iii) the eyes become dull and soft; (iv) the skin becomes pallid and hard.

When Convulsions Are Present.

Convulsions are spasmodic, involuntary contractions or twitchings of the body and limbs.

(*a*) *Epilepsy* is a disease of the brain causing episodes of sudden and complete loss of consciousness. It commences in childhood and may persist till old age.

The usual symptoms are convulsions, perhaps frothing at the mouth, and later quiet stupor, with slow, heavy breathing.

Treatment. Drag the patient from any source of danger, such as a fire-place or a canal bank. Remove from his vicinity light pieces of furniture or similar objects against which he might knock himself. Gently restrain the movements of his limbs. Support his head and put a pencil between his teeth to prevent the tongue being bitten. When the "fit" passes off, cover him up and encourage a natural sleep.

(*b*) *Hysterical Fits* (hysteria). These fits occur in young people, more usually in girls, in consequence of mental excitement.

Signs and Symptoms. The patient throws herself about, clutches at anyone or anything within reach, kicks, cries, and laughs alternately. In some ways hysteria may resemble epilepsy, but complete unconsciousness is never present.

Treatment. Speak sternly to the patient

and threaten a cold water shower. If she persists in her "fit," carry out the threat at once. If such fits are frequent, get medical advice.

(c) *Infantile Convulsions.* These occur in young children. There are generally contortions and twitchings of muscles, blueness of the face, and sometimes froth at the mouth. There may be a single fit followed by some degree of unconsciousness, or a succession of fits. The child should be placed in such a position that it will not injure itself, and medical advice sought without delay.

POISONS AND POISONING. A poison is any substance of which a sufficient quantity, when introduced into the system, is capable of injuring health and destroying life.

Poisoning may be *chronic* or *acute.* The former kind results from small quantities of poison being taken over a long period, and is outside the province of First Aid. The latter occurs after the taking of one or more massive doses of poison, and the life of the poisoned person often depends upon prompt and appropriate first aid treatment.

Acute poisoning usually is the result of:

(a) An accident, such as the eating of tainted food, or the taking of medicine from the wrong bottle, or a wrong dose from the right bottle, or both.

(b) Attempted suicide.

(c) Attempted murder.

Symptoms. Generally speaking, it is suggestive of poisoning if a healthy person is suddenly taken ill soon after taking food or drink, or when a person is found unconscious, perhaps burnt about the lips and mouth or in convulsions, with a suspicious bottle lying near at hand.

In the case of children, who are more prone than adults to sudden illness, suspicious symptoms are vomiting, cramp of the legs and stomach, and pain in the mouth.

General Rules for the Treatment of Poisoning. 1. Send for a doctor, stating what has occurred and the suspected poison.

2. If breathing is not perceptible, start artificial respiration immediately.

3. Preserve any traces of the poison which may exist. Carefully guard any glass,

cup, bottle, packet, or food which may have contained some of the poison; also the patient's vomit, if any, and stained clothing. This may be of legal as well as medical importance.

4. (a) If the patient is conscious, can swallow, and has *no burns or blisters about the lips or mouth,* promote vomiting in order to rid the system of as much as possible of the poison. This can be done as follows:

(i) By tickling the back of the throat with a feather.

(ii) By emetics, i.e., drinks which induce vomiting. Such are two teaspoonfuls of mustard or one tablespoonful of salt in half a tumbler of warm water, or two teaspoonfuls of ipecacuanha wine.

Repeat the doses every five minutes until vomiting begins.

4. (b) If the lips or mouth are burned, *give no emetic.* The poison was either a strong acid or the opposite—an alkali. Discover which and neutralize by administering the other. For *acid* poisoning, give repeated doses of a weak alkali such as baking soda, chalk, magnesia, whitening, or ceiling plaster. For *alkaline* poisoning, give by the tumblerful a weak acid such as vinegar, lime, or lemon juice in an equal quantity of water.

If it is not known which the poison was, give ample draughts of cold water.

5. Administer the proper antidote. This will counteract the poison and render it harmless.

For Acids and Alkalis, *see* paragraph 4 above. For other poisons, *see* TABLE OF ANTIDOTES (page 587).

If there is no clue as to the nature of the poison, give milk, raw eggs beaten up in milk or water, beaten-up cream and flour, strong tea, or even water.

6. Treat any special symptoms.

(a) For shock and collapse, promote warmth and give stimulants.

(b) For drowsiness, keep the patient on the move.

Classification of Poisons. Poisons are classified according to their action in the body. The type of poison largely determines the treatment.

There are four main groups.

Group 1. **Corrosives.** This group comprises all the strong acids and alkalis such as (acids) vitriol or electrolyte (sulphuric acid), spirits of salt (hydrochloric acid), aqua fortis (nitric acid), salts of lemon (oxalic acid), acetic acid, carbolic acid, creosote, and lysol; (alkalis) lime, caustic soda or potash, and ammonia.

These poisons stain, burn, and eat into the tissues of the mouth, throat, gullet and stomach, causing intense pain, suffocation, and collapse.

Treatment. In general no emetic can be given, as the spasm of vomiting might rupture the wall of the stomach, if already corroded, with very serious results. For *oxalic acid* an emetic *may be* given, followed by a weak alkaline solution.

In all cases dilute at once by giving water, after which for carbolic acid, creosote, and lysol give 2 to 3 tablespoonfuls of Epsom or Glauber salts, if readily available. Otherwise, and for all other corrosive acid poisons, neutralize by giving weak alkaline solutions as described in General Rules for Treatment 4 (*b*).

For alkaline poisoning, dilute at once by giving water; if possible neutralize by adding a weak acid as described above in General Rules for Treatment 4 (*b*).

Group 2. Irritants. This group comprises poisonous salts, such as the arsenical derivatives found in weed-killer, rat poison, many coloring substances, etc.; the lead compounds found in paint, hair dye, etc.; mercurial salts used in photography and as disinfectants; copper, phosphorus found in rat poison and matches, paraffin, gasoline, and iodine.

Also included as irritant poisons are poisonous berries, poisonous fungi such as toadstools, and all kinds of tainted food.

Such foods as meat and fish pastes, pork pies, game, canned food, etc., are liable to be infected and thus cause gastroenteritis or food poisoning. If several persons who have partaken of the same food later develop the same symptoms of colicky pain and diarrhea, food poisoning is probable.

Symptoms. All these poisons irritate and inflame the stomach and intestines, causing retching, purging, colicky pains, and ultimately collapse. In iodine and food poisoning there is also great thirst.

Treatment. If able to swallow, give an emetic. Dilute the poison by giving water, tea, or milk in abundance. Keep the pa-

tient warm and give beaten-up eggs or, *except in phosphorus poisoning,* salad oil.

In *iodine* poisoning give starch and water.

N.B. Phosphorus dissolves in oil, and in this form is more readily absorbed into the system. Therefore never give oil in a case of phosphorus poisoning.

Group 3. Narcotics. This group comprises the sleep-producing drugs such as *chloral, veronal, and* various barbiturate drugs; *opium* and its derivative morphia, found in laudanum, paregoric, chlorodyne and many soothing syrups.

Unlike the Corrosives and Irritants, these substances do not directly affect the tissues, but are absorbed into the blood and then act upon the nervous system. They produce drowsiness leading to stupor and insensibility.

Symptoms. The features are generally pale, the pulse slow, the breathing slow, deep and noisy. In opium poisoning the pupils contract to "pin-points."

Treatment. If the patient is able to swallow, give an emetic followed by enough crystals of permanganate of potash to cover a dime in a glass of water. Keep the patient awake by walking him about, flicking his face and chest with a wet towel, and give him plenty of strong black coffee to drink.

If the patient is unconscious, give nothing by mouth, as he cannot swallow. Keep him lying down on his side until the doctor arrives, and be ready to give artificial respiration at once if his breathing shows signs of stopping.

Group 4. Deliriants or Narcotic-irritants. This group comprises a number of poisons possessing the qualities of both Irritants and Narcotics. They irritate the tissues with which they come in contact, as well as reacting after absorption upon the nervous system. Thus they first produce delirium or convulsions, then coma.

The principal poisons in this group are:

(*a*) *Belladonna and Atropine,* found in certain liniments, eyedrops and the poisonous berries of the deadly night-shade. The symptoms are wild excitement, dry, parched mouth and lips, great thirst, widely dilated pupils, delirium, and coma.

Treatment. Give an emetic at once. Combat drowsiness and give strong hot coffee.

(*b*) *Strychnine*, found in vermin-killer. The symptoms are a bitter taste in the mouth, widely dilated pupils, restlessness, convulsive spasms, difficult breathing, and collapse.

Treatment. Give an emetic before spasms commence, followed by large quantities of charcoal or wood cinders.

The antidote is bromide of potassium, of which half an ounce may be administered in water by mouth or injected into the rectum at intervals of 15 minutes while the spasms last. Do not be afraid to give large doses of bromides in a case of strychnine poisoning.

(*c*) *Aconite*, found in neuralgic and rheumatic liniments and in the monkshood, or blue rocket, a common garden flower. The symptoms are a tingling of the mouth and throat which spreads to the whole body; sensation is dulled, especially sight and hearing. Breathing becomes difficult and finally the heart fails.

Treatment. Give an immediate emetic, followed, after the vomiting has ceased, by stimulants such as strong tea or coffee. If they are not retained by the stomach, they must be given per rectum as an enema.

Keep the patient lying down and promote warmth by hot-water bottles and by rubbing the feet and hands. Perform artificial respiration if the breathing fails.

The antidotes are 30 drops of tincture of belladonna (atropine), given by mouth or as an enema, or 20 drops of tincture of digitalis by mouth and repeated in half an hour if necessary.

(*d*) *Prussic Acid and the Cyanides.* These are among the most powerful known poisons and are particularly dangerous, owing to the rapidity of their action. Immediately after the poison is taken giddiness and staggering set in. The eyes stare, the pulse quickly fails, the skin is cold and clammy, the breathing is slow and convulsive, and the patient may lose consciousness within two minutes.

Treatment. This consists of stimulating the patient pending the arrival of a doctor. Instantly dash cold water on the face, chest, and spine. If the patient is still conscious, give an emetic followed by brandy. The latter may be given as an

enema if necessary. Apply ammonia on a handkerchief to the patient's nostrils and carry out artificial respiration.

The antidote is atropine, and may be given as half a teaspoonful of tincture of belladonna.

Alcoholic Poisoning, or Drunkenness. Alcoholic poisoning may be due to excessive drinking over a number of years. In this case it may take the form of delirium tremens ("D.T.'s"), needing medical treatment, not first aid.

Acute alcoholic poisoning is usually the result of a "binge" in an otherwise healthy person. The symptoms are exhilaration and a feeling of well-being followed by drowsiness, and collapse.

Treatment. Alcohol in large quantities is a narcotic poison, and on no account should a person be left to "sleep it off." Give an emetic to get rid of any alcohol in the stomach. Then give strong, hot coffee by mouth or rectum and keep the patient on the move.

When he shows signs of recovery, put him to bed under warm blankets and with hot-water bottles to his feet, and see that he keeps well covered.

INDEX OF POISONS

Copper, *see* IRRITANTS.

Copper Sulphate.

Corrosive Sublimate, *see* IRRITANTS, under MERCURY.

Creosote, *see* CORROSIVE ACIDS.

Cyanides, *see* DELIRIANTS.

Digitalis, *see* DELIRIANTS.

Food Poisoning, *see* IRRITANTS.

Hartshorn, Spirits of, *see* CORROSIVE ALKALIS, under AMMONIA.

Headache Powders, *see* NARCOTICS.

Hemlock, *see* CONIUM (NARCOTICS).

Henbane, *see* DELIRIANTS (HYOSCYAMUS).

Hydrochloric Acid, *see* CORROSIVE ACIDS.

Hydrocyanic Acid, *see* DELIRIANTS, under PRUSSIC ACID.

Hyoscyamus, *see* DELIRIANTS.

Iodine, *see* IRRITANTS.

Laudanum, *see* NARCOTICS.

Lead, *see* IRRITANTS.

Lime, *see* CORROSIVE ALKALIS.

Lunar Caustic, *see* IRRITANTS.

Lysol, *see* CORROSIVE ACIDS.

Meadow Saffron, *see* COLCHICUM.

Medinal, *see* BARBITURATES, under NARCOTICS.

Mercury, *see* IRRITANTS.

Morphia, *see* NARCOTICS.

Muriatic Acid, *see,* CORROSIVE ACIDS, under HYDROCHLORIC.

Mushrooms, *see* IRRITANTS (BAD FOOD).

Nembutal, *see* BARBITURATES, under NARCOTICS.

Nitrate of Silver, *see* IRRITANTS, under LUNAR CAUSTIC.

Nitric Acid, *see* CORROSIVE ACIDS.

Nux Vomica, *see* DELIRIANTS.

Opium, *see* NARCOTICS.

Oxalic Acid, *see* CORROSIVE ACIDS.

Paraffin, *see* IRRITANTS.

Paraldehyde, *see* NARCOTICS.

Paregoric, *see* NARCOTICS.

Petrol, *see* IRRITANTS.

Phenacitin, *see* NARCOTICS, under HEADACHE POWDERS.

Phenobarbitone, *see* BARBITURATES, under NARCOTICS.

Phosphorus, *see* IRRITANTS.

Potash, *see* CORROSIVE ALKALIS.

Prussic Acid, *see* DELIRIANTS.

Ptomaine, *see* IRRITANTS, under FOOD.

Rat Poison, *see* IRRITANTS, under STRYCHNINE.

Salts of Lemon, *see* CORROSIVE ACIDS.

Soda, *see* CORROSIVE ALKALIS.

Spirits of Salt, *see* CORROSIVE ACIDS, under HYDROCHLORIC.

Strychnine, *see* DELIRIANTS.

Sulphonal, *see* NARCOTICS.

Sulphuric Acid, *see* CORROSIVE ACIDS.

Tartar Emetic, *see* IRRITANTS, under ANTIMONY.

Tartaric Acid, *see* CORROSIVE ACIDS.

Veronal, *see* NARCOTICS.

Vitriol, *see* CORROSIVE ACIDS, under SULPHURIC.

Zinc Chloride, *see* CORROSIVE ACIDS.

PULSE. The ordinary method of feeling the pulse is to place the tips of the fingers on the radial artery at the wrist about one and a half inches above the root of the thumb.

The normal pulse-rate is about 72, but the rate varies according to circumstances.

The pulse-rate in infants is high—generally over 120. A person suffering from shock or hemorrhage usually has a fast but feeble pulse.

SEPSIS AND ANTISEPSIS. Sepsis is due to the presence of microorganisms or "germs" in a wound, and is shown by redness and the exudation of matter or pus. Sepsis not only prevents rapid healing, but the germs may pass into the bloodstream and cause *septicemia,* or blood poisoning.

Antisepsis must always be aimed at by washing the hands, by avoiding unnecessary handling of a wound and by the use of antiseptic solutions, such as *weak* solutions of carbolic acid, tincture of iodine, etc., which destroy germs.

SPRAINS. A sudden wrench or twist may tear the ligaments of a joint and the surrounding tissues. If there is no displacement of bones, the injury is called a sprain.

The symptoms are swelling and pain.

Treatment. *For a sprained ankle:*

1. If the accident occurs *out-of-doors.* Cut the laces and remove the shoe. Place the center of an improvised bandage (belt, tie, handkerchief, etc.) under the sole of the foot. Cross the ends over the instep, bring them figure of 8 fashion round the ankle to the front and tie tightly. Saturate with cold water, if available, to tighten the bandage and relieve the pain. On reaching home treat as an indoor accident.

2. If the accident occurs *indoors.* Make

the patient lie down on a couch or bed with his foot supported on a cushion. Remove the shoe and sock, cutting them if necessary. Send for a doctor, and meanwhile keep the foot raised, and wrap it in a towel wrung out in cold water.

STIMULANTS. As a rule, it is wiser not to give a patient alcohol after an accident until a doctor has seen the case.

Strong tea or coffee and hot milk are useful stimulants to give if the patient can swallow. Or smelling salts may be held to his nose, after testing their strength.

STRAINS. The symptoms are a sharp pain and loss of function in the affected muscles. For example, a patient whose back is strained may not be able to stand upright.

Treatment. Rest the injured part by supporting it in the most comfortable position and apply warmth.

WOUNDS, TREATMENT OF.

First, the bleeding must be controlled. In minor injuries this is easy; how to deal with severe bleeding, of hemorrhage, is given under that heading.

Secondly, the wound must be cleaned.

Thirdly, the wound must be dressed to protect it from germs.

Fourthly, the injured part must be rested so that the healing process is not interrupted.

Cleaning a Wound. *Minor Injuries.* It is prudent always to clean even a small cut or abrasion by applying tincture of iodine all over the broken surface immediately. Allow the iodine to dry and do not wash the wound at all.

Larger Wounds. If the wound is dirty and immediate surgical aid is not forthcoming, gently wash away as much dirt as possible by flushing the wound with a weak solution of any household antiseptic. Do not search for foreign bodies you cannot see. Apply tincture of iodine all over the wound and the surrounding skin.

Do not attempt to clean the wound of an open or compound fracture, nor a wound near a fracture; the surgeon will do this. Apply a dressing, or even a clean piece of unprinted paper if nothing better is available.

Dressing a Wound. A dressing should be absorbent and sterile (germ-free), such as pieces of gauze, lint, clean linen handkerchiefs, or towels, which have been baked in an oven, boiled for twenty minutes, or soaked in an antiseptic solution.

Apply the dressing by holding it by one corner and dropping it on to the wound. Then cover with cotton-wool, if available, and a bandage.

Healing of Wounds. The ideal process is called healing *by first intention.* This can only occur if the wound is clean, the edge kept in contact, and the part rested.

If these conditions are not fulfilled, the gap gradually fills with granulation tissue and when level with the surrounding skin, a scar forms.

TABLE OF PRINCIPAL POISONS
AND THEIR ANTIDOTES

Poisons	Signs	Treatment
Corrosive Acids		
Acetic	⎫ Lips and mouth burned and	⎧ *NO EMETIC.* Give water at once
Zinc chloride	⎬ stained.	⎪ to dilute the poison. If possible add
Hydrochloric	⎭	⎪ chalk, magnesia, or ceiling plaster.
Nitric (Aqua Fortis)		⎨ For the pain give oil, milk, or
Sulphuric	⎫ Pain from mouth to stomach.	⎪ beaten-up eggs.
Tartaric	⎭	
Carbolic acid	⎫ ditto	⎧ As above, but use Epsom or Glauber
Creosote	⎬ ditto	⎨ salts.
Lysol	⎭ ditto	
Oxalic acid	⎫ ditto	⎧ An emetic *may* be given, then chalk,
Zinc chloride	⎭	⎨ magnesia, or plaster.
Corrosive Alkalis		
Ammonia	⎫ Lips and mouth burned raw.	⎧ *NO EMETIC.* Give water at once
Lime	⎬ ditto	⎨ to dilute the poison. If possible add
Potash	⎪ ditto	⎩ vinegar, lemon or lime juice.
Soda	⎭	
Irritants		
Antimony	Vomiting, retching, faintness,	*EMETIC.* Water, tea, or milk;
Arsenic	purging, cramps.	beaten-up eggs, salad oil, Keep
Cantharides	ditto	patient warm.
Copper	ditto	ditto
Food, bad	ditto	ditto
Gasoline	ditto	ditto
Iodine	ditto	ditto
Lead	ditto	ditto (starch and
Silver nitrate	ditto	ditto water.)
Mercury	ditto	ditto
Paraffin	ditto	ditto
Phosphorus	ditto	ditto
Silver nitrate	ditto	ditto
		As above, but *NO* oil.
Narcotics		
Opium	Sleepiness, pallor, slow pulse,	*EMETIC.* Solution of potassium per-
Morphia	slow, stertorous breathing,	manganate. Combat sleepiness. Hot
Laudanum	"pinpoint" pupils, musty	coffee. Artificial respiration if breath-
Barbiturates	breath.	ing fails.
Chloral	ditto	ditto
Chlorodyne	ditto	ditto
Conium (Hemlock)	ditto	ditto
Headache powders	ditto	ditto
Paregoric	ditto	ditto
Paraldehyde	ditto	ditto
Phenobarbitone	ditto	ditto
Sulphonal	ditto	ditto
Veronal	ditto	ditto
Cocaine	⎫ Giddiness, pallor, rapid, fee-	⎧ *EMETIC.* Warmth, stimulants, artifi-
	⎭ ble pulse.	⎩ cial respiration.
Deliriants or		
Narcotic Irritants		
Atropine	⎫ Excitement, dry mouth, thirst,	⎧ *EMETIC.* Combat drowsiness, Strong
Belladonna	⎬ dilated pupils.	⎨ coffee.
Hyoscyamus	⎭	
Nux Vomica	⎫ Bitter taste, dilated pupils,	*EMETIC.* Charcoal, wood cinders,
Strychnine	⎭ spasms, difficult breathing.	tincture of iodine, "stewed tea."
		Large doses of potassium bromide.
	Tingling in mouth and throat.	*EMETIC.* Stimulants, warmth, rest.
Aconite	Dulled sight and hearing,	Tincture of belladonna 30 drops, or
	difficult breathing.	tincture of digitalis 20 drops.
Prussic acid	⎫ Giddiness, staggering, coma.	*EMETIC.* Instant cold water douches
Cyanides	⎭ Staring eyes, clammy skin.	on face and back of neck, brandy,
		ammonia to the nostrils.
Digitalis	Green vomit, heart failure.	Stimulants, repose for some hours.
Alcohol	⎫ Drowsiness, deep sleep, col-	⎧ *EMETIC.* Strong coffee, keep mov-
	⎭ lapse.	⎩ ing. Later put into a warm bed.

Table* of Foods
and Their Nutrient Values

The values shown in this table are reasonable averages based on currently available data. Reasonable variations may be expected due to the natural differences in foods, different varieties of the same foods, differences in recipes for prepared foods, differences in chemical analytical methods, and statistical rounding of averages.

Measured in grams (gm): protein (Pro.), total fat (T. Fat), saturated fatty acids (SF), unsaturated fatty acids (UF), polyunsaturated fatty acids (PF) and carbohydrate (CHO).

Measured in milligrams (mg): cholesterol (Chol.).

DAIRY PRODUCTS	Amt.	Cal.	Pro.	T. Fat	SF	UF	PF	CHO	Chol.
Cheese									
cheddar grated	1 tbsp	30	2.0	2.0	1.0	1.0			8
cheddar processed 1 slice	1 oz	105	7.0	9.0	5.0	3.6	0.6		32
cottage, creamed	1 oz	30	3.8	1.4	0.8	0.6	0.1	1	1
cottage, uncreamed	1 oz	25	5.0					1	1
cream	1 tbsp	55	1.0	6.0	3.0	2.7	0.7		9
Swiss Camembert	1 oz	105	7.0	8.0	4.0	3.6	0.6	1	41
Chocolate milk drink	1 oz	24	1.0	0.8	0.4	0.4	0.2	3	
Cocoa									
whole milk	1 oz	29	1.1	1.4	0.8	0.5		3	4
skim milk	1 oz	19	1.2	0.2	0.1	0.1		3	

*oz—ounce, tsp—teaspoon, tbsp—tablespoon, lg—large, sl—slice, med—medium, pc—piece, Cal—calories

(From *Your Heart Has Nine Lives*, by Alton Blakeslee and Jeremiah Stamler, M. D. Reprinted by permission of Prentice-Hall, Inc.)

(Cont. next page)

	Amt.	Cal.	Pro.	T. Fat	SF	UF	PF	CHO	Chol.
Corn starch pudding	½ cup	138	4.5	5.0	3.0	1.8	0.3	20	17
Cream									
half and half (12% fat)	1 tbsp	20		1.8	1.0	0.7	0.1	1	6
light; also sour cream (20% fat)	1 tbsp	35		3.2	1.8	1.3	0.2	1	10
medium (27% fat)	1 tbsp	45		4.9	2.7	1.9	0.3	1	14
heavy (35% fat)	1 tbsp	55		5.8	3.2	2.3	0.4	1	18
restaurant creamer	¾ oz	30		2.7	1.5	1.1	0.1	2	9
Custard, baked or tapioca	½ cup	143	6.5	7.0	3.0	3.7	1.2	14	152
Egg									
whole	1 lg	80	6.0	6.0	2.0	3.7	0.7		234
white	1	15	4.0						
yolk	1	60	3.0	6.0	2.0	3.7	0.7		234
scrambled dry	1 egg	110	6.0	8.0	3.0	5.0	1.0	1	234
Ice cream, plain	½ cup	145	3.0	9.0	5.0	3.6	0.6	15	35
Ice milk	½ cup	143	4.5	5.0	3.0	1.8	0.3	21	6
Metrecal—liquid	1 oz	28	2.2	0.6	0.2	0.4	0.2	4	
Milk									
whole	1 oz	21	1.1	1.2	0.8	0.4		2	4
skim (reconstituted or fortified)	1 oz	11	1.1					2	
evaporated	1 tbsp	22	1.1	1.2	0.7	0.5	0.1	2	9
dry non-fat powder	1 tbsp	18	1.8					3	

(Cont. next page)

	Amt.	Cal.	Pro.	T. Fat	SF	UF	PF	CHO	Chol.
Ovaltine powder	3 tsp	51	2.2	0.3	0.2	0.1		10	1
Pream	1 tsp	11	0.6	0.6	0.3	0.2		1	
Whipped topping (can)	1 tbsp	18	0.1	1.7	0.4	1.3	0.1	1	
Yogurt (partially skimmed milk)	1 oz	15	1.0	0.5	0.2	0.3	0.2	2	

FISH AND SEAFOOD

	Amt.	Cal.	Pro.	T. Fat	SF	UF	PF	CHO	Chol.
Clams, raw	1 oz	23	3.7	0.3	0.1	0.2	0.1	1	35
Crabmeat, canned or cooked	1 oz	30	4.7	0.7	0.2	0.5	0.2		28
Fishsticks, breaded	1 pc	40	3.8	2.0	0.5	1.4	1.0	2	14
Herring	1 pc (25 gm)	53	5.6	3.2	0.7	2.2	1.5		23
Ocean Perch, breaded, deep fat fried	1 oz	65	5.3	3.7	0.8	2.7	0.4	2	18
Oysters, raw (2 or 3 medium)	1 oz	20	2.5	0.5	0.2	0.3	0.2	1	32
Salmon, pink canned	1 oz	40	5.7	1.7	0.3	1.3	1.0		18
Salmon, red smoked	1 oz	50	6.0	2.8	0.8	1.8	0.9		17
Sardines (drained)	1 oz	60	7.3	3.0	0.7	2.2	1.5		23
Shrimps, lobster	1 oz	37	7.7	0.3	0.1	0.2	0.1		42
Tuna, anchovies, caviar	1 oz	57	8.3	2.3	0.7	1.6	1.3		17
Fish: cooked, smoked, lean	1 oz	46	7.0	2.0	0.6	1.3	0.7		18

MIXED DISHES, SOUPS, SALADS, ETC.

	Amt.	Cal.	Pro.	T. Fat	SF	UF	PF	CHO	Chol.
Baked beans canned, with pork	¼ cup	83	4.0	1.8	0.8	1.0	0.3	14	2

(Cont. next page)

591

	Amt.	Cal.	Pro.	T. Fat	SF	UF	PF	CHO	Chol.
with salt pork, homemade	¼ cup	90	3.4	3.9	1.4	2.3	0.6	11	9
with oil, homemade	¼ cup	98	3.1	4.9	0.4	4.4	3.0	11	
Borscht with sour cream	¼ cup	26	0.3	1.8	0.8	1.0	0.2	2	3
Cheese blintzes, baked	1 oz	56	3.1	4.0	2.0	1.9	0.5	2	37
Chicken chow mein, noodles separate	½ cup	132	11.4	8.6	2.4	6.2	1.3	2	28
Chicken livers, chopped	½ oz	28	1.5	2.1	0.7	1.3	0.4	1	28
Chili									
with beans, canned	¼ cup	84	4.8	3.8	1.8	1.8	0.1	8	25
no beans, canned	¼ cup	128	6.5	9.5	4.5	4.6	0.3	4	36
Chop Suey									
lean pork	¼ cup	50	6.2	2.6	0.9	1.7	0.5	1	21
American ground beef	¼ cup	87	6.6	6.5	2.5	3.9	0.3	1	27
Chow mein noodles	⅓ cup	73	2.0	3.5	0.9	2.6	0.3	9	
Corned beef hash, canned	1 oz	40	4.0	1.7	0.7	0.9	0.2	2	12
Denver sandwich: fried eggs, ham	1 sand	318	13.4	18.0	6.8	10.3	2.2	28	274
Dumpling	1 oz	89	2.2	3.8	1.2	2.6	0.2	12	2
Egg roll, deep fat fried	1 pc (1 oz)	83	3.1	6.7	1.2	5.2	3.6	3	16
Gefullte fish	1 oz	37	5.0	1.6	0.5	1.0	0.5	1	19
Gravy									
with beef fat, flour	1 tbsp	34	0.1	3.5	1.7	1.7	0.1	1	4
with oil, flour	1 tbsp	34	0.1	3.5	0.2	3.2	2.2	1	

(Cont. next page)

	Amt.	Cal.	Pro.	T. Fat	SF	UF	PF	CHO	Chol.
Kreplach									
meat, boiled	1 oz	73	5.1	3.0	1.3	1.6	0.1	6	44
cheese, boiled	1 oz	53	4.0	1.5	0.6	0.8	0.2	6	26
Macaroni and cheese	¼ cup	119	4.5	6.3	3.5	2.5	0.5	11	22
Meat loaf	1 oz	101	7.0	7.6	3.7	3.5	0.2	1	45
Noodles and cottage cheese	¼ cup	76	4.6	3.7	1.8	1.8	0.4	6	30
Potato									
pancakes	1 sm (2 oz)	68	1.3	4.8	1.3	3.5	0.4	5	24
patty or cake	2 oz	106	2.0	8.4	3.0	5.1	0.5	6	56
Pot Pie									
beef	½ pie	230	9.0	14.0	5.0	8.3	0.8	16	54
poultry	½ pie	243	8.5	14.0	4.0	9.3	1.8	20	35
Pizza with tomato and cheese	3" wedge	90	4.0	3.0	1.5	1.5		12	2
Rice									
pilaf	¼ cup	64	1.0	2.0	1.0	0.9	0.3	11	7
fried	¼ cup	132	2.0	8.1	2.9	4.8	1.3	12	47
Salad									
chicken	1 oz	64	4.9	4.6	1.1	3.4	1.9		16
kidney bean	¼ cup	87	2.1	6.1	1.1	4.8	3.2	6	5
potato, German	¼ cup	63	2.5	1.5	0.6	1.0	0.2	11	3
potato, with mayonnaise	¼ cup	124	1.0	9.6	1.7	7.4	5.0	8	7
shrimp	1 oz	52	4.8	3.3	0.7	2.5	1.6		37

(Cont. next page)

	Amt.	Cal.	Pro.	T. Fat	SF	UF	PF	CHO	Chol.
tuna or salmon (restaurant)	1 oz	57	4.6	3.4	0.8	2.6	1.9	1	11
Waldorf	¼ cup	57	0.3	4.8	0.8	3.8	2.7	4	3
Salmon loaf	1 oz	49	5.1	2.8	0.9	1.7	0.7	1	36
Soup									
bean	¼ cup	48	2.0	1.3	0.5	0.7	0.2	8	3
beef with meat	¼ cup	25	1.5	1.0	0.5	0.5		3	1
broth: bouillon, consommé, onion	¼ cup	3	0.5						
clam chowder, no milk	¼ cup	21	1.3	0.5		0.5	0.5	3	13
cream, canned (all varieties)	¼ cup	50	1.8	3.0	1.8	1.1	0.1	5	10
cream, homemade	¼ cup	66	2.8	4.4	2.6	1.7	0.3	5	14
noodle or rice	¼ cup	29	1.5	1.0	0.3	0.8	0.3	3	1
pea	¼ cup	35	1.5	0.5	0.3	0.3		6	9
vegetable, tomato	¼ cup	23	0.5	0.5	0.3	0.3	0.2	5	
Spaghetti									
with meat sauce	¼ cup	71	3.3	2.5	0.8	1.7	0.9	9	7
with tomato and cheese	¼ cup	53	1.5	1.3	0.5	0.8	0.5	9	39
Stew									
beef vegetable	¼ cup	46	3.8	2.5	1.3	1.2	0.2	4	27
oyster, made with whole milk and butter	¼ cup	50	2.8	3.0	1.4	1.4	0.2	3	66
Tomato aspic	¼ cup	18	2.0					3	
Veal									
curried	¼ cup	101	12.2	5.8	2.4	3.3	0.3		48

(Cont. next page)

	Amt.	Cal.	Pro.	T. Fat	SF	UF	PF	CHO	Chol.
scallopini (restaurant)	¼ cup	161	10.3	12.2	4.9	6.9	0.5	2	53
VEGETABLES									
Asparagus									
fresh	½ cup	18	2.0					3	
canned	½ cup	20	2.0					3	
Beans									
lima (small)	½ cup	75	4.0	0.5		0.4	0.2	15	
green or wax	½ cup	13	1.0					3	
Beets, diced	½ cup	35	1.0					8	
Broccoli spears	½ cup	23	2.5					4	
Brussels sprouts	½ cup	30	3.0	0.5	0.1	0.4	0.2	6	
Cabbage									
raw shredded	½ cup	13	0.5					3	
sauerkraut or plain cooked	½ cup	20	1.0					5	
coleslaw with dressing	⅛ cup	18	0.1	1.5	0.2	1.2	1.0	1	2
Carrots									
raw (½ medium)	1 oz	10	0.5					3	
diced	½ cup	23	0.5	0.5	0.1	0.4	0.2	5	
Cauliflower	½ cup	15	1.5					3	
Corn									
ear	1	65	2.0	1.0	1.0	1.0	1.0	16	

(Cont. next page)

595

	Amt.	Cal.	Pro.	T.Fat	SF	UF	PF	CHO	Chol.
canned (all varieties)	½ cup	85	2.5	0.5	0.1	0.4	0.2	21	
Greens, all except spinach	½ cup	15	1.5					3	
Lettuce, celery, other salad vegetables	½ cup	6	1.0					2	
Okra	½ cup	30	2.0					6	
Onions	½ cup	40	1.0					9	
Parsnips	½ cup	48	1.0	0.5	0.1	0.4	0.2	11	
Peas									
green fresh or frozen	½ cup	55	4.0	0.5	0.1	0.4	0.2	10	
green canned	½ cup	85	4.0	0.5	0.1	0.4	0.2	16	
Potatoes									
boiled or baked	½ med	45	1.5					11	
French fried in cottonseed oil (5 pc)	1 oz	78	1.0	3.5	0.8	2.7	2.0	10	
French fried in hydrogenated fat (5 pc)	1 oz	78	1.0	3.5	1.2	2.3	0.3	10	
French fried in corn oil (5 pc)	1 oz	78	1.0	3.5	0.3	3.0	2.1	10	
French fried, frozen (5 pc)	1 oz	48	1.0	2.0	0.5	1.5	1.0	8	
mashed with milk and butter	½ cup	58	1.0	3.0	1.8	1.0	1.0	7	11
roasted	½ med	82	1.5	4.0	1.0	3.0	0.3	11	
scalloped	½ cup	120	3.9	5.4	2.4	3.1	0.2	15	8
Potato chips	5 lg pc	55	0.5	3.5	1.0	2.5	1.5	5	
Pumpkin, canned	½ cup	38	1.0	0.5	0.1	0.4	0.2	9	
Spinach	½ cup	23	3.0	0.5	0.1	0.4	0.2	3	

(Cont. next page)

	Amt.	Cal.	Pro.	T. Fat	SF	UF	PF	CHO	Chol.
Soybean sprouts, raw	½ cup	25	3.5	0.5	0.1	0.4	0.2	3	
Squash									
summer diced	½ cup	18	0.5					4	
winter baked or mashed	½ cup	48	2.0	0.5	0.1	0.4	0.2	12	
Sweet potatoes									
boiled	½ med	85	1.0	0.5	0.1	0.4	0.2	20	
candied	½ med	148	1.0	3.0	1.0	2.0	0.5	30	
Tomatoes									
raw	½ med	15	1.0					3	
canned	½ cup	23	1.0					5	
Tomato catsup	1 tbsp	15						4	
Turnips, diced	½ cup	20	0.5					5	
Vegetables, average	½ cup	24	1.4	0.2		0.2		6	
FRUITS									
Apple	1 med	70						18	
Apple juice, also grape, pineapple	½ cup	63						17	
Applesauce, also ½ pear, canned	¼ cup	45						12	
Apricots									
fresh	3	55	1.0					14	
canned (4 with 2 tbsp syrup)	4 halves	105	1.0					27	
dried (¼ cup)	10 halves	98	2.0	0.2		0.2	0.1	25	

(Cont. next page)

	Amt.	Cal.	Pro.	T. Fat	SF	UF	PF	CHO	Chol.
juice, also peach	½ cup	70	0.5					18	
Avocado	¼ cup	65	0.8	6.5	1.2	5.0	2.0	2	
Banana	1 med	85	1.0					23	
Blueberries	½ cup	43	0.5	0.5	0.1	0.4	0.2	11	
Cantaloupe	¼ med	20	0.5					5	
Cherries, raw (8–10 large)	½ cup	33	0.5	0.5	0.1	0.4	0.2	8	
Cranberry sauce	1 tbsp	34		0.1		0.1		9	
Dates, fresh dried (3–4)	1 oz	80	0.6	0.2		0.2		21	
Figs, fresh dried	1 lg	60	1.0					15	
Fruit cocktail, heavy syrup	½ cup	98	0.5	0.5	0.1	0.4	0.2	25	
Grapefruit									
grapefruit	½ med	50	1.0					14	
sections, raw	½ cup	38	0.4					10	
juice, fresh	½ cup	48	0.5					12	
juice, canned sweet	½ cup	65	0.5					16	
Grapes: 15 malaga, 40 green seedless	½ cup	50	0.5					13	
Honeydew melon, fresh pineapple	½ cup	38	0.5					10	
Lemon juice	1 tbsp	5						1	
Lemonade, sweetened	½ cup	56						14	
Orange									
orange	1 med	70	1.0					18	

(Cont. next page)

	Amt.	Cal.	Pro.	T. Fat	SF	UF	PF	CHO	Chol.
juice, canned fresh or frozen	½ cup	56	1.0					14	
Peach, fresh	1 med	35	1.0					10	
Peaches									
canned with juice	1 half	45						12	
dried (4 med halves)	1 oz	75	0.9	0.2		0.2		20	
Pear, fresh	1 lg	100	1.0	1.0		0.8	0.4	25	
Pineapple, canned sliced	1 sl	95			0.2			26	
Plum, fresh	1 lg	30						7	
Prunes, dried	4 med	70	1.0					19	
Raisins	¼ cup	115	1.0					31	
Strawberries									
fresh	½ cup	28	0.5	0.5	0.1	0.4	0.2	7	
frozen	1 oz	30	0.2	0.1		0.1		8	
Watermelon, 4" x 4" wedge	1 pc sm	60	1.0	0.5	0.1	0.4	0.2	15	
Fruit fresh, average	½ cup	58	0.8	0.2		0.2	0.1	15	

CEREALS, BREADS, BAKED GOODS

	Amt.	Cal.	Pro.	T. Fat	SF	UF	PF	CHO	Chol.
Biscuits, baking powder	1 med	130	3.0	4.0	1.0	2.8	0.8	18	2
Bread crumbs, dry grated	1 tbsp	23	0.5	0.5	0.1	0.4	0.1	4	
Bread									
Boston brown	1 sl	100	3.0	1.0	0.2	0.8	0.1	22	1
white enriched	1 sl	60	2.0	1.0	0.2	0.8	0.1	12	1

(Cont. next page)

	Amt.	Cal.	Pro.	T. Fat	SF	UF	PF	CHO	Chol.
white unenriched, raisin, French	1 sl	60	2.0	1.0	0.2	0.8	0.1	12	1
whole wheat	1 sl	55	2.0	1.0	0.2	0.8	0.3	11	1
Brownie, 2" x 2" square	1	124	1.5	8.0	2.9	4.7	1.4	13	39
Cake, without frosting angel food, 2" wedge	1 pc	110	3.0					23	
chiffon cake, 1¼" wedge	1 pc	141	2.8	5.6	1.3	4.1	2.6	19	39
cheese cake, 2" x 3"	1 pc	196	4.6	11.0	6.2	4.3	0.8	18	51
chocolate plain, 2" wedge	1 pc	144	2.7	6.0	3.0	2.7	0.6	21	39
fruit, 2" x 2"	1 pc	105	2.0	4.0	1.0	2.8	0.8	17	22
plain, 2" wedge	1 pc	180	3.9	5.1	0.9	3.9	0.9	30	24
pound, 3" x 3"	1 pc	130	2.0	7.0	2.0	5.0	1.0	15	36
sponge, 2" wedge	1 pc	105	3.0	2.4	0.8	1.5	0.3	17	88
white cake with oil, 1½" wedge	1 pc	210	3.6	5.6	0.3	5.0	3.3	36	
Cereals dry	½ oz	55	1.0					12	
dry sweetened	½ oz	60	1.0					13	
Cookie, small, 1½" med fat	1	35	0.7	1.0	0.3	0.7		6	7
high fat	1	35	0.4	1.4	0.3	1.0	0.1	5	3
chocolate chip	1	31	0.4	1.3	0.5	0.8	0.1	4	4
peanut butter	1	32	0.6	1.4	0.3	1.0	0.2	4	3

(Cont. next page)

	Amt.	Cal.	Pro.	T. Fat	SF	UF	PF	CHO	Chol.
Corn grits									
enriched	¼ cup	30	0.8					7	
unenriched	¼ cup	30	0.8					7	
Corn meal, enriched	2 tbsp	66	1.4	0.2			0.1	14	
Corn muffins, cornbread	1 med	155	4.0	5.0	2.0	2.8	0.8	22	32
Cracker									
graham	1 med	28	0.5	0.5	0.1	0.4	0.1	5	
saltine	1	18	0.5	0.5	0.1	0.4	0.1	3	
Ritz	1	11	0.2	0.5	0.4	0.1		1	1
Doughnut	1	135	2.0	7.0	2.0	5.0	3.0	17	27
Farina, enriched	½ cup	53	1.5					11	
Fig bar	1	55	1.0	1.0	0.2	0.8	0.1	12	
Flour enriched	1 tbsp	25	0.8	0.1		0.1		5	
French toast with butter	1 sl	153	5.0	8.1	3.9	3.8	1.0	15	144
Macaroni, noodles, spaghetti	½ cup	96	3.0	0.6	0.2	0.4		20	
Muffin									
plain	1	135	4.0	5.0	1.0	3.8	0.8	19	23
English, matzo	1 sl	56	2.0	0.2		0.2		12	1
Oatmeal	½ cup	75	2.5	1.5	0.5	1.0	0.5	13	
Pancake									
with hydrogenated fat	1 med	60	2.0	2.0	0.5	1.4	0.9	8	23
with oil	1 med	62	1.9	1.6	0.1	1.4	0.9	10	

(Cont. next page)

	Amt.	Cal.	Pro.	T. Fat	SF	UF	PF	CHO	Chol.
Pie crust with shortening	1/7 crust	94	1.4	5.1	1.1	3.8	0.4	10	
Pies									
custard	1 pc	265	7.0	11.0	4.0	7.0	1.0	34	87
all fruit	1 pc	330	3.0	13.0	4.0	8.4	1.4	53	11
lemon meringue	1 pc	300	4.0	12.0	4.0	7.4	1.4	45	59
mince	1 pc	340	3.0	9.0	2.0	6.6	0.6	62	3
pumpkin	1 pc	265	5.0	12.0	5.0	7.0	1.0	34	87
Popcorn, no fat added	1/2 cup	28	1.0	0.5	0.1	0.4	0.1	6	
Pretzels, small stick	5 sticks	20						4	
Rice	1/2 cup cooked	102	2.0					22	
Roll, hard	1 lg	160	5.0	2.0	1.0	1.0		31	2
Rye wafers, Rye Krisp	2 pc	43	2.0					10	
Strudel, all types	1 small	165	1.5	6.5	2.0	4.2	0.7	27	6
Stuffing									
with hydrogenated fat	1/4 cup	64	0.8	4.6	1.2	3.4	0.5	5	
with oil	1/4 cup	68	0.8	5.2	0.7	4.2	2.5	5	
no added fat	1/4 cup	36	0.8	1.6	0.5	1.1	0.3	5	
Waffle	1 med	240	8.0	9.0	3.0	6.0	1.0	30	128
BEVERAGES AND SPIRITS									
Beer	8 oz	114	1.0					12	

(Cont. next page)

	Amt.	Cal.	Pro.	T. Fat	SF	UF	PF	CHO	Chol.
Carbonated beverages, average	4 oz	53						14	
Cocktails									
Manhattan	1 oz	68						1	
Martini	1 oz	78		0.6	0.1	0.4		1	
Old Fashioned	1 oz	86						1	
Whiskey Sour	1 oz	71						2	
Ginger ale	4 oz	40						11	
Grasshopper	1 oz	99		2.0	1.1	0.8	0.1	7	6
Liqueur or fruit cordial	½ oz	48						4	
Rum	½ oz	48							
Wine									
light dry 12% to 14% alcohol	1 oz	28						2	
dry 20% alcohol	1 oz	41						2	
sweet 20% alcohol	1 oz	45						4	

CANDIES, SWEETS, RELISHES, SAUCES

	Amt.	Cal.	Pro.	T. Fat	SF	UF	PF	CHO	Chol.
Baking chocolate									
bitter	½ oz	73	1.0	7.5	4.0	3.1	0.1	4	
sweet	½ oz	68	0.5	4.0	2.5	1.5		9	
Candy bar, average, chocolate covered	½ oz	73	1.0	3.8	0.7	2.7	1.3	9	
Caramels	½ oz	60	0.5	1.5	1.0	0.5		11	7
Cocoa powder, unsweetened	1 tsp	7	0.2	0.6	0.3	0.2		1	

(Cont. next page)

	Amt.	Cal.	Pro.	T. Fat	SF	UF	PF	CHO	Chol.
Chocolate									
soufflé	¼ cup	123	2.8	6.2	3.1	2.9	0.5	15	74
milk (candy)	½ oz	73	1.0	4.5	2.5	1.8	0.3	8	
syrup	1 tsp	13						4	
Cornstarch	1 tsp	10						2	
Frosting									
boiled, ½ oz	1 tbsp	50						12	
chocolate	⅔ tbsp	60	0.1	2.8	0.8	1.9	0.6	9	5
cream	⅔ tbsp	59	0.1	2.4	0.5	1.8	0.6	10	6
Fudge, plain	½ oz	58		1.5	1.0	0.5		12	1
Gelatin									
powder	1 tbsp	35	9.0						
dessert	½ cup	78	2.0					18	
with fruit	½ cup	86	1.6					22	
Hard candy, non-fat	½ oz	55						14	
Lecithin	1 tbsp	60		5.3	0.7	4.5	3.0		
Macaroon	1 sm	47	1.1	3.0	2.4	0.5	0.1	4	6
Olives									
green	3 lg	16	0.3	1.8	0.3	1.4	0.2		
black	3 lg	21	0.3	2.3	0.3	2.0	0.3	1	
Parfait, chocolate	½ cup	216	0.8	51.6	27.6	21.6	4.0	24	96

(Cont. next page)

	Amt.	Cal.	Pro.	T. Fat	SF	UF	PF	CHO	Chol.
Pickles									
dill	1 oz	4	0.3					1	
sweet	1	20						5	
Postum, Instant	2 tbsp	36	0.6					8	
Sauces									
barbecue with butter	1 tbsp	58		6.0	3.0	2.7	0.7	2	20
chili or mustard	1 tbsp	15						4	
chocolate, rich	1 tsp	46	0.4	2.0	0.7	1.2	0.3	7	3
hollandaise with butter	1 tbsp	68	0.9	7.5	3.6	3.5	1.0		90
meat, restaurant	2 tbsp	41	2.0	3.4	1.3	2.0	0.2	1	9
tomato with oil, no meat	1 tbsp	19		0.9	0.1	0.8	0.1	3	
white with butter	1 tbsp	27	0.6	2.1	1.1	0.9	0.2	1	7
Sherbet	½ cup	118	1.6	1.0	0.6	0.4		28	4
Sugars									
white, brown	1 tsp	17						4	
confectioners	1 tbsp	31						8	
SPREADS, OILS, FATS									
Butter	½ tsp	17		2.0	1.0	0.9	0.2		7
Chicken fat	½ tsp	23		2.5	0.8	1.6	0.6		
Lard, bacon fat	½ tsp	23		2.4	0.9	1.4	0.4		3
Margarine									
average	½ tsp	17		1.9	0.5	1.3	0.2		
modified	½ tsp	17		1.9	0.3	1.5	0.5		

(Cont. next page)

	Amt.	Cal.	Pro.	T. Fat	SF	UF	PF	CHO	Chol.
Mayonnaise	1 tsp	37		4.0	0.7	3.1	2.1		3
Oils									
coconut	½ tsp	21		2.3	2.0	0.2	0.1		
corn	½ tsp	21		2.4	0.2	2.1	1.5		
cottonseed	½ tsp	21		2.4	0.5	1.8	1.3		
olive	½ tsp	21		2.4	0.4	2.0	0.2		
peanut	½ tsp	21		2.3	0.4	1.8	0.6		
safflower	½ tsp	21		2.3	0.2	2.0	1.7		
soy bean	½ tsp	21		2.4	0.4	1.9	1.4		
Salad dressing									
cheese	1 tsp	30	0.3	3.3	0.7	2.4	1.7		37
French	1 tsp	20		2.0	0.3	1.6	1.3	1	
mayonnaise type	1 tsp	20		2.0	0.3	1.6	1.3	1	3
Thousand Island	1 tsp	25		2.7	0.3	2.3	1.6		5
Vegetable fat, hydrogenated	½ tsp	18		2.0	0.5	1.5	0.2		
NUTS AND LEGUMES									
Almonds, shelled (3–4)	⅛ oz	21	0.7	1.9	0.2	1.7	0.4	1	
Beans, dried, canned, Navy, etc.	¼ cup	58	3.8	0.3	0.1	0.2	0.1	11	
Brazil nuts (1)	⅛ oz	23	0.5	2.3	0.5	1.7	0.6		
Cashews, roasted (2)	⅛ oz	20	0.7	1.7	0.3	1.3	0.1	1	
Coconut, shredded	½ tbsp	11	0.1	0.8	0.7	0.1	0.1	1	
Cowpeas, cooked	¼ cup	48	3.3	0.3	0.1	0.2	0.1	9	

(Cont. next page)

	Amt.	Cal.	Pro.	T. Fat	SF	UF	PF	CHO	Chol.
Peanuts, roasted (4)	⅛ oz	21	1.0	1.8	0.4	1.3	0.5	1	
Peanut butter	1 tsp	30	1.3	2.7	0.7	2.0	0.7	1	
Peas, split, cooked	¼ cup	73	5.0	0.3	0.1	0.2	0.1	13	
Pecans, halves (3)	⅛ oz	24	0.3	2.5	0.2	2.2	0.6	1	
Pecans, chopped (tbsp)	¼ oz	50	1.0	5.0	0.4	4.4	1.3	1	
Walnut, halves, shelled (2)	⅛ oz	23	0.5	2.3	0.2	2.0	1.7	1	

MEATS AND POULTRY*

	Amt.	Cal.	Pro.	T. Fat	SF	UF	PF	CHO	Chol.
Cuts of beef, veal and lamb having	2 gms. fat per oz	53	9.4	1.7	0.8	0.8	0.1		36
Trimmed— Sirloin tip roast, heart, all trimmed cuts of veal except breast									
Cuts of beef, veal and lamb having	3 gms. fat per oz	61	9.0	2.8	1.4	1.3	0.1		36
Trimmed— Cube, flank and round steak; leg of lamb									
Untrimmed— Leg and round of veal									
Cuts of beef, veal and lamb having	4 gms. fat per oz	64	7.5	3.8	1.8	1.8	0.1		36

*Nutrient values for meats and poultry are on cooked, edible portions.

(Cont. next page)

	Amt.	Cal.	Pro.	T. Fat	SF	UF	PF	CHO	Chol.
Trimmed— Arm pot roast, rump roast; porterhouse, sirloin, strip and tenderloin steak; loin lamb chops, loin and crown roast of lamb									
Untrimmed— Sirloin tip roast, veal cutlet, rump and shoulder veal roast									
Cuts of beef, veal and lamb having	5 gms. fat per oz	72	7.5	4.7	2.3	2.2	0.1		36
Trimmed— Blade pot roast, rib and T-bone steak, arm and shoulder lamb chop, tongue									
Untrimmed— Leg of lamb, veal blade steak									
Cuts of beef, veal and lamb having	6 gms. fat per oz	82	7.5	5.8	2.8	2.7	0.1		36
Trimmed— Beef brisket, restaurant roast beef, club steak, rib lamb chop, lamb stew meat									
Untrimmed— Round, strip, and tenderloin steak; loin lamb chop, loin and crown lamb roast, rib									

(Cont. next page)

	Amt.	Cal.	Pro.	T. Fat	SF	UF	PF	CHO	Chol.
veal chop, sirloin of veal, arm and sirloin veal steak									
Cuts of beef, veal and lamb having	8 gms. fat per oz	96	6.9	7.6	3.7	3.5	0.2		36
Untrimmed—									
"Barbecue" beef (restaurant)									
Ground beef									
Arm and blade pot roast, Restaurant roast beef, rump roast, sirloin steak, arm and shoulder lamb chops, loin of veal, veal stew meat									
Cuts of beef, veal and lamb having	10 gms. fat per oz	113	5.7	10.0	4.8	4.7	0.2		36
Trimmed—									
Short ribs of beef									
Untrimmed—									
Corned, cured beef; beef club, pinbone sirloin, porterhouse, rib, T-bone steaks; beef chuck stew meat; lamb rib, stew meat, rib chops									
Cuts of beef, veal and lamb having	14 gms. fat per oz	144	5.0	13.8	6.7	6.5	0.3		36

(Cont. next page)

	Amt.	Cal.	Pro.	T. Fat	SF	UF	PF	CHO	Chol.
Untrimmed									
Beef oxtails, plate or boiling beef; rib, rolled or standing roasts; short ribs; Lamb breast									
Cuts of fresh pork having	3 gms. fat per oz	63	9.1	2.9	1.1	1.7	0.5		36
Trimmed—									
Pork chops, butterfly, loin, rib; fresh ham; roasts, crown loin, rib, neck, sirloin; pork steak, tenderloin									
Cuts of fresh pork having	5 gms. fat per oz	77	8.2	4.9	1.8	2.9	0.8		36
Trimmed—									
Pork picnic shoulder, pork Boston butt									
Untrimmed—									
Ham sirloin—if highly marbled; highly marbled chops									
Cuts of fresh pork having	7 gms. fat per oz	95	7.3	7.3	2.8	4.1	0.8		
Untrimmed—									
Pork tenderloin; picnic shoulder; roasts, crown, loin, neck rib; arm and blade steaks									

(Cont. next page)

	Amt.	Cal.	Pro.	T. Fat	SF	UF	PF	CHO	Chol.
Cuts of cured pork having	4 grms. fat per oz	64	7.8	3.6	1.3	2.1	0.6		36
Trimmed—									
Ham-butt and shank									
Untrimmed—									
Canadian bacon									
Cuts of cured pork having	8 grms. fat per oz	95	5.9	7.9	2.9	4.6	1.1		36
Untrimmed—									
Fresh ham, shoulder butt, neck bones									
Cuts of cured pork having	10 grms. fat per oz	116	5.7	10.4	3.8	6.1	1.7		36
Trimmed—									
Pork sausage									
Untrimmed—									
Ham hocks									
Bacon regular sliced	1 sl	48	2.5	4.0	1.5	2.5	0.5	1	8
Beef, chipped or dried	1 oz	58	9.5	2.0	1.0	1.0			36
Bologna, salami	1 oz	86	3.4	7.8	3.2	4.2	0.8		28
Chicken canned	1 oz	57	8.3	2.3	0.7	1.5	0.5		23

(Cont. next page)

	Amt.	Cal.	Pro.	T. Fat	SF	UF	PF	CHO	Chol.
Corned beef, canned	1 oz	60	7.3	3.3	1.7	1.4	0.1		36
Duck, goose, etc.	1 oz	93	4.6	8.2	2.1	5.7	2.0		20
Frankfurter	1 avg	156	6.0	14.0	6.0	7.4	1.4	2	56
Ham, boiled	1 oz	85	6.5	6.5	2.5	3.7	1.2		36
Liver fried in hydrogenated fat	1 oz	60	6.5	2.0	1.0	1.0		3	96
Luncheon meats	1 oz	83	4.0	7.0	2.5	4.2	1.2	1	28
Organ meats	1 oz	41	5.9	1.0	0.3	0.6	0.2	2	96
Poultry with skin	1 oz	62	7.7	3.0	1.0	2.0	0.7		23
no skin	1 oz	34	6.1	0.8	0.3	0.5	0.3		22
Salami, kosher	1 oz	103	3.3	9.9	5.1	4.4	0.2		36
Salt pork	½ oz	102	0.9	10.9	3.9	6.2	1.6		26
Spareribs, 2 av. ribs	1 oz	144	5.0	13.8	5.3	7.8	1.9		36